Biological and Medical Aspects of Electromagnetic Fields

Fourth Edition

Biological Effects of Electromagnetics Series

Series Editors
Frank Barnes
University of Colorado Boulder, Colorado, U.S.A.

Ben Greenebaum
University of Wisconsin–Parkside Somers, Wisconsin, U.S.A.

Electromagnetic Fields in Biological Systems
Edited by James C. Lin

Epidemiology of Electromagnetic Fields
Edited by Martin Röösli

Advanced Electroporation Techniques in Biology and Medicine
Edited by Andrei G. Pakhomov, Damijan Miklavčič, and Marko S. Markov

The Physiology of Bioelectricity in Development, Tissue
Regeneration, and Cancer
Edited by Christine E. Pullar

Handbook of Biological Effects of Electromagnetic Fields, Fourth
Edition – Two Volume Set
Edited by Ben Greenebaum and Frank Barnes

For more information about this series, please visit: https://www.crcpress.com/Biological-Effects-of-Electromagnetics/book-series/CRCBIOEFFOFELE

Biological and Medical Aspects of Electromagnetic Fields

Fourth Edition

Edited by
Ben Greenebaum and Frank Barnes

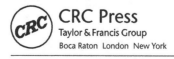

CRC Press
Taylor & Francis Group
Boca Raton London New York

CRC Press is an imprint of the
Taylor & Francis Group, an **informa** business

CRC Press
Taylor & Francis Group
6000 Broken Sound Parkway NW, Suite 300
Boca Raton, FL 33487-2742

First issued in paperback 2022

ISBN-13: 978-1-138-73526-2 (hbk)
ISBN-13: 978-1-03-233877-4 (pbk)
DOI: 10.1201/9781315186641

Visit the Taylor & Francis Web site at
http://www.taylorandfrancis.com

and the CRC Press Web site at
http://www.crcpress.com

Contents

v

Preface

We are honored to have been asked to follow the 2007 3rd Edition of the *Handbook* with this 4th Edition and to carry on the tradition established in the first two editions by Dr. Postow and the late Dr. Polk. In this edition of the *Handbook of Biological Effects of Electromagnetic Fields*, we have added new and newly relevant material on a number of aspects of basic science and on diagnostic and therapeutic applications. While we had to reduce or drop coverage of a few topics that now seem less immediately important, we refer the reader to the material on these in the previous editions. New additions include expanded coverage of brain stimulation, characterization and modeling of epithelial tissue wounds, theoretical models of proposed basic mechanisms giving rise to bioelectromagnetic effects, and dosimetric measurement methods and instrumentation. For the first time in this series we have added coverage of electromagnetic effects in the terahertz region, field effects on plants, and applying electrical engineering concepts of systems engineering and operational amplifiers with feedback to the analysis of biological electromagnetic effects. At the same time, all chapters have been updated in view of what has been learned in the past decade, some receiving relatively minor changes and others being completely revamped.

Research in bioelectromagnetics stems from three sources, all of which are important: Bioelectromagnetics first emerged as a separate scientific subject because of interest in studying possible hazards from exposure to electromagnetic fields and setting human exposure limits. A second interest is in the beneficial use of fields to advance health, both in diagnostics and in treatment, an interest that is as old as the discovery of electricity itself. Finally, the observed interactions between electromagnetic fields and biological systems raise some fundamental, unanswered scientific questions as to how they occur, the answers to which may lead to fields being used as tools to probe basic biology and biophysics. Various chapters treat both basic physical science and engineering aspects and biological and medical aspects of these three. Answering basic bioelectromagnetic questions will not only lead to answers about potential electromagnetic hazards and to better beneficial applications, but they should also contribute significantly to our basic understanding of biological processes. Both strong fields and those on the order of the fields spontaneously generated within biological systems may become tools to perturb the systems, either for experiments seeking to understand how the systems operate or simply to change the systems, such as by injecting a plasmid containing genes whose effects are to be investigated. These three threads are intertwined throughout bioelectromagnetics. Although any specific chapter in this work will emphasize one or another of these threads, the reader should be aware that each aspect of the research is relevant to a greater or lesser extent to all three.

As in previous editions, the authors of the individual chapters were charged with providing the reader, whom we imagine is moderately familiar with one or more of the sciences underlying bioelectromagnetics, though perhaps not in the others or in the interdisciplinary subject of bioelectromagnetics itself, with both an introduction to their topic and a basis for further reading. We asked the chapter authors to imagine and write what they would like to be the first thing they would ask a new graduate student in their laboratory to read. Like its predecessors, this edition is intended to be useful as a reference book but also as a text for introducing the reader to bioelectromagnetics or some of its aspects. For these students and other readers who are not familiar with the basic physical science behind electromagnetic fields, the Introduction ("Chapter 0") and Chapters 5 and 6 are intended to be helpful.

As a "handbook" and not an encyclopedia, this work does not intend to cover all aspects of bioelectromagnetics. Nevertheless, considering the breadth of topics and growth of research, some ideas are unavoidably duplicated in various chapters, sometimes from different viewpoints that could be instructive to the reader and sometimes presenting different aspects or implications. While the amount of material has led to the publication of the handbook as two separate, but interrelated volumes: Biological and Medical Aspects of Electromagnetic Fields (BMA) and Bioengineering and Biophysical Aspects of Electromagnetic Fields (BBA), there is no sharp dividing line, and some topics are dealt with in parts of both volumes. The reader is urged to go beyond a single chapter is researching a specific topic.

The reader should note that the chapter authors have a wide variety of interests and backgrounds. Their work and interests range from safety standards and possible health effects of low-level fields to therapy through applications in biology and medicine to the fundamental physics and chemistry underlying the biology and bioelectromagnetic inter-actions. It is therefore not surprising that the authors may have different and sometimes conflicting points of view on the significance of various results and their potential applica-tions. Thus authors should only be held responsible for the viewpoints expressed in their chapters and not in others. We have tried to select the authors and topics so as to cover the scientific results to date that are likely to serve as a starting point for future work that will lead to the further development of the field. Each chapter's extensive reference section should be helpful for those needing to obtain a more extensive background than is pos-sible from a book of this type.

Some of the material, as well as various authors' viewpoints, are controversial, and their importance is likely to change as the field develops and our understanding of the underlying science improves. We hope that this volume will serve as a starting point for both students and practitioners to understand the various parts of the field of bioelectro-magnetics, as of mid-to-late 2017, when authors contributing to this volume finished their literature reviews.

The editors would like to express their appreciation to all the authors for the extensive time and effort they have put into preparing this edition. It is our wish that it will prove to be of value to the readers and lead to advancing our understanding of this challenging field.

Ben Greenebaum

Frank Barnes

Editors

Ben Greenebaum retired as professor of physics at the University of Wisconsin—Parkside, Kenosha, WI, in May 2001, but was appointed as emeritus professor and adjunct professor to continue research, journal editing, and university outreach projects. He received his PhD in physics from Harvard University in 1965. He joined the faculty of UW—Parkside as assistant professor in 1970 following postdoctoral positions at Harvard and Princeton Universities. He was promoted to associate professor in 1972 and to professor in 1980. Greenebaum is author or coauthor of more than 50 scientific papers. Since 1992, he has been editor in chief of Bioelectromagnetics, an international peer-reviewed scientific journal, and the most cited specialized journal in this field. He spent 1997–1998 as consultant in the World Health Organization's International EMF Project in Geneva, Switzerland. Between 1971 and 2000, he was part of an interdisciplinary research team investigating the biological effects of electromagnetic fields on biological cell cultures. From his graduate student days through 1975, his research studied the spins and moments of radioactive nuclei. In 1977, he became a special assistant to the chancellor and in 1978, associate dean of faculty (equivalent to the present associate vice chancellor position). He served 2 years as acting vice chancellor (1984–1985 and 1986–1987). In 1989, he was appointed as dean of the School of Science and Technology, serving until the school was abolished in 1996, after which he chaired the physics department through 2001. On the personal side, he was born in Chicago and has lived in Racine, WI, since 1970. Married since 1965, he and his wife have three adult sons and two grandchildren.

Frank Barnes received his BS in electrical engineering in 1954 from Princeton University and his MS, engineering, and PhD degrees from Stanford University in 1955, 1956, and 1958, respectively. He was a Fulbright scholar in Baghdad, Iraq, in 1958 and joined the University of Colorado in 1959, where he is currently a distinguished professor emeritus. He has served as chairman of the Department of Electrical Engineering, acting dean of the College of Engineering, and in 1971 as cofounder/director with Professor George Codding of the Political Science Department of the Interdisciplinary Telecommunications Program (ITP). He has served as chair of the IEEE Electron Device Society, president of the Electrical Engineering Department Heads Association, vice president of IEEE for Publications, editor of the IEEE Student Journal, and the IEEE Transactions on Education, as well as president of the Bioelectromagnetics Society and U.S. Chair of Commission K—International Union of Radio Science (URSI). He is a fellow of the AAAS, IEEE, International Engineering Consortium, and a member of the National Academy of Engineering. Dr. Barnes has been awarded the Curtis McGraw Research Award from ASEE, the Leon Montgomery Award from the International Communications Association, the 2003 IEEE Education Society Achievement Award, Distinguished Lecturer for IEEE Electron Device Society, the 2002 ECE Distinguished Educator Award from ASEE, The Colorado Institute of Technology Catalyst Award 2004, and the Bernard M. Gordon Prize from National Academy of Engineering for Innovations in Engineering Education 2004. He was born in Pasadena, CA, in 1932 and attended numerous elementary schools throughout the country. He and his wife, Gay, have two children and two grandchildren.

List of Contributors

Stanislav I. Alekseev
Russian Academy of Sciences
Pushchino, Russian Federation

Somen Baidya
University of Missouri-Kansas City
Kansas City, Missouri

Frank Barnes
University of Colorado Boulder
Boulder, Colorado

Yuri Chizmadzhev
MIT
Cambridge, Massachusetts

C.-K. Chou
C-K. Chou Consulting
Dublin, California

Maria Feychting
Karolinska Institute
Stockholm, Sweden

Ben Greenebaum
University of Wisconsin-Parkside
Kenosha, Wisconsin

D. Haemmerich
Medical University of South
    Carolina
Charleston, South Carolina

Ahmed M. Hassan
University of Missouri-Kansas City
Kansas City, Missouri

Leeka Kheifets
University of California-Los
    Angeles
Los Angeles, California

Raphael C. Lee
Chicago Electrical Trauma Research
    Institute
University of Chicago
Chicago, Illinois

Mei Li
Shanghai Power Hospital
Shanghai, China

Ze Liang
Peking Union Medical College
Beijing, China

Sarah P. Loughran
University of Wollongong
Wollongong, NSW, Australia

Massimo E. Maffei
University of Turin
Turin, Italy

Mats-Olof Mattsson
AIT Austrian Institute of Techololgy
Vienna, Austria

David L. McCormick
IIT Research Institute
Chicago, Illinois

Colin McFaul
University of Chicago
Chicago, Illinois

Junji Miyakoshi
Kyoto University
Kyoto, Japan

Andrew S. Park
University of California-Los Angeles
Los Angeles, California

Charles Polk (Deceased)
Deceased. University of Rhode Island
South Kingstown, Rhode Island

D.B. Rodrigues
University of Maryland School of Medicine
Baltimore, Maryland

Martin Röösli
University of Basel
Basel, Switzerland

Joachim Schüz
International Agency for Research on
    Cancer
Lyon, France

Masaki Sekino
University of Tokyo
Tokyo, Japan

Tsukasa Shigemitsu
Central Research Institute of Electric
    Power Industry
Abiko, Japan

Myrtill Simkó
SciProof International AB
Östersund, Sweden

Joseph A. Spadaro
New York Upstate Medical Center
Syracuse, New York

P.R. Stauffer
Thomas Jefferson University
Philadelphia, Pennsylvania

John Swanson
National Grid
London, United Kingdom

Shoogo Ueno
University of Tokyo
Tokyo, Japan

Ximena Vergara
Electric Power Research Institute
Palo Alto, California
and
University of California-Los Angeles
Los Angeles, California

James C. Weaver
MIT
Cambridge, Massachusetts

Andrew W. Wood
Swinburne University of Technology
Melbourne, VIC, Australia
and
RMIT University
Melbourne, VIC, Australia

Min Zhao
School of Medicine
University of California
Davis, California

Marvin C. Ziskin
Temple University School of Medicine
Philadelphia, Pennsylvania

0

Introduction to Electromagnetic Fields

Frank Barnes
University of Colorado Boulder

Charles Polk*
University of Rhode Island

Ben Greenebaum
University of Wisconsin-Parkside

CONTENTS

0.1 Background

Much has been learned since this handbook's 3rd edition, but a full understanding of biological effects of electromagnetic fields is still to be achieved. The broad range of disciplines that must be studied has to be a factor in the apparent slow progress toward this ultimate end. Understanding how electric and magnetic fields can affect biological systems requires understanding of disciplines that include basic biology, medical science and clinical practice, biological and electrical engineering, basic chemistry and biochemistry, and fundamental physics and biophysics. The subject matter ranges over characteristic lengths and timescales, at one extreme with static fields and low frequencies with wavelengths of tens of kilometers to other extreme with sub-millimeter wavelength fields with periods below 10^{-12} s. Biological systems have response times that range from 10^{-15} s for electronic state transitions in molecules or atoms to many years for generations for humans and other organisms. This chapter is intended to provide a basic review of electric and magnetic fields and the relations between these fields and to define the terms used throughout the rest of these volumes. Maxwell's equations defining these relations have been known for

---

* Deceased.

a long time, however, the solutions to these equations are often complex, as the biological materials can be inhomogeneous, nonlinear, time varying and anisotropic. Additionally, the geometric shapes involved may not lead to simple descriptions. Therefore, a number of approximations which depend on the ratio of the wavelength of the electromagnetic waves to the dimensions of the body being exposed are presented that simplify the calculations of the field strengths at a given location.

0.2 Review of Basic Electromagnetic Theory

The basic force equation for defining electric and magnetic fields is the Lorentz equation.

$$\vec{F} = q(\vec{E} + \vec{v}x\vec{B}) \tag{0.1}$$

where $\vec{F}$ is the force on a charge q. Note $\vec{F}$ is a vector quantity as are the other symbols with arrows over them. $\vec{E}$ is the electric field. $\vec{v}$ is the velocity of the charge and $\vec{B}$ is the magnetic flux density. Thus, $\vec{E}$ is defined as the force on the charge q at a given location due to one or more charges at other locations or

$$\vec{E} = \frac{\vec{F}}{q} \tag{0.2}$$

$\vec{B}$ is similarly defined in the second term of Equation 0.1. In the term $\vec{F} = q(\vec{v}x\vec{B})$, note that $\vec{v}x\vec{B}$ is a vector cross-product so that the force is at right angles to both the velocity of the charge and the magnetic field. The magnetic flux density may also be defined by the incremental force $\vec{F}$ on a current I or charge flowing in an incremental length of a current carrying wire $d\vec{l}$

$$\vec{F} = Id\vec{l}x\vec{B} \text{ and } \left|\vec{F}\right| = I\left|d\vec{l}\right|\left|\vec{B}\right|\sin\theta \tag{0.3}$$

where θ is the angle between $d\vec{l}$ and $\vec{B}$

It is to be noted that the magnetic flux density is related to the magnetic field $\vec{H}$ by the magnetic permeability μ at any given point in space so that $\vec{B} = \mu\vec{H}$ or $\vec{B} = \mu_0\vec{H} + \vec{M}_B$. $\vec{M}_B$ is the magnetic polarization per unit volume and μ_o is the magnetic permeability of free space ($\mu_0 = 4\pi \times 10^{-7}$ H/m or $4\pi \times 10^{-7}$ kg m/A²s²). For many cases the magnetic field $\vec{H}$ is given by

$$\oint \vec{H} \bullet d\vec{l} = \oiint \vec{J} \bullet d\vec{s} = i \tag{0.4}$$

Where $\vec{H}$ is given by the line integral around the current i or integral of the current density $\vec{J}$ over the surface of the conductor. Thus, we have the electric field defined by the force between charges and the magnetic field defined by the forces associated with the rate of change of charge or charge flow.

Time-changing electrical and magnetic fields lead to radiation and they are associated with the acceleration of charges. The power, P_R, emitted by an accelerated charge is given by

$$P_R = \frac{2q^2a^2}{4\pi\varepsilon_0 3c^3} \tag{0.5}$$

where a is the acceleration, ε_0 is the electric permittivity of free space ($\varepsilon_0 = 8.845 \times 10^{-12}$ F/m), and c is the velocity of light. The radiation is at right angles to the motion of the accelerated charge. Electromagnetic waves are also radiated from atoms and molecules undergoing transitions between energy levels. The radiations occurs at frequency, f, such that $hf = \Delta W$ where h is Planck's constant [$h = 6.63 \times 10^{-34}$ J s] and ΔW is the energy difference between energy levels. Transitions between electronic energy states typically lead to radiation at optical wavelengths. Transitions between vibrational levels are often in the infrared and far infrared and rotational transitions in the millimeter and microwave regions. Hyperfine transitions changing the orientation of electron spins in the earth's magnetic field may yield radiations at radio frequencies (RF).

The general relationship between the electric $\vec{E}$ and magnetic fields $\vec{H}$ are given by Maxwell's equations:

$$\vec{\nabla}x\vec{H} = \vec{J} + \frac{\partial \vec{D}}{\partial t} \tag{0.6}$$

$$\vec{\nabla}x\vec{E} = -\frac{\partial \vec{B}}{\partial t} \tag{0.7}$$

$$\vec{D} = \varepsilon_0\vec{E} + \vec{P} \tag{0.8}$$

$$\vec{B} = \mu_0\vec{H} + \vec{M}_B \tag{0.9}$$

where $\vec{D}$ is the displacement vector, related to $\vec{E}$ by the electrical permittivity or dielectric constant ε at a given point in space in Equation 0.8 and ε_0 is the dielectric constant of free space, $\vec{p}$ is the electrical polarlization per unit volume, t is time, $\vec{\nabla}$ is the partial differential operator del, μ_0 is the magnetic permiability of free space and $\vec{M}_B$ is the magnetic polarization per unit volume. $\vec{p}$ and $\vec{M}_B$ are properties of the material and will be discussed in Chapter 4.

Sources of electric and magnetic fields come in a variety of shapes and sizes and different approximations appropriate for describing them are dependent on the distance from the source to the biological systems of interest and the frequency at which these sources are varying in time. For electrical fields common sources include point sources, parallel plates long wires and dipoles; for magnetic fields, long wires, dipoles and coils

See Figure 0.1 for some common electric and magnetic field distributions.

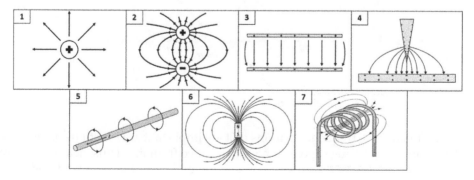

FIGURE 0.1
(1). Electric field of a point charge. (2) Electric field of an electric dipole. (3) Electric field of charge parallel plates. (4) Electric field of a charged probe above a plate. (5) Magnetic field of current carrying wire. (6) Magnetic field of a magnetic dipole. (7) Magnetic field of a current carrying coil.

For point charges the force between two charges is given by Coulomb's Equation

$$\vec{F} = \frac{q_1 q_2}{4\pi \varepsilon \vec{r}^2}$$

(0.10)

where q_1 and q_2 are the two charges, ε is the dielectric constant and $\vec{r}$ is the distance between the two charges.

For a large number of cases the distance from the source to the biological object is much larger than the size of the source of the fields, and the source can be approximated by a dipole, a closely spaced pair of equal positive and negative charges or currents. This particularly true at RF, and it can be a first approximation for the fields generated by current-carrying wires.

Another common approximation is that for many cases we can decompose the signal that is being applied into a sum of sine waves using Fourier analysis. In the case of time-changing fields, different terms in Maxwell's equations dominate when distance from the source to the object is large or small compared to the size of the source; these are the far-field and near-field situations. For the case of a single sine wave driving a dipole source, Maxwell's equations are given by Equations 0.11–0.13 [1].

$$H_\vartheta = \frac{I_o L}{4\pi} e^{-jkr} \left(\frac{jk}{r} + \frac{1}{r^2} \right) \sin\theta$$

(0.11)

Radiated field   Near H Field

$$E_r = \frac{I_o L}{4\pi} e^{-jkr} \left(\frac{2\eta}{r^2} + \frac{2}{j\omega\varepsilon r^3} \right) \cos\theta$$

(0.12)

Induced E Field   Near E Field

$$E_\theta = \frac{I_o L}{4\pi} e^{-jkr} \left(\frac{j\omega\mu}{r} + \frac{1}{j\omega\mu r^3} + \frac{\eta}{r^2} \right) \sin\theta$$

(0.13)

Radiated Field

At radio and microwave frequencies, terms that are important are functions of the ratio L/r of the length of the radiating dipole L and the distance from it, r. Thus, near typical transmitter antennas or close to the antenna of a cell phone, both the near field and far-field terms of Maxwell's equations often need to be taken into account as ω is a large number. At large distances such as are typical for radio, TV, cell phone base stations, and radars, it is the radiated fields that are important.

0.3 Near Fields and Radiation Fields

At low frequencies such as 50 or 60 Hz, we often are interested in the electric and magnetic fields that are generated by two long parallel wires. In this case, it is the near-field terms in Maxwell's equations that are of interest and it is to be noted that the radiation terms are so small that they are usually unimportant. In general radiation from power lines often does not contribute fields that are most likely to be important in affecting biological materials and one only talks about the near fields or the fields induced in the materials by them. In free space, the electromagnetic wavelength $\lambda = c/f$, where c is the velocity of light and f is the frequency in hertz (cycles/s). In vacuum $c = 3 \times 10^8$ m/s. Therefore, the wave length at the power distribution frequency of 60 Hz is approximately 5000 km, and most available human-made structures are much smaller than one wavelength.

The poor radiation efficiency of electrically small structures, that is, structures whose largest linear dimensions l is small compared to λ, can be illustrated easily for linear antennas. In free space the radiation resistance, R_r of a current element, i.e., an electrically short wire of length l carrying uniform current along its length l [2], is given by (Figure 0.2)

$$R_r = 80\pi^2 \left(\frac{l}{\lambda} \right)^2 \tag{0.14}$$

Thus, the R_r of a 0.01 λ antenna, 50 km long at 60 Hz, would be 0.0197 Ω. The radiated power $P_r = I^2 R_r$ where I is the antenna terminal current, whereas the power dissipated as heat in the antenna wire is $I^2 R_d$ where R_d is the resistance of the wire. When I is uniform, the P_r will be very much less than the power used to heat the antenna, given that the ohmic resistance R_d of any practical wire at room temperature will be very much larger than R_r. For example, the resistance of a 50-km long 2-in. diameter solid copper wire could be 6.65 Ω. At DC, of course, no radiation of any sort takes place, as acceleration of charges is a condition for radiation of electromagnetic waves. A second set of circumstances, which guarantees that any object subjected to low frequency E and H fields usually does not experience effects of radiation, is that any configuration that carries electric currents, sets up E and H field components which store energy without contributing to radiation. A short, linear antenna in free space (short electric dipole) generates, in addition to the radiation field E_r, an electrostatic field E_s and an induced field E_i. Neither E_s nor E_i contribute to the P_r [3,4]. Whereas E_r varies as $1/r$, where r is the distance from the antenna, E_i varies as $1/r^2$, and E_s as $1/r^3$. At a distance from the antenna of approximately one-sixth of the wavelength

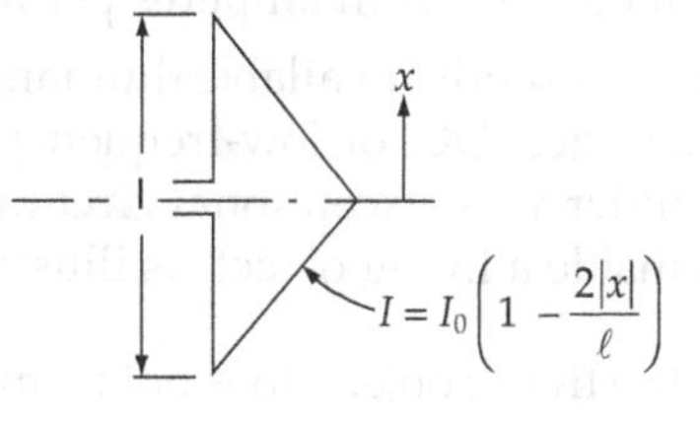

FIGURE 0.2

Current distribution on short, thin, center-fed antenna. $I = I_0 \left(1 - \frac{2|x|}{\ell} \right)$.

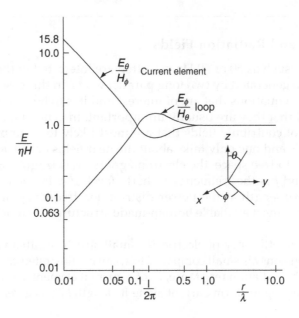

FIGURE 0.3
Ratio of E to H field (divided by wave impedance of free space $\eta = 377\ \Omega$ at $\theta = 90°$; for electric current element at origin along z-axis and for electrically small loop centered at the origin in x–y plane.

($r = \lambda/2\ \pi$), the E_i equals the E_r, and when $r \ll \lambda/6$ the E_r quickly becomes negligible in comparison with E_i and E_s. Similar results are obtained for other antenna configurations [5]. At 60 Hz the distance $\lambda/2\pi$ corresponds to about 800 km and objects at distances of a few kilometers or less from a 60-Hz system are exposed to low frequency near-field components, which are orders of magnitude larger than the part of the field that contributes to radiation.

A living organism exposed to a static (DC) field or to a low frequency near field may extract energy from it, but the quantitative description of the mechanism by which this extraction takes place is very different than at higher frequencies, where energy is transferred by radiation:

1. In the near field, the relative magnitudes of E and H are a function of the current or charge configuration and the distance from the electric system. The E field may be much larger than the H field or vice versa.

2. In the radiation field, the ratio of the E to H is fixed and equal to 377 Ω in free space, if E is given in volts per meter and H in amperes per meter.

3. In the vicinity of most presently available human-made devices or systems carrying static electric charges, DC, or low-frequency (<1000 Hz) currents, the E and H fields will only under very exceptional circumstances be large enough to produce heating effects inside a living object, as illustrated by Figure 0.4.

(This statement assumes that the living object does not form part of a conducting path that permits direct entrance of current from a wire or conducting ground.) However, effects that are not described by changes in the average temperature are possible; thus, an E field of sufficient magnitude may orient dipoles or translate ions or polarizable neutral particles (see Chapter 4 in this volume)

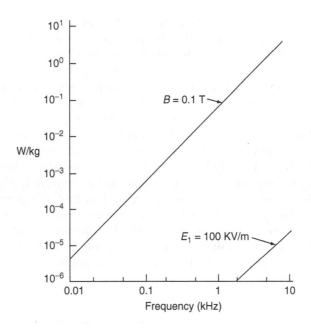

FIGURE 0.4

Top line: Eddy current loss produced in cylinder by sinusoidally time-varying axial *H* field. Cylinder parameters are conductivity $\sigma = 0.1$ S/m, radius 0.1 m, density $D = 1100$ kg/m³, RMS magnetic flux density 0.1 $T = 1000$ G. Watt per kilogram $= \sigma B^2 r^2 w^2/8D$; see Equation 0.29 and use power per volume $= J^2/\sigma$, *Lower line:* Loss produced by 60-Hz E_1 field in Watts per kilogram $= \sigma E_{int}^2/D$, where external field E_1 is related to E_{int} by Equation 0.23 with $\varepsilon_2 = \varepsilon_0 \times 10^5$ at 1 kHz and $\varepsilon_0 = 8 \times 10^4$ at 10 kHz.

The power carried by an electromagnetic wave through space can be calculated by taking the real part of the Poynting vector.

$$\vec{P}_y = \vec{E} \times \vec{H} \tag{0.15}$$

The power emitted through the containing surface of a volume containing a current or accelerated charge can be calculated from.

$$\int_v \left(\vec{H} \bullet \frac{\partial \vec{B}}{\partial t} + \vec{E} \bullet \frac{\partial \vec{D}}{\partial t} + \vec{E} \bullet \vec{J} \right) dV = -\oint_s \left(\vec{E} \bullet \vec{H} \right) \bullet dS \tag{0.16}$$

With radiated power it is relatively easy to produce heating effects in living objects with presently available human-made devices (see Chapter 9 in BMA). This does not imply, of course, that all biological effects of radiated RF power necessarily arise from temperature changes.

The problems we often have are those where a source of electric or magnetic field is specified along with its position with respect to the biological system and we wish to calculate values for $\vec{E}$, $\vec{B}$ or the power density and energy being depoisted in the biological material. Because of the complex geometries and biological material properties, solutions to Equations 0.6–0.9 are often complex. Thus, a large fraction of the time approximations are made to be able to calculate these values and to get insight into how things change with variations in the parameters.

At large distances, the size of a human or other biological system of interest is often small compared to the radius of curvature of the electromagnetic fields and we can approximate the incident fields as plane waves. This greatly simplifies the calculations of the fields interacting with the biological system. Carrying these approximations one step farther in order to get a first approximation to the fields that penetrate or are reflected from the complex shape of a typical biological subject such as a human, we assume that we can approximate the body or biological system with a simple geometric shape. The simplest of these interfaces is the plane sheet of biological material that is infinite in extent.

The results of experiments involving exposure of organic materials and entire living organisms to static E and extremely low frequency (ELF, generally <1 to ~3000 Hz) E fields are described in *BMA*, Chapters 1, 3, and 4.Various mechanisms for the interaction of such fields with living tissue are also discussed there and in *BBA*, Chapter 7. In the present introduction, we shall only point out that one salient feature of static (DC) and ELF E field interaction with living organisms is that the external or applied E field is always larger by several orders of magnitude than the resultant average internal E field [6,7]. This is a direct consequence of the conditions derived from Maxwell's equations (Equations 0.11–0.13).

0.4 Penetration of Direct Current and Low-Frequency Electric Fields into Tissue

Assuming that the two materials illustrated schematically in Figure 0.5 are characterized, respectively, by conductivities σ_1 and σ_2 and dielectric permittivities ε_1 and ε_2, we write E-field components parallel to the boundary as E_P and components perpendicular to the boundary as $E_\perp$. For both static and time-varying fields

$$E_{P1} = E_{P2} \tag{0.17}$$

and for static (DC) fields

$$\sigma_1 E_{\perp 1} = \sigma_2 E_{\perp 2} \tag{0.18}$$

as a consequence of the continuity of current (or conservation of charge). The orientations of the total E fields in media 1 and 2 can be represented by the tangents of the angles between the total fields and the boundary line

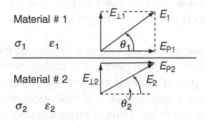

FIGURE 0.5
Symbols used in description of boundary conditions for E-field components.

$$\tan\theta_1 = \frac{E_{\perp 1}}{E_{P1}}, \quad \tan\theta_2 = \frac{E_{\perp 2}}{E_{P2}} \tag{0.19}$$

From these equations it follows that

$$\tan\theta_1 = \frac{\sigma_2}{\sigma_1}\frac{E_{\perp 1}}{E_{P1}} = \frac{\sigma_2}{\sigma_1}\frac{E_{\perp 2}}{E_{P2}} = \frac{\sigma_2}{\sigma_1}\tan\theta_2 \tag{0.20}$$

If material 1 is air with conductivity [8] $\sigma_1 = 10^{-13}$ S/m and material 2 a typical living tissue with $\sigma_2 \approx 10^{-1}$ S/m (compare Chapter 4 in *BBA*), $\tan\theta_1 = 10^{12}\tan\theta_2$, and therefore even if the field in material 2 (the inside field) is almost parallel to the boundary so that $\theta_2 \cong 0.5°$ or $\tan\theta_2 \approx (1/100)$, $\tan\theta_1 = 10^{10}$ or $\theta_1 = (\pi/2 - 10)^{-10}$ rad. Thus, an electrostatic field in air, at the boundary between air and living tissue, must be practically perpendicular to the boundary (See Figure 0.6). The situation is virtually the same at ELF although Equation 0.18 must be replaced by

$$\sigma_1 E_{\perp 1} - \sigma_2 E_{\perp 2} = -j\omega\rho_s \tag{0.21}$$

and

$$\varepsilon_1 E_{\perp 1} - \varepsilon_2 E_{\perp 2} = \rho_s \tag{0.22}$$

where $j = \sqrt{-1}$, ω is the radian frequency (= $2\pi \times$ frequency), and ρ_s is the surface charge density. In Chapter 4 in *BBA* it is shown that at ELF the relative dielectric permittivity of living tissue may be as high as 10^6 so that $\varepsilon_2 = 10^6\,\varepsilon_0$, where ε_0 is the dielectric permittivity of free space $(1/36\,\pi)\,10^{-9}$ F/m; however, it is still valid to assume that $\varepsilon_2 \le 0^{-5}$. Then, from Equations 0.21 and 0.22

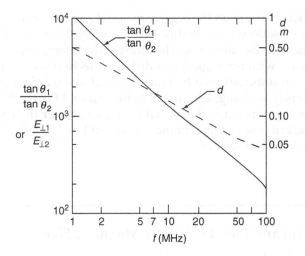

FIGURE 0.6
Orientation of *E*-field components at air–muscle boundary (or ratio of fields perpendicular to boundary); depth (*d*) at which field component parallel to boundary surface decreases by approximately 50% (*d* = 0.6938).

$$E_{\perp 1} = \frac{\sigma_2 + j\omega\varepsilon_2}{\sigma_1 + j\omega\varepsilon_1} E_{\perp 2} \tag{0.23}$$

which gives at 60 Hz with $\sigma_2 = 10^1$ S/m, $\sigma_1 = 10^{-13}$ S/m, $\varepsilon_2 \approx 10^{-5}$ F/m, and $\varepsilon_1 \approx 10^{-11}$ F/m

$$E_{\perp 1} = \frac{10^{-1} + j_4 10^{-3}}{10^{-13} + j_4 10^{-9}} E_{\perp 2} \approx \frac{\sigma_2}{j\omega\varepsilon_1} = -j\left(2.5 \times 10^7\right) E_{\perp 2} \tag{0.24}$$

This result, together with Equations 0.17 and 0.19, shows that for the given material properties, the field in air must still be practically perpendicular to the boundary of a living organism: $\tan\theta_1$: 2.5(10⁷) $\tan\theta_2$.

Knowing now that the living organism will distort the E field in its vicinity in such a way that the external field will be nearly perpendicular to the boundary surface, we can calculate the internal field by substituting the total field for the perpendicular field in Equations 0.18 (DC) and 0.23 (ELF). For the assumed typical material parameters we find that in the static (DC) case

$$\frac{E_{\text{internal}}}{E_{\text{external}}} \approx 10^{-12} \tag{0.25}$$

$$\rho_f = \frac{3(\sigma_2\varepsilon_1 - \sigma_1\varepsilon_2)E_0}{2\sigma_1 + \sigma_2}\cos\vartheta \; \text{C / m}^2$$

and for 60 Hz

$$\frac{E_{\text{internal}}}{E_{\text{external}}} \approx 4(10^{-8}) \tag{0.26}$$

Thus, a 60-Hz external field of 100 kV/m will produce an average E_{internal} field of the order of 4 mV/m.

If the boundary between air and the organic material consists of curved surfaces instead of infinite planes, the results will be modified only slightly. Thus, for a finite sphere (with ε and σ as assumed here) embedded in air, the ratios of the internal field to the undisturbed external field will vary with the angle θ and distance r as indicated in Figure 0.6, but will not deviate from the results indicated by Equations 0.21 and 0.22 by more than a factor of 3 [4,9]. Long cylinders ($L \ll r$) aligned parallel to the external field will have interior fields essentially equal to the unperturbed external field, except near the ends where the field component perpendicular to the membrane surface will be intensified approximately as above (see Chapter 5 in this volume).

0.5 Direct Current and Low-Frequency Magnetic Fields

Direct current and ELF H fields are considered in more detail in Chapters 5 and 6 in this volume. As the magnetic permeability μ of most biological materials is practically equal to the magnetic permeability μ_0 of free space, $4\pi(10^{-7})$ H/m, the DC, or ELF H field "inside" will be practically equal to the H field "outside." The only exceptions are organisms such as the magnetotactic bacteria, which synthesize ferromagnetic material, discussed in Chapter 7 of *BBA*. The known and suggested mechanisms of interaction of DC H fields with living matter are:

1. Orientation of ferromagnetic particles, including biologically synthesized particles of magnetite.

2. Orientation of diamagnetic or paramagnetic anisotropic molecules and cellular elements [10].

3. Generation of potential differences at right angles to a stream of moving ions (Hall effect, also sometimes called a magneto hydrodynamic effect) as a result of the magnetic force $F_m = qvB \sin \theta$, where q is the electric charge, v is the velocity of the charge, B is the magnetic flux density, and $\sin \theta$ is the sine of the angle θ between the directions v and B. One well-documented result of this mechanism is a "spike" in the electrocardiograms of vertebrates subjected to large DC H fields.

4. Changes in intermediate products or structural arrangements in the course of light-induced chemical (electron transfer) reactions, brought about by Zeeman splitting of molecular energy levels or effects upon hyperfine structure. (The Zeeman effect is the splitting of spectral lines, characteristic of electronic transitions, under the influence of an external H field. Hyperfine splitting of electronic transition lines in the absence of an external H field is due to the magnetic moment of the nucleus; such hyperfine splitting can be modified by an externally applied H field.) The magnetic flux densities involved depend upon the particular system and can be as high as 0.2 T (2000 G) but also as low as <0.01 mT (0.1 G). Bacterial photosynthesis and effects upon the visual system are prime candidates for this mechanism [11,12].

5. Induction of E fields with resulting electrical potential differences and currents within an organism by rapid motion through a large static H field. Some magnetic phosphenes are due to such motions [13].

Relatively slow time-varying H fields, which are discussed Chapters 6 and 7 in *BBA*, among others, may interact with living organisms through the same mechanisms that can be triggered by static H fields, provided the variation with time is slow enough to allow particles of finite size and mass, located in a viscous medium, to change orientation or position where required (mechanism 1 and 2) and provided the field intensity is sufficient to produce the particular effect. However, time-varying H fields, including ELF H fields, can also induce electric currents into stationary conducting objects. Thus, all modes of interaction of time-varying E fields with living matter may be triggered by time-varying, but not by static, H fields.

In view of Faraday's law, a time-varying magnetic flux will induce E fields with resulting electrical potential differences and "eddy" currents through available conducting paths. As very large external ELF E fields are required (as indicated by Equations 0.23–0.26) to generate even small internal E fields, many human-made devices and systems generating both ELF E and H fields are more likely to produce physiologically significant internal E fields through the mechanism of magnetic induction.

The induced voltage V around some closed path is given by

$$V = \oint E \cdot d\ell = -\iint \frac{\partial B}{\partial t} \cdot ds \qquad (0.27)$$

where E is the induced E field. The integration $\oint E \cdot dl$ is over the appropriate conduct-ing path, $\partial B/\partial t$ is the time derivative of the magnetic flux density, and the "dot" product with the surface element, ds, indicates that only the component of $\partial B/\partial t$ perpendicular to the surface, i.e., parallel to the direction of the vector ds, enclosed by the conducting path, induces an E field. To obtain an order-of-magnitude indication of the induced current that can be expected as a result of an ELF H field, we consider the circular path of radius r, illus-trated by Figure 0.7. Equation 0.28 then gives the magnitude of the E field as

$$E = \frac{\omega B r}{2} \qquad (0.28)$$

where ω is the $2\pi f$ and f is the frequency. The magnitude of the resulting electric current density J in ampere per square meter is[*]

$$J = \sigma E = \frac{\sigma \omega B r}{2} \qquad (0.29)$$

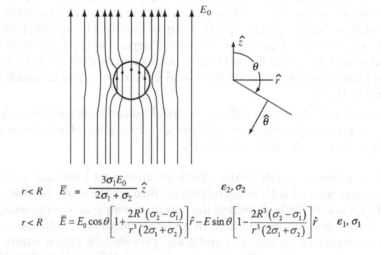

FIGURE 0.7
E field when sphere of radius R, conductivity σ, and dielectric permittivity ε_2 is placed into an initially uniform static field ($E = 2E_0$) within a medium with conductivity σ_1 and permittivity ε_1. The surface charge density is
$\rho_r = \dfrac{3(\sigma_2 \varepsilon_1 - \sigma_1 \varepsilon_2)E_0}{2\sigma_1 + \sigma_2} \cos\theta \; \text{C} / \text{m}^2.$

[*] Equation 0.29 neglects the H field generated by the induced eddy currents. If this field is taken into account, it can be shown that the induced current density in a cylindrical shell of radius r and thickness Δ is given by $\Delta r < 0.01 \; m^2/[1 + j\Delta r/\delta_2]$, where $H_0 = B_0/\mu_0$ and δ is the skin depth defined by Equation 0.28 below. However, for conductivities of biological materials ($\sigma < 5$ s/m) one obtains at audio frequencies $\delta > 1$ m and as for most dimensions of interest $\Delta r < 0.01$ m^2 the term $j\Delta r/\delta_2$ becomes negligible. The result $-jr H_0/\delta_2$ is then identical with Equation 0.29.

where σ is the conductivity along the path in Siemens per meter. In the SI (System International) units used throughout this book, B is measured in tesla ($1T = 10^4$ G) and r in meters. Choosing for illustration a circular path of 0.1 m radius, a frequency of 60 Hz, and a conductivity of 0.1 S/m, Equations 0.28 and 0.29 give $E = 18.85\ B$ and $I = 1.885\ B$. The magnetic flux density required to obtain a current density of 1 mA/m² is 0.53 mT or about 5 G. The E field induced by that flux density along the circular path is 10 mV/m. To produce this same 10 mV/m $E_{internal}$ field by an external 60 Hz $E_{external}$ field would require, by Equation 0.24, a field intensity of 250 kV/m.

As the induced voltage is proportional to the time rate of change of the H field (Equation 0.27), implying a linear increase with frequency (Equation 0.28), one would expect that the ability of a time-varying H field to induce currents deep inside a conductive object would increase indefinitely as the frequency increases or conversely, that the magnetic flux density required to induce a specified E field would decrease linearly with frequency, as indicated in Figure 0.8. This is not true, however, because the displacement current density

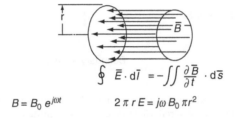

$$\oint \bar{E} \cdot d\bar{l} = -\iint \frac{\partial \bar{B}}{\partial t} \cdot d\bar{s}$$

$$B = B_0\, e^{j\omega t} \qquad 2\pi r E = j\omega B_0 \pi r^2$$

FIGURE 0.8
Circular path (loop) of radius r enclosing uniform magnetic flux density perpendicular to the plane of the loop. For sinusoidal time variation $B = B_0 e^{j\omega t}$.

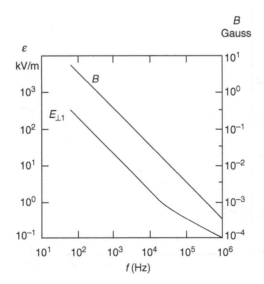

FIGURE 0.9
External E and H field required to obtain an internal E field of 10 mV/m (conductivity and dielectric permittivity for skeletal muscle. (From Foster, K.R., Schepps, J.L., and Schwan, H.P. 1980. *Biophys. J.*, 29, 271–281. H-field calculation assumes a circular path of 0.1-m radius perpendicular to magnetic flux).

$\partial D/\partial t$, where $D = \varepsilon E$, must also be considered as the frequency increases. This leads to the wave behavior discussed in Part 3, implying that at sufficiently high frequencies the effects of both external E and H fields are limited by reflection losses (Figures 0.9–0.11) as well as by skin effect [14], i.e., limited depth of penetration d in Figure 0.6.

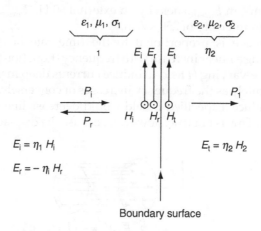

FIGURE 0.10
Reflection and transmission of an electromagnetic wave at the boundary between two different media, perpendicular incidence; P_i = incident power, P_r = reflected power, P_t = transmitted power.

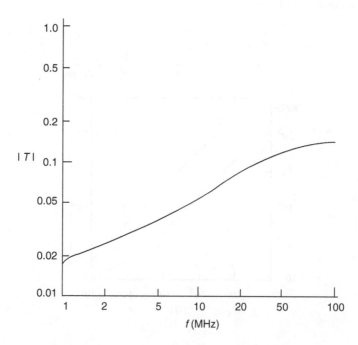

FIGURE 0.11
Magnitude of transmission coefficient T for incident E field parallel to boundary surface. $T = E_t/E_i$: reflection coefficient $r = E_r/E_i = T - 1$. Γ and T are complex numbers; ε_r and σ for skeletal muscle from Chapter 4 in *BBA*.

0.6 RF Fields

At frequencies well below those where most animals and many field-generating systems have dimensions on the order of one free-space wavelength, e.g., at 10 MHz where $\lambda = 30$ m, the skin effect limits penetration of the external field. This phenomenon is fundamentally different from the small ratio of internal to external E fields described in Equation 0.18 (applicable to DC) and Equation 0.23.

Equation 0.23 expresses a "boundary condition" applicable at all frequencies, but as the angular frequency ω increases and in view of the rapid decrease with frequency of the dielectric permittivity ε_2 in biological materials (see Chapter 4 of *BBA*), the ratio of the normal component of the external to the internal E field at the boundary decreases with increasing frequency. This is illustrated by Figure 0.6 where $\tan \theta_1 / \tan \theta_2$ is also equal to $E_{\perp_1}/E_{\perp_2}$ in view of Equations 0.17, 0.19, and 0.23. However, at low frequencies the total field inside the boundary can be somewhat larger than the perpendicular field at the boundary; and any field variation with distance from the boundary is not primarily due to energy dissipation, but in a homogeneous body it is a consequence of shape. At RF, on the other hand, the E and H fields of the incoming electromagnetic wave, after reflection at the boundary, are further decreased due to energy dissipation. Both E and H fields decrease exponentially with distance from the boundary

$$g(z) = Ae^{-\frac{z}{\delta}} \tag{0.30}$$

where $g(z)$ is the field at the distance z and A is the magnitude of the field just *inside* the boundary. As defined by Equation 0.30 the skin depth δ is the distance over which the field decreases to $1/e$ (= 0.368) of its value just *inside* the boundary. (Due to reflection, the field A just inside the boundary can already be very much smaller than the incident external field; see Figures 0.9 and 0.10.)

Expressions for δ given below were derived [3,4,14,15] for plane boundaries between infinite media. They are reasonably accurate for cylindrical structures if the ratio of radius of curvature to skin depth (r_0/δ) is larger than about five [14]. For a good conductor

$$\delta = \frac{1}{\sqrt{\pi f \mu \sigma}} \tag{0.31}$$

where a good conductor is one for which the ratio p of conduction current, $J = \sigma E$, to displacement current, $\partial D/\partial t = \varepsilon(\partial E/\partial t) = j\omega \varepsilon E$ is large:

$$p = \frac{\sigma}{\omega \varepsilon} \gg 1 \tag{0.32}$$

Since for most biological materials p is of the order of one ($0.1 < p < 10$) over a very wide frequency range (see Chapter 4 of *BBA*), it is frequently necessary to use the more general expression [14]

$$\delta = \frac{1}{\omega \left[\frac{\mu \varepsilon}{2} (\sqrt{1+p^2} - 1) \right]^{1/2}} \tag{0.33}$$

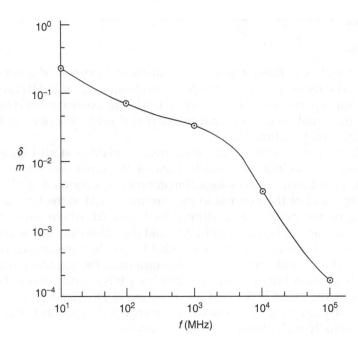

FIGURE 0.12
Electromagnetic skin depth in muscle tissue from plane wave expression (Equation 0.33, Table 0.1).

The decrease in field intensity with distance from the boundary surface indicated by Equation 0.30 becomes significant for many biological objects at frequencies where $r_0/\delta \geq 5$ is not satisfied. However, the error resulting from the use of Equations 0.30 and 0.31 or Equation 0.33 with curved objects is less when $z < \delta$. Thus, at $z = 0.693\,\delta$, where $g(z) = 0.5$ A from Equations 0.30 and 0.31, the correct values of $g(z)$, obtained by solving the wave equation in cylindrical coordinates, differs only by 20% (it is 0.6 A) even when r_0/δ is as small as 2.39 [15]. Therefore, Figure 0.12 shows the distance $d = 0.693\,\delta$, at which the field decreases to half of its value just inside the boundary surface, using Equation 0.33 with typical values for σ and ε for muscle. It is apparent that the skin effect becomes significant for humans and larger vertebrates at frequencies >10 MHz.

Directly related to skin depth, which is defined for fields varying sinusoidally with time, is the fact that a rapid transient variation of an applied magnetic flux density constitutes an exception to the statement that the DC H field inside the boundary is equal to the H field outside. Thus, from one viewpoint one may consider the rapid application or removal of a DC H field as equivalent to applying a high-frequency field during the switching period, with the highest frequencies present of the order of $1/\tau$, where τ is the rise time of the applied step function. Thus, if $\tau < 10^{-8}$ s, the skin effect will be important during the transient period, as d in Figure 0.6 is <5 cm above 100 MHz. It is also possible to calculate directly the magnetic flux density inside a conducting cylinder as a function of radial position r and time t when a magnetic pulse is applied in the axial direction [16,17]. Assuming zero rise time of the applied field B_0, i.e., a true step function, one finds that the field inside a cylinder of radius a is

$$B = B_0\left[1 - \sum_{k=1}^{\infty} J_0\left(r\frac{v_k}{a}\right)e^{-t/T_k}\right] \qquad (0.34)$$

where J_0 $(r\,v_k/a)$ is the zero-order Bessel function of argument $r\,v_k/a$ and the summation is over the nulls of J_0 designated v_k (the first four values of v_k are 2.405, 5.520, 8.654, and 11.792).* T_k is the rise time of the kth term in the series and is given by

$$T_k = \frac{\mu_0 \sigma a^2}{v_k} \qquad (0.35)$$

As v_k increases, the rise time decreases and therefore the longest delay is due to the first term in the summation with $k = 1$

$$T_1 = \frac{\mu_0 \sigma a^2}{2.405} \qquad (0.36)$$

For a cylinder with 0.1 m radius and a conductivity $\sigma \approx 1$ S/m, which is a typical value for muscle between 100 and 1000 MHz, Equation 0.36 gives $T_1 = 2.6 \times 10^{-8}$ s. This finite rise time (or decay time in case of field removal) of the internal H field may be of some importance when pulsed H fields are used therapeutically [18]. It might also be used to measure non-invasively the conductivity of biological substances *in vivo* through determination of the final decay rate of the voltage induced into a probe coil by the slowly decaying internal field after the applied field is removed [17].

The properties of biological substances in the intermediate frequency range, above ELF (>300 Hz), and below the higher RFs, where wave behavior and skin effect begin to be important (~20 MHz), are discussed in Chapter 4 of *BBA*. However, many subsequent chapters are concerned with biological effects at DC and ELF frequencies below a few kilohertz, while others deal primarily with the higher RFs >50 MHz. One reason for this limited treatment of the intermediate frequency range is that very little animal data are available for this spectral region in comparison with the large number of experiments performed at ELF and microwave frequencies in recent years.† Another reason is that most electrical processes known to occur naturally in biological systems—action potentials, EKG, EEG, ERG, etc.—occur at DC and ELF frequencies. Therefore, one might expect some physiological effects from external fields of appropriate intensity in the same frequency range, even if the magnitude of such fields is not large enough to produce thermal effects. As illustrated by Figures 0.4 and 0.8, most E fields below 100 kHz set up by currently used human-made devices, and most H fields below 10 kHz except the very strongest, are incapable of producing thermal effects in living organisms, excluding, of course, fields accompanying currents directly introduced into the organism via electrodes. Thus, the frequencies between about 10 and 100 kHz have been of relatively little interest because they have not been seen to be very likely to produce thermal or other biological effects. On the other hand, the higher RFs are frequently generated at power levels where enough energy may be introduced into living organisms to produce local or general heating. In addition, despite skin effect and the reflection loss to be discussed in more detail below, microwaves modulated at an ELF rate may serve as a vehicle for introducing ELF fields into a living organism of at least the same order of magnitude as would be introduced by direct exposure to ELF. Any effect of such ELF-modulated microwaves would, of course, require the existence of some amplitude-dependent demodulation mechanism to extract the ELF from the microwave carrier.

---

* This result is based on solution of $\partial B/\partial t = (1/\mu_0)\nabla^2 B$, which is a consequence of Ampere's and Faraday's laws when displacement is disregarded. Equations 0.20–0.22 are therefore only correct when $p \gg 1$.

† Though this statement was written for the second edition in 1995, it continues to be true.

Among the chapters dealing with RF, Chapters 5, 9, and 10 of *BBA* give the necessary information for establishing the magnitude of the fields present in biological objects: (1) experimental techniques and (2) analytical methods for predicting field intensities without construction of physical models made with "phantom" materials, i.e., dielectric materials with properties similar to those of living objects which are to be exposed. As thermal effects at microwave frequencies are certainly important, although one cannot assume *a priori* that they are the only biological effects of this part of the spectrum, and as some (but not all) thermal effects occur at levels where the thermoregulatory system of animals is activated. Thermoregulation in the presence of microwave fields is discussed in Chapters 9 and 11 of *BMA*, as well as in Chapter 9 of *BBA*. Not only are most therapeutic applications of microwaves based upon their thermal effects, but also it is now experimentally established that there are biological effects for exposure levels that are below the levels where significant changes expected to occur as a result of heating and changes in temperature. See Chapters 7 and 11 in *BBA* and many in *BMA*. Effects at the threshold of large-scale tissue heating in particular living systems also requires thorough understanding of thermoregulatory mechanisms. The vast amount of experimental data obtained on animal systems exposed to microwave is discussed in Chapter 5 in *BMA*. Both non-modulated fields and modulated fields, where the type of modulation had no apparent effect other than modification of the average power level, are considered. These chapters and the Chapters 6 and 7 in *BMA* consider very new extensions of experiments into exposures to ultra-short and to ultra-high-power pulses.

At the higher RF frequencies, the external E field is not necessarily perpendicular to the boundary of biological materials (see Figures 0.5 and 0.11), and the ratio of the total external E field to the total internal field is not given by Equation 0.23. However, the skin effect (Equations 0.30–0.33) and reflection losses still reduce the E field within any biological object below the value of the external field. As pointed out in Chapter 4, dielectric permittivity and electrical conductivity of organic substances both vary with frequency. At RF, most biological substances are neither very good electrical conductors nor very good insulators, with the exception of cell membranes, which are good dielectrics at RF but at ELF can act as intermittent conductors or as dielectrics and are ion-selective [19–21]. The ratio p (Equation 0.32) is neither much smaller nor very much larger than values shown for typical muscle tissue [22,23] in Table 0.1.

Reflection loss at the surface of an organism is a consequence of the difference between its electrical properties and those of air. Whenever an electromagnetic wave travels from one material to another with different electrical properties, the boundary conditions

TABLE 0.1

Ratio p of Conduction Current to Displacement as a Function of Frequency For Typical Muscle Tissue

f (MHz)	σ	ε_r	$p = \dfrac{\sigma}{\omega\varepsilon_0\varepsilon_r}$
1	0.40	2000	3.6
10	0.63	160	7.1
100	0.89	72	2.2
10^3	1.65	50	0.59
10^4	10.3	40	0.46
10^5	80	6	2.4

(Equations 0.17 and 0.22) and similar relations for the H field require the existence of a reflected wave. The expressions for the reflection coefficient

$$\Gamma = \frac{E_r}{E_i} \tag{0.37}$$

and the transmission coefficient

$$T = \frac{E_t}{E_i} \tag{0.38}$$

becomes rather simple for loss-free dielectrics ($p \ll 1$) and for good conductors ($p \gg 1$). As biological substances are neither the most general expressions for Γ and T, applicable at plane boundaries, are needed [4,14]. For perpendicular incidence, illustrated by Figure 0.9,

$$\Gamma = \frac{\eta_2 - \eta_1}{\eta_2 + \eta_1} \tag{0.39}$$

$$T = \frac{2\eta_2}{\eta_2 + \eta_1} = 1 + \Gamma \tag{0.40}$$

where η_1 and η_2 are the wave impedances, respectively, of mediums 1 and 2. The wave impedance of a medium is the ratio of the E to the H field in a plane wave traveling through that medium; it is given by [14]

$$\eta = \left(\frac{j\omega\mu}{\sigma + j\omega\varepsilon} \right)^{1/2} \tag{0.41}$$

Clearly, Γ and T are in general complex numbers, <u>even</u> when medium 1 is air for which Equation 0.41 reduces to the real quantity $\eta_0 = \sqrt{\mu_0 / \varepsilon_0}$, because medium 2, which here is living matter, usually has a complex wave impedance at RFs.

The incident, reflected, and transmitted powers are given by [14]

$$P_i = R_1 |E_i|^2 \frac{1}{\eta_1^*} = \frac{|E_i|^2}{|\eta_1|^2} R_1 \tag{0.42}$$

$$P_r = R_1 |E_r|^2 \frac{1}{\eta_1^*} = \frac{|E_r|^2}{|\eta_1|^2} R_1 \tag{0.43}$$

$$P_t = R_1 |E_t|^2 \frac{1}{\eta_2^*} = \frac{|E_t|^2}{|\eta_2|^2} R_2 \tag{0.44}$$

where the E fields are effective values ($E_{eff} = E_{peak}/\sqrt{2}$) of sinusoidal quantities, R_1 signifies "real part of," η^*. It is the complex conjugate of η, and R_1 and R_2 are the real parts of η_1 and η_2. If medium 1 is air, $\eta_1 = R_1 = 377 \ \Omega$, it follows from Equations 0.37, 0.38, and 0.42–0.44 and conservation of energy that the ratio of the transmitted to the incident real power is given by

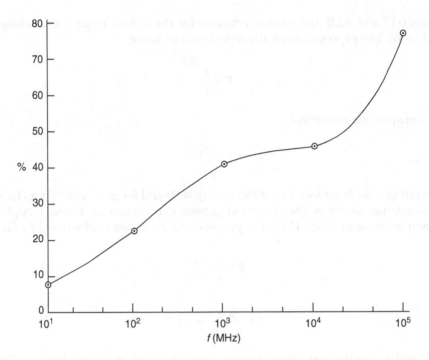

FIGURE 0.13
Ratio of transmitted to incident power expressed as percent of incident power. Air–muscle interface, perpendicular incidence (Equation 0.45, Table 0.1).

$$\frac{P}{P_1} = |T|^2 \, \frac{\eta_1 \eta_2^* + \eta_1^* \eta_2}{2|\eta_2|^2} = 1 - \frac{P_r}{P_i} = 1 - |\Gamma|^2 \tag{0.45}$$

The magnitude of the transmission coefficient T for the air–muscle interface over the 1- to 100-MHz frequency range is plotted in Figure 0.10, which shows that the magnitude of the transmitted E field in muscle tissue is considerably smaller than the E field in air. The fraction of the total incident power that is transmitted (Equation 0.45) is shown in Figure 0.13, indicating clearly that reflection loss at the interface decreases with frequency. However, for deeper lying tissue this effect is offset by the fact that the skin depth δ (Equation 0.33) also decreases with frequency (Figure 0.12) so that the total power penetrating beyond the surface decreases rapidly.

In addition to reflection at the air–tissue boundary, further reflections take place at each boundary between dissimilar materials. For example, the magnitude of the reflection coefficient at the boundary surface between muscle and organic materials with low-water content, such as fat or bone, is shown in Table 0.2.

The situation is actually more complicated than indicated by Figures 0.10 and 0.12, because the wave front of the incident electromagnetic wave may not be parallel to the air–tissue boundary. Two situations are possible: the incident E field may be polarized perpendicular to the plane of incidence defined in Figure 0.14 (perpendicular polarization, Figure 0.14a) or parallel to the plane of incidence (parallel polarization, Figure 0.14b). The transmission and reflection coefficients [9] are different for the two types of polarization and also become functions of the angle of incidence α_1:

TABLE 0.2

Reflection Coefficient "Capital Gamma" for Low–Water-Content Materials

f (MHz)	σ (S/m)	ε_r	Muscle[a]–Fat (Γ)
	Fat or Bone		
10^2	0.048	7.5	0.65
10^3	0.101	5.6	0.52
10^4	0.437	4.5	0.52

[a] σ and ε_r for muscle from Table 0.1.

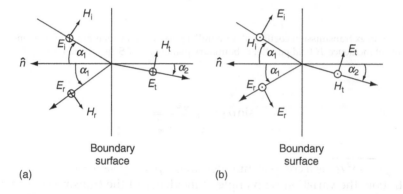

(a)   (b)

FIGURE 0.14

Oblique incidence of an electromagnetic wave at the boundary between two different media. (a) Perpendicular polarization (E vector perpendicular to plane of incidence); (b) parallel polarization (E vector parallel to plane of incidence). The plane of incidence is the plane formed by the surface normal (unit vector n and the direction of the incident wave); $\otimes$ indicates a vector into the plane of the paper; $\odot$ indicates a vector out of the plane of the paper. The orientation of the field vectors in the transmitted field is shown for loss-free dielectrics. For illustration of the transmitted wave into a medium with finite conductivity, where the wave impedance η_2 becomes a complex number, see Stratton, J.A., *Electromagnetic Theory*, McGraw-Hill, New York, 1941, p. 435.

$$\text{Perpendicular polarization} \begin{cases} T_\perp = \dfrac{2\eta_2 \cos\alpha_1}{\eta_2 \cos\alpha_1 + \eta_1 \cos\alpha_2} \\[2em] \Gamma_\perp = \dfrac{\eta_2 \cos\alpha_1 - \eta_1 \cos\alpha_2}{\eta_2 \cos\alpha_1 + \eta_1 \cos\alpha_2} \end{cases} \quad\quad (0.46 \text{ and } 0.47)$$

$$\text{Parallel polarization} \begin{cases} T_p = \dfrac{2\eta_2 \cos\alpha_1}{\eta_2 \cos\alpha_2 + \eta_1 \cos\alpha_1} \\[2em] \Gamma_p = \dfrac{\eta_1 \cos\alpha_1 - \eta_2 \cos\alpha_2}{\eta_2 \cos\alpha_2 + \eta_1 \cos\alpha_1} \end{cases} \quad\quad (0.48 \text{ and } 0.49)$$

where α_2 is given by the generalized Snell's law (when both the media have the magnetic permeability of free space) by [a]σ and ε_r for muscle from Table 0.1.

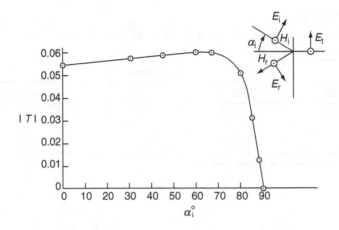

FIGURE 0.15
Magnitude of complex transmission coefficient for parallel polarization versus angle of incidence α_1 at 10 MHz (E field in plane of incidence, H field parallel to boundary plane; $\sigma_2 = 0.7$ S/m, $\varepsilon_{r2} = 150$, $T = E_t/E_r$).

$$\sin \alpha_2 = \frac{\sqrt{\varepsilon_1}}{\sqrt{\varepsilon_2 - j\frac{\sigma_2}{\omega}}} \tag{0.50}$$

so that $\alpha_2 = \sqrt{1 - \sin^2 \alpha_2}$ is a complex number unless $\rho_2 = (\sigma_2/\omega\varepsilon_2) = 1$.

As illustration, the variation with angle of incidence of the transmission coefficient for parallel polarization at the air–muscle interface at 10 MHz, is shown in Figure 0.15. It is apparent that the transmitted field is not necessarily maximized by perpendicular incidence in the case of parallel polarization. Furthermore, whenever $p \approx 1$ or $p > 1$ (see Table 0.1, above), α_2 is complex, which causes the waves entering the tissue to be inhomogeneous— they are not simple plane waves, but waves where surfaces of constant phase and constant amplitude do not coincide [4,24]; only the planes of constant amplitude are parallel to the boundary surface.

Analytical solutions for non-planar structures taking into account size and shape of entire animals have been given [25] and are also described in the RF modeling Chapter 9 of *BBA*.

0.7 Biophysical Interactions of Fields: Ionization, Ionizing Radiation, Chemical Bonds, and Excitation

RF fields can be characterized as nonionizing radiation. By this, we mean that there is not enough energy in a single quantum of RF energy, hf, to ionize an atom or a molecule, where h is Planck's constant and f is the frequency. By comparison radiation in the UV or x-ray regions often lead to ionization. It is desirable to begin by reviewing the differences between ionizing and nonionizing radiations, to explain ionization phenomena and also to discuss related excitation phenomena, which require less energy than ionization; a number of proposed models concerning atomic or molecular-level interactions of fields will be introduced. A number of these theories will be discussed and their predictions compared with experimental results in many later chapters. Heating, cell excitation, electroporation, and other results of high-intensity fields have been accepted as explanations for many bioelectromagnetic phenomena. For low-intensity exposure, however, no theory is widely accepted as a general explanation for bioelectromagnetic phenomena, and few specific phenomena have accepted explanations. It is quite possible that no general explanation exists and that more than one mechanism of interaction between fields will be found to be operating, depending on the situation. Chapter 7 of BBA has a summary of many proposed mechanisms, including discussion of the possible role of radicals' and other molecular structures' rotational, electronic, and nuclear angular momenta in explaining a number of types of biological effects. Binhi's book [26] contains a good summary of many theoretical proposals, including comparisons with data and critiques of their strong and weak points, as well as his own theory.

We note first that the energy of electromagnetic waves is quantized with the quantum of energy (in joules) being equal to Planck's constant ($h = 6.63 \times 10^{-34}$ J s) times the frequency. This energy can also be expressed in electron volts, i.e., in multiples of the kinetic energy acquired by an electron accelerated through a potential difference of 1 V (1 eV $\approx 1.6 \times 10^{-19}$ J). Energy quanta for a few frequencies are listed in Table 0.3.

Quantized energy can "excite" molecules; appropriate frequencies can couple to vibrational and rotational oscillation; and if the incident energy quantum has sufficient magnitude it can excite other changes in the electron configuration, such as changing an electron to another (unoccupied) energy level or tearing an electron away from one of the constituent atoms. The latter process called as ionization. The energy required to remove one electron from the highest energy orbit of a particular chemical element is called its "ionization potential." Typical ionization potentials are of the order 10 eV; for example, for the hydrogen atom it is 13.6 eV and for gaseous sodium, 5.1 eV. As chemical binding forces are essentially electrostatic, ionization implies profound chemical changes. Therefore, ionization by any outside agent of the complex compounds that make up a living system leads to profound and often irreversible changes in the operation of that system.

Table 0.3 shows that even the highest RF (millimeter waves) has quantum energies well below the ionization potential of any known substance; thus, one speaks of nonionizing radiation when referring to electromagnetic waves below UV light frequencies. Ionizing radiation includes UV and higher frequency electromagnetic waves (x-rays, γ-rays).

This explanation of the difference between ionizing and nonionizing radiation should not imply that nonionizing electromagnetic radiation cannot have profound effects upon

TABLE 0.3

Wave and Quantum Characteristics of Various Types of Radiation

Name of Radiation or Application	Frequency (Hz)	Wavelength (m)	Energy of 1 Quantum of Radiation (eV)
UHF TV	7×10^8	0.43	2.88×10^{-6}
Microwave radar	10^{10}	3×10^{-2}	4.12×10^{-5}
Millimeter wave	3×10^{11}	1×10^{-3}	1.24×10^{-3}
Visible light	6×10^{14}	5×10^{-7}	2.47
Ionizing UV	10^{16}	3×10^{-4}	41.2
Soft x-ray	10^{18}	3×10^{-10}	4120
Penetrating x-ray	10^{20}	3×10^{-12}	4.12×10^5

inorganic and organic substances. As excitation of coherent vibrational and rotational modes requires considerably less energy than ionization, it could occur at RF; this will be discussed in later chapters. In addition, many other possible biological effects require energies well below the level of ionizing potentials. Examples are tissue heating, dielectrophoresis, depolarization of cell membranes, mechanical stress due to piezoelectric transduction, or dielectric saturation, resulting in the orientation of the polar side chains of macromolecules and leading to the breaking of hydrogen bonds. These and other mechanisms will be discussed by the authors of several chapters (see especially Chapter 7 of *BBA*). Returning to the discussion of ionization, it is important to note that ionization of a chemical element can be brought about not only by absorption of electromagnetic energy, but also by collision either with foreign (injected) atoms, molecules, or subatomic particles of the requisite energy, or by sufficiently violent collision among its own atoms. The latter process constitutes ionization by heating, or thermal breakdown of a substance, which will occur when the kinetic energy of the colliding particles exceeds the ionization potential. As the average thermal kinetic energy of particles is related to temperature [27] by $W = kT$ where k is Boltzmann's constant (= 1.38×10^{-23} J/K), we find that the required temperature is

$$1.38(10^{-23})\, T \approx 5\,\text{eV} \approx (5)1.6(10^{-19})\,\text{J}$$

$$T \approx 5(10^4)\,\text{K}$$

which is about twice the temperature inside a lightning stroke [28] and orders of magnitude higher than any temperature obtainable from electromagnetic waves traveling through air.

Actually, initiation of lightning strokes is an example of ionization by collision with injected energetic particles. The few free electrons and ions always present in the air due to ionization by cosmic rays are accelerated by the E fields generated within clouds to velocities corresponding to the required ionization energy. Only when the field is large enough to impart this energy over distances shorter than the mean free path of the free electrons or ions at atmospheric pressure can an avalanche process take place: an accelerated electron separates a low-energy electron from the molecule with which it collides and in the process loses most of its own energy; thus, one high-energy free electron is exchanged for two free low-energy electrons and one positive ion. Both the electrons are in turn accelerated again by the field, giving them high kinetic energy before they collide with neutral molecules; their collision produces four free electrons and the multiplication process continues. The breakdown field strength for air at atmospheric pressure is approximately 3×10^6 V/m, implying a mean free path of electrons

$$\Delta \ell \approx \left[5\text{eV} \,/\, 3 \times 10^6\,\text{V/m} \right] \approx 10^{-6}\,\text{m}$$

However, this model is not entirely accurate because the actual mean free path corresponds to energies of the order of 0.1 eV, which is only sufficient to excite vibrational modes in the target molecule. Apparently such excitation is sufficient to cause ionization if the collision process lasts long enough [29].

Except for some laboratory conditions where a sufficiently high potential difference can be applied directly across a biological membrane to bring about its destruction, collisional ionization is generally not a factor in the interaction of electromagnetic waves with tissue: The potential difference required for membrane destruction [30] is between 100 nV and 300 mV, corresponding to a field strength of the order of 2×10^7 V/m, assuming a membrane thickness ($d = 100$ Å; $E = V/d$). However, there is a third mechanism of ionization that is particularly important in biological systems. When a chemical compound of the type wherein positive and negative ions are held together by their electrostatic attraction, such as the ionic crystal NaCl, is placed in a suitable solvent, such as H_2O, it is separated into its ionic components. The resulting solution becomes an electrolyte, i.e., an electrically conducting medium in which the only charge carriers are ions.

In this process of chemical ionization, the Na^+ cations and Cl^- anions are separated from the original NaCl crystal lattice and individually surrounded by a sheet of solvent molecules, the "hydration sheath." If the solvent is H_2O, this process is called "hydration," or more generally, for any solvent, "solvation."

A dilute solution of NaCl crystals in H_2O is slightly cooler than the original constituents before the solvation process, indicating that some internal energy of the system was consumed. Actually energy is consumed in breaking up the original NaCl bonds and some, but less, is liberated in the interaction between the dipole moment of the solvent molecule (H_2O in our example) and the electric charges on the ions. Thus, solvents with higher relative dielectric constant ε_r, indicating higher inherent electric dipole moment per unit volume (P), solvate ions more strongly ($\varepsilon_r = 1 + P/[\varepsilon_o E]$, where E is the electric field applied during the measurement of ε_r). For example, H_2O with $\varepsilon_r \approx 80$ solvates more strongly than methanol with $\varepsilon_r \approx 33$. For biological applications, it is worth noting that solvation may affect not only ionic substances, but also polar groups, i.e., molecular components which have an inherent dipole moment, such as $-C=O$, $-NH$, or $-NO_2$. Details of the process are discussed in texts on electrochemistry [31,32].

In biological processes not only chemical ionization and solvation of ionic compounds, but also all kinds of chemical reactions take place. One of the central questions in the study of biological effects of E and H fields is therefore not only whether they can cause or influence ionization, but also whether they can affect—speed up, slow down, or modify—any naturally occurring biologically important chemical reaction.

In Table 0.4 typical energies for various types of chemical bonds are listed. For comparison, the thermal energy per elementary particle at 310 K is also shown. Complementing the numbers in Table 0.4 one should also point out that:

1. The large spread in the statistical distribution of energies of thermal motion guarantees that at physiological temperatures some molecules always have sufficient energy to break the strongest weak bonds [33].

2. The average lifetime of a weak bond is only a fraction of a second.

3. The weak binding forces (Van der Waals) are effective only between the surfaces in close proximity and usually require complementary structures such as a (microscopic) plug and hole, such as are thought to exist, between antigen and antibody, for instance [34].

4. Most molecules in aqueous solution form secondary bonds.

5. The metabolism of biological systems continuously transforms molecules and therefore also changes the secondary bonds that are formed.

Comparison of the last columns in Tables 0.3 and 0.4 shows that millimeter waves have quantum energies which are only about one order of magnitude below typical Van der Waals energies (waves at a frequency of 10^{12} Hz with a quantum energy of 0.004 eV

TABLE 0.4

Bond and Thermal Energies

Type of Bond	Change in Free Energy (Binding Energy) kcal/mol	eV/ Molecule
Covalent	50–100	2.2–4.8
Van der Waals	1–2	0.04–0.08
Hydrogen	3–7	0.13–0.30
Ionic[a]	5	0.2
Avg. thermal energy at 310K	0.62	0.027

[a] For ionic groups of organic molecules such as COO–, NH3$_{\overline{3}}$ in aqueous solution.

have a wavelength of 0.3 mm and can still be classified as millimeter waves). One might expect therefore that such waves could initiate chemically important events, such as configurational changes, e.g., multiple transitions between closely spaced vibrational states at successively high-energy levels [47].

Energies associated with transition from one to another mode of rotation of a diatomic molecule are given by $W = \ell(\ell + 1)A$ [26,33], where $\ell = 0, 1, 2, 3\ldots$ and $A = 6 \times 10^{-5}$ eV; thus, an electromagnetic wave with a frequency as low as 29 GHz—still in the microwave region—can excite a rotational mode. Vibrational modes of diatomic molecules [27,34] correspond to energies of the order of 0.04 eV, requiring excitation in the IR region. Vibrational frequencies in a typical H-bonded system [35] are of the order of 3000 GHz; however, attenuation at this frequency by omnipresent free H_2O may prevent any substantial effect [35].

Kohli et al. [36] predict that longitudinal and torsional modes of double helical DNA should not be critically damped at frequencies >1 GHz, although relaxation times are of the order of picoseconds, and Kondepudi [37] suggests the possibility of an influence of millimeter waves at approximately 5×10^{11} Hz upon oxygen affinity of hemoglobin due to the resonant excitation of heme plane oscillations. Although Furia et al. [38] did not find resonance absorption at millimeter waves in yeast, such was reported by Grundler et al. [39,48]. The latter experiment has been interpreted [40,41] as supporting Fröhlich's theory of cooperative phenomena in biological systems. That theory postulates "electric polarization waves" in biological membranes which are polarized by strong biologically generated [19] fields (10^7 V/m). Fröhlich [42,43] suggests that metabolically supplied energy initiates mechanical vibrations of cell membranes. The frequency of such vibrations is determined by the dimensions and the elastic constants of the membranes; based on an estimate of the sound velocity in the membrane of 10^3 m/s and a membrane thickness of 100 Å (equal to one half wavelength) one obtains a frequency of $5(10^{10})$ Hz. Individual molecules within and outside the membrane may also oscillate, and frequency estimates vary between 10^9 Hz for helical RNA [44] and 5×10^{13} Hz for hydrogen-bonded amide structures [45]. As the membranes and molecules involved are strongly polarized, the mechanically oscillating dipole electromagnetic fields those are able to transmit energy, at least in some situations, over distances much larger than the distance to the next adjacent molecule.

Electromagnetic coupling of this type may produce long-range cooperative phenomena. In particular, Fröhlich [46] has shown that two molecular systems may exert strong forces upon each other when their respective oscillation frequencies are nearly equal, provided the dielectric permittivity of the medium between them is strongly dispersive or excitation is supplied by pumping, i.e., by excitation at the correct frequency from an external source. The mechanism is nonlinear in the sense that it displays a step-like dependence on excitation intensity. Possible long-range effects may be, for example, attraction between enzyme and substrate [43]. These and related topics have been discussed in detail by Illinger [35] and are reviewed in Chapters 5 and 7 in this volume.

References

1. Ramo, S., Whinnery, J.R., and Van Duzer, T., *Fields and Waves in Communication Electronics*, John Wiley & Sons, New York, 1965, p. 644.
2. Jordan, E.C., *Electromagnetic Waves and Radiating Systems*. Prentice-Hall, Englewood Cliffs, NJ, 1950.
3. Schelkunoff, S.A., *Electromagnetic Waves*, D Van Nostrand, New York, 1943, p. 133.
4. Stratton, J.A., *Electromagnetic Theory*, McGraw-Hill, New York, 1941, p. 435.
5. Van Bladel, J., *Electromagnetic Fields*, McGraw-Hill, New York, 1964, p. 274.
6. Kaune, W.T. and Gillis, M.F., General properties of the interaction between animals and ELF electric fields, *Bioelectromagnetics*, 2, 1, 1981.
7. Bridges, J.E. and Preache, M., Biological influences of power frequency electric fields—a tutorial review from a physical and experimental viewpoint, *Proc. IEEE*, 69, 1092, 1981.
8. Iribarne, J.V. and Cho, H.R., *Atmospheric Physics*, D. Reidel, Boston, MA, 1980, p. 134.
9. Zahn, M., *Electromagnetic Field Theory, A Problem Solving Approach*, John Wiley & Sons, New York, 1979.
10. Schulten, K., Magnetic field effects in chemistry and biology, in *Festkörperprobleme/Advances in Solid State Physics*, Vol. 22, Heyden, Philadelphia, 1982, p. 61.
11. Raybourn, M.S., The effects of direct-current magnetic fields on turtle retina in vitro, *Science*, 220, 715, 1983.
12. Blankenship, R.E., Schaafsma, T.J., and Parson, W.W., Magnetic field effects on radical pair intermediates in bacterial photosynthesis, *Biochim. Biophys. Acta*, 461, 297, 1977.
13. Sheppard, A.R., Magnetic field interactions in man and other mammals: An overview, in *Magnetic Field Effect on Biological Systems*, Tenforde, T.S., Ed., Plenum Press, New York, 1979, p. 33.
14. Jordan, E.C., *Electromagnetic Waves and Radiating Systems*, Prentice-Hall, Englewood Cliffs, NJ, 1950, p. 132.
15. Ramo, S., Whinnery, J.R., and Van Duzer, T., *Fields and Waves in Communication Electronics*, John Wiley & Sons, New York, 1965, p. 293.
16. Smyth, C.P., *Static and Dynamic Electricity*, McGraw-Hill, New York, 1939
17. Bean, C.P., DeBlois, R.W., and Nesbitt, L.B., Eddy-current method for measuring the resistivity of metals, *J. Appl. Phys.*, 30(12), 1959, 1976.
18. Bassett, C.A.L., Pawluk, R.J., and Pilla, A.A., Augmentation of bone repair by inductively coupled electromagnetic fields, *Science*, 184, 575, 1974.
19. Plonsey, R. and Fleming, D., *Bioelectric Phenomena*, McGraw-Hill, New York, 1969, p. 115.
20. Houslay, M.D. and Stanley, K.K., *Dynamics of Biological Membranes*, John Wiley & Sons, New York, 1982, p. 296.
21. Wilson, D.F., Energy transduction in biological membranes, in *Membrane Structure and Function*, Bittar, E.D., Ed., John Wiley & Sons, New York, 1980, p. 182.
22. Johnson, C.C. and Guy, A.W., Nonionizing electromagnetic wave effects in biological materials and systems, *Proc. IEEE*, 60, 692, 1972.
23. Schwan, H.P., Field interaction with biological matter, *Ann. NY Acad. Sci.*, 303, 198, 1977.
24. Kraichman, M.B., *Handbook of Electromagnetic Propagation in Conducting Media*, NAVMAT P-2302, U.S. Superintendent of Documents, U.S. Government Printing Office, Washington, DC, 1970.

25. Massoudi, H., Durney, C.H., Barber, P.W., and Iskander, M.F., Postresonance electromagnetic absorption by man and animals, *Bioelectromagnetics*, 3, 333, 1982.
26. Binhi, V.N., *Magnetobiology: Understanding Physical Problems*, Academic Press, London, 473 pp.
27. Sears, F.W., Zemansky, M.W., and Young, H.D., *University Physics*, 5th ed., Addison-Wesley, Reading, MA, 1976, p. 360.
28. Uman, M.A., *Lightning*, McGraw-Hill, New York, 1969, p. 162.
29. Coelho, R., *Physics of Dielectrics for the Engineer*, Elsevier, Amsterdam, 1979, p. 155.
30. Schwan, H.P., Dielectric properties of biological tissue and biophysical mechanisms of electromagnetic field interaction, in *Biological Effects of Nonionizing Radiation*, Illinger, K.H., Ed., ACS Symposium Series 157, American Chemical Society, Washington, DC, 1981, p. 121.
31. Koryta, J., *Ions, Electrodes and Membranes*, John Wiley & Sons, New York, 1982.
32. Rosenbaum, E.J., *Physical Chemistry*, Appleton-Century-Crofts, Education Division, Meredith Corporation, New York, 1970, p. 595.
33. Watson, J.D., *Molecular Biology of the Gene*, W.A. Benjamin, Menlo Park, CA, 1976, p. 91.
34. Rosenbaum, E.J., *Physical Chemistry*, Appleton-Century-Crofts, Education Division, Meredith Corporation, New York, 1970, p. 595.
35. Illinger, K.H., Electromagnetic-field interaction with biological systems in the microwave and far-infrared region, in *Biological Effects of Nonionizing Radiation*, Illinger, K.H., Ed., ACS Symposium Series 157, American Chemical Society, Washington, DC, 1981, p. 1.
36. Kohli, M., Mei, W.N., Van Zandt, L.L., and Prohofsky, E.W., Calculated microwave absorption by double-helical DNA, in *Biological Effects of Nonionizing Radiation*, Illinger, K.H., Ed., ACS Symposium Series 157, American Chemical Society, Washington, DC, 1981, p. 101.
37. Kondepudi, D.K., Possible effects of 10^{11} Hz radiation on the oxygen affinity of hemoglobin, *Bioelectromagnetics*, 3, 349, 1982.
38. Furia, L., Gandhi, O.P., and Hill, D.W., Further investigations on resonant effects of mm-waves on yeast, Abstr. 5th Annu. Sci. Session, Bioelectromagnetics Society, University of Colorado, Boulder, June 12–17, 1983, p. 13.
39. Grundler, W., Keilman, F., and Fröhlich, H., Resonant growth rate response of yeast cells irradiated by weak microwaves, *Phys. Lett.*, 62A, 463, 1977.
40. Fröhlich, H., Coherent processes in biological systems, in *Biological Effects of Nonionizing Radiation*, Illinger, K.H., Ed., ACS Symposium Series 157, American Chemical Society, Washington, DC, 1981, p. 213.
41. Fröhlich, H., What are non-thermal electric biological effects? *Bioelectromagnetics*, 3, 45, 1982.
42. Fröhlich, H., Coherent electric vibrations in biological systems and the cancer problem, *IEEE Trans. Microwave Theory Tech.*, 26, 613, 1978.
43. Fröhlich, H., The biological effects of microwaves and related questions, in *Advances in Electronics and Electron Physics*, Marton, L. and Marton, C., Eds., Academic Press, New York, 1980, p. 85.
44. Prohofsky, E.W. and Eyster, J.M., Prediction of giant breathing and rocking modes in double helical RNA, *Phys. Lett.*, 50A, 329, 1974.
45. Careri, J., Search for cooperative phenomena in hydrogen-bonded amide structures, in *Cooperative Phenomena*, Haken, H. and Wagner, W., Eds., Springer-Verlag, Basel, 1973, p. 391.
46. Fröhlich, H., Selective long range dispersion forces between large systems, *Phys. Lett.*, 39A, 153, 1972.
47. Barnes, F.S. and Hu, C.-L.J., Nonlinear Interactions of electromagnetic waves with biological materials, in *Nonlinear Electromagnetics*, Uslenghi, P.L.E., Ed., Academic Press, New York, 1980, p. 391.
48. Grundler, W., Keilmann, F., Putterlik, V., Santo, L., Strube, D., and Zimmermann, I., Nonthermal resonant effects of 42 GHz microwaves on the growth of yeast cultures, in *Coherent Excitations of Biological Systems*, Frölich, H. and Kremer, F., Eds., Springer-Verlag, Basel, 1983, p. 21.

1

Experimental Results on Cellular and Subcellular Systems Exposed to Low-Frequency and Static Magnetic Fields

Myrtill Simkó
SciProof International AB

Mats-Olof Mattsson
AIT Austrian Institute of Technology

CONTENTS

1.1 Introduction

Many studies have investigated whether there are responses to different kinds of electromagnetic field (EMF) exposure regimes in different cell types *in vitro*, showing both the presence and absence of effects. The reasons for the diverse outcomes can be based on various factors such as that there are no effects to detect at all, the effects are too subtle and difficult to detect in comparison to effects caused by other stressors (chemicals, UV, or ionizing radiation), or there are too many experimental variables that are not well controlled. This list can be expanded; however, the main problem is that no generally accepted mechanism or hypothesis exists that explains the mode of interaction between living matter and EMF at low levels.

In this chapter, we are discussing effects caused by exposure to static magnetic fields (SMFs) and extremely low frequency (ELF) magnetic fields (ELF-MFs) (sine wave and pulsed). Furthermore, we have grouped the relevant literature using a concept based on known cell-biological/physiological mechanisms. We infer that the initial interaction, which takes place within a very short time frame, affects a very basic cellular characteristic or process. This initial interaction is causing secondary and even tertiary effects "downstream" of the initial interaction, in a cell-specific manner (Figure 1.1). It is not clear how the first interaction takes place, although there are some hypotheses available (see, e.g., Valberg et al. 1997). We suggest that the interaction can take place at the cell membrane and/or at an organelle's membrane (on its inner or outer side), such as the membranes of mitochondria or the endoplasmic reticulum (ER). Since it is known that MF has too low energy to break molecules, the interaction can possibly be via heat development in the form of intracellular "hot spots" by induced electric fields that change the conformations of molecules such as receptors and ion channels, by radical pair mechanisms, or by a combination of these or other mechanisms, which can start a reaction. Very fundamental processes that are affected immediately by any external stimulation include intracellular/mitochondrial calcium ions (Ca^{2+}) concentrations and redox homeostasis.

Mitochondrial Ca^{2+} transport fosters the energy metabolism stimulation of the respiratory chain. This induces an increase in the level of reactive oxygen species (ROS). Recent findings show that mitochondrial Ca^{2+} modulates the matrix redox state, promoting the redox signaling via oxidation reactions (Santo-Domingo 2015). If there is a molecular signal(s) which is "strong" enough to affect redox signaling, signal transduction mechanisms can be triggered leading to different activities within the cell. These can be on the gene level, starting a gene activation or suppression, but also on the protein level starting with phosphorylation/activation processes that initiate a cascade of pathway/s leading to different cellular functions. Such functions can be identified and measured, which is especially "easy" if the activities are outside of the normal range. We call such cellular functions "biological endpoints," which include cell-cycle regulation, apoptosis, immune cell reaction, differentiation, nerve cell transmission, etc. Epigenetic effects can also occur due to the initial external signal, with different outcomes that are more difficult to identify. These changes include DNA methylation and histone modification, which affect the gene expression, and are normal occurrences also during development/differentiation (see Reik 2007).

The continuation of this chapter will first focus on immediate reactions to external stimuli. We will provide the necessary mainstream biological knowledge and follow up with references to relevant studies that have investigated the effects of ELF-MF. Studies related to SMF will also be referred to, when available. Further sections in the chapter deal with certain secondary events and more complex biological endpoints.

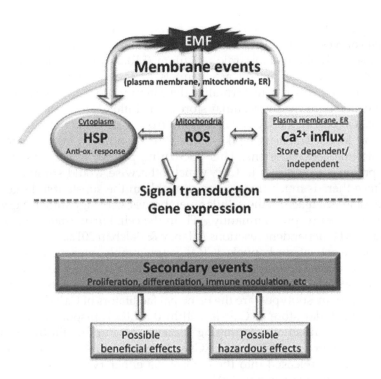

FIGURE 1.1

A summary cartoon depicting the cellular/subcellular events that can be triggered by exposure to static magnetic fields or extremely low-frequency magnetic fields. This model supposes that initial interactions between fields and a cell take place at or near cellular membranes, which trigger very rapid changes in radical homeostasis (ROS levels) and/or ion concentrations (Ca^{2+}). These changes have the potential to influence "downstream" events, which may or may not influence the physiology of the cell. Whether such an influence is beneficial or detrimental is dependent on the functional state of the cell.

1.2 Membrane Interaction

The cell's semipermeable plasma membrane is a glycerophospholipid bilayer, with embedded (trans)membrane proteins. Some substances pass the cell membrane by diffusion, others by specific protein channels and transporters such as the plasma membrane Ca^{2+} ATPase (PMCA). Other active membrane translocating processes include endocytosis and exocytosis. Besides transport functions, membrane-bound proteins also function as receptors, as enzymes, and as adhesion molecules. Many of these aspects have been the subject of studies into biological effects of MF.

1.2.1 Ca²⁺ Transport

Calcium ions have many functions in intracellular signaling, regulating processes involved in metabolism, motility, gene expression, intercellular communication, cell death, etc. (see, *inter alia*, Berridge et al. 1998). Normally, the intracellular concentrations are very low (around 100 nM in most eukaryotic cells) compared to the extracellular levels that exceed 1 mM. This is important since small changes in intracellular Ca^{2+} concentration can influence many cellular processes. The causes for an increased intracellular level are either from external sources, via Ca^{2+}-permeable plasma membrane channels, or from intracellular stores, primarily the endoplasmic reticulum (ER), mitochondria, and sarcoplasmic reticulum (SR), that also express Ca^{2+}-channels in their membranes. ATP-dependent enzymes ("pumps") then strive to normalize the concentrations by transporting Ca^{2+} back to the cell's outside or to the intracellular stores. The influx events are acting on very different time scales (Berridge et al. 2003), ranging from µs to events that need many hours of elevated Ca^{2+} levels. Transient "spikes" in Ca^{2+}-concentration increase are followed by periods at baseline concentrations. This fluctuating pattern is very important, since it counteracts prolonged increases in Ca^{2+}, which otherwise would stimulate induction of apoptosis. Since there is much free energy available in the substantial large gradients of Ca^{2+} that are established across the cellular membranes, Ca^{2+} signaling is very sensitive to the available free energy, predominantly ATP, in the cell. Furthermore, the Ca^{2+} ion itself regulates many ATP-dependent reactions (Glancy & Balaban 2012).

Calcium release-activated channels (CRAC) are mainly present in electrically non-excitable cells where they open as a reaction to low cytoplasmic Ca^{2+} levels and allow influx of extracellular Ca^{2+} (see, e.g., Parekh & Putney Jr 2005). In excitable cells, voltage-gated Ca^{2+}-channels (VGCC; many subtypes) are the principal facilitators of Ca^{2+} entry (Dolphin 2006).

The main intracellular store of Ca^{2+} is within the ER. Transport across the ER membrane occurs in both directions, "pumping" excess Ca^{2+} into the ER by means of sarco/endoplasmic reticulum Ca^{2+} ATPases (SERCAs; (Strehler & Treiman 2004). In the opposite direction, Ca^{2+} can be released into the cytosol via either ryanodine receptors (RyR) or Ins3P receptors (Strehler & Treiman 2004).

Since the Ca^{2+} ion plays such a central role in the physiology of all cells, studies focused on the cell's Ca^{2+} homeostasis have been considered relevant to answer the question if there are any rapidly occurring effects of MF exposure. In this context, it is important to realize that any findings of immediate changes in intracellular Ca^{2+} concentration do not automatically imply that other downstream events will be affected so that the cell's normal physiology is influenced.

Here, we discuss studies that are reporting effects on Ca^{2+} homeostasis after exposure to low-frequency MF and static MF. As can be expected, there are also studies that do not find any effects. However, we are not listing "positive" versus "negative" studies; instead, we provide examples of effects seen in studies that are performed according to reasonably strict criteria.

1.2.1.1 Extremely Low Frequency-Magnetic Field

A pioneering study was published by Conti et al. (1985) who used human lymphocytes that were exposed to a 3 Hz, 6 mT pulsed MF for 72 h. The Ca^{2+} flux was studied as uptake of radio-labeled Ca^{2+} and cannot indicate any changes that are occurring on a short-term basis. However, the authors reported that exposure caused decreased uptake of Ca^{2+}. A similar approach was employed by Walleczek and Liburdy (1992) who exposed rat thymocytes to a 60 Hz MF (22 mT, 1 h exposure duration). The results showed increased uptake of $^{45}Ca^{2+}$ in activated thymocytes, but not in resting ones.

Later studies have used fluorescent markers for intracellular Ca^{2+} and measured either fluctuations in real time or the concentrations of the ion. Many such studies have been published, and Golbach et al. (2016) made a meta-analysis of their results. Forty-two studies were identified that were further looked into regarding relevance and appropriate methodologies. Twelve of the studies focused on intracellular Ca^{2+} oscillation, and 24 studies were measuring the Ca^{2+} ion concentrations. Their meta-analyses found a correlation between MF exposure and a higher frequency of oscillations and also for higher intracellular Ca^{2+} concentrations.

A series of studies from one laboratory used single Jurkat E6-1 human T-cell leukemia cells with the fluorochrome Fura-2 as Ca^{2+} indicator. Consistently, the studies found that ELF-MF exposure caused increased fluctuations of intracellular Ca^{2+} levels, comparable to treatment with the positive control, an anti-CD3 antibody. The exposures were to a vertical MF and responses to the MF were seen within seconds, and disappearing shortly after exposure termination. Specifically, the responses were seen after exposure to a 50 Hz MF at 0.10 mT (Lindström et al. 1993); to different frequencies (in the interval 5–100 Hz, with a peak at 50 Hz) and flux density dependent (threshold found at 0.04 mT and no further response increases above 0.15 mT) (Lindström et al. 1995). Expression of the membrane protein CD45 was necessary for effects to occur (Lindström et al. 1995). In further studies, the group also documented that different clones of the cell line responded differently (Mattsson et al. 2001) but that expression of a range of cell surface markers was not crucial for the response. Furthermore, this study also investigated the possible importance of the local geomagnetic field for the response to the ELF-MF. The response was the same, however, if the local static field was present as well as when it was backed away.

These studies seem to support that exposure to a low-level ELF-MF cause replicable change in Ca^{2+} levels in individual Jurkat T-cell leukemia cells, but not in all cells. Furthermore, the responses are "physiological" in the sense that they are comparable to the positive controls used (response magnitude, time for response appearance and disappearance, and oscillation frequency). However, when the authors tested the hypothesis that the Ca^{2+} changes also triggered Ca^{2+}-dependent downstream events, the outcome was negative. Cells that were transfected with Ca^{2+}-dependent gene constructs ("reporter genes") responded to positive controls as expected, but not to 50 Hz, 0.10 mT MF (Still 2002). This is in contrast to their finding that the exposure triggered immediate phosphorylation events at the T-cell receptor complex in these cells (Lindström et al. 2001).

Loschinger et al. (1999) exposed human skin fibroblasts to a 20 Hz MF, 8 mT. On average, 30% of the investigated cells responded to this MF with Ca^{2+} fluctuations within 40 min. Further analysis revealed that it was primarily mitotic progenitor cells that were responding, whereas post-mitotic cells were unresponsive.

Cardiomyocytes from rats have also been used for fluorescence-microscope-based investigations of intracellular Ca^{2+} (Wei et al. 2015). The study found that a rectangular pulse-shaped MF (2 mT) at various frequencies (15, 50, 75, 100 Hz) all increased cytosolic Ca^{2+} fluctuations (both frequencies and amplitudes) with a significant contribution of Ca^{2+} from the SR.

The individual cell's response to MF exposure suggested by the studies mentioned above is also suggested by others, who showed the importance of selection of test cells and test conditions for the outcome of exposure (Walleczek & Budinger 1992; Loschinger et al. 1999). In more detail, the inconsistencies in outcomes regarding real-time cytosolic Ca^{2+} fluctuations after ELF-MF exposures were addressed by McCreary et al. (2002). Jurkat E6.1 cells were exposed to different types and flux densities of MFs of which one ELF-MF was employed (60 Hz; 100 μT). A reduction of cytosolic Ca^{2+} was seen in all exposure situations, including the ELF field, if co-variates (pH, cell cycle stage, response to a Ca^{2+} agonist) were taken into account. The authors stressed that the MF effects may be difficult to detect unless specific consideration is made regarding the biological material's characteristics. This has also been pointed out by other authors (Lindström et al. 1995; Loschinger et al. 1999; Mattsson et al. 2001).

There are also a number of other studies where Ca^{2+} measurements or events dependent on Ca^{2+} signaling have been documented. These studies include the work by Morgado-Valle et al. (1998) who documented an increased Ca^{2+} influx under influence of a 60 Hz MF (0.7 mT; 2 h/day for 6 days) in primary cultures of adrenal chromaffin cells from rats. By using whole-cell patch-clamp recordings, the authors found that the MF treatment as well as the control (the neurotrophin nerve growth factor (NGF)) caused 2.4-fold higher inward Ca^{2+}-current. Furthermore, by using various inhibitors, they found that the effect was on L-type Ca^{2+}-channels. Another study employing bovine adrenal chromaffin cells was published by Ikehara et al. (2002). The exposure setup generated a 1.51 T MF that was switched on and off automatically every 3 s. Cells were exposed for 30 min or 2 h and investigated for concentration of intracellular Ca^{2+}. The control experiments used bradykinin, which causes release of Ca^{2+} from intracellular stores and thus increases cytosolic concentrations of Ca^{2+}. This effect was inhibited transiently by the MF, whereas exposure had no effect on transmembrane fluxes of Ca^{2+}.

In contrast to the acute effects of Ca^{2+} fluxes reported in several studies, other authors have documented Ca^{2+}-related effects of ELF-MF on cell survival and cell differentiation in the absence of effects on Ca^{2+}-channel gating. Two studies from the same group (Grassi et al. 2004; Piacentini et al. 2008) found that long-term (24–96 h) exposure to 50 Hz MF (0.5–1.0 mT) caused lower rates of apoptosis and higher degrees of differentiation in human IMR32 neuroblastoma cells, rat pituitary GH3 cells, and mouse cortical neuronal stem cells. The exposures were leading to higher levels of intracellular Ca^{2+} and larger Ca^{2+}-currents, without the properties of individual Ca^{2+}-channels being modified. Instead, the effects on Ca^{2+} homeostasis were suggested to be due to increased levels of the VGCC-subunit a1 (Grassi et al. 2004) leading to an increased activity of the specific Ca_v1-channel system (Piacentini et al. 2008).

1.2.1.2 Static Magnetic Field

Bekhite et al. (2013) performed experiments that were similar in design to studies using ELF-MF as the exposure. The authors established an embryonic stem (ES) cell line of cardiovascular cells from the inner cell mass of mouse embryos. The cells were exposed to an SMF acutely or for 2–4 days, and intracellular Ca^{2+} levels in real time were measured. A number of other endpoints were also analyzed, including ROS formation, expression of genes and transcription factors typically involved in cardiac muscle cell differentiation, and morphological signs of myocyte differentiation. Exposure caused an immediate (within seconds) increase in cytosolic Ca^{2+}, in a flux density-dependent manner (between 0.3 and 5 mT). The Ca^{2+} increase was absent if Ca^{2+}-free medium and the chelator 1,2-*bis*(o-aminophenoxy)ethane-*N,N,N',N'*-tetraacetic acid (BAPTA) was used, indicating that the cytosolic increase had extracellular origin. Furthermore, the inhibitor thapsigargin, which blocks uptake of Ca^{2+} into the ER and thus increases Ca^{2+} levels in the cytosol, did not affect the MF-induced Ca^{2+} rise, strengthening the case for a Ca^{2+} influx. Importantly, the MF treatment combined with the absence of extracellular Ca^{2+} did not result in either ROS increase or any signs of cardiomyocyte differentiation.

Several other studies have also seen MF-induced increases in intracellular Ca^{2+} concentration after exposures to static MF. Flipo et al. (1998) found increased concentrations in Concanavalin A-stimulated mouse lymphocytes at flux densities ranging from 0.8 to 1.5 mT, in a dose-dependent fashion. Similarly, primary porcine granulosa cells exposed to a 2 mT SMF immediately displayed Ca^{2+} increases during exposure (Bodega et al. 2005). In this study, the MF effects were abolished if the cell culture medium contained the

Ca^{2+}-chelator ethylenediaminetetraacetic acid (EDTA), supporting that extracellular Ca^{2+} was the main source for the concentration increase. A more refined approach was used in a study on human histiocytic lymphoma U937 cells (Cerella et al. 2011) where real-time recording of intracellular Ca^{2+} was performed during exposure to 6 mT. The authors used the Ca^{2+}-ATPase inhibitor thapsigargin and found that the MF did not increase the rising levels of Ca^{2+}, but caused a "second wave" of Ca^{2+} increase, which was originating from the outside. The authors referred to this as a non-capacitative influx of Ca^{2+}.

The results from Surma et al. (2014) using skeletal muscle cells from newborn Wistar rats exposed to SMFs (0.2 and 0.4 mT) point to internal stores (SR) being the main sources for MF-induced increases in cytoplasmic Ca^{2+} concentration. Exposure led to Ca^{2+} levels increasing 1.5–3.5-fold, depending on muscle cell size and thus degree of maturation. The effect remained when the cells were bathed in medium lacking Ca^{2+} but with EDTA as chelator, or treated with an inhibitor to VGCC. However, treatment with Dantrolene, a ryanodine receptor blocker inhibiting Ca^{2+} release from the SR, inhibited any SMF effect.

ELF-MF exposures have been repeatedly shown to affect Ca^{2+} fluxes, fluctuations, and cytoplasmic concentrations at MF levels from 0.10 mT up to several mT. Several studies suggest that not all cells, even in a seemingly homogenous population, are responding, but that a certain state of "preparedness" needs to be present. Different membrane-bound proteins have been indicated as necessary components of the response to ELF-MF, but no coherent picture has emerged.

The effect of SMF on intracellular Ca^{2+} is also shown in several studies, at flux densities ranging from tenths of mT up to several mT. The studies are not consistent regarding the Ca^{2+} source. There is evidence for both influx from the extracellular space as well as release from ER/SR being relevant. The two-step model suggested by Cerella et al. (2011) can possibly accommodate both these observations. Initially, the MF triggers release from the ER/SR, thus leading to a non-capacitative influx from the cells' exterior, which serves as a means to provide enough Ca^{2+} to be pumped back into the ER/SR.

1.2.2 Reactive oxygen species/Oxidative Stress

Reactive oxygen species (ROS) are molecules containing oxygen that are highly chemically reactive because they contain free radicals. ROS refer to both prooxidants and oxygen-free radicals. The generation of ROS is a naturally occurring process in cell metabolism, and normally, specific enzymes and antioxidants are controlling the ROS level.

Oxidative stress is the imbalance between the production of prooxidants and antioxidants. Oxidative stress is recognized as a main mechanism by which MF might induce toxicity. Reactive nitrogen species (RNS), derived from nitric oxide (NO), and superoxide are produced via the enzymatic activity of inducible nitric oxide synthase 2 (NOS2) and NADPH oxidase, respectively. The formation and release of ROS is closely connected to the immune defense system and especially to phagocytic processes. Thus, ROS formation is part of the cascade of events in the antimicrobial action of phagocytic cells, called oxidative burst, which results from the assembly of a complex electron transport system in the plasma membrane. High levels of ROS can lead to a number of damaging pathological consequences in cells and the organism, including lipid peroxidation, protein damage, deactivation of enzymatic activities, and DNA modification and pro-inflammatory processes. In the normal cellular biochemistry, there is a balance between free radical formation and the action of an antioxidative system. A number of primary antioxidant enzymes such as different dismutases, catalases, reductases, or peroxidases are known to neutralize the amounts of ROS. Irregularity or disturbance in the redox homeostasis by increased quantities of ROS or by the inhibition of the action of antioxidants can lead to cellular oxidative stress causing direct oxidative damages in cells and tissues, and may also initiate inflammatory processes. Other modulations in cell functions via signal transduction processes can furthermore be induced. Therefore, oxidative stress caused by the formation of radical oxygen and nitrogen species plays a decisive role in cytotoxicity and inflammation, eventually leading to the onset of pathophysiological alterations and pathogenesis.

1.2.2.1 Extremely Low Frequency-Magnetic Field

Despite numerous investigations that have shown the presence of a multitude of biological effects of ELF-MF exposure, the first point of interaction between MF and cells, and the underlying molecular mechanisms, are still not clear. However, the release of ROS or other oxidative processes is often connected to the investigated effects. Scientists have investigated ROS production directly and also indirectly by detecting DNA damage in different cell types by various exposure conditions. Therefore, we assume that oxidative processes triggered by MF play a key role for the effectiveness of MF (Simko 2007; Simkó et al. 2004). In a recent review (Mattsson & Simkó 2014), a total of 41 scientific original publications were analyzed to test the hypothesis that ELF-MF exposure *in vitro* causes changes in oxidative status as an early response. The authors suggested that the strongest association between MF exposure and effects occurs at 0.1 or 1 mT, the effects are not dependent on cell type or on exposure duration, and they are modest in comparison with the corresponding positive controls. Since then, several other scientists have investigated the induction of ROS after MF exposure. Zeng et al. (2017) applied repeated exposure to 50 Hz, 2 mT ELF-MF for 8 h/day on primary cultured hippocampal neurons to investigate oxidative stress among other endpoints and detected increased ROS levels.

Mannerling et al. (2010) reported that 0.025–0.10 mT MF (50 Hz, 1 h exposure) increased (30%–40%) the levels of the superoxide radical anion, comparable to the positive control phorbol 12-myristate 13-acetate (PMA) in the human leukemia cell line K562, and increased two-fold the level of the heat stress protein HSP70. MF exposure together with the free radical scavengers melatonin or 1,10-phenanthroline inhibited the MF-induced increase in HSP70 and superoxide radical anion release. These findings were recently confirmed by Pooam et al. (2017) using RAW264 macrophages. The authors showed similar effects, namely that 50 Hz MF diminished the mitochondrial membrane potential leading to the increase in the production of O^{2-} and the expression of HSP70 protein.

Calcabrini et al. (2016) investigated ROS levels in human keratinocytes exposed for 1 h to 50 Hz ELF-MF from 0.025 to 0.2 mT and detected significant ROS increases at 0.05 and 0.1 mT. Moreover, glutathione content, antioxidant defense activity, and lipid peroxidation markers were assessed for different exposure lengths. The authors detected that there was a greater sensitivity of the cells exposed to 0.05 mT.

Protective effects of MF exposure on the human microglial cell line, HMO6, against ischemic cell death induced by *in vitro* oxygen-glucose deprivation (OGD) was investigated by Duong and Kim (2016). OGD caused significant elevation of intracellular Ca^{2+} and ROS levels as well as cell death, and 50 Hz 1 mT MF reduced these effects more effectively than 10 Hz and 1 mT.

It is hypothesized that MF might influence certain neurodegenerative diseases. Reale et al. (2014) evaluated the effects of MF (50 Hz, 1 mT) on a neuronal cell model, human SH-SY5Y cells, on NOS and oxygen radicals release and detected increased levels of these intermediates accompanied by changes in antioxidant catylase (CAT) activity and enzymatic kinetic parameters related to CYP-450 and CAT activity.

1.2.2.2 Static Magnetic Field

Regarding *in vitro* investigations after exposure to SMF, studies have been carried out on different cell models, applying a wide range of exposure protocols in terms of magnetic field strengths and exposure durations.

Synowiec-Wojtarowicz et al. (2017) investigated the redox homeostasis in mouse fibroblasts co-exposed to static magnetic fields (0.4, 0.55, and 0.7 T for 72 h) and the antioxidants dihydrochalcones phloretin and phloridzin. SMF alone did not change the homeostasis of the cells. Co-exposed cells showed a different reaction, namely an increased activity of antioxidant enzymes (SOD, GPx, GST) and in the concentration of malondialdehyde (MDA). The strongest interaction, leading to an intensification of the lipid peroxidation process, was observed in cells co-exposed to aglycone, phloretin, and an SMF with a magnetic flux density of 0.7 T. The authors reason that SMF has an influence on the dihydrochalcones properties that disturbs the antioxidative capacity of the cells. In an earlier study (Pawłowska-Góral et al. 2016), they investigated the mRNA content of some antioxidant enzymes after treatment to similar exposure conditions. Neither SMF alone nor in co-exposure with phloretin did influence the mRNA levels in the used human dermal fibroblasts. The antioxidant system with SMF alone or in co-exposure with fluoride ions (0.12 mM) was investigated in human fibroblasts as well (Kurzeja et al. 2013). Here, the authors detected that SMFs reduce the oxidative stress caused by the fluoride ions and normalize the activities of antioxidant enzymes.

A decrease of the membrane mitochondrial potential up to 30% was detected after 24 h of exposure to SMF (2.2 mT) in human SH-SY5Y neuronal-like cells, and this effect was associated with an ROS production increase (Calabrò et al. 2013). The authors proposed that moderate SMF causes alteration in the cell homeostasis, via changes in protein structures.

A further study showed that the exposure to SMF (60 mT, for 15, 30, or 45 min) of human neutrophils induced statistically significant changes in ROS production in non-stimulated and PMA-stimulated cells after 45 min of exposure (Poniedziałek et al. 2013).

Chondro-osteogenesis and vasculogenesis in embryonic stem (ES) cells and bone mineralization of mouse fetuses were detected by an ROS-dependent upregulation of vascular endothelial growth factor (VEGF) expression as described by Bekhite et al. (2010). Interestingly, SMFs of 1 mT (low MF level) increased and 10 mT (higher MF level) decreased the VEGF expression, which was abolished by diphenyleneiodonium (DPI) and radical scavengers.

Ishisaka et al. (2000) studied ROS generation in oral polymorphonuclear leukocytes exposed to strong SMF (0.6–20 T) and detected a decrease in ROS production in comparison to the control. The authors concluded that the SMF inhibits the activity of NADPH oxidase. Remarkably, even a respiratory burst was detected by Noda et al. (2000) in rat peritoneal neutrophils after exposure to SMFs of 2.5 and 20 mT (400–2,000 sec).

The exposure to strong SMF (8.5 T, 3 h) in different cell types was investigated for different endpoints in the presence or absence of specific inhibitors by Zhao et al. (2011). No effects on CD59 mutation frequency and the cell cycle distribution were detected, but the cellular ATP-content was reduced, and here accompanied by an increased ROS level.

1.2.3 The Function of Chaperones—the Dual Face of HSPs

Heat shock proteins (HSPs) are belonging to the most conserved proteins present in prokaryotes and eukaryotes. Some of the HSPs expression can be induced by a variety of physiological, physical, and environmental factors such as heat, oxidative stress, or anticancer drugs; for recent reviews, see Radons (2016). HSPs act as molecular chaperones; these proteins play an essential role to refold stress-induced misfolded proteins to prevent protein aggregation and thus to tolerate and "repair" certain lethal conditions and restore the balance of protein homeostasis. Therefore, intracellular HSPs have cell protective functions. According to their molecular size, HSP are classified into five groups: HSP100, HSP90, HSP70, HSP60, and the small HSPs. While HSP90 is constitutively expressed, HSP70 and HSP27 are not or very little expressed in non-stressed cells. HSP70 and HSP27 are highly inducible by different kinds of stresses and can be targeted at different cellular compartments. However, once they are induced, these proteins can modulate many different cellular functions to protect the cell or to be involved in the apoptotic-signaling pathway. HSP70s are powerful antiapoptotic proteins and block apoptosis at a number of different levels (Stankiewicz et al. 2005; Yang et al. 2012). It has to be pointed out that the basal level of HSPs is strongly cell and tissue dependent. It has been shown that certain cancer cells "rely" on the HSP70-based buffering system for survival, with high basal levels of HSP70 leading to the activation of antiapoptotic mechanisms, enhanced cell growth, suppression of senescence, but also to the sensitivity to cytostatic drugs and ionization radiation (Gehrmann et al. 2008). However, while intracellular HSP70s play a key role in proteomic homeostasis, extracellular or membrane-bound HSPs mediate immunological functions, and stimulate innate and adaptive immunity (for review, see Jacob et al. 2017). Thus, HSPs have a dual role: intracellular cell protective and extracellular cell signaling for immune modulation.

1.2.3.1 Extremely Low Frequency-Magnetic Field

In EMF research, HSPs have often been investigated as a "hazardous" marker protein. Many studies also investigated the induction of HSPs on the DNA or RNA level using different exposure conditions, however, with inconsistent outcomes. However, considering that the basal expression levels of HSPs are cell type dependent and findings after MF exposure are diverse, here we scrutinize the responses by cell type.

In some studies, no HSP-related effects were detected after ELF-MF exposure ranging from a few µT to mT and from minutes to 24 h using different cell types such as astroglial cells (Bodega et al. 2005), HL-60, H9c2, Girardi heart cells (Gottwald et al. 2007; Morehouse & Owen 2000), and human keratinocytes (Shi et al. 2003). Also in human leukocytes, no changes on the gene level were detected (Coulton et al. 2004). An interesting study investigated the expression of the luciferase gene contained in a plasmid labeled as electromagnetic field-plasmid (pEMF). The pEMF vector was transfected into two different cell lines (INER-37 and RMA E7) that were later exposed to MF. An increased luciferase gene expression was observed in INER-37 cells exposed to MF compared to controls, but MF exposure had no effect in the RMA E7 cell line (Heredia-Rojas et al. 2010).

However, studies showed the induction of HSPs or genes after ELF-MF exposure in primary or non-transformed ("primary-like") cell lines such as human primary osteoarthritic chondrocytes (Corallo et al. 2014), mouse macrophages (Frahm et al. 2010), transfected rat primary fibroblast (RAT1) cells (Frisch et al. 2013), transfected rat primary cells (Laramee et al. 2014), or cardiomyocytes isolated from neonatal Sprague-Dawley rats (Wei et al. 2016), porcine aortic endothelial cells (Bernardini et al. 2007), endothelial cells (SPAE, HUVECs), and human fibroblasts (HuDe, WI-38) (Alfieri et al. 2006). Considering that the basal level of HSPs expression is strongly cell type dependent, it can be hypothesized that primary cells or primary-like cell lines have a lower basal HSP level; thus, HSPs are rather inductive in non-cancer cells than cancer cell lines. As mentioned above, in a number of cancers such as breast cancer, ovarian cancer, osteosarcoma, endometrial cancer, and leukemias, an increased level of HSP27, and in high-grade malignant tumors such as endometrial cancer, osteosarcoma, and renal cell tumors, HSP70 has been detected, relative to its level in non-transformed cells; see review by Schmitt et al. (2006). Thus, investigations using transformed or tumor cell lines possibly do not show any change after ELF-MF exposure.

In immune relevant cell lines, increases in HSP expression level were detected, such as in macrophages (RAW264 cell line) (Pooam et al. 2017) and in human leukemia and lymphoma cells (CEM, HL-60, U937, K562 cells, THP-1 cells) (Alfieri et al. 2006; Mannerling et al. 2010; Garip & Akan 2010; Akan et al. 2010; Tokalov & Gutzeit 2004). Immune relevant cells or cell lines produce also extracellular HSPs as a signal molecule for immune response. Since so far no investigation has been performed on extracellular HSPs expression/release after ELF-MF exposure, it can be hypothesized that in immune relevant cells HSP is inducible both extracellularly and intracellularly.

The hypothesis that non-stressed cells or organisms are rather responsive to HSP induction after ELF-MF exposure has been demonstrated in some *in vivo* studies in invertebrates: the expression of HSP70 was elevated after ELF-MF exposure or in co-exposure to mild heat in *Mytilus galloprovincialis* (Malagoli et al. 2004), in the planarian *Dugesia dorotocethala* (Goodman et al. 2009), in *Drosophila melanogaster* (Zhang et al. 2016), and also in *Dictyostelium discoideum* cells (Amaroli et al. 2013). Using *Escherichia coli* (Del Re et al. 2006; Nakasono & Saiki 2000), significantly higher levels of DnaK and GroE proteins (corresponding to HSP) as well as changes in HSP-related protein synthesis were detected.

1.2.3.2 Static Magnetic Field

HSP induction was also investigated in a few studies after exposure to SMF. In rat primary fibroblasts (RAT1) transfected with a HSP70 promoter-linked luciferase reporter gene, a 3.5-fold increase of HSP70 was detected after SMF (1–440 mT) exposure (Laramee et al. 2014). The response to SMF exposure was at 48 h duration, starting at 48 h post-transfection. This effect was, according to the authors, non-linearly increasing with magnitude, but peaked for 10 and 100 mT exposures.

In another study, a HSP70/luciferase reporter gene was again used to transfect mouse fibroblast NIH3T3 cells to test the hypothesis that oxidative stress induced by glutathione depletion would act to increase HSP70 levels and that the addition of a 100 mT SMF exposure in the absence or presence of heat would further increase these levels (Belton et al. 2011). The hypothesis was rejected since no effects were detected. The authors discussed that the HSP70 protein and/or mRNA response is specific to and dependent on the cell type that was used. Also in cultured astroglial cells, no differences on the expression level of the proteins HSP25, HSP60, and HSP70 were detected after 1 mT sinusoidal, static, or combined magnetic field for 1 h (Bodega et al. 2005).

In a study by Tenuzzo et al. (2009), the gene expressions of bcl-2, bax, p53, and HSP70 in freshly isolated and culture-aged human lymphocytes were investigated after exposure to 6 mT SMF for up to 24 h and in the presence or absence of the apoptosis inducer cycloheximide. HSP70 gene product levels decreased progressively with cell age and with time of SMF exposure. However, HSP70 increased when cells were challenged with cycloheximide alone but decreased when SMF was applied concomitantly with the apoptotic inducer.

These and other studies show similar outcomes for SMF as with using ELF-MF, namely that the induction of HSPs on the protein or at the mRNA level is inconsistent and can be dependent on the cell types used.

1.3 Secondary Events

1.3.1 Cell Proliferation and Apoptosis

Cell proliferation, apoptosis, and differentiation are fundamental processes in multicellular organisms and are tightly connected to each other. Increased cell numbers may result from increased proliferation or from decreased cell death. Cell proliferation can be stimulated by physiological and pathological conditions, and is largely controlled by signals from the microenvironment that either stimulate or inhibit proliferation. Alteration in cell proliferation is a very sensitive indicator of cellular stress.

As Ca^{2+} plays a pivotal role in promoting cell proliferation and apoptosis but also in cell differentiation (for review, see Roderick & Cook 2008), it is clear that this section will cover all these endpoints. Furthermore, ROS plays a similarly central role for these endpoints; thus, Ca^{2+} and/or ROS seem to be the connecting bridge by which the cellular mechanisms are affected by ELF-EMF.

1.3.1.1 Extremely Low Frequency-Magnetic Field

The effects of ELF-MF on cell growth/proliferation are still controversial, since it seems to depend on experimental conditions like exposure intensity and duration, modulation of intracellular signals, and cell types used (Zwirska-Korczala et al. 2005; Köbbert et al. 2008; Huo et al. 2010). Many studies investigated these effects with different outcomes (inhibition or promotion of cell proliferation); however, molecular studies show dependency of these effects on cell type and exposure condition. The majority of the recent studies aim to use the effects in medical applications such as wound healing. Thus, Patruno et al. (2015) used HaCaT cells to investigate the molecular mechanism after short ELF-MF (50 Hz, 1 mT, 1 h) exposure. The authors detected the modulation of gene expression that is involved in cell proliferation and in the cell cycle regulation, and hypothesized that applied fields "may induce a rearrangement of membrane surface proteins and/or activation of membrane receptors (e.g., EGFR, Kit, Fms, Flt–3) resulting in Ras/Raf/EK/ERK and PI3K/PTEN/Akt signaling pathways activation…." Thus, the increases of mTOR regulation (PI3K/Akt) and activation of ERK signaling pathways were detected. Earlier studies by the same group showed that ELF-MF exposure enhances keratinocyte proliferation and early NOS activities, decreases O_2, and induces AP-1 activation and nuclear translocation (Patruno et al. 2010).

In another study, the effects of ELF-MF (50 Hz, 0.4 mT) on hippocampal neural progenitor cells (NPCs) cultured from embryonic and adult ischemic brains were investigated by Cheng et al. (2015). Significantly enhanced cell proliferation both in embryonic NPCs and in ischemic NPCs was detected, accompanied by neuronal differentiation enhancement (after 7 days of exposure), whereas glial differentiation was not influenced. Moreover, the expression of phosphorylated Akt was increased during the proliferation process. The authors suggested that these data show that ELF-MF promotes neurogenesis of ischemic NPCs and that this effect may occur through the Akt pathway.

On the other hand, for example, Buckner et al. (2017) presented results on exposure to a so-called Thomas-EMF, a burst of pulses with varying spacing in time. This field inhibits cell proliferation (by 40% after 5 days) and promotes calcium uptake of B16-BL6 melanoma cells if EMF is set to 3 ms (point duration for the waveform generator) for 1 h/day, while setting the point duration to 1, 2, 4, or 5 ms, it had no effect on cell proliferation.

Ma et al. (2014) examined the gene expression that regulates neuronal differentiation in embryonic neural stem cells (eNSCs) after exposure to 50 Hz MF at various intensities and exposure duration. They suggested that molecular changes during eNSCs differentiation were induced, which might be compensated for by post-transcriptional mechanisms to support cellular homeostasis.

This list of modulation of cell proliferation can be enlarged (e.g., Salimi et al. 2013; Ross et al. 2015; Wócik-Piotrowicz et al. 2014; Delle Monache et al. 2013; Bae et al. 2013); however, it is obvious that the modest findings are especially cell type but also exposure condition dependent. It is also clear that this effect is more like a "second" event after the first interaction between MF and the cell that could be the membrane, Ca^{2+} concentration, and also redox modulations leading to the modulation of cell proliferation via the Ras/Raf/EK/ERK and PI3K/Akt signaling pathway.

Apoptosis is a normal physiological process essential for the balanced tissue homeostasis and is thus part of cell growth. There are several lines of evidence that apoptosis and proliferation are strongly connected. Nevertheless, apoptosis can also be induced by a variety of pathologic stimuli. Differentiation is a common process whereby, e.g., stem cells divide and generate fully differentiated daughter cells during tissue repair and during normal cell turnover. Apoptosis is an important process during the differentiation process. Thus, cell proliferation, apoptosis, and differentiation are strongly connected to each other.

Apoptosis, or programmed cell death, is an evolutionary conserved mechanism for the selective removal of aging, damaged, or otherwise unwanted cells. It is an essential component of many normal physiological processes such as embryogenesis, normal tissue development, and the immune response. Unintentional cellular insults may also trigger cell death such as those caused by ultraviolet light or chemical or physical agents. Apoptosis is distinguishable from cell death by necrosis, which is considered as a random event causing a potentially damaging or inflammatory response. The biochemical features of apoptosis include DNA fragmentation, protein cleavage at specific locations, increased mitochondrial membrane permeability, and the appearance of phosphatidylserine (PE) on the cell membrane surface. There is no doubt that mitochondrial Ca^{2+} overload is one of the pro-apoptotic ways to induce the swelling of mitochondria, with perturbation or rupture of the outer membrane, and in turn cause the release of mitochondrial apoptotic factors into the cytosol (for review, see Giorgi et al. 2012). Apoptosis can be triggered by intracellular or extracellular signals, whereby two main pathways exist: the intrinsic or mitochondrial pathway that transmits intracellular received death signals and the extrinsic or death receptor pathway relaying apoptotic messages via receptors. ROS and mitochondria play an important role in apoptosis induction also, via the mitochondria-associated membranes; at the same time, ROS have also antiapoptotic effects. Although these pathways act independently to initiate the death machinery, there is a subtle coordination between the extrinsic and intrinsic pathways, which leads to the activation of a caspase (cysteinyl, aspartate-specific proteases) cascade. As described in Section 1.2.3, HSPs play a crucial role in apoptosis induction/inhibition as well.

A number of studies investigated apoptosis induction together with cell proliferation and differentiation but also in connection to oxidative stress. Zeng et al. (2017) investigated all parameters in cultured hippocampal cells but detected no significant effects on DNA damage, apoptosis, or autophagy, after repeated exposure to 50 Hz, 2 mT ELF-MF for 8 h/day. Benassi and colleagues (2016) also detected no effects on survival, shape, and morphology of either proliferating or differentiated SH-SY5Y cells after ELF-MF exposure, but they found significantly impaired redox homeostasis and thiol content, triggering an increase in protein carbonylation. In Balb/c 3T3 cells (2.3 mT for 2 h/day, 5 days/week, 11 weeks), cell morphology, apoptosis, cell migration ability, and cell transformation did not change, but cell viability decreased and cell cycle distribution was changed after 11 weeks of exposure accompanied by the decrease in proliferating cell nuclear antigen and CyclinD1 protein levels (An et al. 2015). On the other hand, in oxygen-glucose deprivation (OGD)-induced microglial cells, 50 Hz, 1 mT MF reduced the OGD-induced cell death, intracellular Ca^{2+}, and ROS levels (Duong & Kim 2016) showing protective effect against OGD. Similarly, the expression of the antiapoptotic protein BAG3 was induced in the human melanoma cell line M14, *in vitro* and in orthotopic xenografts exposed for 6 h or 4 weeks, respectively, without any variation of HSP70/72 protein levels or apoptosis (Basile et al. 2011).

However, molecular analysis on glioblastoma cells (U87) using ELF-pulsed electromagnetic fields (ELF-PEMFs) showed that after 24 h exposure, the cell viability and Cyclin-D1 expression were increased at 50 Hz (10, 1.5 mT; 30%, 45%), but were decreased at 100 Hz (29%, 31%). P53 and Caspase-3, both typical proteins for apoptosis induction, were elevated after 100 Hz, 10 or 1.5 mT, and no significant differences were observed at 50 Hz, at 5 or 1 mT (Akbarnejad et al. 2016).

There is a large body of literature showing that ELF-MF exposure alters cell proliferation and differentiation (Gaetani et al. 2009; Falone et al. 2007; Kang et al. 2013; Tsai et al. 2009; Chen et al. 2000). It was shown by Mayer-Wagner et al. (2010) that 15 Hz, 5 mT, for 21 days increased the collagen type II expression and glycosaminoglycan content of cultures in human mesenchymal stem cells (hMSCs), and thereby stimulated the chondrogenic differentiation of stem cells (for review, see Tamrin et al. 2016). Gaetani and coworkers (2009) showed the increase in cardiac markers expression after 5 days of ELF-MF exposure (7 Hz, 2.5 µT) in cardiac stem cells. Modulation of osteogenesis in human mesenchymal stem cells to a daily PEMF (pulse duration of 300 µs, constant rate of 7.5 Hz) showed that the PEMF stimulation modulated the osteogenic differentiation of human MSCs (Tsai et al. 2009).

ELF-MF has often been shown to be effective in the enhancement of osteogenesis at 7.5 Hz, 1 mT and 15 Hz, 2 mT, and chondrogenesis at 15 Hz, 5 mT, showing that specific EMF frequencies enhance human mesenchymal stem/stromal cell (hMSC) adherence, proliferation, differentiation, and viability, whereby Ca^{2+} always plays a central role in signal transduction pathways (for review, see Fathi & Farahzadi 2017). In earlier studies, it was shown that short-term exposure (1 and 6 h) to PEMF (2.3 mT at 75 Hz) of chondrocytes from healthy patients did not result in an increased DNA synthesis, although longer durations (9 and 18 h) did (De Mattei et al. 2001). Also in porcine chondrocytes, it was detected that long-term PEMF exposure (1.8–3 mT, 75 Hz for 2 h/day for 3 weeks) was more effective than 1 week to the similar exposure (Chang et al. 2011).

Ca^{2+} is the most relevant molecule in osteogenic differentiation, where human bone marrow mesenchymal stem cells (hBMSCs) differentiate to bone, and Ca^{2+} has been connected to EMF-induced cell differentiation (D'Souza et al. 2001). Li et al. (2006) reported that PEMF exposure led to an increase in cytosolic Ca^{2+} and activation of calmodulin, which is also the mechanism of the osteogenesis process, whereas Hou et al. (2006) indicated that EMF activates the extracellular signal-regulated kinase mitogen-activated protein kinase (ERK-MAPK) and p38 pathways. However, it was also shown by Yong et al. (2016) that 15 Hz, 1 mT furthered MSCs osteogenesis mediated by both the protein kinase A and MAPK signaling pathways. Molecular studies showed the production of key osteogenic regulatory genes, RUNX2/CBFA1, and alkaline phosphatase that were stimulated in hMSCs by PEMF (daily PEMF stimulation with single, narrow 300 µs quasi-rectangular pulses, repetition rate of 7.5 Hz). Hinsenkamp and Collard (2011) and Collard et al. (2013) presented gene and protein modifications (up- and down-regulations), specifically the expression of BMP-2 that was significantly increased at day 12 of exposure. Yan et al. (2015) used 50 Hz PEMF (0.6 mT) and showed that the fields stimulate both proliferation and osteogenic differentiation of rat calvarial osteoblasts.

1.3.1.2 Static Magnetic Field

Increasing evidence shows that static magnetic fields (SMFs) can affect cell proliferation and apoptosis when using different cell types and exposure conditions. Many of the recent studies are interested in whether SMF can be used in medical applications or if these fields are interfering with certain types of, e.g., pharmacologic cancer treatment or other combinations using physical agents. Thus, an interesting study by Naarala et al. (2017) showed that the direction of the SMF (vertical 60 or 120 μT) in relation to, in this case, ELF-MF direction is relevant for bio-effects. They measured cell proliferation and ROS release after different combinations of the two fields and found the following: SMF combined with ELF (18 Hz, 30 μT) induced a decreased proliferation by a horizontal, but not by a vertical ELF field. ROS level was increased in glioma C6 cells exposed to the vertical 33 μT SMF and a horizontal 50 Hz (30 μT) ELF-MF but not affected by a vertical 50 Hz MF, suggesting that ELF-MF may interact with the static geomagnetic field in producing biological effects.

In some studies, the molecular pathway by which SMF influences the cell proliferation was investigated. It was documented by Zhang et al. (2017) that 1 T SMF does not have an apparent impact on cell cycle or cell death as tested in 15 different cell lines, including 12 human and 3 rodent cell lines. However, the authors also tested whether cell density is influencing these endpoints and found that exposure at higher cell density reduces the cell numbers in six out of seven solid human cancer cell lines: The authors identified that the EGFR-Akt-mTOR pathway seems to be involved by using specific inhibitors. Moreover, it was shown that SMF also increases the efficacy of Akt inhibitors on the inhibition of some cancer cell growth. So, fast-growing human glioblastoma multiforme U87MG and U251MG cell lines were used for the exposure to 0.2 mT SMF, and a significant decrease in cell proliferation accompanied by the protein expression level modulation of cyclin B1 and cyclin-dependent kinase 1 was detected (Kim et al. 2016). Luo et al. (2016) were interested in the influence of SMF on tubulin *in vitro* because of the diamagnetic anisotropy of this molecule and its importance during mitosis. The authors detected that after 1 T SMF exposure to HeLa, HCT116, CNE-2Z, and MCF7 cell lines, the mitotic spindles were abnormal, and at the same time, an increased mitotic index was detected, caused by a delayed mitotic exit. Interestingly, it was detected that co-exposure to the antitumor drugs Paclitaxel (Taxol), 5-Fluorouracil (5-FU), and Cisplatin increased the antitumor efficacy of 5-FU or 5-FU/Taxol, but not of Cisplatin.

Lin et al. (2014) investigated whether a combination of SMF and a tumor necrosis factor-related apoptosis-inducing ligand (TRAIL) could have synergistic effects on human breast cancer cells, MDA-MB-468 and T47D. They found that SMF (3.0 mT, 24 h) sensitized transformed cancer cells to TRAIL-mediated apoptosis via the repression of a cell cycle-related protein, Cdc2, and the subsequent downregulation of the antiapoptotic protein survivin. It was also pointed out that SMF did not sensitize non-transformed human mammary epithelial cells to TRAIL-mediated apoptosis.

SMF (0.5 T) also enhanced the viability and proliferation rate of adipose tissue-derived mesenchymal stem cells through the activation of the PI3K/Akt pathway, as shown by Maredziak et al. (2017), and also in rat bone marrow stem cells after 15 mT exposure (Mo et al. 2013).

After exposure to 0.4 T SMF, cell proliferation and anisotropy of the lipid bilayer of dental pulp stem cells (DPSCs) were examined by Lew et al. (2016). The authors detected a higher proliferation rate, an increased anisotropy value, and the activation of intracellular calcium ions. Furthermore, F-actin cytoskeletal structure changes were detected. It was summarized that SMF may activate the p38 mitogen-activated protein kinase signaling, and thus reorganize the cytoskeleton, which contributes to the increased cell proliferation.

SMFs have also been shown to inhibit cancer cell proliferation in several studies (Wang et al. 2016; Li et al. 2012; Kim & Im 2010; Aldinucci et al. 2003; Rosen & Chastney 2009; Strelczyk et al. 2009; Raylman et al. 1996). For example, Zhang et al. (2016) investigated whether it is possible to influence the activity of the EGFR by SMF (1–9 T, 0–60 min or up to 3 days). The authors showed that the kinase activity of isolated EGFR was effectively inhibited by SMFs at 0.7 T. In *in vitro* investigations, the expression and phosphorylation levels of EGFR were analyzed in a number of cell lines. EGFR was highly expressed and phosphorylated in HCT116 and CNE-2Z cancer cells but not in CHO cells. The inhibition on cell proliferation in transfected CHO cells (overexpressing EGFR) was also documented. Molecular dynamics simulation indicated that strong SMFs affect the orientation of EGFR kinase domain proteins. By applying certain EGFR inhibitors, it was shown that 1 T SMF suppresses the mTOR inhibitor-induced EGFR reactivation and enhances the antitumor efficacy of mTOR inhibitor and EGFR inhibitor afatinib. The authors suggested that SMFs directly affect the EGFR kinase domain protein orientation to inhibit its activity in a magnetic field intensity-dependent way.

In a comprehensive study by Wang et al. (2016), 0.5 T SMF was used to investigate several endpoints in adipose-derived stem cells (ASCs). After 7 days of exposure, the authors detected a slight inhibition of cell viability and proliferation. Also the reduction of certain surface antigens expression (CD49d, CD54, and CD73) was detected, as well as the downregulation of cytokine secretion (VEGF, IGF-1, TGF-β1), stem cell genetic marker expression, and adipogenic and osteogenic differentiation without affecting the DNA integrity.

In a recent investigation using human fetal lung fibroblasts (MRC-5) and 370 mT SMF exposure, the absence of any effects on cell viability, ROS levels, and DNA integrity was reported (Romeo et al. 2016).

1.3.2 Neuronal Differentiation

The adult nervous system in vertebrates has a very limited capacity to renew its population of neurons, which has strongly negative consequences for the individual in the case of certain medical conditions. Thus, spinal cord injury, stroke, traumatic brain injury, Parkinson's disease, Huntington's disease, Alzheimer's disease, and multiple sclerosis, which all are conditions where nerve cells degenerate and die, have very severe effects. Until recently, almost all treatments for these conditions have aimed at inhibiting further degeneration of nervous tissue, with very little hope for restoring original function. The advent of technologies for stem cell culture and differentiation has changed this scenario, and currently, considerable optimism has arisen regarding treatment of many neurological disorders and diseases.

Stem cells are undifferentiated, karyotypically normal cells with capacity for self-renewal. These cells, during certain circumstances, can also generate differentiated cells (Forostyak et al. 2016; Takahashi et al. 2007). Generation of stem cells with neuronal differentiation potential is possible from several adult tissues (see, e.g., Kanno 2013), but for most practical purposes, cells from mesenchymal tissues are especially suitable (mesenchymal stem cells, MSC). Especially good results have been obtained with cells from adipose tissues, which are available as autologous sources. These cells are also easy to expand *in vitro*, do not confer any immunological complications, and can be manipulated to differentiate into several different cell populations, including nerve cells (Drela et al. 2013; Pei et al. 2010).

Several signaling pathways lead to neuronal differentiation of stem cells. These pathways include the stimulation of receptor tyrosine kinases by ligand binding, which activates among other pathways also the inositol-triphospahte/diacyl-glycerol (InsP3/DAG) pathway. In turn, a major feature is the downstream opening of ion channels in the ER, which allows Ca^{2+} to flow into the cytosol (Salehi et al. 2016). The resulting increase in intracellular Ca^{2+} seems to be crucial for nerve cell differentiation of stem cells. Typically, neuronal differentiation from adult stem cells is very much dependent on Ca^{2+} release from the endoplasmic reticulum, whereas embryonic stem cells rely on Ca^{2+} influx through the cell membrane via voltage-gated Ca^{2+}-channels (see Forostyak et al. (2016) for a comprehensive review).

There is considerable interest in investigating the potential of MF exposure, alone or in combination with chemical treatment, to promote neuronal differentiation. This process is actually more of a tertiary event than a secondary event after MF exposure. It is dependent on that control of cell proliferation and cell survival and apoptosis is functioning normally and thus that any MF effects are not negatively influencing those functions.

1.3.2.1 Extremely Low Frequency-Magnetic Field

A number of studies employing ELF-MF have used human bone marrow mesenchymal stem cells as a model for induction of differentiation. One of these studies was a comprehensive piece of work where 50 or 100 Hz, 1 mT, vertical MF was used (Park et al. 2013). Cells were treated with differentiation promoting medium with or without simultaneous MF exposure for 4 or 8 days. MF exposure (both frequencies) improved viability of cells and also promoted differentiation. The MF exposure caused phosphorylation of the cyclic adenosine monophosphate (cAMP) response element binding protein (CREB), which is associated with neuronal survival, development, and differentiation. The study could also show that upstream activating events involved in CREB phosphorylation by the MF involved activation of the EGF receptor. The scenario was further elucidated by findings that exposure caused elevated ROS levels and that antioxidant treatment not only decreased ROS levels but also strongly inhibited neuronal differentiation by MF. The study thus strongly suggests that MF exposure of stem cells leads to initial ROS formation, which in turn causes a cascade of events that can trigger the cells to differentiate into, in this case, cells with a neuronal phenotype.

A similar study with the same cells and the same exposure setup and protocol focused on proteomic effects and Ca^{2+} homeostasis (Kim et al. 2013). Once again, the MF caused increased neuronal differentiation. The scientists also documented proteins that were uniquely affected by ELF-MF. Five of the proteins were increasing their expression, and three proteins had decreased expression levels. Calcium measurements showed a 30% increase in intracellular Ca^{2+} compared to controls. Whether this increase was involved in the induced neuronal differentiation was not studied. In summary, both these studies showed a positive MF effect at 1 mT on neuronal differentiation of MSC. Furthermore, parts of the involved signal transduction pathways were elucidated, and the results strongly suggest that an initial and necessary event is induction of ROS production.

The same stem cells and ELF-MF exposure protocol was recently used in a study where the aim was to find out if MF exposure can induce astrocyte differentiation (Jeong et al. 2017). The stem cells respond differently to different chemical inducers, and by using other media additives, an astrocyte differentiation pathway can be initiated. Cells were exposed for 12 days to the 50 Hz field (1 mT). Compared to controls, MF-exposed cells displayed lower proliferation (−39%) and lower expression levels of the markers nestin and OCT3/4, whereas the levels of the astrocyte-specific intermediate filament protein glial fibrillary acidic protein (GFAP) were strongly increased. Intracellular ROS levels were increased by 76% as a consequence of exposure. The levels of the ROS-dependent sirtuin protein (SIRT1) were increased on both mRNA and protein levels, as well as some SIRT1 downstream proteins (TLE1, HES1, MASH1).

A recent study used embryonic neural stem cells isolated from the telencephali of embryonic day 13.5 BALB/c mice (Ma et al. 2014). The cells were exposed to a 50 Hz 1 mT MF (4 h/day) for 1, 2, or 3 days. Cells cultured in normal medium responded to the MF exposure with increased proliferation. When stimulated to differentiate, the exposure enhanced differentiation characteristics (Tuj1 expression, neurite outgrowth, proneural gene expression, expression of the TRPC1 membrane channel and its function). Also intracellular Ca^{2+} concentration was increased. By using siRNA, the gene for TRPC1 was silenced, which as expected led to that the MF-induced Ca^{2+} increase was inhibited. This treatment also prevented neuronal differentiation and neurite outgrowth. Thus, the study brings more support for that ELF-MF can promote neuronal differentiation by acting on the membrane-bound TRPC1 channel, which mediates increased cytosolic levels of Ca^{2+}.

Further investigations into MF-induced neuronal differentiation include a study using both human bone marrow MSC and mouse embryonal neuronal precursor cells (Seong et al. 2014). A 50 Hz MF (also 100 and 200 Hz were used in occasional experiments) at 1 mT for up to 8 days induced neuronal differentiation both in cell cultures raised in normal medium (the human cells) and after embryonic stem cells were induced (induction medium) to develop into the neuronal precursor cells. The study focused on gene expression and found that MF treatment strongly increased levels of nerve cell markers, whereas markers typical for glia cells were decreased or at the same levels as before MF exposure. An investigation into global gene expression revealed that >50 genes were increased (>1.5-fold) in their expression levels. Most of these genes belonged to the transcription factor category. One such gene, the transcription factor Egr1, stood out particularly in both investigated cell types. In order to investigate its importance further, a lentivirus construct was made and introduced to the stem cells, which caused overexpression of the gene. This overexpression itself did not cause nerve cell differentiation, but both cell types responded strongly to MF exposure with neuronal differentiation in this condition. Finally, the reverse situation was constructed where the Egr1 gene was knocked down in the human cells, which then did not respond to the MF exposure with differentiation.

Thus, the study supports that Egr1 is necessary but not sufficient for neural differentiation and that ELF-MF acts via a pathway involving this protein, which is associated with neuronal activity. The tyrosine kinase c-Abl is involved in its induction via the MEK/ERK signaling pathway, which in turn is responding to oxidative stress (Stuart et al. 2005).

Other studies have also used different types of stem cells and investigated if ELF-MFs have any effects on neuronal differentiation. Examples include Bai et al. (2013) who employed rat bone marrow MSC and found facilitation of nerve cell differentiation after a 50 Hz, 5 mT exposure for 12 days. Stem cells obtained from mice brain have also been used, and similar results regarding positive effects on neuronal gene expression and morphological features were obtained (Ma et al. 2014; Cheng et al. 2015). The studies are not identical, e.g., different cell-specific markers were investigated, but still provide a fairly coherent picture that the MF exposure at least enhances the effects of the differentiation-promoting cell culture medium that has been used and in some cases even causes differentiation when normal cell culture medium has been employed. Furthermore, the exposures were primarily to 50 Hz fields, with flux densities in the mT range and duration over days.

As discussed in more detail in Section 1.2.1, the work by Piacentini et al. (2008) and Cuccurazzu et al. (2010) showed that MF effects on neuronal differentiation both *in vivo* and *in vitro* are dependent on the MF exposure causing intracellular Ca^{2+} concentration increase. Also in these studies, a number of neuronal markers were identified that were expressed at a higher level after exposure, allegedly as a consequence of the noted increase in intracellular Ca^{2+} concentrations.

1.3.2.2 Static Magnetic Field

The use of SMFs for the purpose of inducing differentiation of nervous system components (neurons and glial cells) with focus on subcellular and cellular events has been investigated in only a few studies. A number of different endpoints have been in focus in these studies, with either direct or indirect connection to the differentiation process.

One of the earlier studies employed primary cultures of hippocampal neurons from embryonic day 18 Wistar rat embryos (Hirai & Yoneda 2004). The cells were exposed for 3–9 days to a 100 mT static MF, which resulted in increasing expression levels of a more mature phenotype of neurons, whereas markers for earlier stage neurons such as MAP-2, NeuN, and GAP-43 were either decreasing or remained at the original expression level. In contrast, 3-day exposures caused significant increases in the levels of mRNAs encoding subunits of the N-Methyl-D-aspartic acid (NMDA) glutamate receptor. The exposed cells furthermore responded to addition of NMDA to the culture medium with enhanced influx of Ca^{2+}, which indicates that exposure caused physiological effects that are typical for more mature neurons. No changes in cell number or cell survival were noted in this study, which is in line with most of the other studies examining these endpoints in the context of nervous system differentiation.

A continuation and expansion of the study was later published (Nakamichi et al. 2009) where cells at an earlier differentiation stage were investigated. Neural progenitor cells were isolated from rat embryos and investigated with antibodies against markers of differentiation into neural or glial cell lineages. A 12-day exposure (100 mT) reduced proliferation but did not change the viability of the cells. Concomitantly, astrocyte markers among the progenitor cells decreased, and markers for the neuronal lineage were increased. mRNA analyses indicated that this was brought about by an initial SMF-mediated decrease in *Hes5* expression, causing the proneural genes *Mash1*, *Math1*, and *Math3* to be activated.

Further studies of gene expression as a marker for differentiation have been performed. Thus, a global mRNA profiling study on human embryoid body derived lymphatic vascular endothelial cells (LVEC) (a stem cell line) showed that MF at 0.23–0.28 T for 24 h affected expression levels of hundreds of genes (Wang et al. 2009). The authors identified nine different signaling networks that were directly involved and were selected to further characterize effects linked to the inflammatory IL-6 pathway. Proliferation was suppressed by the exposure, but there were no indications of any toxic effects. Microscopic investigations showed that the cells developed dendrite-like outgrowths, which can be found in both neural and glial precursors. However, on the protein levels, the cells increased their expression levels of vimentin and Gal-C, suggesting that the exposure had stimulated the stem cells to develop along an oligodendrocyte pathway, whereas markers for neurons and for astrocytes were downregulated. That the IL-6 signaling network was induced suggests that the initial events are effects of changing Ca^{2+} levels, since IL-6 signaling is modulated by Ca^{2+} influx.

Also a study from Prasad et al. (2017) found that induced human pluripotent stem cells responded to SMF exposure with differentiation toward oligodendrocytes. The stem cells were initially having the phenotype of oligodendrocyte precursors, and 0.3 T exposure (2 h/day for 2 weeks) promoted the differentiation to mature oligodendrocytes. This was seen as changes in gene expression where the activating gene c-fos was strongly expressed, accompanied by downregulation of early oligodendrocyte precursor genes and increases in the levels of markers for mature oligodendrocytes (CNT, MBP). Furthermore, both gene expression and secretion of the neurotrophic factors (brain-derived neurotrophic factor [BDNF] and neurotrophin-3 [NT3]) were seen as a result of exposure, supporting that the differentiation leads to a physiologically relevant phenotype. Finally, the exposed cells displayed enhanced levels of the mRNAs for the VGCC subunits Cav1.2 and Cav1.3, and also higher intracellular levels of Ca^{2+}. Also primary neuronal cells from cortex and hippocampus (in 1-day-old Sprague-Dawley rats) display these types of ion channels (Yakir-Blumkin et al. 2014), which were activated during acute exposures to fields from 0.8 to 5 mT.

1.4 Immune Response

The immune system is a complex network of cells, tissues, and organs, which protects the organism against invading pathogens and diseases. This defense system comprises many biological structures and processes including different organs and cell types. Investigating bio-effects after MF exposure on the immune system *in vitro* means that many different "primary" or "secondary" endpoints can be considered. Therefore, here we consider the immune system and its cells as an extra sub-chapter, even though it is clear that some effects can be primary and others, secondary effects.

1.4.1 Extremely Low Frequency-Magnetic Field

The human immune system can be classified into subsystems, such as the innate immune system and the adaptive immune system, or humoral immunity and cell-mediated immunity. Multiple defense mechanisms have evolved to recognize and neutralize pathogens, such as phagocytosis, the release of antimicrobial peptides (defensins), the production of intermediates (ROS, interleukins), and the complement system. Adaptive immunity creates immunological memory after an initial response to a specific pathogen. However, some pathogens can rapidly evolve and adapt and thereby avoid detection and neutralization by the immune system.

The protection is based on that the immune system can differentiate between "self" and "nonself" cells, organisms, and substances. However, the immune system can be activated by many "nonself" substances; these are called antigens, which are proteins on the surfaces of the pathogens (bacteria, fungi, and viruses). After binding of antigens to a special receptor(s) on the defense cells, a series of cell activation processes and signaling pathways is started and the immune system is activated. However, Matzinger (1994, 2002) proposed the so-called "danger theory," which postulates that self-components could also trigger an immune response if they are dangerous. Hence, nonself "safe" antigens would be tolerated by the immune system, as (normally) they occur together with commensal bacteria and food antigens. Danger signals are therefore signals of stress from cells under the attack of invading pathogens or the effect of endogenous factors. Toll-like receptors (TLRs) induce a cascade of events leading to activation of innate immune cells, especially dendritic cells, which in turn induce the adaptive immune response. It has also been demonstrated that the innate and adaptive immune systems are not two separate entities, but work together (Janeway & Medzhitov 2002).

Heat shock proteins (HSP), interferon-γ (IFN-γ), interleukin-1ß (IL-1ß), uric acid, ATP, adenosine, and many other molecules have been classified as "damage signals." HSPs have been extensively discussed before (Section 1.2.3), but it should be noticed that HSPs play an important role in the immune response. Extracellular HSPs activate antigen-presenting cells and take part in the induction of the adaptive immune response by carrying peptides for cross-presentation. HSPs have also been described to act as danger signals (likewise in the absence of pathogens) because, once released in the extracellular milieu during cell damage processes (necrosis), they are able to modulate the pathogen-associated molecular patterns (PAMP)-induced responses and induce the secretion of inflammatory cytokines in dendritic cells and macrophages (Basu et al. 2000). Thus, HSPs work as damage signal during physiological conditions but can also prime and modulate danger signals.

Adenosine receptors (ARs) expression, at different levels and in different cell types, plays an important role in inflammatory processes, especially in cartilage and bone pathologies. In the context of the bone physiology, there is strong evidence that PEMFs exert an anti-inflammatory effect through the upregulation of specific ARs, namely A2A and A3 (Vincenzi et al. 2013; Ochaion et al. 2008). PEMF exposure increased A2A adenosine receptors not only on human neuronal cancer cells, osteoblasts, and chondrocyte cell lines, but also in *ex vivo* isolated peripheral blood neutrophils. Neutrophils treated with PEMF showed significant increase of the A2A adenosine receptor signaling and in the capability, upon treatment with adenosine agonists, to inhibit the generation of superoxide anion production. Also the role of adenosine analogues and MF stimulation for PGE2 release and COX-2 expression in bovine synovial fibroblasts (SFs) has been investigated (De Mattei et al. 2009). MF exposure (75 Hz, 1.5 mT) of bovine monolayer synovial fibroblasts reduced PGE2 production and potentiated PGE2 inhibition caused by the presence of adenosine agonists. Changes in PGE2 levels were associated with modification of COX-2 expression. This study supports the anti-inflammatory activity of adenosine receptors and MFs in bovine SFs. In a more recent study (Ongaro et al. 2012), human SFs from osteoarthritis patients were treated with IL-1ß and PEMF (peak intensity of the magnetic field was 1.5 mT, 75 Hz) to investigate a possible involvement of adenosine receptors (ARs) in limiting cartilage degradation and in controlling inflammation. EMF exposure induced a selective increase in A2A and A3 ARs, which were associated with changes in cAMP levels, indicating that ARs were functionally active. Additional data showed that in the presence of adenosine agonists and antagonists, PEMF inhibited the release of PGE2 and of the pro-inflammatory cytokines IL-6 and IL-8, while stimulating the release of the anti-inflammatory cytokine IL-10, an effect partially mediated by the adenosine pathway through A2A and A3 activation. Hence, PEMF may interfere with neutrophil pro-inflammatory abilities by modulating the expression and function of adenosine receptors (Varani et al. 2002). A recent review (Varani et al. 2017) reported that PEMF exposure mediates a significant upregulation of A2A and A3ARs expressed in various cells or tissues involving a reduction in most of the pro-inflammatory cytokines and hypothesized the anti-inflammatory effect of PEMF.

Neutrophils are empowered with sophisticated machineries to perform migration (Nourshargh et al. 2010) and produce granules containing either chemokines and cytokines or other innate antimicrobial proteins to be released upon appropriate stimulus (Borregaard et al. 2007). Thus, in addition to the traditional phagocytic function, neutrophils may fight microbes by delivering granules with enzymatic functions (Reeves et al. 2002) and by what has been defined in 2004 as neutrophil extracellular traps (NETs) (Brinkmann et al. 2004). NETs are extracellular traps that capture and destroy extracellular microbes and are basically a backbone of nuclear decondensed chromatin mixed with neutrophil-derived antimicrobial proteins. The generation of NET results, for the neutrophil, in a unique form of cell death called NETosis followed by autophagy or phagocytosis by macrophages (Parker et al. 2012).

The role that neutrophils play in immune response and their high reactivity, mobility, and sensitivity made them putative targets to investigate possible cell modulation effects by ELF-MF exposure. The first study investigating ELF-MF impact on NET formation, *ex vivo*, was performed by Golbach et al. (2015) and showed that ELF-MF exposure alone induced NETs. ELF-MF significantly enhanced NET formation in freshly isolated peripheral blood neutrophils that were pre-activated with PMA. In fact, PMA is a potent activator of NADPH oxidase that triggers the generation of ROS, which are key elements for the formation of NET. ROS is needed for the dissociation of peptide complexes containing neutrophil-derived antimicrobial proteins. Golbach and colleagues used selective pharmacological oxidase inhibitors, demonstrating that the NADPH pathway is critical for ELF-MF-enhanced NET formation, possibly by increasing ROS production (Golbach et al. 2015).

Calcium plays an important role as receptor-mediated intracellular second messenger in neutrophils and in the immune system. Since the Ca^{2+} involvement of MF-related cellular reactions has already been extensively elaborated in Section 1.2.1 of this chapter, we dispense with a further discussion here.

In line with neutrophils as phagocytic cells, we find other professional phagocytes like monocytes, dendritic cells (DCs), and macrophages. Monocytes are the precursors of macrophages and DCs. They are generated in the bone marrow, stored in the spleen as immature monocytes, released in circulation, and within days they seed in tissues. Once monocytes leave the circulation through the endothelium, they differentiate into macrophages or dendritic cells depending on the signals received from the tissue microenvironment (Geissmann et al. 2010).

Macrophages are antigen-presenting phagocytes releasing both antimicrobial mediators and pro-inflammatory factors to stimulate other cells of the immune system and are partly responsible for the redox homeostasis. Macrophages are involved in both innate and adaptive immune responses. Depending on the types of cytokines they are exposed to, macrophages can be activated by the classical (Th1) or the alternative (Th2) pathway. The classically activated M1 macrophages are activated by T-helper (Th)-1 cytokine interferon gamma (IFN-γ), tumor necrosis factor (TNF-α), lipopolysaccharide (LPS) or endogenous danger signals (Laskin et al. 2011) and they require priming. After phagocytic uptake, these cells have the capacity to produce reactive oxygen radicals or NO to destroy the remaining pathogens and induce pro-inflammatory cytokines, such as TNF-α, IL-1ß, iNOS, and IL-12 as an acute inflammatory response. The alternative pathway does not require any priming. M2 macrophages (alternative pathway activated) are activated by Th2 cytokines such as IL-4, IL-10, or IL-13 (Gordon 2003) and act as anti-inflammatory cells. These cells produce low-level oxygen intermediates, polyamines, and proline, which induce proliferation and collagen production, respectively, being involved in resolving inflammation, activating tissue repair, wound healing, and increasing fibrogenesis (Gordon & Martinez 2010; Mosser & Edwards 2008; Song et al. 2000).

Oxidative stress is a very important player in the immune response (see Section 1.2.2). It has been suggested that ELF-MF influences immune cells by membrane-associated components leading to moderate ROS release and changes in radical homeostasis (Lupke et al. 2004;

Lantow et al. 2006; Mattsson & Simkó 2014). This, in turn, causes downstream events including changes in gene expression leading to the activation of the alternative pathway of human monocytes. ROS release and cytokine production, such as IL-1β, are common cell activation markers in immune relevant cells. So, for example, Frahm et al. (2006) detected a time-dependent IL-1ß formation increase after 4 h to exposure 1 mT MF with a maximum of 12.3-fold increase after 24 h compared to controls. Cossarizza and colleagues described the increased release of IL-2, IL-1, and IL-6 in peritoneal lymphocytes after long-term exposure to ELF-MF (Cossarizza et al. 1989). On the other hand, investigation on cytokine production by Pessina and Aldinucci (1998) showed no effects after EMF on peritoneal blood cells. Gomez-Ochoa et al. (2011) exposed fibroblast-like cells derived from peripheral blood mononuclear cells (PBMCs) to PEMF (15 min on days 7, 8, and 9 of culture). The authors detected a decrease in the pro-inflammatory cytokines IL-1 and TNF, and the increase of IL-10. In another study, the effects of 45 mT PEMF were investigated on cytokine production in PBMC from healthy donors and from Crohn's disease (CD) patients (Kaszuba-Zwoińska et al. 2008). Exposed and stimulated PBMCs from CD patients showed a decrease in IFN-γ and an increase in IL-10 production, whereas PEMF exposure had minimal effect on peripheral blood mononuclear cells (PBMCs) from controls. *Ex vivo* stimulation of PBMC and spleen cells with PHA induced a higher IL-6 secretion in the exposed group compared to controls; none of the other assessed cytokines were significantly different between the two groups. The authors suggested that long-term exposure to low dose of MF alters the cytokine profile toward the downregulation of Th1-type and upregulation of Th17-type cytokines but which cell types are sensitive/modulated by EMF remains to be determined (Salehi et al. 2013).

Falone et al. (2007) found changes in the redox and differentiation status in neuroblastoma cells after short-term MF exposure. The authors detected modulations of the redox status of the cells, without any oxidative damage, by a positive modulation of antioxidant enzyme expression and a significant increase in glutathione level.

1.4.2 Static Magnetic Field

It has often been stated and shown that also SMFs are physical stimulators that have anti-inflammatory effects in human macrophages (Flipo et al. 1998; Vergallo et al. 2013) and lymphocytes (Salerno et al. 1999) and in human peripheral blood mononuclear cells (PBMC) (Aldinucci et al. 2003). It has also been shown that SMF attenuates LPS-induced neuroinflammatory effects in LPS-challenged BV-2 microglia cells (Shen et al. 2014).

In an interesting study, Hsieh et al. (2015) investigated whether SMF (0.4 T) can attenuate inflammatory response of LPS-challenged dental pulp cells (DPCs). The authors detected a 25% enhancement of proliferation and a 15% increase in cell viability 3 days after initiating cell culture. SMF-pre-treated LPS-challenged (to mimic infection) cells' viability was even 25% higher than in sham controls. In addition, SMF increased the cell membrane rigidity and, in LPS-challenged condition, a higher tolerance to LPS-induced inflammatory response was observed.

Salerno et al. (2006) exposed human CD4$_+$ T cells for 2 h to 0.5 mT SMF and subsequently stimulated the cells with the mitogen phytohemaglutinin (PHA). The co-exposure caused bio-effects such as a decrease of interferon-γ production, cell proliferation, expression of CD25 and a decrease of the cytosolic free calcium concentration in exposed CD4$_+$ T cell lines. In a follow-up study, the same group (Salerno et al. 2009) investigated whether specific subsets of the CD4$_+$ T cells, namely CD45RA$_+$ and CD45RA$_-$, have different sensitivities to 0.5 mT SMF. The effects of SMF after 24 and 48 h of cell culture were analyzed, and it was found that the CD4$_+$CD45RA2$_-$ was more sensitive than CD45RA$_+$. The release of IFN-γ from exposed CD4$_+$CD45RA2$_-$ T cells was significantly decreased compared to that released by PHA-stimulated CD4$_+$CD45RA2$_-$ T cells. It was also pointed out that the effects of SMF are transient and are completely reversed after 48 h. In an earlier study of Salerno et al. (1999), the effect of 0.5 T SMF exposure on interleukin release in PBMC was investigated. No effect on PHA-dependent TNF-α, IL-6, and IL-10 secretion was detected.

In another study, Onodera et al. (2003) exposed PBMCs to 10 T SMF in the presence or absence of lymphocyte stimulation with PHA and investigated the viability of CD4$_+$ T cells, CD8$_+$ T cells, B cells, and natural killer (NK) cells. Non-stimulated cells did not show any difference, but stimulated ones reduced the viability of CD4$^+$ and CD8$^+$ T cells. Also, a significantly increased apoptosis of PHA-stimulated lymphocytes was observed.

Lin et al. (2008) demonstrated that fibroblasts exposed for 12 h to 400 mT SMF were characterized by a higher cell viability and lower levels of LPS-induced IL-1ß. SMF tended also to increase the level of LPS-induced IL-1 receptor antagonist (IL-1Ra) and IL-6, a pro-inflammatory cytokine. Gruchlik et al. (2012) showed that 300 mT SMF (6, 12, 24 h) inhibited TNF-α-dependent IL-6 secretion of normal human colon myofibroblasts CCD-18Co cells but triggered the cell proliferation, whereas it did not alter the cell viability.

An early study by Flipo and coworkers (1998) applied *in vitro* exposure of C57Bl/6 murine macrophages, spleen lymphocytes, and thymic cells to 25–150 mT SMF for 24 h. The exposure led to a decreased macrophage phagocytic activity, enhanced the apoptotic death of thymocytes, and inhibited the lymphocyte mitogenic response to Con A. The latter was associated with an increased Ca^{2+} influx in the SMF-exposed cells.

1.5 Gene-Related Studies

1.5.1 Gene Expression

Over the years, many studies have investigated the possibility that ELF-MFs affect gene expression on mRNA and protein levels. Historically, most of these studies have focused on the expression of single genes and their products. Some of these studies are also discussed in other sections of this chapter dealing with specific cellular processes.

Another approach to gene expression analysis employs a more global approach, where smaller or larger subsets of the available mRNAs and proteins are investigated. Such large-scale approaches are often referred to as high-throughput or high-content screening and take advantage of modern molecular biology techniques, which can detect even minute amounts of biomolecules. Applications of such "omics" technologies allow the scientist to simultaneously investigate the expression levels of thousands of genes, mRNAs, proteins, or metabolic intermediates. This is a tremendous discovery tool which when combined with hypothesis-driven experiments can produce totally new and meaningful knowledge. Omics-approaches have made a great impact in mainstream biology and medicine as well as in toxicology, but have not been adopted to any larger extent when investigating biological effects of magnetic fields.

Sinclair et al. (2006) published one of the earliest studies using ELF-MF exposure and evaluating the effects with a proteomics approach. The authors applied both mass spectroscopy and 2D gel electrophoresis in a study investigating the effects of a 50 Hz, 1 mT, MF for 1 h on the yeast *Saccharomyces pombe*. If the authors used changes larger than or equal to 1.5-fold compared to control cells, a total of six different proteins appeared either up- or downregulated by the field. However, the authors were exposing cells at different days of culture and could not find any consistency in the responses.

Also more recent papers report very weak or inconsistent responses when applying either proteomics or transcriptomics tools. Using three different cell lines, Kuzniar and co-authors (2017) performed a proteome-wide investigation on the effects of a 50 Hz, 2 mT MF exposure. Exposure was 15 h intermittent, with 5 min on and 15 min off cycles. The data suggested that <1% of the proteome in the cell lines responded to exposure, and with modest changes in expression (mostly <1.5-fold). Consistently, the data from all three cell lines indicated that an up-regulated protein was the DNA mismatch protein MLH1. A follow-up study in order to validate this change was done using quantitative immunoblotting. However, this approach could not corroborate the changes seen with mass spectroscopy.

In contrast, statistically significant effects of 50 Hz exposure were seen in two papers exposing the human neuroblastoma SH-SY5Y cell line to 0.5, 1, and 2 mT for 3 h (Hasanzadeh et al. 2014; Rezaie-Tavirani et al. 2017). The authors used 2D gel electrophoresis to find changes in protein expression and reported that they found alterations in a dose-dependent fashion. At the highest flux density, 189 proteins were changed relative to the control cells.

Gene expression profiling (whole-genome cDNA array) was performed by Lupke et al. (2006) on human monocytes after exposure to 1 mT MF for 45 min. The authors detected alteration of 986 genes involved in metabolism, cellular physiological processes, signal transduction, and immune responses. Further RT-PCR analysis of the kinetics of the expression of some genes (IL15RA, IL10RA) indicated the regulation of monocyte activation via the alternative pathway, whereas the delayed gene expression of FOS, IL2RA, and the enzyme HIOMT suggests the suppression of inflammatory processes.

A reanalysis of transcriptomics data from several studies on human cell lines was recently published (Parham et al. 2016). Results from five studies with complete microarray data and from three studies with a list of significantly changed mRNAs were analyzed from the viewpoint of signal transduction and metabolic pathways. The ambition was further to see if the data could suggest ELF-MF effects on the development of any specific diseases. The authors found several examples of exposure effects, but the individual data sets could not provide any coherent picture suggesting that ELF-MF leads to a specific disease.

In summary, there are the occasional studies where either mRNA or protein data have been obtained using omics-technologies. However, the studies are few and have not presented any support for consistent exposure effects that can be used for further hypothesis-driven research.

More recently, another aspect of gene regulation has received considerable attention. This is the field of epigenetic control of the expression of genes, which includes how modifications of the DNA affect how "easy" or "difficult" it is for a gene to be transcribed and thus translated into a useful protein. The phenomenon has been known for decades to influence the potency of cells, i.e., to what degree a cell can further differentiate and acquire a specific phenotype. It is thus of utmost importance for stem cells (see, e.g., Reik (2007) for a useful overview), where epigenetic mechanisms such as histone modifications and DNA methylation provide the genes with short- or long-term silencing.

Environmental conditions have recently been strongly associated with epigenetic regulation of gene expression. This includes ionizing radiation where it has been suggested that genomic instability caused by radiation is due to changes in methylation patterns of the DNA (Aypar et al. 2011). Also other environmental toxicants have been shown to influence DNA methylation (Kim et al. 2012). These authors showed that several toxicants caused both global hypomethylation and specific hypermethylation of various tumor suppressor genes. The latter phenomenon, in turn, leads to the tumor suppressor genes being more difficult to transcribe and therefore tumor development including cancer is facilitated. Interestingly, the normal cellular metabolism, when producing redox intermediates, can have a direct effect on epigenetic signaling (Cyr & Domann 2011). These authors have pointed to a strong link between metabolism and epigenetics in the pathogenesis of cardiovascular disease, Alzheimer's disease, certain types of cancer, and environmental toxicology.

Still another epigenetic feature is the transposable elements that are present in the genome. These elements are repetitive DNA sequences, which are considered to be critical regulators of gene expression (Miousse et al. 2015). They are controlled by epigenetic mechanisms such as DNA methylation and histone modifications, but environmental stressors for example, can decrease the inhibiting effects of these modifications, which will allow the transposable elements to be activated and possibly be transcribed and produce various faulty proteins. This can, in turn, also lead to various disease states, including cancer (Miousse et al. 2015).

During recent years, a number of studies have attempted to study the influence of ELF-MF on markers for epigenetic mechanisms of gene expression. Two studies employed the mouse spermatocyte-derived GC-2 cell line for experiments using 50 Hz MF exposure (1, 2, and 3 mT; 5 min on and 10 min off; 72 h exposure duration) (Liu et al. 2015 a,b). The first of the studies (Liu et al. 2015a) found that exposure had flux density-dependent effects on global DNA methylation (decrease at 1 mT, increase at 3 mT) and on expression of the DNA methyltransferases DNMT1 and DNMT3b, which catalyze methylation of the CpG dinucleotides in the genome. In accordance with the global methylation changes, the expression of the enzymes decreased at 1 mT and increased at 3 mT. The second study (Liu et al. 2015b) focused on microRNA (miRNA), which are small noncoding RNAs that regulate gene expression at the post-transcriptional level by binding to the 3′-untranslated region of mRNAs. This binding causes inhibition of translation and/or increased degradation of the mRNA and is considered an important aspect of epigenetic control of gene expression. Aberrant expression of miRNA is associated with certain disease states, including cancer. The results from the study pointed to differential expression of a number of miRNAs after exposure. More miRNAs were affected at 3 mT ($n=27$) than at 1 mT ($n=19$). These changes were not reflected in any changes in growth, apoptosis, or cell cycle distribution.

Several studies related to induction of nerve cell differentiation were discussed in Section 1.3.2. As a follow-up to earlier findings of the research group on induction of hippocampal neuronal differentiation after ELF-MF exposure, investigations of gene expression in neuronal stem cells were done (Leone et al. 2014). The cell cultures were exposed to a 50 Hz MF (1 mT, 2 days) after which a number of genes were studied with quantitative RT-PCR. Key genes such as the pro-proliferative gene HES1 and the neuronal determination genes NeuroD1 and Neurogenin1 were enhanced in expression levels after exposure, which was preceded by increased acetylation of the amino acid lysine in position 9 of the histone H3 and binding of the phosphorylated form of the transcription factor CREB to the promoter regions of the genes. This is another example of how ELF-MF influences epigenetic mechanisms. Interestingly, the effects on neuronal differentiation and also on histone acetylation were inhibited in the presence of the Ca^{2+}-channel blocker nifedipine.

Other examples of studies finding effects on epigenetic processes include a study on mouse tail-tip fibroblasts that were reprogrammed into induced pluripotent stem cells (Baek et al. 2014). Stem cell reprogramming was initiated with treatment with a cocktail of transcription factors, which led to colonies of cells with stem cell markers. This transformation from fibroblasts to stem cells was enhanced if cells were simultaneously exposed to a 50 Hz MF, 1 mT for 15 days. The treatment also led to induction of the histone lysine M-methyltransferase (MII2), which contributes to methylation of the histone H3. Histone marks and DNA methylation were also investigated by Manser et al. (2017) who studied the influence of a 50 Hz MF (1 mT; 5 min on and 10 min off; 72 h) on the Jurkat leukemia cell line and hematopoietic stem cells undergoing differentiation to neutrophilic granulocytes. For most of the endpoints (various histone modifications, global DNA methylation), exposure did not produce any significant effects. However, the exposure was statistically correlated to increased variability of epigenetic modifications between experiments, which the authors suggest was due to different chromatin structure in the cells in the different experiments.

A considerable part of the human (and most other species') genome consists of repetitive noncoding elements such as long interspersed nuclear elements (LINE-1). These elements can be inserted via reverse transcription into other genomic sites and cause a number of DNA-related problems including mutagenesis and DNA-breaks. The activity of the LINE-1 elements is controlled by, e.g., methylation levels of its promoter region. The hypomethylated state has been shown to be a marker in several cancer forms, and recent research has shown that environmental factors affect the methylation state (Klutstein et al. 2016). A pulsed MF (square wave; 50 Hz; 1 mT; 0.6 ms rise time; 24 or 48 h exposure duration) was used to expose human BE(2)C neuroblastoma cells, either alone or in combination with oxidative stress (Giorgi et al. 2017). The MF exposure alone did not affect DNA methylation levels at different CpG islands of the LINE-1 element. However, in combination with the oxidative stress, a significant decrease in DNA methylation was observed. This decrease was present only in some of the available CpG units and was found to be transient.

1.5.2 Genotoxicity

It is currently accepted that damage to DNA in cells that undergo cell divisions plays a contributory role in development of cancer. This damage can occur spontaneously but can also be the result of exposure to environmental agents (physical, chemical, biological). Such environmental "stress" can either have a direct "genotoxic" effect or act indirectly, either as a co-factor to another directly genotoxic agent or via cellular processes (e.g., radical formation) that generate conditions that are negatively influencing the integrity of DNA. A direct genotoxic effect by static or LF MF is not physically plausible, but an indirect effect of MF exposure has been investigated in many studies. It is not the objective of this chapter to analyze available literature regarding DNA effects of MF, but a brief overview of the current state of knowledge is provided.

Performed studies have investigated DNA from various sources, including humans (primarily occupational exposure), animals (*in vivo* exposures), and cells in culture (both primary cells and established cell lines). Investigated endpoints have included DNA strand breaks, micronucleus formation, sister chromatid exchanges, chromosomal aberrations, DNA repair, and gene mutations.

A very comprehensive review of ELF-MF effects on mammalian cells was published by Vijayalaxmi and Obe (2005). The authors scrutinized relevant papers published 1990–2003 and categorized the outcome according to whether exposure caused an increase in DNA damage, had no effects, or were inconclusive. In summary, the review reported that 14 of 63 investigated studies (23%) found increased damages in exposed cells compared to control material, whereas 46% found no effects. An additional 32% of the studies generated inconclusive results. The authors concluded that the studies suggested that MF exposure did not cause any direct genotoxic effects, and that there was little evidence for indirect effects. Vijayalaxmi and Obe stressed in their conclusions that many studies reporting the absence of effects reported exposure conditions and experimental protocols in sufficient detail, whereas this was lacking in many of the other studies.

Shortcomings in study quality were also stressed by Maes and Verschaeve (2016) in a recent review. The focus of this analysis was on human cytogenetic biomonitoring studies where tissue samples (peripheral blood lymphocytes and cells from the buccal epithelium) from people occupationally exposed to electric and/or magnetic fields. Although many of the studies reported exposure effects, a firm conclusion was still difficult to draw.

1.6 Conclusions

In this chapter, data from *in vitro* studies after ELF-MF and SMF exposures were compiled based on known cell biology mechanisms to see if MF exposure is acting by the stimulation of common cell physiological processes. Since the very first interaction between fields and cell is still unknown, we followed the route starting with an interaction on or at the cell membrane or any of the intracellular membrane organelles, leading to primary events such as changes in the levels of Ca^{2+}, ROS, and HSP expression, since these are very immediate processes. Modulations in the levels of these compounds lead to the activation of signal transduction pathways. These can, in turn, activate secondary processes, such as modulation of cell proliferation, differentiation, and other molecular and cellular processes.

Although the available data are inconsistent, the studies show no general difference between SMF and ELF-MF when causing effects. If cellular activation was detected after exposure to any of the types of MF, similar findings were reported also for the other modality. Therefore, here we do not differentiate between the two MF variants any further in this discussion, even though there are differences in the efficacy seemingly depending on the physical parameters.

Regarding the interactions on or at the membrane, most studies report an interaction between MF and intracellular Ca^{2+} levels. There is evidence that both influx from the extracellular space as well as release from ER/SR can be relevant. The two-step model suggested by Cerella et al. (2011) can possibly accommodate both these observations. Thus, initially the MF triggers release from the ER/SR, leading to a non-capacitative influx from the cells exterior, which serves as a means to provide enough Ca^{2+} to be pumped back into the ER/SR.

Another cellular event that occurs immediately during exposure is the effect on radical homeostasis. Thus, MF seems to induce moderate oxidative stress *in vitro*. Since this effect is modest, around 30% increase compared to controls, it initiates signal transduction pathways, leading more likely to protective effects for the cell by inducing, e.g., antioxidant enzymes and/or HSPs, than hazardous effects. The induction of antioxidants and HSPs can be activated directly by ROS, but also via changes in the intracellular Ca^{2+} concentration. On the basis of the available data dealing with exposure to MF causing HSP expression modulations, no (co)relation to MF dose, specific exposure conditions, or cell type could be identified. There is some evidence that MF might act as a mild stressor, which induces HSPs. Such HSP induction might produce secondary responses, such as cell proliferation modulation.

Many studies have investigated modulations in proliferation, apoptosis induction, and differentiation, where mostly the induction of proliferation or differentiation was observed. Some molecular studies showed evidence that MF induces cell proliferation indirectly via Ras/ERK and PI3K/Akt pathways. If cells are in a differentiating state, they can be triggered to differentiate via EGFR/Akt/mTOR and the p38 mitogen-activated protein kinase signaling. On the other hand, apoptosis has not generally been detected as a direct or indirect effect after MF exposure. Regarding neuronal differentiation, there is some evidence that the field exposure causes changes in gene expression that corresponds to differentiation toward both neural and glial cell types. There also seems to be an involvement of VGCC of the L-type in the differentiation process.

An interesting outcome is the potential of the fields to modulate the immune system. It emerges that MFs activate immune cells to release moderate amounts of free radicals via the alternative pathway, which then can lead to the consumption of the intracellular antioxidants. In general, pro-inflammatory factors are downregulated and anti-inflammatory cytokines are upregulated as a result of the moderate oxidative stress caused by MF exposure. This leads to cell activation of the immune cells by shifting them toward pro-oxidative states, which seems to stimulate the anti-inflammatory pathways. This stimulation appears stronger in the presence of other stimuli such as LPS or PHA.

Studies of gene expression based on high-throughput screening technologies are few in the area of bioelectromagnetics research. Most of them show that changes on both mRNA and protein levels occur, but that the significance of the findings is unclear at this point. Also studies that are focusing on gene regulation from the point of view of DNA methylation and other forms of "epigenetic" gene regulation are too few to allow any far-reaching conclusions. At most, the studies so far suggest that ELF-MF exposures may influence the genome's ability to be expressed in a controlled manner.

Taking it together, both SMF and ELF-MFs can interact with cellular systems and activate cell physiological processes. These can lead to that cells are in a kind of "activated state" and better suited to handle stress. Since the majority of the described findings are not explicitly signs of hazardous effects, this "activated state" might have more advantageous consequences that deserve more attention and elucidation of potential practical use.

References

Akan, Z. et al., 2010. Extremely low-frequency electromagnetic fields affect the immune response of monocyte-derived macrophages to pathogens. *Bioelectromagnetics*, 31(8), pp. 603–612.

Akbarnejad, Z. et al., 2016. Effects of extremely low-frequency pulsed electromagnetic fields (ELF-PEMFs) on glioblastoma cells (U87). *Electromagnetic Biology and Medicine*, 36, pp. 1–10.

Aldinucci, C. et al., 2003. The effect of strong static magnetic field on lymphocytes. *Bioelectromagnetics*, 24(2), pp. 109–117.

Alfieri, R.R. et al., 2006. Increased levels of inducible HSP70 in cells exposed to electromagnetic fields. *Radiation Research*, 165(1), pp. 95–104.

Amaroli, A. et al., 2013. Effects of an extremely low-frequency electromagnetic field on stress factors: a study in Dictyostelium discoideum cells. *European Journal of Protistology*, 49(3), pp. 400–405.

An, G.Z. et al., 2015. Effects of long-term 50Hz power-line frequency electromagnetic field on cell behavior in Balb/c 3T3 cells. *PLoS ONE*, 10(2), pp. 1–13.

Aypar, U., Morgan, W.F. & Baulch, J.E. 2011. Radiation-induced genomic instability: Are epigenetic mechanisms the missing link? *International Journal of Radiation Biology*, 87(2), pp. 179–191.

Bae, J.E. et al., 2013. Electromagnetic field-induced converse cell growth during a long-term observation. *International Journal of Radiation Biology*, 89(12), pp. 1–10.

Baek, S. et al., 2014. Electromagnetic fields mediate efficient cell reprogramming into a pluripotent state. *ACS Nano*, 8(10), pp. 10125–10138.

Bai, W.F. et al., 2013. Fifty-Hertz electromagnetic fields facilitate the induction of rat bone mesenchymal stromal cells to differentiate into functional neurons. *Cytotherapy*, 15(8), pp. 961–970.

Basile, A. et al., 2011. Exposure to 50 Hz electromagnetic field raises the levels of the anti-apoptotic protein BAG3 in melanoma cells. *Journal of Cellular Physiology*, 226(11), pp. 2901–2907.

Basu, S. et al., 2000. Necrotic but not apoptotic cell death releases heat shock proteins, which deliver a partial maturation signal to dendritic cells and activate the NF-kappa B pathway. *International Immunology*, 12(11), pp. 1539–1546.

Bekhite, M.M. et al., 2010. Static electromagnetic fields induce vasculogenesis and chondro-osteogenesis of mouse embryonic stem cells by reactive oxygen species-mediated up-regulation of vascular endothelial growth factor. *Stem Cells and Development*, 19(5), pp. 731–743.

Bekhite, M.M. et al., 2013. Static magnetic fields increase cardiomyocyte differentiation of Flk-1+ cells derived from mouse embryonic stem cells via Ca^{2+} influx and ROS production. *International Journal of Cardiology*, 167(3), pp. 798–808.

Belton, M., Prato, F.S. & Carson, J.J.L., 2011. Effect of glutathione depletion, hyperthermia, and a 100-mT static magnetic field on an hsp70/luc reporter system. *Bioelectromagnetics*, 32(6), pp. 453–462.

Benassi, B. et al., 2016. Extremely low frequency magnetic field (ELF-MF) exposure sensitizes SH-SY5Y cells to the pro-Parkinson's disease toxin MPP+. *Molecular Neurobiology*, 53(6), pp. 4247–4260.

Bernardini, C. et al., 2007. Effects of 50 Hz sinusoidal magnetic fields on Hsp27, Hsp70, Hsp90 expression in porcine aortic endothelial cells (PAEC). *Bioelectromagnetics*, 28(3), pp. 231–237.

Berridge, M.J., Bootman, M.D. & Lipp, P., 1998. Calcium—a life and death signal. *Nature*, 395(6703), pp. 645–648.

Berridge, M.J., Bootman, M.D. & Roderick, H.L., 2003. Calcium signalling: dynamics, homeostasis and remodelling. *Nature Reviews Molecular Cell Biology*, 4(7), pp. 517–529.

Bodega, G. et al., 2005. Acute and chronic effects of exposure to a 1-mT magnetic field on the cytoskeleton, stress proteins, and proliferation of astroglial cells in culture. *Environmental research*, 98(3), pp. 355–362.

Borregaard, N., Sørensen, O.E. & Theilgaard-Mönch, K., 2007. Neutrophil granules: a library of innate immunity proteins. *Trends in Immunology*, 28(8), pp. 340–345.

Brinkmann, V. et al., 2004. Neutrophil extracellular traps kill bacteria. *Science*, 303(5663), pp. 1532–1535.

Buckner, C.A. et al., 2017. The effects of electromagnetic fields on B16-BL6 cells are dependent on their spatial and temporal character. *Bioelectromagnetics*, 38(3), pp. 165–174.

Calabrò, E. et al., 2013. Effects of low intensity static magnetic field on FTIR spectra and ROS production in SH-SY5Y neuronal-like cells. *Bioelectromagnetics*, 34(8), pp. 618–629.

Calcabrini, C. et al., 2016. Effect of extremely low-frequency electromagnetic fields on antioxidant activity in the human keratinocyte cell line NCTC 2544. *Biotechnology and Applied Biochemistry*, 64(3), pp. 415–422.

Cerella, C. et al., 2011. Magnetic fields promote a pro-survival non-capacitative Ca^{2+} entry via phospholipase C signaling. *The International Journal of Biochemistry & Cell Biology*, 43(3), pp. 393–400.

Chang, S.-H., Hsiao, Y.-W. & Lin, H.-Y., 2011. Low-frequency electromagnetic field exposure accelerates chondrocytic phenotype expression on chitosan substrate. *Orthopedics*, 34(1), pp. 20–20.

Chen, G. et al., 2000. Effect of electromagnetic field exposure on chemically induced differentiation of friend erythroleukemia cells. *Environmental Health Perspectives*, 108(10), pp. 967–972.

Cheng, Y. et al., 2015. Extremely low-frequency electromagnetic fields enhance the proliferation and differentiation of neural progenitor cells cultured from ischemic brains. *Neuroreport*, 26(15), pp. 896–902.

Collard, J.-F. et al., 2013. Statistical validation of the acceleration of the differentiation at the expense of the proliferation in human epidermal cells exposed to extremely low frequency electric fields. *Progress in Biophysics and Molecular Biology*, 111, pp. 37–45.

Conti, P. et al., 1985. A role for Ca²⁺ in the effect of very low frequency electromagnetic field on the blastogenesis of human lymphocytes. *FEBS Letters*, 181(1), pp. 28–32.

Corallo, C. et al., 2014. Proteomics of human primary osteoarthritic chondrocytes exposed to extremely low-frequency electromagnetic fields (ELF EMFs) and to therapeutic application of musically modulated electromagnetic fields (TAMMEF). *Electromagnetic Biology and Medicine*, 33(1), pp. 3–10.

Cossarizza, A. et al., 1989. Extremely low frequency pulsed electromagnetic fields increase interleukin-2 (IL-2) utilization and IL-2 receptor expression in mitogen-stimulated human lymphocytes from old subjects. *FEBS Letters*, 248(1–2), pp. 141–144.

Coulton, L.A. et al., 2004. Effect of 50 Hz electromagnetic fields on the induction of heat-shock protein gene expression in human leukocytes. *Radiation Research*, 161(4), pp. 430–434.

Cuccurazzu, B. et al., 2010. Exposure to extremely low-frequency (50 Hz) electromagnetic fields enhances adult hippocampal neurogenesis in C57BL/6 mice. *Experimental Neurology*, 226(1), pp. 173–182.

Cyr, A.R. & Domann, F.E., 2011. The redox basis of epigenetic modifications: from mechanisms to functional consequences. *Antioxidants & Redox Signaling*, 15(2), pp. 551–589.

Delle Monache, S. et al., 2013. Inhibition of angiogenesis mediated by extremely low-frequency magnetic fields (ELF-MFs). *PLoS ONE*, 8(11), p. e79309. doi:10.1371/journal.pone.0079309.

Dolphin, A.C., 2006. A short history of voltage-gated calcium channels. *British Journal of Pharmacology*, 147(Suppl 1), pp. S56–S62.

Drela, K. et al., 2013. Human mesenchymal stem cells in the treatment of neurological diseases. *Acta Neurobiologiae Experimentalis*, 73(1), pp. 38–56.

D'Souza, S.J.A. et al., 2001. Ca²⁺ and BMP-6 signaling regulate E2F during epidermal keratinocyte differentiation. *Journal of Biological Chemistry*, 276(26), pp. 23531–23538.

Duong, C.N. & Kim, J.Y., 2016. Exposure to electromagnetic field attenuates oxygen-glucose deprivation-induced microglial cell death by reducing intracellular Ca²⁺ and ROS. *International Journal of Radiation Biology*, 92(4), pp. 195–201.

Falone, S. et al., 2007. Fifty hertz extremely low-frequency electromagnetic field causes changes in redox and differentiative status in neuroblastoma cells. *International Journal of Biochemistry and Cell Biology*, 39(11), pp. 2093–2106.

Fathi, E. & Farahzadi, R., 2017. Enhancement of osteogenic differentiation of rat adipose tissue-derived mesenchymal stem cells by zinc sulphate under electromagnetic field via the PKA, ERK1/2 and Wnt/β-catenin signaling pathways B. O. Williams, ed. *PLoS ONE*, 12(3), p. e0173877.

Flipo, D. et al., 1998. Increased apoptosis, changes in intracellular Ca²⁺, and functional alterations in lymphocytes and macrophages after in vitro exposure to static magnetic field. *Journal of Toxicology and Environmental Health A*, 54(1), pp. 63–76.

Forostyak, O. et al., 2016. Physiology of Ca²⁺ signalling in stem cells of different origins and differentiation stages. *Cell Calcium*, 59(2–3), pp. 57–66.

Frahm, J. et al., 2006. Alteration in cellular functions in mouse macrophages after exposure to 50 Hz magnetic fields. *Journal of Cellular Biochemistry*, 99(1), pp. 168–177.

Frahm, J. et al., 2010. Exposure to ELF magnetic fields modulate redox related protein expression in mouse macrophages. *Toxicology Letters*, 192(3), pp. 330–336.

Frisch, P. et al., 2013. Induction of heat shock gene expression in RAT1 primary fibroblast cells by ELF electric fields. *Bioelectromagnetics*, 34(5), pp. 405–413.

Gaetani, R. et al., 2009. Differentiation of human adult cardiac stem cells exposed to extremely low-frequency electromagnetic fields. *Cardiovascular Research*, 82(3), pp. 411–420.

Garip, A.I. & Akan, Z., 2010. Effect of ELF-EMF on number of apoptotic cells; correlation with reactive oxygen species and HSP. *Acta Biologica Hungarica*, 61(2), pp. 158–167.

Gehrmann, M. et al., 2008. The therapeutic implications of clinically applied modifiers of heat shock protein 70 (Hsp70) expression by tumor cells. *Cell Stress and Chaperones*, 13(1), pp. 1–10.

Geissmann, F. et al., 2010. Development of monocytes, macrophages, and dendritic cells. *Science,* 327(5966), pp. 656–661.

Giorgi, C. et al., 2012. Mitochondrial Ca²⁺ and apoptosis. *Cell Calcium,* 52(1), pp. 36–43.

Giorgi, G. et al., 2017. Assessing the combined effect of extremely low-frequency magnetic field exposure and oxidative stress on LINE-1 promoter methylation in human neural cells. *Radiation and Environmental Biophysics,* 56(2), pp. 193–200.

Glancy, B. & Balaban, R.S., 2012. Role of mitochondrial Ca²⁺ in the regulation of cellular energetics. *Biochemistry,* 51(14), pp. 2959–2973.

Golbach, L.A. et al., 2015. Low-frequency electromagnetic field exposure enhances extracellular trap formation by human neutrophils through the NADPH pathway. *Journal of Innate Immunity,* 7(5), pp. 459–465.

Golbach, L.A. et al., 2016. Calcium homeostasis and low-frequency magnetic and electric field exposure: a systematic review and meta-analysis of in vitro studies. *Environment International,* 92–93, pp. 695–706.

Gómez-Ochoa, I. et al., 2011. Pulsed electromagnetic fields decrease proinflammatory cytokine secretion (IL-1β and TNF-α) on human fibroblast-like cell culture. *Rheumatology International,* 31(10), pp. 1283–1289.

Goodman, R. et al., 2009. Extremely low frequency electromagnetic fields activate the ERK cascade, increase hsp70 protein levels and promote regeneration in Planaria. *International Journal of Radiation Biology,* 85(10), pp. 851–859.

Gordon, S., 2003. Alternative activation of macrophages. *Nature Reviews Immunology,* 3(1), pp. 23–35.

Gordon, S. & Martinez, F.O., 2010. Alternative activation of macrophages: mechanism and functions. *Immunity,* 32(5), pp. 593–604.

Gottwald, E. et al., 2007. Expression of HSP72 after ELF-EMF exposure in three cell lines. *Bioelectromagnetics,* 28(7), pp. 509–518.

Grassi, C. et al., 2004. Effects of 50 Hz electromagnetic fields on voltage-gated Ca²⁺ channels and their role in modulation of neuroendocrine cell proliferation and death. *Cell Calcium,* 35(4), pp. 307–315.

Gruchlik, A. et al., 2012. Effects of 300 mT static magnetic field on IL-6 secretion in normal human colon myofibroblasts. *Acta Poloniae Pharmaceutica - Drug Research,* 69(6), pp. 1320–1324.

Hasanzadeh, H. et al., 2014. Effect of ELF-EMF exposure on human neuroblastoma cell line: a proteomics analysis. *Iranian Journal of Cancer Prevention,* 7(1), pp. 22–27.

Heredia-Rojas, J.A. et al., 2010. Effect of 60 Hz magnetic fields on the activation of hsp70 promoter in cultured INER-37 and RMA E7 cells. *In Vitro Cellular & Developmental Biology-Animal,* 46(9), pp. 758–763.

Hinsenkamp, M. & Collard, J.-F., 2011. Bone Morphogenic Protein—mRNA upregulation after exposure to low frequency electric field. *International Orthopaedics,* 35(10), pp. 1577–1581. Available at: http://link.springer.com/10.1007/s00264-011-1215-9.

Hirai, T. & Yoneda, Y., 2004. Functional alterations in immature cultured rat hippocampal neurons after sustained exposure to static magnetic fields. *Journal of Neuroscience Research,* 75(2), pp. 230–240.

Hou, X. et al., 2006. [Effects of magnetic field on MAPK signaling pathways of human retinal pigment epithelial cells bound with beads in vitro]. *[Zhonghua yan ke za zhi] Chinese Journal of Ophthalmology,* 42(12), pp. 1103–1108.

Hsieh, S.C. et al., 2015. Static magnetic field attenuates lipopolysaccharide-induced inflammation in pulp cells by affecting cell membrane stability. *Scientific World Journal,* 2015, 9 pp. doi:10.1155/2015/492683.

Huo, R. et al., 2010. Noninvasive electromagnetic fields on keratinocyte growth and migration. *Journal of Surgical Research,* 162(2), pp. 299–307.

Ikehara, T. et al., 2002. Effects of a time varying strong magnetic field on release of cytosolic free Ca²⁺ from intracellular stores in cultured bovine adrenal chromaffin cells. *Bioelectromagnetics,* 23(7), pp. 505–515.

Ishisaka, R. et al., 2000. Effects of a magnetic fields on the various functions of subcellular organelles and cells. *Pathophysiology*, 7(2), pp. 149–152.

Jacob, P., Hirt, H. & Bendahmane, A., 2017. The heat-shock protein/chaperone network and multiple stress resistance. *Plant Biotechnology Journal*, 15(4), pp. 405–414.

Janeway, C.A. & Medzhitov, R., 2002. Innate immune recognition. *Annual Review of Immunology*, 20(2), pp. 197–216.

Jeong, W.-Y. et al., 2017. Extremely low-frequency electromagnetic field promotes astrocytic differentiation of human bone marrow mesenchymal stem cells by modulating SIRT1 expression. *Bioscience, Biotechnology, and Biochemistry*, 8451, pp. 1–7.

Kang, K.S. et al., 2013. Regulation of osteogenic differentiation of human adipose-derived stem cells by controlling electromagnetic field conditions. *Experimental & Molecular Medicine*, 45(1), p. e6.

Kanno, H., 2013. Regenerative therapy for neuronal diseases with transplantation of somatic stem cells. *World Journal of Stem Cells*, 5(4), pp. 163–171.

Kaszuba-Zwoińska, J. et al., 2008. Magnetic field anti-inflammatory effects in Crohn's disease depends upon viability and cytokine profile of the immune competent cells. *Journal of Physiology and Pharmacology*, 59(1), pp. 177–187.

Kim, H.-J. et al., 2013. Extremely low-frequency electromagnetic fields induce neural differentiation in bone marrow derived mesenchymal stem cells. *Experimental Biology and Medicine*, 238, pp. 923–931.

Kim, M. et al., 2012. Environmental toxicants—induced epigenetic alterations and their reversers. *Journal of Environmental Science and Health. Part C, Environmental Carcinogenesis & Ecotoxicology Reviews*, 30(4), pp.323–67.

Kim, S.C. et al., 2016. Static magnetic field controls cell cycle in cultured human glioblastoma cells. *Cytotechnology*, 68(6), pp.2745–2751.

Kim, S. & Im, W., 2010. Static magnetic fields inhibit proliferation and disperse subcellular localization of gamma complex protein3 in cultured C2C12 myoblast cells. *Cell Biochemistry and Biophysics*, 57(1), pp. 1–8.

Klutstein, M. et al., 2016. DNA methylation in cancer and aging. *Cancer Research*, 76(12), pp. 3446–3450.

Köbbert, C. et al., 2008. Low-energy electromagnetic fields promote proliferation of vascular smooth muscle cells. *Electromagnetic Biology and Medicine*, 27(1), pp. 41–53.

Kurzeja, E. et al., 2013. Effect of a static magnetic fields and fluoride ions on the antioxidant defense system of mice fibroblasts. *International Journal of Molecular Sciences*, 14(7), pp. 15017–15028.

Kuzniar, A. et al., 2017. Semi-quantitative proteomics of mammalian cells upon short-term exposure to nonionizing electromagnetic fields. *PLoS ONE*, 12(2), p. e0170762. doi:10.1371/journal.pone.0170762.

Lantow, M. et al., 2006. ROS release and Hsp70 expression after exposure to 1,800 MHz radiofrequency electromagnetic fields in primary human monocytes and lymphocytes. *Radiation and Environmental Biophysics*, 45(1), pp. 55–62.

Laramee, C.B. et al., 2014. Elevation of heat shock gene expression from static magnetic field exposure in vitro. *Bioelectromagnetics*, 35(6), pp. 406–413. Available at: http://doi.wiley.com/10.1002/bem.21857.

Laskin, D.L. et al., 2011. Macrophages and tissue injury: agents of defense or destruction? *Annual Review of Pharmacology and Toxicology*, 51, pp. 267–288.

Leone, L. et al., 2014. Epigenetic modulation of adult hippocampal neurogenesis by extremely low-frequency electromagnetic fields. *Molecular Neurobiology*, 49(3), pp. 1472–1486.

Lew, W.-Z. et al., 2016. Static magnetic fields enhance dental pulp stem cell proliferation by activating the p38 MAPK pathway as its putative mechanism. *Journal of Tissue Engineering and Regenerative Medicine*, 12(1), pp. 19–29. doi:10.1002/term.2333.

Li, J.K.J. et al., 2006. Comparison of ultrasound and electromagnetic field effects on osteoblast growth. *Ultrasound in Medicine and Biology*, 32(5), pp. 769–775.

Li, Y. et al., 2012. Low strength static magnetic field inhibits the proliferation, migration, and adhesion of human vascular smooth muscle cells in a restenosis model through mediating integrins β1-FAK, Ca^{2+} signaling pathway. *Annals of Biomedical Engineering*, 40(12), pp. 2611–2618.

Liburdy, R.P., 1992. Calcium signaling in lymphocytes and ELF fields evidence for an electric field metric and a site of interaction involving the calcium ion channel. *FEBS Letters*, 301(1), pp. 53–59.

Lin, C.-P.C.-T. et al., 2008. Long-term continuous exposure to static magnetic field reduces popolysaccharide-induced cytotoxicity of fibroblasts. *International Journal of Radiation Biology*, 84(3), pp. 219–226.

Lin, T. et al., 2014. A moderate static magnetic field enhances TRAIL-induced apoptosis by the inhibition of Cdc2 and subsequent downregulation of survivin in human breast carcinoma cells. *Bioelectromagnetics*, 35(5), pp. 337–346.

Lindström, E. et al., 1993. Intracellular calcium oscillations induced in a T-cell line by a weak 50 Hz magnetic field. *Journal of Cellular Physiology*, 156(2), pp. 395–398.

Lindström, E. et al., 1995. CD45 phosphatase in Jurkat cells is necessary for response to applied ELF magnetic fields. *FEBS Letters*, 370(1–2), pp. 118–122.

Lindström, E. et al., 1995. Intracellular calcium oscillations in a T-cell line after exposure to extremely-low-frequency magnetic fields with variable frequencies and flux densities. *Bioelectromagnetics*, 16(1), pp. 41–47.

Lindström, E. et al., 2001. ELF magnetic fields initiate protein tyrosine phosphorylation of the T cell receptor complex. *Bioelectrochemistry (Amsterdam, Netherlands)*, 53, pp. 73–78.

Liu, Y. et al., 2015a. Effect of 50 Hz extremely low-frequency electromagnetic fields on the DNA methylation and DNA methyltransferases in mouse spermatocyte-derived cell line GC-2. *BioMed Research International*, 2015, 10 pp. doi:10.1155/2015/237183.

Liu, Y. et al., 2015b. Extremely low-frequency electromagnetic fields affect the miRNA-mediated regulation of signaling pathways in the GC-2 cell line M. R. Scarfi, ed. *PLoS ONE*, 10(10), p. e0139949.

Loschinger, M. et al., 1999. Induction of intracellular calcium oscillations in human skin fibroblast populations by sinusoidal extremely low-frequency magnetic fields (20 hz, 8 mT) is dependent on the differentiation state of the single cell. *Radiation Research*, 151(2), pp. 195–200.

Luo, Y. et al., 2016. Moderate intensity static magnetic fields affect mitotic spindles and increase the antitumor efficacy of 5-FU and Taxol. *Bioelectrochemistry*, 109, pp. 31–40.

Lupke, M. et al., 2006. Gene expression analysis of ELF-MF exposed human monocytes indicating the involvement of the alternative activation pathway. *Biochimica et Biophysica Acta - Molecular Cell Research*, 1763(4), pp. 402–412.

Lupke, M., Rollwitz, J. & Simkó, M., 2004. Cell activating capacity of 50 Hz magnetic fields to release reactive oxygen intermediates in human umbilical cord blood-derived monocytes and in Mono Mac 6 cells. *Free Radical Research*, 38(9), pp. 985–993.

Ma, Q. et al., 2014. Extremely low-frequency electromagnetic fields affect transcript levels of neuronal differentiation-related genes in embryonic neural stem cells. *PLoS ONE*, 9(3), p. e90041. doi:10.1371/journal.pone.0090041.

Maes, A. & Verschaeve, L., 2016. Genetic damage in humans exposed to extremely low-frequency electromagnetic fields. *Archives of Toxicology*, 90(10), pp. 2337–2348.

Malagoli, D. et al., 2004. 50 Hz magnetic fields activate mussel immunocyte p38 MAP kinase and induce HSP70 and 90. *Comparative Biochemistry and Physiology. Toxicology & Pharmacology : CBP*, 137(1), pp. 75–79.

Mannerling, A.C. et al., 2010. Effects of 50-Hz magnetic field exposure on superoxide radical anion formation and HSP70 induction in human K562 cells. *Radiation and Environmental Biophysics*, 49(4), pp. 731–741.

Manser, M. et al., 2017. ELF-MF exposure affects the robustness of epigenetic programming during granulopoiesis. *Scientific Reports*, 7, p. 43345.

Maredziak, M. et al., 2017. Static magnetic field enhances the viability and proliferation rate of adipose tissue-derived mesenchymal stem cells potentially through activation of the phosphoinositide 3-kinase/Akt (PI3K/Akt) pathway. *Electromagnetic Biology and Medicine*, 36(1), pp. 45–54.

De Mattei, M. et al., 2009. Adenosine analogs and electromagnetic fields inhibit prostaglandin E2 release in bovine synovial fibroblasts. *Osteoarthritis and Cartilage*, 17(2), pp. 252–262.

De Mattei, M. et al., 2001. Effects of pulsed electromagnetic fields on human articular chondrocyte proliferation. *Connective Tissue Research*, 42(4), pp. 269–279.

Mattsson, M.-O. & Simkó, M., 2014. Grouping of experimental conditions as an approach to evaluate effects of extremely low-frequency magnetic fields on oxidative response in in vitro studies. *Frontiers in Public Health*, 2(September), p. 132.

Mattsson, M.-O. et al., 2001. [Ca^{2+}]i rise in jurkat e6-1 cell lines from different sources as a response to 50hz magnetic field exposure is a reproducible effect and independent of poly- l-lysine treatment. *Cell Biology International*, 25(9), pp. 901–907.

Matzinger, P., 1994. Tolerance, danger, and the extended family. *Annual Review of Immunology*, 12, pp. 991–1045.

Matzinger, P., 2002. The danger model: a renewed sense of self. *Science*, 296(2002), pp. 301–305.

Mayer-Wagner, S. et al., 2010. Effects of low frequency electromagnetic fields on the chondrogenic differentiation of human mesenchymal stem cells. *Bioelectromagnetics*, 290, pp. 283–290.

McCreary, C.R., Thomas, A.W. & Prato, F.S., 2002. Factors confounding cytosolic calcium measurements in Jurkat E6.1 cells during exposure to ELF magnetic fields. *Bioelectromagnetics*, 23(4), pp. 315–328.

Miousse, I.R. et al., 2015. Response of transposable elements to environmental stressors. *Mutation Research - Reviews in Mutation Research*, 765, pp. 19–39.

Mo, W.C. et al., 2013. Magnetic shielding accelerates the proliferation of human neuroblastoma cell by promoting G1-phase progression K. Roemer, ed. *PLoS ONE*, 8(1), p. e54775. Available at: http://dx.plos.org/10.1371/journal.pone.0054775.

Morehouse, C.A. & Owen, R.D., 2000. Exposure to low-frequency electromagnetic fields does not alter HSP70 expression or HSF-HSE binding in HL60 cells. *Radiation Research*, 153(5 Pt 2), pp. 658–662.

Morgado-Valle, C. et al., 1998. The role of voltage-gated Ca^{2+} channels in neurite growth of cultured chromaffin cells induced by extremely low frequency (ELF) magnetic field stimulation. *Cell & Tissue Research*, 291(2), pp. 217–230.

Mosser, D.M. & Edwards, J.P., 2008. Exploring the full spectrum of macrophage activation. *Nature Reviews Immunology*, 8(12), pp. 958–969.

Naarala, J. et al., 2017. Direction-dependent effects of combined static and ELF magnetic fields on cell proliferation and superoxide radical production. *BioMed Research International*, 2017, p. 5675086.

Nakamichi, N. et al., 2009. Possible promotion of neuronal differentiation in fetal rat brain neural progenitor cells after sustained exposure to static magnetism. *Journal of Neuroscience Research*, 87(11), pp. 2406–2417.

Nakasono, S. & Saiki, H., 2000. Effect of ELF magnetic fields on protein synthesis in Escherichia coli K12. *Radiation Research*, 154(2), pp. 208–216.

Noda, Y. et al., 2000. Magnetic fields and lipoic acid influence the respiratory burst in activated rat peritoneal neutrophils. *Pathophysiology*, 7, pp. 137–141.

Nourshargh, S., Hordijk, P.L. & Sixt, M., 2010. Breaching multiple barriers: leukocyte motility through venular walls and the interstitium. *Nature Reviews. Molecular Cell Biology*, 11(5), pp. 366–378.

Ochaion, A. et al., 2008. The A3 adenosine receptor agonist CF502 inhibits the PI3K, PKB/Akt and NF-κB signaling pathway in synoviocytes from rheumatoid arthritis patients and in adjuvant-induced arthritis rats. *Biochemical Pharmacology*, 76(4), pp. 482–494.

Ongaro, A. et al., 2012. Electromagnetic fields (EMFs) and adenosine receptors modulate prostaglandin E 2 and cytokine release in human osteoarthritic synovial fibroblasts. *Journal of Cellular Physiology*, 227(6), pp. 2461–2469.

Onodera, H. et al., 2003. Effects of 10-T static magnetic field on human peripheral blood immune cells. *Radiation Research*, 159(6), pp. 775–779.

Parekh, A.B. & Putney Jr, J.W., 2005. Store-operated calcium channels. *Physiological Reviews*, 85(2), pp. 757–810.

Parham, F. et al., 2016. The use of signal-transduction and metabolic pathways to predict human disease targets from electric and magnetic fields using in vitro data in human cell lines. *Front Public Health*, 4, p. 193.

Park, J.-E. et al., 2013. Electromagnetic fields induce neural differentiation of human bone marrow derived mesenchymal stem cells via ROS mediated EGFR activation. *Neurochemistry
International*, 62(4), pp. 418–424.

Parker, H. et al., 2012. Requirements for NADPH oxidase and myeloperoxidase in neutrophil extracellular trap formation differ depending on the stimulus. *Journal of Leukocyte Biology*, 92(4),
pp. 841–849.

Patruno, A. et al., 2010. Extremely low frequency electromagnetic fields modulate expression of
inducible nitric oxide synthase, endothelial nitric oxide synthase and cyclooxygenase-2 in the
human keratinocyte cell line HaCat: potential therapeutic effects in wound healing. *British
Journal of Dermatology*, 162(2), pp. 258–266.

Patruno, A. et al., 2015. MTOR activation by PI3K/Akt and ERK signaling in short ELF-EMF exposed
human keratinocytes. *PLoS ONE*, 10(10), pp. 1–15.

Pawłowska-Góral, K. et al., 2016. Effect of static magnetic fields and phloretin on antioxidant
defense system of human fibroblasts. *Environmental Science and Pollution Research*, 23(15),
pp. 14989–14996.

Pei, D. et al., 2010. Induced pluripotent stem cell technology in regenerative medicine and biology.
Advances in Biochemical Engineering/Biotechnology, 123, pp. 127–141.

Pessina, G.P. & Aldinucci, C., 1998. Pulsed electromagnetic fields enhance the induction of
cytokines by peripheral blood mononuclear cells challenged with phytohemagglutinin.
Bioelectromagnetics, 19(8), pp. 445–451.

Piacentini, R. et al., 2008. Extremely low-frequency electromagnetic fields promote in vitro neurogenesis via upregulation of Cav1-channel activity. *Journal of Cellular Physiology*, 215(1), pp. 129–139.

Poniedziałek, B. et al., 2013. Reactive oxygen species (ROS) production in human peripheral blood
neutrophils exposed *in vitro* to static magnetic field. *Electromagnetic Biology and Medicine*, 32(4),
pp. 560–568.

Pooam, M. et al., 2017. Effect of 50-Hz sinusoidal magnetic field on the production of superoxide
anion and the expression of heat-shock protein 70 in RAW264 cells. *International Journal of
Chemistry*, 9(2), p. 23.

Prasad, A. et al., 2017. Static magnetic field stimulation enhances oligodendrocyte differentiation
and secretion of neurotrophic factors. *Scientific Reports*, 7(1), p. 6743.

Radons, J., 2016. The human HSP70 family of chaperones: where do we stand? *Cell Stress and
Chaperones*, 21(3), pp. 379–404.

Raylman, R.R., Clavo, A.C. & Wahl, R.L., 1996. Exposure to strong static magnetic field slows the
growth of human cancer cells in vitro. *Bioelectromagnetics*, 17, pp. 358–363.

Del Re, B. et al., 2006. Synthesis of DnaK and GroEL in Escherichia coli cells exposed to different
magnetic field signals. *Bioelectrochemistry (Amsterdam, Netherlands)*, 69(1), pp. 99–103.

Reale, M. et al., 2014. Neuronal cellular responses to extremely low frequency electromagnetic field
exposure: implications regarding oxidative stress and neurodegeneration. *PLoS ONE*, 9(8),
p. e104973. doi:10.1371/journal.pone.0104973.

Reeves, E.P. et al., 2002. Killing activity of neutrophils is mediated through activation of proteases
by K+ flux. *Nature*, 416(6878), pp. 291–297.

Reik, W., 2007. Stability and flexibility of epigenetic gene regulation in mammalian development.
Nature, 447(7143), pp. 425–432.

Rezaie-Tavirani, M. et al., 2017. Proteomic analysis of the effect of extremely low-frequency electromagnetic fields (ELF-EMF) with different intensities in SH-SY5Y Neuroblastoma cell line.
Journal of Lasers in Medical Sciences, 8(2), pp. 79–83.

Roderick, H.L. & Cook, S.J., 2008. Ca^{2+} signalling checkpoints in cancer: remodelling Ca^{2+} for cancer
cell proliferation and survival. *Nature Reviews Cancer*, 8(5), pp. 361–375.

Romeo, S. et al., 2016. Lack of effects on key cellular parameters of MRC-5 human lung fibroblasts
exposed to 370 mT static magnetic field. *Scientific Reports*, 6, p. 19398.

Rosen, A.D. & Chastney, E.E., 2009. Effect of long term exposure to 0.5 T static magnetic fields on
growth and size of GH3 cells. *Bioelectromagnetics*, 30(2), pp. 114–119.

Ross, C.L. et al., 2015. The effect of low-frequency electromagnetic field on human bone marrow stem/progenitor cell differentiation. *Stem Cell Research*, 15(1), pp. 96–108.

Salehi, H. et al., 2016. An overview of neural differentiation potential of human adipose derived stem cells. *Stem Cell Reviews and Reports*, 12(1), pp. 26–41.

Salehi, I., Sani, K.G. & Zamani, A., 2013. Exposure of rats to extremely low-frequency electromagnetic fields (ELF-EMF) alters cytokines production. *Electromagnetic Biology and Medicine*, 32(1), pp. 1–8.

Salerno, S. et al., 1999. Static magnetic fields generated by a 0.5 T MRI unit affects in vitro expression of activation markers and interleukin release in human peripheral blood mononuclear cells (PBMC). *International Journal of Radiation Biology*, 75(4), pp. 457–463.

Salerno, S. et al., 2006. Reversible effect of MR and ELF magnetic fields (0.5 T and 0.5 mT) on human lymphocyte activation patterns. *International Journal of Radiation Biology*, 82(2), pp. 77–85. Available at: www.ncbi.nlm.nih.gov/pubmed/16546906.

Salerno, S. et al., 2009. Reversible effect of magnetic fields on human lymphocyte activation patterns: different sensitivity of naive and memory lymphocyte subsets. *Radiation Research*, 450(4), pp. 444–450.

Salimi, M. et al., 2013. Effect of extremely low-frequency (50 hz) field on proliferation rate of human adipose-derived mesenchymal stem cells. *Journal of Isfahan Medical School*, 31(232), pp. 1–17.

Santo-Domingo, J., 2015. Modulation of the matrix redox signaling by mitochondrial Ca^{2+}. *World Journal of Biological Chemistry*, 6(4), p. 310.

Schmitt, E. et al., 2006. Intracellular and extracellular functions of heat shock proteins: repercussions in cancer therapy. *Journal of Leukocyte Biology*, 81(1), pp. 15–27.

Seong, Y., Moon, J. & Kim, J., 2014. Egr1 mediated the neuronal differentiation induced by extremely low-frequency electromagnetic fields. *Life Sciences*, 102(1), pp. 16–27.

Shen, L.-K. et al., 2014. A static magnetic field attenuates lipopolysaccharide-induced neuro-inflammatory response via IL-6-mediated pathway. *Electromagnetic Biology and Medicine*, 33(2), pp. 132–138.

Shi, B. et al., 2003. Power-line frequency electromagnetic fields do not induce changes in phosphory-lation, localization, or expression of the 27-kilodalton heat shock protein in human keratino-cytes. *Environmental Health Perspectives*, 111(3), pp. 281–288.

Simko, M., 2007. Cell type specific redox status is responsible for diverse electromagnetic field effects. *Current Medicinal Chemistry*, 14, pp. 1141–1152. Available at: www.ingentaconnect.com/content/ben/cmc/2007/00000014/00000010/art00008.

Simkó, M. & Mattsson, M.-O., 2004. Extremely low frequency electromagnetic fields as effectors of cellular responses in vitro: possible immune cell activation. *Journal of Cellular Biochemistry*, 93(1), pp. 83–92. Available at: www.ncbi.nlm.nih.gov/pubmed/15352165.

Sinclair, J. et al., 2006. Proteomic response of Schizosaccharomyces pombe to static and oscillating extremely low-frequency electromagnetic fields. *Proteomics*, 6(17), pp. 4755–4764.

Song, E. et al., 2000. Influence of alternatively and classically activated macrophages on fibrogenic activities of human fibroblasts. *Cellular Immunology*, 204(1), pp. 19–28.

Stankiewicz, A.R. et al., 2005. Hsp70 inhibits heat-induced apoptosis upstream of mitochondria by preventing Bax translocation. *Journal of Biological Chemistry*, 280(46), pp. 38729–38739.

Still, M., 2002. Inability of 50Hz magnetic fields to regulate Pkc- and Ca^{2+}-dependent gene expression in Jurkat cells. *Cell Biology International*, 26(2), pp. 203–209.

Strehler, E.E. & Treiman, M., 2004. Calcium pumps of plasma membrane and cell interior. *Current Molecular Medicine*, 4(June), pp. 323–335.

Strelczyk, D. et al., 2009. Static magnetic fields impair angiogenesis and growth of solid tumors in vivo. *Cancer Biology & Therapy*, 8(18), pp. 1756–1762.

Stuart, J.R. et al., 2005. c-Abl regulates early growth response protein (EGR1) in response to oxidative stress. *Oncogene*, 24(55), pp. 8085–8092.

Surma, S.V. et al., 2014. Effect of weak static magnetic fields on the development of cultured skeletal muscle cells. *Bioelectromagnetics*, 35(8), pp. 537–546.

Synowiec-Wojtarowicz, A. et al., 2017. Influence of static magnetic fields up to 700 mT and dihydrochalcones on the antioxidant response in fibroblasts. *Journal of Environmental Science and Health, Part A*, 52(4), pp. 385–390.

Takahashi, K. et al., 2007. Induction of pluripotent stem cells from fibroblast cultures. *Nature Protocols*, 2(12), pp. 3081–3089.

Tamrin, S.H. et al., 2016. Electromagnetic fields and stem cell fate: when physics meets biology. *Reviews of Physiology Biochemistry and Pharmacology*, 171, pp. 63–97.

Tenuzzo, B., Vergallo, C. & Dini, L., 2009. Effect of 6mT static magnetic field on the bcl-2, bax, p53 and hsp70 expression in freshly isolated and in vitro aged human lymphocytes. *Tissue & Cell*, 41(3), pp. 169–179.

Tokalov, S.V. & Gutzeit, H.O., 2004. Weak electromagnetic fields (50 Hz) elicit a stress response in human cells. *Environmental Research*, 94(2), pp. 145–151.

Tsai, M.-T. et al., 2009. Modulation of osteogenesis in human mesenchymal stem cells by specific pulsed electromagnetic field stimulation. *Journal of Orthopaedic Research : Official Publication of the Orthopaedic Research Society*, 27(9), pp. 1169–1174.

Valberg, P.A., Kavet, R. & Rafferty, C.N., 1997. Can low-level 50/60 Hz electric and magnetic fields cause biological effects? *Radiation Research*, 148(1), p. 2.

Varani, K. et al., 2002. Effect of low frequency electromagnetic fields on A2A adenosine receptors in human neutrophils. *British Journal of Pharmacology*, 136(1), pp. 57–66.

Varani, K. et al., 2017. Adenosine receptors as a biological pathway for the anti-inflammatory and beneficial effects of low frequency low energy pulsed electromagnetic fields. *Mediators of Inflammation*, 2017, p. 2740963.

Vergallo, C. et al., 2013. In vitro analysis of the anti-inflammatory effect of inhomogeneous static magnetic field-exposure on human macrophages and lymphocytes. *PLoS ONE*, 8(8), p. e72374. doi:10.1371/journal.pone.0072374.

Vijayalaxmi & Obe, G., 2005. Controversial cytogenetic observations in mammalian somatic cells exposed to extremely low frequency electromagnetic radiation: a review and future research recommendations. *Bioelectromagnetics*, 26(5), pp. 412–430.

Vincenzi, F. et al., 2013. A2A adenosine receptors are differentially modulated by pharmacological treatments in rheumatoid arthritis patients and their stimulation ameliorates adjuvant-induced arthritis in rats. *PLoS ONE*, 8(1).

Walleczek, J. & Budinger, T.F., 1992. Pulsed magnetic field effects on calcium signaling in lymphocytes: dependence on cell status and field intensity. *FEBS Letters*, 314(3), pp. 351–355.

Wang, J. et al., 2016. Inhibition of viability, proliferation, cytokines secretion, surface antigen expression, and adipogenic and osteogenic differentiation of adipose-derived stem cells by seven-day exposure to 0.5 T static magnetic fields. *Stem Cells International*, 2016, p. 12. doi:10.1155/2016/7168175.

Wang, Z. et al., 2009. Moderate strength (0.23–0.28 T) static magnetic fields (SMF) modulate signaling and differentiation in human embryonic cells. *BMC genomics*, 10, p. 356.

Wei, J. et al., 2015. Effects of extremely low frequency electromagnetic fields on intracellular calcium transients in cardiomyocytes. *Electromagnetic Biology and Medicine*, 34(1), pp. 77–84.

Wei, J. et al., 2016. EMF protects cardiomyocytes against hypoxia-induced injury via heat shock protein 70 activation. *Chemico-Biological Interactions*, 248, pp. 8–17.

Wócik-Piotrowicz, K. et al., 2014. Influence of static and alternating magnetic fields on U937 cell viability. *Folia medica Cracoviensia*, 54(4), pp. 21–33.

Ben Yakir-Blumkin, M. et al., 2014. Neuroprotective effect of weak static magnetic fields in primary neuronal cultures. *Neuroscience*, 278, pp. 313–326.

Yan, J.-L. et al., 2015. Pulsed electromagnetic fields promote osteoblast mineralization and maturation needing the existence of primary cilia. *Molecular and Cellular Endocrinology*, 404, pp. 132–140.

Yang, X. et al., 2012. Hsp70 promotes chemoresistance by blocking Bax mitochondrial translocation in ovarian cancer cells. *Cancer Letters*, 321(2), pp. 137–143.

Yong, Y. et al., 2016. Electromagnetic fields promote osteogenesis of rat mesenchymal stem cells through the PKA and ERK1/2 pathways. *Journal of Tissue Engineering and Regenerative Medicine*, 10(10), pp. E537–E545.

Zeng, Y. et al., 2017. Effects of single and repeated exposure to a 50-Hz 2-mT electromagnetic field on primary cultured hippocampal neurons. *Neuroscience Bulletin*, 33(3), pp. 299–306.

Zhang, L. et al., 2016. Moderate and strong static magnetic fields directly affect EGFR kinase domain orientation to inhibit cancer cell proliferation. *Oncotarget*, 7(27), pp. 41527–41539.

Zhang, L. et al., 2017. Cell type- and density-dependent effect of 1 T static magnetic field on cell proliferation. *Oncotarget*, 8(8), pp. 13126–13141.

Zhang, Z.-Y. et al., 2016. Coupling mechanism of electromagnetic field and thermal stress on drosophila melanogaster. *PLoS ONE*, 11(9), p. e0162675.

Zhao, G. et al., 2011. Cellular ATP content was decreased by a homogeneous 8.5 T static magnetic field exposure: role of reactive oxygen species. *Bioelectromagnetics*, 32(2), pp. 94–101.

Zwirska-Korczala, K. et al., 2005. Effect of extremely low frequency electromagnetic fields on cell proliferation, antioxidative enzyme activities and lipid peroxidation in 3T3-L1 preadipocytes - an in vitro study. *Journal of Physiology and Pharmacology*, 56(Suppl. 6), pp. 101–108.

2

Cellular Effects of Radio Frequency, Millimeter, and Terahertz Waves

Junji Miyakoshi
Kyoto University

CONTENTS

2.1 Introduction

From the end of the twentieth century to the present century, our living environment became more densely filled with electromagnetic waves. The main cause of this phenomenon has been the rapid development of cell phones and wireless LANs, along with the establishment of mobile phone base stations worldwide. Furthermore, acceleration of communication technologies and rapid spread of wireless power supplies (wireless energy transmission) by radio waves are anticipated in the coming years. Consequently, in the society of the near future, in addition to static magnetic fields (SMFs), extremely low-frequency waves (ELFWs), and radio frequency waves (RFWs), a wide variety of electromagnetic changes will occur in our environment in the regions of intermediate-frequency waves (IFWs), millimeter waves (MMWs), and terahertz waves (THWs). As in the case of ionizing radiation (IR), the electromagnetic environment is invisible, and many people are concerned about the influence of electromagnetic waves on health. The history of full-scale research on this topic is very shallow in comparison to the literature on health effects of IR. Here, we focus on cellular research on the biological effects of high-frequency electromagnetic waves, and summarize the results of published research, mainly in regard to RFWs. We also describe reports of research on the cellular effects of MMWs and THWs, which have received increasing attention in recent years. In order to classify the frequency range of these electromagnetic waves in a simple manner, RFWs are defined as several hundred MHz to 10 GHz, MMWs as 10–100 GHz, and THWs as 100 GHz (0.1 THz) or more.

2.2 Positioning of Cellular Research and Its Evaluation Index

The main approaches for assessing safety are (1) human epidemiological studies and volunteer research, (2) animal studies, and (3) cellular studies. It is impossible to decide which research subject (i.e., humans, animals, or cells) is superior to the others. In general, however, when evaluating the influence on humans, epidemiological studies should be given the greatest weight, followed by animal studies and cellular studies in that order. On the other hand, cellular studies are the most accurate and reproducible, followed by animal and epidemiological studies in that order. Epidemiological studies take the longest, followed by animal and cellular studies. In recent years, research in the field of molecular biology has progressed markedly, and studies targeting DNA and genes are developing rapidly. Consequently, the weight of cellular studies is greater than it once was.

Evaluation of the influence of RFW using cells is progressing according to multiple experimental criteria (Miyakoshi, 2006; 2009; 2013). Table 2.1 summarizes the main criteria for cellular experiments, which can be classified as genotoxic or nongenotoxic studies. Genotoxic studies include assays of micronucleus (MN) formation, chromosomal aberration (CA), primary DNA damage assessed using alkaline and neutral comet assays, sister chromatid exchange, and mutation. Nongenotoxic studies include measurements of cell proliferation and cell-cycle distribution, gene expression (mRNA and protein), the

TABLE 2.1

Experimental Criteria for Evaluation of the Cellular Effects of Electromagnetic Fields

Research Category	Evaluation Criteria
Genotoxic study	Micronucleus formation, chromosomal aberration, sister chromatid exchange, primary DNA damage assessed using alkaline and neutral comet assays, mutation, transformation, DNA migration
Nongenotoxic study	Cell proliferation, cell-cycle distribution, DNA synthesis, gene expression, transcriptomics (microarray analysis), signal transduction, ion channels, cell differentiation, apoptosis, immune system, reactive oxygen species, Alzheimer's disease, gap junction intercellular communication, endoplasmic reticulum

immune system, transcriptomics (microarray analysis), apoptosis, and reactive oxygen species (ROS).

2.3 Cellular Studies

2.3.1 Radio Frequency Waves

2.3.1.1 Genotoxic Studies

2.3.1.1.1 MN Formation

In the case of DNA damage or cell division, if an abnormality occurs during chromosome separation, a MN separated from the nucleus may be formed. The MN test, in which these structures are observed under a microscope, is frequently used to study genotoxicity following exposure to electromagnetic waves. Because MN formation rarely occurs spontaneously, it is useful as an indicator of genotoxicity. In addition, it has recently been proposed to be associated with cancer and consequently has attracted attention as an important experimental method (Crasta et al., 2012).

Multiple studies have reported no effect on MN formation in cells exposed to RFWs at a specific absorption rate (SAR) of 10 W/kg or less (Bisht et al., 2002; McNamee et al., 2002). In addition, many recent studies reported that exposure to RFWs in the 900–2450 MHz band has no effect on cells (Speit et al., 2007; Sannino et al., 2009; Vijayalaxmi et al., 2013). Even when cells were exposed to 2.45 GHz RFWs at 50 W/kg or less, the MN formation frequency did not differ from that in controls (Koyama et al., 2003; 2004). When the SAR was 78 W/kg or more, the frequency of MN formation increased in comparison with controls, but was almost the same as the frequency due to the temperature increase under this condition. Therefore, MN formation is thought to occur as a result of thermal effects accompanying rising temperature. On the other hand, some previous studies reported that the frequency of MN formation increased with low SAR (Garaj-Vrhovac et al., 1992), and Schwarz et al. (2008) reported that exposure to 1950 MHz RFWs at 0.05–0.1 W/kg increased the MN frequency in fibroblasts. However, at the same time, Schwarz et al. (2008) also published results showing that lymphocytes do not exhibit any change in the MN formation. Therefore, further research is required. Although many studies have reported that low SAR has no effect on MN formation, combined exposure to RFWs and X-rays decreases MN formation due to an adaptive response to RFW exposure following irradiation with X-rays (Sannino et al., 2014). Cao et al. (2009) showed that an amplification effect is observed upon combined exposure to IR and RFW. Thus, it is possible that some biological effects are not seen with RFW alone. It is unlikely that the output energy used in mobile phones will have an immediate effect on health, but considering the results of combined exposure, it is undeniable that these waves have some biological effect.

2.3.1.1.2 Chromosomal Aberrations

Cleavage of DNA strands by IR is well known to result in formation of CAs, and accordingly CAs have been used for many years as typical indicators of genotoxicity. CAs can occur naturally in cultured cells, but only very rarely.

In a CA assay, the observer identifies CAs and chromatid aberrations such as *ctg* (chromatid gap), *ctb* (chromatid cleavage), *cte* (chromatid exchange), *frag* (fragmentation), *min* (minute chromosome), and *dic* (dicentric under a microscope). An early study (Garaj-Vrhovac et al., 1991) reported that RFW exposure affects CAs. In recent years, one study reported that exposure of leukocytes to RFWs had some positive effects (Mazor et al., 2008), whereas other studies reported no positive results (Mashevich et al., 2003; Stronati et al., 2006; Bourthoumieu et al., 2010). RFW exposure at 2.45 GHz for 2 h did not induce CAs, even at CW exposure levels of 5–100 W/kg and PW exposure at a peak power of 900 W/kg (an average SAR of 100 W/kg) (Komatsubara et al., 2005).

It is reported that RFWs have no effect on chromatid aberration (Maes et al., 2001). Antonopoulos et al. (1997) investigated the effects of RFWs on human lymphocytes *in vitro*. Specifically, human peripheral lymphocytes were incubated in the presence of RFWs of 380, 900, and 1800 MHz. The measured endpoints were cell-cycle progression and the frequencies of sister-chromatid exchanges. No differences between treated and control cultures were observed.

In many experiments, formation of MN and CA were monitored in parallel. Many studies reported no influence on either endpoint. It is important to note, however, that some positive reactions were observed. Since these tests also require skilled observation, it is necessary to find a way to detect effects more easily.

2.3.1.1.3 DNA Strand Breaks (Comet Assay)

DNA strand breaks indicate whether DNA strands have been destroyed directly due to toxicity to cells, and the comet assay method is often used to assess genotoxicity. As an example of positive results, RFW exposure of MOLT-4 lymphoblasts resulted in DNA strand breaks (Phillips et al., 1998), and RFW exposure from cellular phones caused single-strand DNA breakage (Çam and Seyhan, 2012). In particular, Diem et al. (2005) reported a significant influence of intermittent exposure, not mediated by thermal effects, as follows. Cultured human diploid fibroblasts and cultured rat granulosa cells were exposed to intermittent and continuous RFWs used in mobile phones, with different SAR and mobile phone modulations. RFW exposure (1800 MHz; SAR 1.2 or 2 W/kg; different modulations; duration of 4, 16, and 24 h; intermittent 5 min on/10 min off or continuous wave) induced DNA single- and double-strand breaks, and the intermittent exposure had a stronger effect than continuous exposure.

When cells are exposed to combined treatment with RFWs and mitomycin C (MMC), an alkylating agent for DNA, DNA stand breaks occur more frequently than when RFWs are applied alone (Zhang et al., 2002). Although some papers have reported that DNA strand breaks are induced by RFW exposure, many others report no such effect (Miyakoshi et al., 2002; Tice et al., 2002; Lagroye et al., 2004). In general, this is consistent with the idea that RFW exposure does not directly sever DNA strands. Accordingly, there is a consensus that DNA strands are not broken by RFW exposure.

2.3.1.1.4 Mutation

Mutation is a genotoxic effect that cannot be detected by experimental methods designed to assess MN formation, CAs, or DNA strand breaks. Human cells harbor approximately 30,000 genes. Because the number of whole genes is very large, it is difficult to investigate mutations in all genes. A single gene is composed of several thousands to tens of thousands of bases, and it is difficult to find a mutation in sequences of this size. Therefore, instead of searching for any mutation, a method has been established that focuses on a specific gene, used as a marker, and determines whether the gene has undergone a mutation. If the frequency of this specific mutation rises following exposure to a chemical substance or physical phenomenon, it can be inferred that mutations will also occur in other genes. When a mutation occurs in a gene on a DNA strand, it may affect the gene function, potentially exerting fatal effects on the cell.

Although a few experiments have examined the influence of RFW exposure on mutation, to date most studies have reported no effect (Meltz et al., 1990; Koyama et al., 2007). However, because the body of literature is small, it is difficult to reach an unequivocal conclusion. Therefore, further research is necessary.

2.3.1.2 Nongenotoxic Studies

2.3.1.2.1 Cell Proliferation and Cell-Cycle Distribution

Proliferation is a fundamental dynamic feature of cells, and an important endpoint to evaluation in experiments. Under normal culture conditions, the proliferation rate is almost constant for each cell. However, changes in the cell-cycle distribution or the speed of DNA synthesis will affect cell proliferation. Multiple studies have reported that RFW exposure alters the proliferation rate, resulting in a change in the cell-cycle distribution (Velizarov et al., 1999; Marinelli et al., 2004).

On the other hand, multiple studies have reported that RFW exposure has no effect on cell proliferation or cell-cycle distribution (Pacini et al., 2002; Gurisik et al., 2006; Sanchez et al., 2006). As the SAR of RFWs increases, temperature also increases. Consequently, some apparent effects of RFWs described in the following study can be attributed to heat.

Fundamental cellular responses such as cell growth, survival, and cell-cycle distribution were examined following RFW exposure at a wide range of SAR values. When cells were exposed a continuous RFW at an SAR of 0.05–100 W/kg for 2 h, growth rate, survival, and cell-cycle distribution were not affected. At 200 W/kg, the growth rate was suppressed, and cell survival decreased. Exposure to RFWs resulted in heating of the medium, and the magnitude of the thermal effect depends on the mean SAR. Therefore, these results suggest that decrease in proliferation was caused by thermal effect (Takashima et al., 2006).

Even in studies reporting positive effects, it is thought that issues related to the environment of the RFW system and temperature control cannot be completely eliminated. Consequently, the effect of RFWs on cell proliferation is not supported by clear evidence.

2.3.1.2.2 Apoptosis

Apoptosis, also called programmed cell death, is a defense mechanism that removes damaged cells, thereby maintaining the tissue, organ, or body in homeostasis. Cell death that occurs as a result of serious damage or being placed in an unfavorable cellular environment is called necrosis, which is distinct from apoptosis. Apoptosis, which occurs in response to DNA damage following exposure to chemical substances and IR, is a consequence of signal transduction via p53 or caspase-3. Two reports showed that RFW exposure has little effect on apoptosis (Hirose et al., 2006; Palumbo et al., 2008). However, several recent papers have reported that RFW exposure increases apoptosis due to reactive oxygen species mediated by caspase-3, as described below (Liu et al., 2012; Çiğ and Nazıroğlu, 2015). Although there is no consensus regarding the effects of RFW exposure on apoptosis, recent positive results are noteworthy and should be explored in future work.

2.3.1.2.3 Gene Expression

Gene expression is a metabolic process in a cell in which the DNA sequence (genetic information) is transcribed into mRNA, and ultimately translated into protein. Research on the effect of RFW exposure on gene expression has focused on heat shock proteins (HSPs). Generally, increased expression of HSPs, including HSP70 and HSP27, is seen as a stress reaction to heat and cytotoxic chemical substances. The effect of RFW exposure on HSP has been investigated by various laboratories, and it has been observed that HSP expression is increased by the temperature rise due to high SARs of 20 W/kg or more. Another study investigated whether exposure to 2450 MHz RFWs could act as an environmental insult and evoke a stress response in A172 cells, using HSP70 and HSP27 as stress markers. The cells were exposed to 2450 MHz RFWs with a wide range of SAR values (5–200 W/kg) or sham conditions. Expression of HSP70 increased in a time- and dose-dependent manner at >50 W/kg SAR for 1–3 h. A similar effect was also observed in the corresponding heat controls. There was no significant change in HSP27 expression following exposure to RFWs at 5–200 W/kg or comparable heating for 1–3 h (Wang et al., 2006).

Several studies have reported that HSP expression increases in response to a so-called nonthermal effect of RFW exposure with low SAR not accompanied by a temperature rise (Leszczynski et al., 2002; Miyakoshi et al., 2005; Sanchez et al., 2006). Furthermore, some reports (Leszczynski et al., 2002; Buttiglione et al., 2007) showed that the increase in HSP affects signal transduction. One study (Calabrò et al., 2012) reported an increase in HSP20 and HSP70 expression with no change in survival rate, HSP27 expression, or caspase-3 activation. In many other studies, however, RFW exposure did not increase HSP expression (Cotgreave, 2005; Simkó et al., 2006; Hirose et al., 2007). The exposure system, cell type, frequency, SAR, exposure time, etc. differed considerably among these papers. Therefore, it is difficult to reach a deterministic conclusion. Gene expression experiments are valuable in studies of the cellular influences of RFW exposure, and future studies should address the reproducibility of these measurements.

A study was performed focusing on oncogenes, such as c-*myc*, c-*fos*, and c-*jun*, which react initially during cell proliferation. Expression of c-*fos* and c-*jun* after RFW exposure was monitored by northern blotting as follows (Ivaschuk et al., 1997). Rat PC12 pheochromocytoma cells were treated with nerve growth factor, and then exposed to athermal levels of packet-modulated RFW at 836.55 MHz. Exposures were for 20, 40, and 60 min, and included an intermittent exposure regimen (20 min on/20 min off). No change in c-*fos* transcript levels was detected after 20 min exposure at each field intensity (20 min was the only time period at which c-*fos* mRNA could be detected consistently). Transcript levels for c-*jun* were altered only after a 20 min exposure to RFWs at 9 mW/cm^2 (average decrease of 38%). mRNA expression of c-*jun* was reduced, but returned to control levels after longer exposure. These results suggest that RFW exposure temporarily inhibits c-*jun* gene expression. However, Goswami et al. (1999) observed no change in the expression of c-*myc*, c-*fos*, and c-*jun* after RFW exposure of C3H 10T 1/2 cells, as determined by reverse transcription polymerase chain reaction (RT-PCR), although c-*fos* mRNA levels increased in cells exposed to frequency-modulated continuous wave (FMCW) and code division multiple access (CDMA). On the other hand, several reports showed RFW exposure does not affect HSP27, HSP70, FOS, JUN, or MYC protein level (Chauhan et al., 2006). Overall, at present, the results regarding the effect of RFW exposure on gene expression are not consistent, and future research should continue to address this issue.

2.3.1.2.4 *Transcriptomics (Microarray Analysis)*

Complete sequencing of the human genome and the dramatic development of methods such as microarray analysis made it possible to comprehensively examine the expression level of mRNA. The effects of RFW exposure have also been investigated by this method, although in current microarray analyses, it is sometimes difficult to accurately identify responsive genes due to the possibility of false positive detection; consequently, candidates must be confirmed by RT-PCR.

Intermittent RFW exposure affects gene expression including various cellular functions (cytoskeleton, signal transduction, and metabolism) (Zhao et al., 2007). Several studies have also reported on gene expression following RFW exposure in various cell types (Nylund and Leszczynski, 2006) and shown that the expression of genes encoding ribosomal proteins differs according to cell type (Remondini et al., 2006). On the other hand, no effect on gene expression following RFW exposure can be detected by microarray analysis (Hirose et al., 2006). Sakurai et al. (2011) used microarrays to examine the effects of exposure to RFWs (2.45 GHz, continuous wave) at SARs of 1, 5, and 10 W/kg for 1, 4, or 24 h on gene expression in the normal human glial cell line SVGp12. Their analysis revealed 23 assigned gene spots and 5 nonassigned gene spots as potentially altered. To validate the microarray results, 22 out of the 23 identified gene spots were analyzed by RT-PCR in order but no significant alterations in gene expression were observed.

These reports indicate that it will remain difficult to detect the effect of RFW exposure by microarray analysis unless the analytical method can be improved by further technical innovation. Based on other research results, it is very likely that even if there is a biological effect of RFW exposure, it is very minute; consequently, the technical accuracy is so far insufficient for exhaustive analysis. Thus, this method may not be optimal. In recent years, technological innovations aimed at comprehensive gene expression have advanced, and new research results are anticipated.

2.3.1.2.5 *Immune System*

The immune system protects the host from infection and cancer. When bacteria or other microorganisms intrude into the body, immune cells attack them in self-defense. This system also produces substances involved in self-defense, such as cytokines. Immune cells play very important roles, and accordingly the effect of RFW exposure on immune cells has been studied extensively. One study reported that pulse RFW affects leukocyte immune activity (Dabrowski et al., 2003), and another study showed that mitogenic factors and immunogenic activities are enhanced by RFW exposure (Stankiewicz et al., 2006).

On the other hand, Tuschl et al. (2006) reported negative results as follows. Their study aimed at investigating whether global system for mobile communications (GSM)-modulated RFWs have adverse effects on the functional competence of human immune cells. Exposure was performed at GSM signal with basic 1950 MHz at an SAR of 1 mW/g in an intermittent mode (5 min on/10 min off), with a maximum ΔT of 0.06°C, for a duration of 8 h. Exposure had no statistically significant effects on production of interleukin 2 (IL-2), interferon γ (INF-γ) IL-1, or tumor necrosis factor α (TNF-α), and there is no indication that emissions from mobile phones are associated with adverse effects on the human immune system.

Another study reported that there was no change in immune-related TNF-α or interleukin levels as a result of RFW exposure in microglial cells (Hirose et al., 2010). A similar result was obtained by another group (Thorlin et al., 2006). Furthermore, Koyama et al. (2015) reported that immune function is not affected by RFW exposure. They examined the effect of 2.45 GHz RFW at SARs of 2 and 10 W/kg for 4 or 24 h on neutrophil chemotaxis and phagocytosis in differentiated human HL-60 cells. Neutrophil chemotaxis was not affected by RFW exposure, nor was subsequent phagocytosis, in comparison with sham exposure conditions. Based on these results, the currently available evidence is not sufficient to draw conclusions about the response of the immune function to RFW exposure. Further research is needed.

2.3.1.2.6 Reactive Oxygen Species

Stress caused by aging, exercise, ultraviolet, and other causes increases the production of ROS in the body. ROS include oxygen ions, radicals, and organic and inorganic peroxides; in general usage, the term refers to four types of oxygen molecules: superoxide anion radical, hydroxyl radical, hydrogen peroxide, and singlet oxygen. Intracellular DNA and lipoproteins are altered by reaction with ROS, causing changes in cell functions. Although few studies have examined the production of ROS following RFW exposure, several reports have shown that RFW exposure has no effect on free radical production, and that there is no increase in superoxide concentration following combined exposure to phorbol 12-myristate 13-acetate (PMA) and RFW (Lantow et al., 2006). When RFW exposure was performed in the presence or absence of 3-chloro-4-(dichloromethyl)-5-hydroxy-2-(5H)-furanone, a compound produced during the chlorination of drinking water, no ROS production was observed under any circumstances tested (Zeni et al., 2007a). In recent years, however, several studies have reported that RFW exposure increases ROS production, resulting in damage to DNA (Liu et al., 2014; Çiğ and Nazıroğlu, 2015), and that a ROS amplification effect can be seen (Luukkonen et al., 2008).

Another study suggested that ROS play an important role in apoptosis in human peripheral blood mononuclear cells, which is induced by RFW at 900 MHz at an SAR of ~0.4 W/kg for exposures lasting longer than 2 h. Although human peripheral blood mononuclear cells have a self-protective mechanism (i.e., release of carotenoid in response to oxidative stress) that prevents a further increase in ROS levels, the imbalance between antioxidant defenses and ROS formation still results in an increase in cell death under these exposure times; about 37% of human peripheral blood mononuclear cells died within 8 h (Lu et al., 2012). Also, the remarkable result that induces the cytosolic Ca^+ influx together with ROS by exposure to 2.45 GHz RFW is reported (Nazıroğlu et al., 2012). On the other hand, no ROS production or amplification effects have been observed under these conditions (Brescia et al., 2009; Luukkonen et al., 2010). Thus, the mechanism underlying the induction of ROS production by RFW exposure has not yet been elucidated.

2.3.1.3 Other Cellular Studies

Other cellular studies, including some interesting reports on DNA migration, Alzheimer's disease, and transformation, are described below.

A 24 h intermittent exposure (5 min on/10 min off) was administered to the mouse spermatocyte-derived GC-2 cell line on an 1800 MHz GSM signals, in GSM-Talk mode, at an SAR of 1, 2, or 4 W/kg. The extent of DNA migration was significantly increased at an SAR of 4 W/kg. However, no detectable DNA strand breakage was observed by the alkaline comet assay. Taking together, these findings imply that RFW with insufficient energy to directly induce DNA strand breaks may produce genotoxicity through oxidative DNA base damage in male germ cells (Liu et al., 2013).

The study was designed to determine the effects of 2.45 GHz RFW on the antioxidant redox system, calcium ion signaling, cell count, and viability in HL-60 cells. In these cells, the average SAR on the top of the flask surface during exposure to radiation was 0.1 W/kg, and the electric field density was set to 10 V/m. These conditions appeared to induce proliferative effects through oxidative stress and Ca^{2+} influx although blocking of transient receptor potential melastatin 2 channels by 2-aminoethyl diphenylborinate seemed to counteract the effects on Ca^{2+} influx (Nazıroğlu et al., 2012).

The cells were then exposed to RFWs at a wide range of SARs of 5–200 W/kg for 2 h, either alone or in combination with a known initiating chemical, methylcholanthrene

(MC) (2.5 µg/ml). No significant differences were observed in the frequency of malignant transformation (Type II + Type III) between controls and RFW-exposed cells, with or without 12-O-tetradecanoylphorbol-13-acetate (TPA) (0.5 ng/ml). However, in response to RFW at an SAR of more than 100 W/kg with MC or MC + TPA, the transformation frequency was increased in comparison with MC alone or MC + TPA. Thus, 2450 MHz RFW does not contribute to the initiation stage of tumor formation, but may contribute to the promotion stage at extremely high SAR values (≥100 W/kg) (Wang et al., 2005).

The effect of RFW exposure was investigated in *in vitro* models of neurodegenerative disease (Vecchio et al., 2009). The aim of that study was to investigate whether prolonged exposure to 900 MHz GSM-modulated RFWs affects viability and vulnerability of two neural cultures, primary cortical neurons and the SN56 cell line, exposed to 25–35AA beta-amyloid (related to Alzheimer's disease), glutamate, or H_2O_2. The results indicated that mobile phone–like exposure worsened SN56 cell vulnerability to oxidative stress, but no effects on glutamate or beta-amyloid–dependent cell death were detected.

In addition, the effects of mobile phone RFW (910 and 940 MHz) on the structure and function of hemoglobin A (HbA) were investigated. Oxygen affinity was measured by sodium dithionite on a UV–vis spectrophotometer. Structural changes were studied by circular dichroism and fluorescence spectroscopy. The results revealed that mobile phone RFW altered the oxygen affinity and tertiary structure of HbA (Mousavy et al., 2009).

The production of spindle disturbances in FC2 cells, a human-hamster hybrid (AL) cell line, was studied using RFW with a field strength of 90 V/m at a frequency of 835 MHz. Spindle disturbances did not change the fraction of mitotic cells with exposures times up to 2 h (Schrader et al., 2008).

The possible biological effects of mobile phone RFW (940 MHz, 15 V/m, and SAR at 40 mW/kg) on the structure of calf thymus DNA (ctDNA) were evaluated immediately and 2 h after a 45 min exposure, using a diverse range of spectroscopic instruments. The results revealed that 940 MHz altered the structure of DNA. The displacement of electrons in DNA by RFW may lead to conformational changes of DNA and DNA disaggregation (Hekmat et al., 2013).

Studies using cells are conducted by genotoxic (MN formation, CA, comet assay, mutation, etc.) and nongenotoxic examinations (immune function, gene expression [mRNA, protein], transcriptomics, apoptosis, ROS, etc.). Although some studies have reported positive results, at the present time, we do not believe that clear evidence has been obtained regarding the mechanism of RFW action on cells under nonthermal (or athermal) conditions (Miyakoshi, 2013).

2.4 Millimeter and Terahertz Waves

In recent years, various technical applications of MMWs and THWs have been developed. These include localization techniques, military applications, medical imaging devices, security scanners, communication equipment, and monitoring devices for industrial production processes. Furthermore, in Fifth Generation (5G) high-speed communication technology, which will be released widely within a few years, the MMW domain is a strong candidate frequency for 5G technology. Therefore, like ELFWs and RFWs, the biological effects of MMWs and THWs are of social concern. The number of studies that have evaluated how MMWs and THWs affect living organisms at the cellular level is gradually increasing, but these wavelengths have been studied far less extensively than ELFWs and RFWs. The *in vitro* study of MMWs and THWs is introduced below. In addition, the issue has been the subject of several reviews (Pakhomov et al., 1998; Ramundo-Orlando and Gallerano, 2009).

2.4.1 Millimeter Waves

2.4.1.1 Genotoxic Effects

Human corneal epithelial (HCE-T) and human lens epithelial (SRA01/04) cells derived from the human eye were exposed to 60 GHz MMW at 1 mV/cm^2 for 24 h. There was no statistically significant increase in the MN frequency in exposed cells in comparison with sham-exposed controls and incubator controls. In addition, neither the comet assay, used to detect DNA strand breaks, nor HSP expression exhibited any statistically significant effects of exposure (Koyama et al., 2016b).

2.4.1.2 Cell Growth

The biological effects produced by low-power MMWs were studied on the RPMI 7932 human melanoma cell line. Three different frequency-type exposure modes were used: the 53.57–78.33 GHz wide-band frequency range and two monochromatic frequencies, 51.05 and 65.00 GHz. The mean power at the output of the generator was less than 1 μW. The results provided evidence of antiproliferative effects on tumor cells induced by low-power MMWs in the 50–80 GHz frequency range (Wu et al., 2012).

The cellular effects of MMWs were also investigated in the U-2 OS human osteosarcoma cell line. The results revealed that MMWs induced morphological changes and reduced cell viability in a dose- and time-dependent manner. MMWs inhibited the growth of these cells and induced apoptosis via the mitochondrion-dependent pathway (Wu et al., 2012).

2.4.1.3 Gene Expression

The ability of low-power MMWs to modulate cytokine production, including RANTES and IP-10, was analyzed *in vitro* in keratinocytes (HaCaT cells). The same study investigated whether low-power MMW exposure induces a heat-stress reaction in keratinocytes, and specifically whether it stimulates HSP70 production. No harmful effect of low-power MMW exposure was observed on either keratinocyte function or structure *in vitro*, although the cells were sensitive to higher MMW power resulting in heat stress and cellular damage (Szabo et al., 2003).

The effect of 60 GHz on expression of a set of stress-sensitive genes encoding molecular chaperones, namely clusterin (CLU) and HSP70, was examined in a human brain cell line. The U-251 MG glial cell line was sham-exposed or exposed to MMW at 60 GHz for different durations (1–33 h) at two different power densities (5.4 or 0.54 mW/cm^2). The data revealed no significant modifications in transcription, mRNA levels, or protein levels of these genes under the conditions examined (Zhadobov et al., 2007).

2.4.1.4 Gap Junction Intercellular Communication (GJIC)

The effect of 30.16 GHz MMW exposure at 1.0 and 3.5 mW/cm^2 was studied on gap junction intercellular communication (GJIC) in cultured HaCaT keratinocytes. While MMW exposure alone for 1 h at either 1.0 or 3.5 mW/cm^2 did not affect GJIC, MMW exposure in combination with 5 ng/ml TPA treatment reversed TPA-induced suppression of GJIC (Chen et al., 2004).

2.4.1.5 Apoptosis

A KFA-100A MMW therapeutic instrument was manufactured, and wavelengths of 7.5–10.0 mm, a power density of 4 mW/cm^2, and an exposure area 45.6 ± 4.0 mm long × 33.2 ± 3.0 mm wide were used in experiments. In SW1353 human chondrosarcoma cells, MMF exposure induced apoptosis by affecting the ratio of Bax/Bcl-2 (Li et al., 2012).

2.4.1.6 Endoplasmic Reticulum

To investigate the potential effects of low-power MMW exposure on cellular physiology, the human glial cell line, U-251 MG, was exposed to 60.4 GHz MMWs at a power density of 0.14 mW/cm^2, and the effect of MMW exposure on ER stress was examined. Exposure to 60.4 GHz MMWs did not modify ER protein folding and secretion, nor did it induce maturation of the XBP1 and ATF6 transcription factors (Nicolas Nicolaz et al., 2009a).

To study the potential biological effects of low-power MMW on the ER, the human glial cell line, U-251 MG, was exposed or sham-exposed for 24 h with a peak incident power density of 0.14 mW/cm^2. The average SAR within the cell monolayer ranged from 2.64 ± 0.08 to 3.3 ± 0.1 W/kg, depending on the location of the exposed cell. Exposure to low-power MMWs did not significantly affect the mRNA levels of stress-sensitive genes (Nicolas Nicolaz et al., 2009b).

To investigate the potential effects of MMW exposure on the cellular ER stress, human skin cell lines were exposed to 60.4 GHz MMWs at incident power densities ranging between 1 and 20 mW/cm^2. The data revealed that MMW exposures did not change basal mRNA levels of ER-stress sensors (BIP or ORP150) (Le Quément et al., 2014).

2.4.1.7 Microarray Analysis

Primary human skin cells were exposed for 1, 6, or 24 h to 60.4 GHz with an average incident power density of 1.8 mW/cm^2 at an average SAR of 42.4 W/kg. Gene expression microarrays containing over 41,000 unique human transcript probe sets were used, and data were compared between exposed and sham-exposed cells. No significant difference in gene expression was observed when the data were subjected to a stringent statistical analysis such as the Benjamini–Hochberg procedure. However, when a *t*-test was employed to analyze microarray data, 130 transcripts were identified. Five of them, namely, CRIP2, PLXND1, PTX3, SERPINF1, and TRPV2, were confirmed to be differentially expressed after 6 h of exposure (Le Quément et al., 2012).

To evaluate the biocompatibility of MMW at 60 GHz, a whole-genome expression approach was used to assess the effect of acute 60 GHz exposure on primary cultures of human keratinocytes. Cells were exposed to 60.4 GHz MMWs for 3 h. Average and peak SARs over the cell monolayer were 594 and 1233 W/kg, respectively. By RT-PCR, seven genes were validated as differentially expressed: ADAMTS6, NOG, IL7R, FADD, JUNB, SNAI2, and HIST1H1A (Habauzit et al., 2014).

Modifications to the whole genome were analyzed in a human keratinocyte model exposed to MMWs at 60.4 GHz and an incident power density of 20 mW/cm^2 for 3 h under athermic conditions. No transcriptome modifications were observed. In addition, the effect of MMWs on cell metabolism was tested by co-treating MMW exposed cells with a glycolysis inhibitor, 2-deoxyglucose (2dG, 20 mM for 3 h), and whole-genome expression was evaluated along with adenosine triphosphate (ATP) content. RT-PCR-based validation confirmed six MMW-sensitive genes (SOCS3, SPRY2, TRIB1, FAM46A, CSRNP1, and PPP1R15A) under 2dG treatment. These genes encode transcription factors or inhibitors of cytokine pathways, raising questions regarding the potential impact of long-term or chronic MMW exposure on metabolically stressed cells (Mahamoud et al., 2016).

2.4.2 Terahertz Waves

2.4.2.1 Genotoxic Effects

Human whole blood samples from healthy donors were exposed to THWs for 20 min. Frequencies of 120 and 130 GHz were chosen; the first one was tested at an SAR of 0.4 mWg^{-1}, and the second was tested at SARs of 0.24, 1.4, and 2 mW/g. The results revealed that THW exposure, under the electromagnetic conditions tested, is not able to induce either genotoxicity (MN formation and DNA strand breaks) or alteration of cell-cycle kinetics in human blood cells from healthy subjects (Zeni et al., 2007b).

Another study investigated the genotoxic effect of THW in human peripheral blood lymphocytes following 20 min exposure to 1 mW average power Free Electron Laser radiation in the frequency range of 120–140 GHz. Material from nine healthy donors was tested, and the cytokinesis block technique was applied to study MN frequency and cell proliferation. None of the electromagnetic conditions adopted altered the investigated parameters (Scarfì et al., 2003).

Cells were exposed to 0.106 THz THWs for 2, 8, or 24 h at power intensities ranging from 0.04 to 2 mW/cm^2, representing levels below, at, and above current safety limits. THWs did not induce manifest genomic damage (MN formation or DNA strand breaks) *in vitro* (Hintzsche et al., 2012).

To investigate the cellular effects of THW, human corneal epithelial cells (HCE-T) derived from the human eye were exposed to 0.12 THz THWs at 5 mW/cm^2 for 24 h. There was no statistically significant increase in the MN frequency, morphological changes, or HSP expression (HSP27, HSP70, and HSP90α) in cells exposed to 0.12 THz in comparison with sham-exposed and incubator controls (Koyama et al., 2016a).

Continuous-wave THW (0.1 THz, 0.031 mW/cm^2) was applied to dividing lymphocytes for 1, 2, and 24 h. Changes in chromosome number of chromosomes 1, 10, 11, and 17, as well as changes in the replication timing of their centromeres using interphase fluorescence *in situ* hybridization, were examined. Chromosomes 11 and 17 were most vulnerable (about 30% increase in aneuploidy after 2 and 24 h of exposure), whereas chromosomes 1 and 10 were not affected. Changes were also observed in the asynchronous mode of replication of centromeres 1, 11, and 17 after 2 h of exposure (40%) and of all four centromeres after 24 h of exposure (50%). Based on these results, exposure of lymphocytes *in vitro* to a low power density at 0.1 THz may induce genomic instability (Korenstein-Ilan et al., 2008).

Human embryonic stem cells are extremely sensitive to environmental stimuli. Therefore, this model was used to investigate the nonthermal effects of THW exposure. DNA damage and transcriptome responses were studied in cells exposed to narrowband THWs (2.3 THz) under strict temperature control. THW exposure did not induce the formation of cH2AX foci or structural chromosomal aberrations in the cells. In addition, no effect on mitotic index or morphology was observed following THW exposure (Bogomazova et al., 2015).

2.4.2.2 Molecular Interactions

The effect of THW (100 GHz) exposure was examined on two defined molecular interactions: the interaction of soluble or immobilized calf alkaline phosphatase with its substrate p-nitrophenylphosphate, and the interaction between an antibody (mouse monoclonal anti-dinitrophenyl (DNP)) and its antigen DNP. The power density of the exposure at the bottom of the microplate wells was measured at 0.08 W/m^2 using an HP423A power meter. Exposure of both enzymes, either prior to addition of substrate or during the enzymatic reaction, resulted in small but significant reductions in enzyme activity (Homenko et al., 2009).

2.4.2.3 Heat Shock Proteins

The cellular response was evaluated in mesenchymal mouse stem cells exposed to low-power THWs from both a pulsed broadband (centered at 10 THz) source and a CW laser (2.52 THz) source. Differential expression of the heat shock proteins HSP105, HSP90, and CPR was unaffected, whereas expression of certain other genes (adiponectin, GLUT4, and PPARG) showed clear effects after prolonged, broadband THW exposure (Alexandrov et al., 2011).

2.4.2.4 THWs and Heat

THW exposure of human dermal fibroblasts was performed in a temperature-controlled chamber using a molecular gas THz laser (2.52 THz; 84.8 mW/cm^2; durations: 5, 10, 20, 40, or 80 min). Cellular temperatures increased by 3°C during all THW exposures. For each exposure duration tested, the THW and hyperthermic exposure groups exhibited equivalent levels of cell survival (~90%) and heat shock protein expression (~3.5-fold increases). Human dermal fibroblasts exhibited comparable cellular and molecular effects when exposed to THWs and hyperthermic stress (Wilmink et al., 2011).

2.4.2.5 Gene Chip Survey

Mouse stem cells were exposed to broad-spectrum THWs (centered at ~10 THz) for 2 and 6 h at an average power density of ~1 mW/cm^2. A gene chip survey revealed that while 89% of protein-coding genes in mouse stem cells did not respond to the applied THW exposure, certain genes were activated and certain others were repressed. The response was not only gene-specific but also dependent on exposure conditions. The applied THW exposure accelerated cell differentiation toward an adipose phenotype by activating the transcription factor peroxisome proliferator–activated receptor gamma (Bock et al., 2010).

2.5 Conclusion and Future Prospects

There have been remarkable advances in communication technology, including mobile phones, wireless power supply system, and the engineering techniques used in the fields of medicine and security. On the other hand, electromagnetic waves must also be considered as new environmental factors worthy of social attention. RFWs, MMWs, and THWs have no ionization ability, but in general society, the possibility that the term "nonionizing electromagnetic wave" would be accepted in the same way as "ionizing radiation" cannot be denied.

The use of electromagnetic waves is increasing all over the world. Human epidemiological studies and animal experiment research are also important in considerations of the future electromagnetic environment. On the other hand, the development of cellular and genetic level research in the past few decades has been remarkable. In order to assess safety based on scientific data, it is necessary to promote further research on areas not yet thoroughly elucidated, using advanced life sciences technology.

Meanwhile, research on the effects of electromagnetic waves on living organisms, cells, and macromolecular polymers at intensities far above their environmental levels are also important for the future development of this field. The results of research ranging from low to high intensities are based on electromagnetic waves' dose–response relationship. (Currently, dose for ELFW is defined in terms of magnetic intensity and induction current, whereas dose for RFW is defined in terms of exposure time and SAR. It is possible to estimate appropriate threshold dose based on these research outcomes). It is conceivable that electromagnetic waves could be used as research tools in life science. Furthermore, from the standpoint of applications, results from the life sciences should be actively utilized in a wide range of fields, including engineering, agriculture, and medicine.

Abbreviation List

ATP:	adenosine triphosphate
CA:	chromosomal aberration
CDMA:	code division multiple access
CLU:	clusterin
ELFW:	extremely low frequency wave
ER:	endoplasmic reticulum
FMCW:	frequency-modulated continuous wave
5G:	Fifth Generation
GJIC:	gap junction intercellular communication
GSM:	global system for mobile communication
HbA:	hemoglobin A
HSP:	heat shock protein
IFW:	intermediate-frequency wave
IL-2:	interleukin 2
INF-γ:	interferon γ
IR:	ionizing radiation
MC:	methylcholanthrene
MMC:	mitomycin C
MMW:	millimeter wave
MN:	micronucleus
PMA:	phorbol 12-myristate 13-acetate
RFW:	radio frequency wave
ROS:	reactive oxygen species
RT-PCR:	reverse transcription polymerase chain reaction
SAR:	specific absorption rate
SMF:	static magnetic field
THW:	terahertz, wave

TNF-α: tumor necrosis factor α
TPA: 12-O-tetradecanoylphorbol-13-acetate

References

Alexandrov, B.S., Rasmussen, K.Ø., Bishop, A.R., Usheva, A., Alexandrov, L.B., Chong, S., Dagon, Y., Booshehri, L.G., Mielke, C.H., Phipps, M.L., Martinez, J.S., Chen, H.T. and Rodriguez, G. (2011) Non-thermal effects of terahertz radiation on gene expression in mouse stem cells. *Biomed Opt Express*, 2(9), 2679–2689.

Antonopoulos, A., Eisenbrandt, H. and Obe, G. (1997) Effects of high-frequency electromagnetic fields on human lymphocytes in vitro. *Mutat Res*, 395, 209–214.

Bisht, K.S., Moros, E.G., Straube, W.L., Baty, J.D. and Roti, J.L.R. (2002) The effect of 835.62 MHz FDMA or 847.74 MHz CDMA modulated radiofrequency radiation on the induction of micronuclei in C3H 10T(1/2) cells. *Radiat Res*, 157(5), 506–515.

Bock, J., Fukuyo, Y., Kang, S., Phipps, M.L., Alexandrov, L.B., Rasmussen, K.Ø., Bishop, A.R., Rosen, E.D., Martinez, J.S., Chen, H.-T., Rodriguez, G., Alexandrov, B.S. and Usheva, A. (2010) Mammalian stem cells reprogramming in response to terahertz radiation. *PLoS One*, 5(12), e15806.

Bogomazova, A.N., Vassina, E.M., Goryachkovskaya, T.N., Popik, V.M., Sokolov, A.S., Kolchanov, N.A., Lagarkova, M.A., Kiselev, S.L. and Peltek, S.E. (2015) No DNA damage response and negligible genome-wide transcriptional changes in human embryonic stem cells exposed to terahertz radiation. *Sci Rep*, 5, Article number: 7749.

Bourthoumieu, S., Joubert, V., Marin, B., Collin, A., Leveque, P., Terro, F. and Yardin, C. (2010) Cytogenetic studies in human cells exposed in vitro to GSM-900 MHz radiofrequency radiation using R-banded karyotyping. *Radiat Res*, 174(6a), 712–718.

Brescia, F., Sarti, M., Massa, R., Calabrese, M.L., Sannino, A. and Scarfì, M.R. (2009) Reactive oxygen species formation is not enhanced by exposure to UMTS 1950 MHz radiation and co-exposure to ferrous ions in Jurkat cells. *Bioelectromagnetics*, 30, 525–535.

Buttiglione, M., Roca, L., Montemurno, E., Vitiello, F., Capozzi, V. and Cibelli, G. (2007) Radiofrequency radiation (900 MHz) induces Egr-1 gene expression and affects cell-cycle control in human neuroblastoma cells. *J Cell Physiol*, 213, 759–767.

Calabrò, E., Condello, S., Currò, M., Ferlazzo, N., Caccamo, D., Magazù, S. and Ientile, R. (2012) Modulation of heat shock protein response in SH-SY5Y by mobile phone microwaves. *World J Biol Chem*, 3(2), 34–40.

Çam, S.T. and Seyhan, N. (2012) Single-strand DNA breaks in human hair root cells exposed to mobile phone radiation. *Int J Radiat Biol*, 88, 420–424.

Cao, Y., Zhang, W., Lu, M.X., Xu, Q., Meng, Q.Q., Nie, J.H. and Tong, J. (2009) 900-MHz microwave radiation enhances gamma-ray adverse effects on SHG44 cells. *J Toxicol Environ Health A*, 72, 727–732.

Chauhan, V., Mariampillai, A., Bellier, P.V., Qutob, S.S., Gajda, G.B., Lemay, E., Thansandote, A. and McNamee, J.P. (2006) Gene expression analysis of a human lymphoblastoma cell line exposed in vitro to an intermittent 1.9 GHz pulse-modulated radiofrequency field. *Radiat Res*, 165(4), 424–429.

Chen, Q., Zeng, Q.L., Lu, D.Q. and Chiang, H. (2004) Millimeter wave exposure reverses TPA suppression of gap junction intercellular communication in HaCaT human keratinocytes. *Bioelectromagnetics*, 25(1), 1–4.

Çiğ, B. and Nazıroğlu, M. (2015) Investigation of the effects of distance from sources on apoptosis, oxidative stress and cytosolic calcium accumulation via TRPV1 channels induced by mobile phones and Wi-Fi in breast cancer cells. *Biochim Biophys Acta*, 1848, 2756–2765.

Cotgreave, I.A. (2005) Biological stress responses to radio frequency electromagnetic radiation: are mobile phones really so (heat) shocking? *Arch Biochem Biophys*, 435(1), 227–240.

Crasta, K., Ganem, N.J., Dagher, R., Lantermann, A.B., Ivanova, E.V., Pan, Y., Nezi, L., Protopopovm, A., Chowdhury, D. and Pellman, D. (2012) DNA breaks and chromosome pulverization from errors in mitosis. *Nature*, 482(7383), 53–58.

Dabrowski, M.P., Stankiewicz, W., Kubacki, R., Sobiczewska, E. and Szmigielski, S. (2003) Immunotropic effects in cultured human blood mononuclear cells pre-exposed to low-level 1300 MHz pulse-modulated microwave field. *Electromagn Biol Med*, 22(1), 1–13.

Diem, E., Schwarz, C., Adlkofer, F., Jahn, O. and Rüdiger, H. (2005) Non-thermal DNA breakage by mobile-phone radiation (1800 MHz) in human fibroblasts and in transmed GFSH-R17 rat granulosa cells in vitro. *Mutat Res*, 583(2), 178–183.

Garaj-Vrhovac, V., Horvat, D. and Koren, Z. (1991) The relationship between colony-forming ability, chromosome aberrations and incidence of micronuclei in V79 Chinese hamster cells exposed to microwave radiation. *Mutat Res*, 263(3), 143–149.

Garaj-Vrhovac, V., Fucić, A. and Horvat, D. (1992) The correlation between the frequency of micronuclei and specific chromosome aberrations in human lymphocytes exposed to microwave radiation in vitro. *Mutat Res*, 281(3), 181–186.

Goswami, P.C., Albee, L.D., Parsian, A.J., Baty, J.D., Moros, E.G. and Pickard, W.F. (1999) Proto-oncogene mRNA levels and activities of multiple transcription factors in C3H 10T 1/2 murine embryonic fibroblasts exposed to 835.62 and 847.74 MHz cellular phone communication frequency radiation. *Radiat Res*, 151(3), 300–309.

Gurisik, E., Warton, K., Martin, D.K. and Valenzuela, S.M. (2006) An in vitro study of the effects of exposure to a GSM signal in two human cell lines: monocytic U937 and neuroblastoma SK-N-SH. *Cell Biol Int*, 30, 793–799.

Habauzit, D., Le Quément, C., Zhadobov, M., Martin, C., Aubry, M., Sauleau, R. and Le Dréan, Y. (2014) Transcriptome analysis reveals the contribution of thermal and the specific effects in cellular response to millimeter wave exposure. *PLoS One*, 9(10), e109435.

Hekmat, A., Saboury, A.A. and Moosavi-Movahedi, A.A. (2013) The toxic effects of mobile phone radiofrequency (940 MHz) on the structure of calf thymus DNA. *Ecotoxicol Environ Saf*, 88, 35–41.

Hintzsche, H., Jastrow, C., Kleine-Ostmann, T., Karst, U., Schrader, T. and Stopper, H. (2012) Terahertz electromagnetic fields (0.106 THz) do not induce manifest genomic damage in vitro. *PLoS One*, 7(9), e46397.

Hirose, H., Sakuma, N., Kaji, N., Suhara, T., Sekijima, M., Nojima, T. and Miyakoshi, J. (2006) Phosphorylation and gene expression of p53 are not affected in human cells exposed to 2.1425 GHz band CW or W-CDMA modulated radiation allocated to mobile radio base stations. *Bioelectromagnetics*, 27(6), 494–504.

Hirose, H., Sakuma, N., Kaji, N., Nakayama, K., Inoue, K., Sekijima, M., Nojima, T. and Miyakoshi, J. (2007) Mobile phone base station-emitted radiation does not induce phosphorylation of Hsp27. *Bioelectromagnetics*, 28(2), 99–108.

Hirose, H., Sasaki, A., Ishii, N., Sekijima, M., Iyama, T., Nojima, T. and Ugawa, Y. (2010) 1950 MHz IMT-2000 field does not activate microglial cells in vitro. *Bioelectromagnetics*, 31(2), 104–112.

Homenko, A., Kapilevich, B., Kornstein, R. and Firer, M.A. (2009) Effects of 100 GHz radiation on alkaline phosphatase activity and antigen-antibody interaction. *Bioelectromagnetics*, 30, 167–175.

Ivaschuk, O.I., Jones, R.A., Ishida-Jones, T., Haggren, W., Adey, W.R. and Phillips, J.L. (1997) Exposure of nerve growth factor-treated PC12 rat pheochromocytoma cells to a modulated radiofrequency field at 836.55 MHz: effects on c-jun and c-fos expression. *Bioelectromagnetics*, 18(3), 223–229.

Komatsubara, Y., Hirose, H., Sakurai, T., Koyama, S., Suzuki, Y., Taki, M. and Miyakoshi, J. (2005) Effect of high-frequency electromagnetic fields with a wide range of SARs on chromosomal aberrations in murine m5S cells. *Mutat Res*, 587(1–2), 114–119.

Korenstein-Ilan, A., Barbul, A., Hasin, P., Eliran, A., Gover, A. and Korenstein, R. (2008) Terahertz radiation increases genomic instability in human lymphocytes. *Radiat Res*, 170, 224–234.

Koyama, S., Nakahara, T., Wake, K., Taki, M., Isozumi, Y. and Miyakoshi, J. (2003) Effects of high frequency electromagnetic fields on micronucleus formation in CHO-K1 cells. *Mutat Res*, 541(1–2), 81–89.

Koyama, S., Isozumi, Y., Suzuki, Y., Taki, M. and Miyakoshi, J. (2004) Effects of 2.45-GHz electromagnetic fields with a wide range of SARs on micronucleus formation in CHO-K1 cells. *Sci World J*, 4(S2), 29–40.

Koyama, S., Takashima, Y., Sakurai, T., Suzuki, Y., Taki, M. and Miyakoshi, J. (2007) Effects of 2.45 GHz electromagnetic fields with a wide range of SARs on bacterial and HPRT gene mutations. *J Radiat Res*, 48(1), 69–75.

Koyama, S., Narita, E., Suzuki, Y., Taki, M., Shinohara, N. and Miyakoshi, J. (2015) Effect of a 2.45-GHz radiofrequency electromagnetic field on neutrophil chemotaxis and phagocytosis in differentiated human HL-60 cells. *J Radiat Res*, 56(1), 30–36.

Koyama, S., Narita, E., Shimizu, Y., Shiina, T., Taki, M., Shinohara, N. and Miyakoshi, J. (2016a) Twenty four-hour exposure to a 0.12 THz electromagnetic field does not affect the genotoxicity, morphological changes, or expression of heat shock protein in HCE-T cells. *Int J Environ Res Public Health*, 13(8), 793.

Koyama, S., Narita, E., Shimizu, Y., Suzuki, Y., Shiina, T., Taki, M., Shinohara, N. and Miyakoshi, J. (2016b) Effects of long-term exposure to 60 GHz millimeter-wavelength radiation on the genotoxicity and heat shock protein (Hsp) expression of cells derived from human eye. *Int J Environ Res Public Health*, 13(8), 802.

Lagroye, I., Hook, G.J., Wettring, B.A., Baty, J.D., Moros, E.G., Straube, W.L. and Roti, L.R. (2004) Measurements of alkali-labile DNA damage and protein-DNA crosslinks after 2450 MHz microwave and low-dose gamma irradiation in vitro. *Radiat Res*, 161(2), 201–214.

Lantow, M., Lupke, M., Frahm, J., Mattsson, M.O., Kuster, N. and Simko, M. (2006) ROS release and Hsp70 expression after exposure to 1,800 MHz radiofrequency electromagnetic fields in primary human monocytes and lymphocytes. *Radiat Environ Biophys*, 45(1), 55–62.

Le Quément, C., Nicolas Nicolaz, C., Zhadobov, M., Desmots, F., Sauleau, R., Aubry, M., Michel, D. and Le Dréan, Y. (2012) Whole-genome expression analysis in primary human keratinocyte cell cultures exposed to 60 GHz radiation. *Bioelectromagnetics*, 33(2), 147–158.

Le Quément, C., Nicolaz, C.N., Habauzit, D., Zhadobov, M., Sauleau, R. and Le Dréan, Y. (2014) Impact of 60-GHz millimeter waves and corresponding heat effecton endoplasmic reticulum stress sensor gene expression. *Bioelectromagnetics*, 35, 444–451.

Leszczynski, D., Joenväärä, S., Reivinen, J. and Kuokka, R. (2002) Non-thermal activation of the hsp27/p38MAPK stress pathway by mobile phone radiation in human endothelial cells: molecular mechanism for cancer-and blood-brain barrier-related effects. *Differentiation*, 70(2–3), 120–129.

Li, X., Ye, H., Cai, L., Yu, F., Chen, W., Lin, R., Zheng, C., Xu, H., Ye, J., Wu, G. and Liu, X. (2012) Millimeter wave radiation induces apoptosis via affecting the ratio of Bax/Bcl-2 in SW1353 human chondrosarcoma cells. *Oncol Rep*, 27(3), 664–672.

Liu, Y.X., Tai, J.L., Li, G.Q., Zhang, Z.W., Xue, J.H., Liu, H.S., Zhu, H., Cheng, J.D., Liu, Y.L., Li, A.M. and Zhang, Y. (2012) Exposure to 1950-MHz TD-SCDMA electromagnetic fields affects the apoptosis of astrocytes via caspase-3-dependent pathway. *PLoS One*, 7(8), e42332.

Liu, C., Duan, W., Xu, S., Chen, C., He, M., Zhang, L., Yu, Z. and Zhou, Z. (2013) Exposure to 1800 MHz radiofrequency electromagnetic radiation induces oxidative DNA base damage in a mouse spermatocyte-derived cell line. *Toxicol Lett*, 218(1), 2–9.

Liu, K., Zhang, G., Wang, Z., Liu, Y., Dong, J., Dong, X., Liu, J., Cao, J., Ao, L. and Zhang, S. (2014) The protective effect of autophagy on mouse spermatocyte derived cells exposure to 1800MHz radiofrequency electromagnetic radiation. *Toxicol Lett*, 228(3), 216–224.

Lu, Y.S., Huang, B.T. and Huang, Y.X. (2012) Reactive oxygen species formation and apoptosis in human peripheral blood mononuclear cell induced by 900MHz mobile phone radiation. *Oxid Med Cell Longev*, 2012, Article ID 740280, 8 pages.

Luukkonen, J., Hakulinen, P., Mäki-Paakkanen, J., Juutilainen, J. and Naarala, J. (2008) Enhancement of chemically induced reactive oxygen species production and DNA damage in human SH-SY5Y neuroblastoma cells by 872 MHz radiofrequency radiation. *Mutat Res*, 662(1–2), 54–58.

Luukkonen, J., Juutilainen, J. and Naarala, J. (2010) Combined effects of 872 MHz radiofrequency radiation and ferrous chloride on reactive oxygen species production and DNA damage in human SH-SY5Y neuroblastoma cells. *Bioelectromagnetics*, 31(6), 417–424.

Maes, A., Collier, M. and Verschaeve, L. (2001) Cytogenetic effects of 900 MHz (GSM) microwaves on human lymphocytes. *Bioelectromagnetics*, 22(2), 91–96.

Mahamoud, Y.S., Aite, M., Martin, C., Zhadobov, M., Sauleau, R., Le Dréan, Y. and Habauzit, D. (2016) Additive effects of millimeter waves and 2-deoxyglucose co-exposure on the human keratinocyte transcriptome. *PLoS One*, 11(8), e0160810.

Marinelli, F., La Sala, D., Cicciotti, G., Cattini, L., Trimarchi, C., Putti, S., Zamparelli, A., Giuliani, L., Tomassetti, G. and Cinti, C. (2004) Exposure to 900 MHz electromagnetic field induces an unbalance between pro-apoptotic and pro-survival signals in T-lymphoblastoid leukemia CCRF-CEM cells. *J Cell Physiol*, 198(2), 324–332.

Mashevich, M., Folkman, D., Kesar, A., Barbul, A., Korenstein, R., Jerby, E. and Avivi, L. (2003) Exposure of human peripheral blood lymphocytes to electromagnetic fields associated with cellular phones leads to chromosomal instability. *Bioelectromagnetics*, 24(2), 82–90.

Mazor, R., Korenstein-Ilan, A., Barbul, A., Eshet, Y., Shahade, A., Jerbu, E. and Korenstein, R. (2008) Increased levels of numerical chromosome aberrations after in vitro exposure of human peripheral blood lymphocytes to radiofrequency electromagnetic fields for 72 hours. *Radiat Res*, 169(1), 28–37.

McNamee, J.P., Bellier, P.V., Gajda, G.B., Miller, S.M., Lemay, E.P., Lavallée, B.F., Marro, L. and Thansandote, A. (2002) DNA damage and micronucleus induction in human leukocytes after acute in vitro exposure to a 1.9 GHz continuous-wave radiofrequency field. *Radiat Res*, 158(4), 523–533.

Meltz, M.L., Eagan, P. and Erwin, D.N. (1990) Proflavin and microwave radiation: absence of a mutagenic interaction. *Bioelectromagnetics*, 11(2), 149–157.

Miyakoshi, J., Yoshida, M., Tarusawa, Y., Nojima, T., Wake, K. and Taki, M. (2002) Effects of high-frequency electromagnetic fields on DNA strand breaks using comet assay method. *Electr Eng Jpn*, 141(4), 9–15.

Miyakoshi, J., Takemasa, K., Takashima, Y., Ding, G.R., Hirose, H. and Koyama, S. (2005) Effects of exposure to a 1950 MHz radio frequency field on expression of Hsp70 and Hsp27 in human glioma cells. *Bioelectromagnetics*, 26(4), 251–257.

Miyakoshi, J. (2006) Radiofrequency biology: in vitro, In *Electromagnetics in Biology*, Kato, M. (Ed.), Japan: Springer, 305–316.

Miyakoshi, J. (2009) Cellular biology aspect of mobile phone radiation, In *Advances in Electromagnetic Fields in Living Systems*, vol. 5, Health Effects of Cell Phone Radiation, Lin, J. (Ed.), New York: Springer, 1–33.

Miyakoshi, J. (2013) Cellular and molecular responses to radio-frequency electromagnetic fields. *Proc IEEE*, 101(6), 1494–1502.

Mousavy, S.J., Riazi, G.H., Kamarei, M., Aliakbarian, H., Sattarahmady, N., Sharifizadeh, A., Safarian, S., Ahmad, F. and Moosavi–Movahedi, A. (2009) Effects of mobile phone radiofrequency on the structure and function of the normal human hemoglobin. *Int J Biol Macromol*, 44(33), 278–285.

Nazıroğlu, M., Cığ, B., Doğan, S., Cihangir Uğuz, A., Dilek, S. and Faouzi, D. (2012) 2.45-Gz wireless devices induce oxidative stress and proliferation through cytosolic Ca^{2+} influx in human leukemia cancer cell. *Int J Radiat Biol*, 88(6), 449–456.

Nicolas Nicolaz, C., Zhadobov, M., Desmots, F., Sauleau, R., Thouroude, D., Michel, D. and Le Dréan, Y. (2009a) Absence of direct effect of low-power millimeter-wave radiation at 60.4 GHz on endoplasmic reticulum stress. *Cell Biol Toxicol*, 25(5), 471–478.

Nicolas Nicolaz, C., Zhadobov, M., Desmots, F., Ansart, A., Sauleau, R., Thouroude, D., Michel, D. and Le Dréan, Y. (2009b) Study of narrow band millimeter-wave potential interactions with endoplasmic reticulum stress sensor genes. *Bioelectromagnetics*, 30(5), 365–373.

Nylund, R. and Leszczynski, D. (2006) Mobile phone radiation causes changes in gene and protein expression in human endothelial cell lines and the response seems to be genome-and proteome-dependent. *Proteomics*, 6(17), 4769–4780.

Pacini, S., Ruggiero, M., Sardi, I., Aterini, S., Gulisano, F. and Gulisano, M. (2002) Exposure to global system for mobile communication (GSM) cellular phone radiofrequency alters gene expression, proliferation, and morphology of human skin fibroblasts, *Oncol Res*, 13, 19–24.

Pakhomov, A.G., Akyel, Y., Pakhomova, O.N., Stuck, B.E. and Murphy, M.R. (1998) Current state and implications of research on biological effects of millimeter waves: a review of the literature. *Bioelectromagnetics*, 19(7), 393–413.

Palumbo, R., Brescia, F., Capasso, D., Sannino, A., Sarti, M., Capri, M., GErassilli, E. and Scarfi, M.R. (2008) Exposure to 900 MHz radiofrequency radiation induces caspase 3 activation in proliferating human lymphocytes. *Radiat Res*, 170(3), 327–334.

Phillips, J.L., Ivaschuk, O., Ishida-Jones, T., Jones, R.A., Campbell-Beachler, M. and Haggren, W. (1998) DNA damage in Molt-4 T-lymphoblastoid cells exposed to cellular telephone radiofrequency fields in vitro. *Bioelectrochem Bioenerg*, 45(1), 103–110.

Ramundo-Orlando, A. and Gallerano, G.P. (2009) Terahertz radiation effects and biological applications. *J Infrared Millimeter Terahertz Waves*, 30, 1308–1318.

Remondini, D., Nylund, R., Reivinen, J., Poulletier de Gannes, F., Veyret, B., Lagroye, I., Haro, E., Trillo, M.A., Capri, M., Franceschi, C., Schlatterer, K., Gminski, R., Fitzner, R., Tauber, R., Schuderer, J., Kuster, N., Leszczynski, D., Bersani, F. and Maercker, C. (2006) Gene expression changes in human cells after exposure to mobile phone microwaves. *Proteomics*, 6(17), 4745–4754.

Sakurai, T., Kiyokawa, T., Narita, E., Suzuki, Y., Taki, M. and Miyakoshi, J. (2011) Analysis of gene expression in a human-derived glial cell line exposed to 2.45 GHz continuous radiofrequency electromagnetic fields. *J Radiat Res*, 52(2), 185–192.

Sanchez, S., Milochau, A., Ruffie, G., Poulletier de Gannes, F., Lagroye, I., Haro, E., Surleve-Bazeille, J.E., Billaudel, B., Lassegues, M. and Veyret, B. (2006) Human skin cell stress response to GSM-900 mobile phone signals. In vitro study on isolated primary cells and reconstructed epidermis. *FEBS J*, 273(24), 5491–5507.

Sannino, A., Di Costanzo, G., Brescia, F., Sarti, M., Zeni, O., Juutilainen, J. and Scarfi, M.R. (2009) Human fibroblasts and 900 MHz radiofrequency radiation: evaluation of DNA damage after exposure and co-exposure to 3-chloro-4-(dichloromethyl)-5-hydroxy-2(5h)-furanone (MX). *Radiat Res*, 171(6), 743–751.

Sannino, A., Zeni, O., Romeo, S., Massa, R., Gialanella, G., Grossi, G. Manti, L., Vijayalaxmi and Scarfi, M.R. (2014) Adaptive response in human blood lymphocytes exposed to non-ionizing radiofrequency fields: resistance to ionizing radiation-induced damage. *J Radiat Res*, 55(2), 210–217.

Scarfi, M.R., Romanò, M., Di Pietro, R., Zeni, O., Doria, A., Gallerano, G.P., Giovenale, E., Messina, G., Lai, A., Campurra, G., Coniglio, D. and D'Arienzo, M. (2003) THz exposure of whole blood for the study of biological effects on human lymphocytes. *J Biol Phys*, 29(2–3), 171–176.

Schrader, T., Münter, K., Kleine-Ostmann, T. and Schmid, E. (2008) Spindle disturbances in human-hamster hybrid (A_L) cells induced by mobile communication frequency range signals. *Bioelectromagnetics*, 29(8), 626–639.

Schwarz, C., Kratochvil, E., Pilger, A., Kuster, N., Adlkofer, F. and Rüdiger, H.W. (2008) Radiofrequency electromagnetic fields (UMTS, 1,950 MHz) induce genotoxic effects in vitro in human fibroblasts but not in lymphocytes. *Int Arch Occup Environ Health*, 81(6), 755–767.

Simkó, M., Hartwig, C., Lantow, M., Lupke, M., Mattsson, M.O., Rahman, Q. and Rollwitz, J. (2006) Hsp70 expression and free radical release after exposure to non-thermal radio-frequency electromagnetic fields and ultrafine particles in human Mono Mac 6 cells. *Toxicol Lett*, 161(1), 73–82.

Speit, G., Schütz, P. and Hoffmann, H. (2007) Genotoxic effects of exposure to radiofrequency electromagnetic fields (RF-EMF) in cultured mammalian cells are not independently reproducible. *Mutat Res*, 626(1–2), 42–47.

Stankiewicz, W., Dabrowski, M.P., Kubacki, R., Sobiczewska, E. and Szmigielski, S. (2006) Immunotropic influence of 900 MHz microwave GSM signal on human blood immune cells activated in vitro. *Electromagn Biol Med*, 25(1), 45–51.

Stronati, L., Testa, A., Moquet, J., Edwards, A., Cordelli, E., Villani, P., Marino, C., Fresegna, A.M., Appolloni, M. and Lloyd, D. (2006) 935 MHz cellular phone radiation. An in vitro study of genotoxicity in human lymphocytes. *Int J Radiat Biol*, 82(5), 339–346.

Szabo, I., Manning, M.R., Radzievsky, A.A., Wetzel, M.A., Rogers, T.J. and Ziskin. M.C. (2003) Low power millimeter wave irradiation exerts no harmful effect on human keratinocytes in vitro. *Bioelectromagnetics*, 24(3), 165–173.

Takashima, Y., Hirose, H., Koyama, S., Suzuki, Y., Taki, M. and Miyakoshi, J. (2006) Effects of continuous and intermittent exposure to RF fields with a wide range of SARs on cell growth, survival, and cell cycle distribution. *Bioelectromagnetics*, 27(5), 392–400.

Thorlin, T., Rouquette, J.M., Hamnerius, Y., Hansson, E., Persson, M., Björklund, U., Rosengren, L., Rönnbäck, L. and Persson, M. (2006) Exposure of cultured astroglial and microglial brain cells to 900 MHz microwave radiation. *Radiat Res*, 166(2), 409–421.

Tice, R.R., Hook, G.G., Donner, M., McRee, D.I. and Guy, A.W. (2002) Genotoxicity of radiofrequency signals. I. Investigation of DNA damage and micronuclei induction in cultured human blood cells. *Bioelectromagnetics*, 23(2), 113–126.

Tuschl, H., Novak, W. and Molla-Djafari, H. (2006) In vitro effects of GSM modulated radiofrequency fields on human immune cells. *Bioelectromagnetics*, 27(3), 188–196.

Vecchio, G.D., Giuliani, A., Fernandez, M., Mesirca, P., Bersani, F., Pinto, R., Ardoino, L., Lovisolo, G.A., Giardino, L. and Calza, L. (2009) Effect of radiofrequency electromagnetic field exposure on in vitro models of neurodegenerative disease. *Bioelectromagnetics*, 30(7), 564–572.

Velizarov, S., Raskmark, P. and Kwee, S. (1999) The effects of radiofrequency fields on cell proliferation are non-thermal. *Bioelectrochem Bioenerg*, 48(1), 177–180.

Vijayalaxmi, Reddy, A.B., McKenzie, R.J., McIntosh, R.L., Prihoda, T.J. and Wood, A.W. (2013) Incidence of micronuclei in human peripheral blood lymphocytes exposed to modulated and unmodulated 2450 MHz radiofrequency fields. *Bioelectromagnetics*, 34(7), 542–548.

Wang, J., Sakurai, T., Koyama, S., Komay, Yukiubara, Y., SUZUKI, Y., Taki, M. and Miyakoshi, J. (2005) Effects of 2450 MHz electromagnetic fields with a wide range of SARs on methylcholanthrene-induced transformation in C3H10T1/2 cells. *J Radiat Res*, 46(3), 351–361.

Wang, J., Koyama, S., Komatsubara, Y., Suzuki, Y., Taki, M. and Miyakoshi, J. (2006) Effects of a 2450 MHz high-frequency electromagnetic field with a wide range of SARs on the induction of heat-shock proteins in A172 cells. *Bioelectromagnetics*, 27(6), 479–486.

Wilmink, G.J., Rivest, B.D., Roth, C.C., Ibey, B.L., Payne, J.A., Cundin, L.X., Grundt, J.E., Peralta, X., Mixon, D.G. and Roach, W.P. (2011) In vitro investigation of the biological effects associated with human dermal fibroblasts exposed to 2.52THz radiation. *Laser Surg Med*, 43(2), 152–163.

Wu, G., Chen, X., Peng, J., Cai, Q., Ye, J., Xu, H., Zheng, C., Li, X., Ye, H. and Liu, X. (2012) Millimeter wave treatment induces apoptosis via activation of the mitochondrial-dependent pathway in human osteosarcoma cells. *Int J Oncol*, 40(5), 1543–1552.

Zeni, O., Di Pietro, R., d'Ambrosio, G., Massa, R., Capri, M., Naarala, J., Juutilainen, J. and Scarfi, M.R. (2007a) Formation of reactive oxygen species in L929 cells after exposure to 900 MHz RF radiation with and without co-exposure to 3-chloro-4-(dichloromethyl)-5-hydroxy-2(5H)-furanone. *Radiat Res*, 167(3), 306–311.

Zeni, O., Gallerano, G.P., Perrotta, A., Romano, M., Sannino, A., Sarti, M., Arienzo, M.D., Doria, A., Giovenale, E., Lai, A., Messina, G. and Scarfı, M.R. (2007b) Cytogenetic observations in human peripheral blood leukocytes following in vitro exposure to THz radiation: a pilot study. *Health Phys*, 92(4), 349–357.

Zhadobov, M., Sauleau, R., Le Coq, L., Debure, L., Thouroude, D., Michel, D. and Le Dréan, Y. (2007) Low-power millimeter wave radiations do not alter stress-sensitive gene expression of chaperone proteins. *Bioelectromagnetics*, 28(3), 188–196.

Zhang, M.B., He, J.L., Jin, L.F., Lu, D.Q. (2002) Study of low-intensity 2450-MHz microwave exposure enhancing the genotoxic effects of mitomycin C using micronucleus test and comet assay in vitro. *Biomed Environ Sci*, 15(4), 283–290.

Zhao, R., Zhang, S., Xu, Z., Ju, L., Lu, D. and Yao, G. (2007) Studying gene expression profile of rat neuron exposed to 1800MHz radiofrequency electromagnetic fields with cDNA microassay. *Toxicology*, 235(3), 167–175.

3

Plant Responses to Electromagnetic Fields

Massimo E. Maffei

University of Turin

CONTENTS

3.1 Introduction

During evolution, all living organisms experienced the action of the Earth's magnetic field (MF) (also called geomagnetic field, GMF), which is a natural component of the environment. GMF is steadily acting on living systems, and influences many biological processes. There are significant local differences in the strength and direction of the GMF. For instance, at the surface of the Earth, the vertical component is maximal at the magnetic pole, amounting to about $67\,\mu T$ and is zero at the magnetic equator. The horizontal component is maximal at the magnetic equator, about $33\,\mu T$, and is zero at the magnetic poles (Kobayashi et al., 2004). The MF strength at the Earth's surface ranges from less than $30\,\mu T$ in an area including most of South America and South Africa (the so-called south Atlantic anomaly) to almost $70\,\mu T$ around the magnetic poles in northern Canada and southern Australia and in part of Siberia (Maffei, 2014; Occhipinti et al., 2014; Bertea et al., 2015). Most of the magnetic field observed at the Earth's surface has an internal origin. It is mainly produced by the dynamo action of turbulent flows in the fluid metallic outer core of the planet, while little is due to external magnetic fields located in the ionosphere and the magnetosphere (Qamili et al., 2013). The GMF, through the magnetosphere, protects the Earth, together with its biosphere, from the solar wind deflecting most of its charged particles (Maffei, 2014).

The literature related to MF effects on living systems contains a plethora of contradictory reports, few successful independent replication studies, and a dearth of plausible biophysical interaction mechanisms. Most such investigations have been unsystematic, devoid of testable theoretical predictions and, ultimately, unconvincing (Harris et al., 2009). The progress and status of research on the effect of magnetic field on plant life have been reviewed in the past years (Phirke et al., 1996; Abe et al., 1997; Volpe, 2003; Belyavskaya, 2004; Bittl and Weber, 2005; Galland and Pazur, 2005; Minorsky, 2007; Vanderstraeten and Burda, 2012; Maffei, 2014; Occhipinti et al., 2014; Teixeira da Silva and Dobranszki, 2015; Teixeira da Silva and Dobranszki, 2016).

The first report on MF effects on plants dates back to the sixties, with the pioneering work of Krylov and Tarakonova (1960). They proposed an auxin-like effect of the MF on germinating seeds, by calling this effect magnetotropism. The auxin-like effect of MF was also suggested to explain ripening of tomato fruits (Boe and Salunkhe, 1963). Because of the insufficient understanding of the biological action of magnetic fields and its mechanism, it is rare to document the magnetic environment as a controlled factor for scientific experiment. Two experimental approaches aimed to evaluate the physiological responses of plant exposed to MF: response to weak or strong magnetic fields. This chapter updates data of a previously published review (Maffei, 2014).

3.2 Exposure of Plants to Low MF

The term weak or low magnetic field generally refers to the intensities from 100 nT to 0.5 mT, whereas superweak, near-null, or conditionally zero (the so called magnetic vacuum) is related to magnetic fields below 100 nT. Investigations of low MF effects on biological systems have attracted attention of biologists for several reasons. For instance, interplanetary navigation will introduce man, animals, and plants in magnetic environments where the magnetic field is near 1 nT. It is known that a galactic MF induction does not exceed 0.1 nT, in the vicinity of the Sun (0.21 nT), and on the Venus surface (3 nT) (Belov and Bochkarev, 1983). This brought a new wave of interest in MF role in regulating plant growth and development (Belyavskaya, 2004). In the laboratory, low MFs have been created by different methods, including shielding (surrounding the experimental zone by ferromagnetic metal plates with high magnetic permeability, which deviate MF and concentrate it in the metal) and compensating (by using Helmholtz coils) (Bertea et al., 2015). In general, developmental studies on plant responses have been performed at various MF intensities.

3.2.1 Effects of Low MF on Plant Development

Sunflower (*Helianthus annuus*) seedlings exposed to 20 μT vertical MF showed small, but significant increases in total fresh weights, shoot fresh weights, and root fresh weights, whereas dry weights and germination rates remained unaffected (Fischer et al., 2004).

Pea (*Pisum sativum*) epicotyls were longer in low magnetic field (11.2 ± 4.2 mm, n = 14) when compared to normal geomagnetic conditions (8.8 ± 4.0 mm, n = 12) (Yamashita et al., 2004). Elongation of pea epicotyl was confirmed, by microscopic observation of sectioned specimen, to result from the elongation of cells and osmotic pressure of seedlings was significantly higher in low MF than controls. This observation suggests that the promotion of cell elongation under low MF may relate to an increase of osmotic pressure in the cells (Negishi et al., 1999). Furthermore, pea seedlings showed ultrastructural peculiarities such as a noticeable accumulation of lipid bodies, development of a lytic compartment (vacuoles, cytosegresomes, and paramural bodies), and reduction of phytoferritin in plastids. Mitochondria were the most sensitive organelles to low MF treatment; and their size and relative volume in cells increased, matrix was electron-transparent, and cristae reduced. It was also observed that low MF effects on ultrastructure of root cells were due to disruptions in different metabolic systems including effects on Ca^{2+} homeostasis (Belyavskaya, 2001).

In broad bean (*Vicia faba*) seedlings, low MF intensities of 10 and 100 μT at 50 or 60 Hz were observed to alter membrane transport processes in root tips (Stange et al., 2002), whereas seeds of soybean (*Glycine max*) exposed to pulsed MF of 1500 nT at 0.1, 1.0 10.0, and 100.0 Hz for 5 h per day for 20 days, induced by enclosure coil systems, significantly increased the rate of seed germination, while 10 and 100 Hz pulsed MFs showed the most effective response (Radhakrishnan and Kumari, 2013). Treatment with MF also improved germination-related parameters like water uptake, speed of germination, seedling length, fresh weight, dry weight, and vigor indices of soybean seeds under laboratory conditions (Shine et al., 2011).

Controversial data have also been reported. The exposure to near null magnetic field of different *in vitro* cultures of various species of the genus *Solanum* was either stimulating or inhibiting the growth of *in vitro* plants. The effect was apparently also dependent on the species, genotype, type of initial explant, treatment duration, or even culture medium (Rakosy-Tican et al., 2005).

By using ferromagnetic shields, the influence of weak, alternating magnetic field, which was adjusted to the cyclotron frequency of Ca^{2+} and K^+ ions, was studied on the fusion of tobacco (*Nicotiana tabacum*) and soybean protoplasts. It was observed that in these conditions protoplasts fusion increased its frequency 2–3 times with the participation of calcium ions in the induction of protoplast fusion (Nedukha et al., 2007). The observations of the increase in the $[Ca^{2+}]_{cyt}$ level after exposure to very low MF suggest that Ca^{2+} entry into the cytosol might constitute an early MF sensing mechanism (Belyavskaya, 2001).

When wheat (*Triticum aestivum*) seeds were treated with low-frequency MF at the stage of esterase activation during seed swelling, the activation of esterases was enhanced by changing qualitatively the time course of the release of reaction products into the medium. These results helped to explain unusual dependences of biological effects on the amplitude of the electromagnetic field (EMF), including the atypical enhancement of these effects by the action of weak low-frequency fields (Aksenov et al., 2000). A two-layer Permalloy magnetic screen was used to test the effects of a wide range of low MF (from 20 nT to 0.1 mT) on 3–5 day old wheat seedlings. It was observed that seedlings grew slower than controls (Bogatina et al., 1978).

Barley (*Hordeum vulgare*) seedlings grown in Helmholtz coils with a 10 nT MF intensity showed a decrease in fresh weight of shoots (by 12%) and roots (by 35%), as well as dry weight of shoots (by 19%) and roots (by 48%) in comparison with GMF controls. From this pioneer study, it was concluded that very low MF was capable of delaying both organ formation and development (Lebedev et al., 1977).

The effect of a combined magnetic field at the resonance frequency of Ca^{2+} ions inside a μ-metal shield and the altered gravitropic reaction of cress (*Lepidium sativum*) roots was performed to evaluate the structure and functional organization of root cap statocytes.

The experimented conditions were observed to change normally positively gravitropic cress root to exhibit negative gravitropism (Kordyum et al., 2005).

Artificial shielding of GMF caused a significant decrease in the cell number with enhanced DNA content in root and shoot of onion (*Allium cepa*) meristems. Furthermore, the uncytokinetic mitosis with formation of binuclear and then tetranuclear cells, as well as a fusion of normal nuclei resulting in appearance of giant cells with vast nuclei, seems to dominate in very low MF conditions (Nanushyan and Murashov, 2001).

Gibberellin (GA) levels and expressions of GA biosynthetic and signaling genes have been studied in wild type Arabidopsis plants and cryptochrome double mutant, *cry1/cry2*, grown in near-null magnetic field. Wild-type GA_4, GA_9, GA_{34}, and GA_{51} levels were significantly decreased in near-null conditions compared with local GMF controls whereas the GA levels in the *cry1/cry2* mutants were similar to controls. Expressions of some GA20-oxidase and GA3-oxidase genes in wild type plants were significantly reduced in the near-null MF compared with controls. In contrast, expressions of all the detected GA biosynthetic and signaling genes in *cry1/cry2* mutants were not affected by near-null magnetic field. Based on these consideration, Xu and co-workers (Xu et al., 2017a) suggest that the effect of near-null magnetic field on Arabidopsis flowering is GA-related, which is caused by cryptochrome-involved suppression of GA biosynthesis. However, this work did not provide any proteomic or metabolomic evidence in support of the conclusions.

Changes in the ultrastructural organization of some organelles and cellular compartments, alterations in condensed chromatin distribution and reduction in volume of granular nucleolus component with the appearance of nucleolus vacuoles were also found in several other species exposed to very low MF, indicating a decrease in activities of rRNA synthesis in some nucleoli (Belyavskaya, 2004 and references cited therein).

The exposure of *Lemna minor* plants to reduced GMF significantly stimulated growth rate of the total frond area in the magnetically treated plants and suggest that the efficiency of photosystem II is not affected by variations in GMF (Jan et al., 2015).

3.2.2 Effects of Low MF on Transition to Flowering

Near-null magnetic field can be produced by three mutually perpendicular couples of Helmholtz coils and three sources of high-precision direct current power, which can counteract the vertical, north–south and east–west direction components of the geomagnetic field (Xu et al., 2012; Bertea et al., 2015).

Perilla plants (*Perilla nankinensis* Lour. Decne.) grown in weak permanent horizontal magnetic field (PHMF) of $500\,\mu T$ flux density under controlled illumination, temperature, and humidity retarded plant flowering as compared to control. This treatment increased total lipid content, including polar lipids, among them glycolipids and phospholipids; however, it did not affect the content of neutral lipids. These studies indicate that PHMF stimulated synthesis of membrane lipids of chloroplasts, mitochondria, and cytoplasm in Perilla leaves (Novitskii et al., 2016).

Although the functions of cryptochrome have been well demonstrated for *Arabidopsis thaliana*, the effect of the GMF on the growth of Arabidopsis and its mechanism of action are poorly understood. In Arabidopsis, seedlings grown in a near-null magnetic field show a flowering delay of ca. 5 days compared with those grown in the GMF. Moreover, PCR analyses of three cryptochrome-signaling-related genes, *PHYB*, *CO*, and *FT* also changed; the transcript level of *PHYB* was elevated ca. 40%, and that of *CO* and *FT* was reduced ca. 40% and 50%, respectively. These data suggest that the effects of a near-null magnetic field on Arabidopsis might be cryptochrome-related, which may be revealed by a modification of the active state of cryptochrome and the subsequent signaling cascade (Xu et al., 2012). Moreover, the biomass accumulation of plants in the near-null magnetic field was significantly suppressed at the time when plants were switching from vegetative growth to reproductive growth compared with that of plants grown in the local GMF, which was caused by the delay in the flowering of plants in the near-null magnetic field conditions. These resulted in a significant reduction of about 20% in the harvest index of plants in the near-null magnetic field compared with that of the controls. Therefore, the removal of the local geomagnetic field negatively affects the reproductive growth of Arabidopsis, which thus affects the yield and harvest index (Xu et al., 2013).

To further demonstrate that the effect of near-null magnetic field on Arabidopsis flowering is associated with CRY, Arabidopsis wild type and *cry* mutant plants were grown in the near-null magnetic field under blue or red light with different light cycle and photosynthetic photon flux density. Arabidopsis flowering was significantly suppressed by near-null magnetic field in blue light with lower intensity and shorter cycle (12 h period: 6 h light/6 h dark). However, flowering time of *cry1/cry2* mutants did not show any difference between plants grown in near-null magnetic field and in local geomagnetic field under detected light conditions. In red light, no significant difference was shown in Arabidopsis flowering between plants in near-null magnetic field and local geomagnetic field under detected light cycles and intensities. According to Xu and co-workers (Xu et al., 2015), these results suggest that changes of blue light cycle and intensity alter the effect of near-null magnetic field on Arabidopsis flowering, which is mediated by CRY. However, much more is still to be understood and a thorough proteomic and transcriptomic analysis is needed to better understand the involvement of photoreceptors in GMF perception.

3.3 Exposure of Plants to MF Intensities Higher than the Geomagnetic Filed

A consistent number of papers described the effect of MF intensities higher than the GMF levels. In general, intensities higher than the GMF relate to values higher than 100 µT. Experimental values can reach very high MF levels, ranging from 500 µT up to 15 T. Most of the attention has been focused on seed germination of important crops like wheat, rice, and legumes. However, many other physiological effects of high MF on plants described plant responses in terms of growth, development, photosynthesis, and redox status.

3.3.1 Effects of High MF on Germination

Standardization of magnetic field was done for maximum enhancement in germination characteristics of maize seeds. Seeds of maize were exposed to static magnetic fields of strength 50, 100, 150, 200, and 250 mT for 1, 2, 3, and 4 h for all field strengths. MF application enhanced percentage germination, speed of germination, seedling length, and seedling dry weight compared to unexposed control. 200 mT for 1 h exposure was found to provide the best results. Furthermore, MF exposure improved seed coat membrane integrity by reducing cellular leakage and, consequently, electrical conductivity. Experiments conducted at a research farm showed that exposure to 200 mT for 1 h prompted higher values of leaf area index, shoot length, number of leaves, chlorophyll content, shoot/root dry weight, and increased seed yield as compared to corresponding values in untreated control (Vashisth and Joshi, 2017).

Aged green pea seeds were magnetoprimed by exposure to pulsed MF of 100 mT for 1 h in three pulsed modes. The 6 min on and off MF showed significant improvement in germination (7.6%) and vigor (84.8%) over aged seeds (Bhardwaj et al., 2016).

In soybean, exposure to 100 and 200 mT MF effectively slowed the rate of biochemical degradation and loss of cellular integrity in seeds stored under conditions of accelerated aging and thus, protected the deterioration of seed quality (Kumar et al., 2015).

The speed of germination was in general increased for *Pinus taeda* L. seeds treated with a static MF of 150 mT for 10, 30, and 60 min, whereas a negative impact was found in seeds treated for 24 and 48 h (Yao and Shen, 2015).

A magnetic field applied to dormant seeds was found to increase the rate of subsequent seedling growth of barley, corn (*Zea mays*), beans, wheat, certain tree fruits, and other tree species. Moreover, a low-frequency magnetic field (16 Hz) can be used as a method of post-harvest seed improvement for different plant species, especially for seeds of temperature sensitive species germinating at low temperatures (Rochalska and Orzeszko-Rywka, 2005).

Seeds of hornwort (*Cryptotaenia japonica*) exposed to sinusoidally time-varying extremely low-frequency (ELF) magnetic fields (AC fields) in combination with the local GMF showed a promoted activity of cells and enzymes in germination stage of the seed. This suggests that an optimum ELF MF might exist for the germination of hornwort seeds under the local GMF (Kobayashi et al., 2004). The application of AC field also promoted the germination of bean (*Phaseolus vulgaris*) seeds (Sakhnini, 2007).

In seeds of mung bean (*Vigna radiata*), exposed in batches to static magnetic fields of 87–226 mT intensity for 100 min, a linear increase in germination magnetic constant with increasing intensity of MF was found. Calculated values of mean germination time, mean germination rate, germination rate coefficient, germination magnetic constant, transition time, and water uptake indicate that the impact of applied static MF improves the germination of mung beans seeds even in off-season (Mahajan and Pandey, 2014).

The seeds of pea exposed to full-wave rectified sinusoidal nonuniform MF of strength 60, 120, and 180 mT for 5, 10, and 15 min prior to sowing showed significant increase in germination. The emergence index, final emergence index, and vigor index increased by 86%, 13%, and 205%, respectively. Furthermore, it was found that exposure of 5 min for MF strengths of 60 and 180 mT significantly enhanced the germination parameters of the pea and these treatments could be used practically to accelerate the germination in pea (Iqbal et al., 2012).

MF application with a strength from 0 to 250 mT in steps of 50 mT for 1–4 h significantly enhanced speed of germination, seedling length, and seedling dry weight compared to unexposed control in chickpea (*Cicer arietinum*). It was also found that magnetically treated chickpea seeds may perform better under rainfed (un-irrigated) conditions where there was a restrictive soil moisture regime (Vashisth and Nagarajan, 2008).

Different intensities of static MF (4 or 7 mT) were tested on seed germination and seedling growth of bean or wheat seeds in different media having 0, 2, 6, and 10 atmospheres osmotic pressure prepared with sucrose or salt. The application of both MFs promoted the germination ratios, regardless of increasing osmotic pressure of sucrose or salt. The greatest germination and growth rates in both plants were from the test groups exposed to 7 mT (Cakmak et al., 2010).

Wheat seeds were imbibed in water overnight and then treated with or without a 30 mT static magnetic field (SMF) and a 10 kHz electromagnetic field (EMF) for 4 days, each 5 h.

Exposure to both MF increased the speed of germination, compared to the control group, suggesting promotional effects of EMFs on membrane integrity and growth characteristics of wheat seedlings (Payez et al., 2013).

Pre-sowing treatment of corn seeds with pulsed electromagnetic fields for 0, 15, 30, and 45 min improved germination percentage, vigor, chlorophyll content, leaf area, plant fresh and dry weight, and finally yields. Seeds that have been exposed to magnetic field for 30 and 45 min have been found to perform the best results with economic impact on producer's income in a context of a modern, organic, and sustainable agriculture (Bilalis et al., 2012).

Various combinations of MF strength and exposure time significantly improved tomato (*Solanum lycopersicum*) cv. Lignon seed performance in terms of reduction of time required for the first seeds to complete germination, time to reach 50% germination, time between 10 and 90% germination with increasing germination rate, and increased germination percentage at 4 and 7 days, seedling shoot and root length compared to the untreated control seeds. The combinations of 160 mT for 1 min and 200 mT for 1 min gave the best results (De Souza et al., 2010). Higher germination (about 11%) was observed in magnetically exposed tomato var. MST/32 seed than in non-exposed ones, suggesting a significant effect of non-uniform MFs on seed performance with respect to relative humidity (RH) (Poinapen et al., 2013a).

The effect of pre-sowing magnetic treatments was investigated on germination, growth, and yield of okra (*Abelmoschus esculentus* cv. Sapz paid) with an average magnetic field exposure of 99 mT for 3 and 11 min. A significant increase ($P < 0.05$) was observed in germination percentage, number of flowers per plant, leaf area, plant height at maturity, number of fruits per plant, pod mass per plant, and number of seeds per plant. The 99 mT for 11 min exposure showed better results as compared to control (Naz et al., 2012).

However, contrasting results have also been reported. For instance, the mean germination time of rice (*Oryza sativa*) seeds exposed to one of two magnetic field strengths (125 or 250 mT) for different times (1 min, 10 min, 20 min, 1 h, 24 h, or chronic exposure) was significantly reduced compared to controls, indicating that this type of magnetic treatment clearly affects germination and the first stages of growth of rice plants (Florez et al., 2004).

3.3.2 Effects of High MF on Cryptochrome

The blue light receptor cryptochrome can form radical pairs after exposure to blue light and has been suggested to be a potential magnetoreceptor based on the proposition that radical pairs are involved in magnetoreception. Nevertheless, the effects of MF on the function of cryptochrome are poorly understood. When Arabidopsis seedlings were grown in a 500 μT magnetic field and a near-null MF it was found that the 500 μT MF enhanced the blue light-dependent phosphorylations of CRY1 and CRY2, whereas the near-null magnetic field weakened the blue light-dependent phosphorylation of CRY2 but not CRY1. Dephosphorylations of CRY1 and CRY2 in the darkness were slowed down in the 500 μT MF, whereas dephosphorylations of CRY1 and CRY2 were accelerated in the near-null MF. These results suggest that MF with strength higher or weaker than the local geomagnetic field affects the activated states of cryptochromes, which thus modifies the functions of cryptochromes (Xu et al., 2014). Moreover, the magnitude of the hyperfine coupling constants ($A_{max}^{(iso)} = 1.75$ mT) suggests that artificial magnetic fields (0.1–0.5 mT) involved in experiments with Arabidopsis can affect the signal transduction rate. On the other hand, hyperfine interactions in the FADH$^{\bullet}$-Trp$^{\bullet+}$ biradicals are much stronger than the Zeeman interaction with the magnetic field of the Earth (≈0.05 mT). Therefore, an alternative mechanism for the bird avian compass has been proposed recently. This mechanism involves radicals with weaker hyperfine interactions ($O_2^{\bullet-}$ and $FADH^{\bullet}$), and thus, it could be more plausible for explaining incredible sensitivity of some living species to even tiny changes in the MF (Izmaylov et al., 2009).

Contrasting results were obtained when the intensity of the ambient magnetic field was varied from 33–44 to 500 μT. According to Ahmad et al. (2007), there was an enhanced growth inhibition in Arabidopsis under blue light, when cryptochromes are the mediating photoreceptor, but not under red light when the mediating receptors are phytochromes, or in total darkness. Hypocotyl growth of Arabidopsis mutants lacking cryptochromes was unaffected by the increase in magnetic intensity. Additional cryptochrome-dependent responses, such as blue-light-dependent anthocyanin accumulation and blue-light-dependent degradation of CRY2 protein, were also enhanced at the higher magnetic intensity. On the contrary, Harris et al. (2009), by using the experimental conditions chosen to match those of the Ahmad study, found that in no case consistent, statistically significant magnetic field responses were detected. For a more comprehensive discussion on cryptochromes, see below.

3.3.3 Effects of High MF on Roots and Shoots

Increased growth rates have been observed in different species when seeds where treated with increased MF. Treated corn plants grew higher and heavier than control, corresponding with increase of the total fresh weight. The greatest increases were obtained for plants continuously exposed to 125 or 250 mT (Florez et al., 2007). A stimulating effect on the first stages of growth of barley seeds was found for all exposure times studied. When germinating barley seeds were subjected to a magnetic field of 125 mT for different times (1, 10, 20, and 60 min, 24 h, and chronic exposure), increases in length and weight were observed (Martinez et al., 2000). Pants of pea exposed to 125 or 250 mT stationary MF generated by magnets under laboratory conditions for 1, 10 and 20 min, 1 and 24 h and continuous exposure were longer and heavier than the corresponding controls at each time of evaluation. The major increases occurred when seeds were continuously exposed to the MF (Carbonell et al., 2011).

Z. *mays* plants exposed to modulated continuous wave homogenous MF at specific absorption rate (SAR) of $1.69 \pm 0.0 \times 10^{-1}$ W kg^{-1} for A1/2, 1, 2, and 4 h for 7 days revealed that short-term exposure did not induce any significant change, while longer exposure of 4 h caused significant growth and biochemical alterations. Maize plants showed a reduction in the root and coleoptile length with more pronounced effect on coleoptile growth (23% reduction on 4 h exposure) (Kumar et al., 2016).

By treating with twice-gradient MF *Dioscorea opposita*, it was found that they could grow best in the seedling stage. Compared with the control, the rate of emergence increased by 39%, root number increased by 8%, and the average root length increased by 2.62 cm (Li, 2000). The 16 Hz frequency and 5 mT MF as well as alternating MF influence increased sugar beet (*Beta vulgaris* var. *saccharifera*) root and leaf yield (Rochalska, 2008), while a dramatic increase in root length, root surface area, and root volume was observed in chickpea exposed in batches to static MF of strength from 0 to 250 mT in steps of 50 mT for 1–4 h (Vashisth and Nagarajan, 2008). In the same conditions, seedlings of sunflower showed higher seedling dry weight, root length, root surface area, and root volume. Moreover, in germinating seeds, enzyme activities of α-amylase, dehydrogenase, and protease were significantly higher in treated seeds than controls (Vashisth and Nagarajan, 2010).

3.3.4 Effects of High MF on Gravitropic Responses

The growth response that is required to maintain the spatial orientation is called gravitropism and consists of three phases: reception of a gravitational signal, its transduction to a biochemical signal that is transported to the responsive cells and finally the growth response, or bending of root or shoot. Primary roots exhibit positive gravitropism, i.e., they grow in the direction of a gravitational vector. Shoots respond negatively gravitropic and grow upright opposite to the gravitational vector. However, lateral roots and shoots branches are characterized by intermediate set-point angles and grow at a particular angle that can change over time (Firn and Digby, 1997). Gravitropism typically is generated by dense particles that respond to gravity. Experimental stimulation by high-gradient MF provides a new approach to selectively manipulate the gravisensing system.

High-gradient MF has been used to induce intracellular magnetophoresis of amyloplasts and the obtained data indicate that a magnetic force can be used to study the gravisensing and response system of roots (Kuznetsov and Hasenstein, 1996). The data reported strongly support the amyloplast-based gravity-sensing system in higher plants and the usefulness of high MF to substitute gravity in shoots (Kuznetsov and Hasenstein, 1997; Kuznetsov et al., 1999). For example, in shoots of the lazy-2 mutant of tomato that exhibit negative gravitropism in the dark, but respond positively gravitropically in (red) light, induced magnetophoretic curvature showed that lazy-2 mutants perceive the displacement of amyloplasts in a similar manner than wild type and that the high MF does not affect the graviresponse mechanism (Hasenstein and Kuznetsov, 1999). Arabidopsis stems positioned in a high MF on a rotating clinostat demonstrate that the lack of apical curvature after basal amyloplast displacement indicates that gravity perception in the base is not transmitted to the apex (Weise et al., 2000). The movement of corn, wheat, and potato (*Solanum tuberosum*) starch grains in suspension was examined with videomicroscopy during parabolic flights that generated 20–25 s of weightlessness. During weightlessness, a magnetic gradient was generated by inserting a wedge into a uniform, external MF that caused repulsion of starch grains. Magnetic gradients were able to move diamagnetic compounds under weightless or microgravity conditions and serve as directional stimulus during seed germination in low-gravity environments (Hasenstein et al., 2013). The response of transgenic seedlings of Arabidopsis, containing either the CycB1-GUS proliferation marker or the DR5-GUS auxin-mediated growth marker, to diamagnetic levitation in the bore of a superconducting solenoid magnet was evaluated. Diamagnetic levitation led to changes that are very similar to those caused by real [i.e., on board the International Space Station (ISS)] or mechanically simulated microgravity [i.e., using a random positioning machine (RPM)]. These changes decoupled meristematic cell proliferation from ribosome biogenesis, and altered auxin polar transport (Manzano et al., 2013). Arabidopsis *in vitro* callus cultures were also exposed to environments with different levels of effective gravity and MF strengths simultaneously. The MF itself produced a low number of proteomic alterations, but the combination of gravitational alteration and MF exposure produced synergistic effects on the proteome of plants (Herranz et al., 2013). However, MF leads to redistribution of the cellular activities and this is why application of the proteomic analysis to the whole organs/plants is not so informative.

3.3.5 Effects of High MF on Redox Status

Effects of MFs have been related to uncoupling of free radical processes in membranes and enhanced ROS generation. It has been experimentally proven that MF can change activities of some scavenging enzymes such as catalase (CAT), superoxide dismutase (SOD), glutathione reductase (GR), glutathione transferase (GT), peroxidase (POD), ascobtate peroxidase (APX), and polyphenoloxidase (POP). Experiments have been performed on several plant species, including pea, land snail (*Helix aspesa*), radish (*Raphanus sativus*), *Leymus chinensis*, soybean, cucumber (*Cucumis stivus*), broad bean, corn, parsley (*Petroselinum crispum*), and wheat (Xia and Guo, 2000; Regoli et al., 2005; Baby et al., 2011; Polovinkina et al., 2011; Anand et al., 2012; Bhardwaj et al., 2012; Jouni et al., 2012; Radhakrishnan and Kumari, 2012; Shine and Guruprasad, 2012; Shine et al., 2012; Payez et al., 2013; Radhakrishnan and Kumari, 2013; Rajabbeigi et al., 2013; Serdyukov and Novitskii, 2013; Aleman et al., 2014; Haghighat et al., 2014). The results suggest that exposure to increased MF causes accumulation of reactive oxygen species and alteration of enzyme activities.

The effects of continuous, low-intensity static MF (7 mT) and EF (20 kV/m) on antioxidant status of shallot (*Allium ascalonicum*) leaves, increased lipid peroxidation and H_2O_2 levels in EF applied leaves. These results suggested that apoplastic constituents may work as potentially important redox regulators sensing and signaling MF changes. Static continuous MF and EF at low intensities have distinct impacts on the antioxidant system in plant leaves, and weak MF is involved in antioxidant-mediated reactions in the apoplast, resulting in overcoming a possible redox imbalance (Cakmak et al., 2012).

In mung bean seedlings treated with 600 mT MF followed by cadmium stress the concentration of malondialdehyde, H_2O_2 and O_2^-, and the conductivity of electrolyte leakage decreased, while the NO concentration and NOS activity increased compared to cadmium stress alone, showing that magnetic field compensates for the toxicological effects of cadmium exposure are related to NO signal (Chen et al., 2011).

Superoxide and hydrogen peroxide production increased in green pea germinating primed seeds by 27% and 52%, respectively, over aged seeds when exposed to 100 mT MF. In particular, NADH peroxidase and superoxide dismutase involved in generation of H_2O_2 showed increased activity in MF primed seeds. Increase in catalase, ascorbate peroxidase and glutathione reductase activity after 36 h of imbibition in primed seeds demonstrated its involvement in seed recovery during magnetopriming. An increase in total antioxidants also helped in maintaining the level of free radicals for promoting germination of magnetoprimed seeds. A 44% increase in the level of protein carbonyls after 36 h indicated involvement of protein oxidation for counteracting and/or utilizing the production of ROS and faster mobilization of reserve proteins. Higher production of free radicals in primed seeds did not cause lipid peroxidation as malondialdehyde content was low. Lipoxygenase was involved in the germination-associated events as the magnitude of activity was higher in primed aged seeds compared to aged seeds. This study elucidated that MF-mediated improvement in seed quality of aged pea seeds was facilitated by fine tuning of free radicals by the antioxidant defense system and protein oxidation (Bhardwaj et al., 2016).

3.3.6 Effects of High MF on Photosynthesis

Photosynthesis, stomatal conductance, and chlorophyll content increased in corn plants exposed to static MFs of 100 and 200 mT, compared to control under irrigated and mild stress condition (Anand et al., 2012).

Pre-seed electromagnetic treatments have been used to minimize the drought-induced adverse effects on different crop plants. Pretreatment of seeds of two corn cultivars with different magnetic treatments significantly alleviated the drought-induced adverse effects on growth by improving chlorophyll *a* (Chl *a*) and photochemical quenching and non-photochemical quenching. Of all magnetic treatments, 100 and 150 mT for 10 min were most effective in alleviating the drought-induced adverse effects (Javed et al., 2011).

Polyphasic Chl *a* fluorescence transients from magnetically treated soybean plants gave a higher fluorescence yield. The total soluble proteins of leaves showed increased intensities of the bands corresponding to a larger subunit (53 KDa) and smaller subunit (14 KDa) of Rubisco in the treated plants. Therefore, pre-sowing magnetic treatment was found to improve biomass accumulation in soybean (Shine et al., 2011).

Other general effects on MF application on chlorophyll content have been documented for several plant species (Voznyak et al., 1980; Rochalska, 2005; Turker et al., 2007; Radhakrishnan and Kumari, 2013).

The CO_2 uptake rate of MF exposed radish seedlings was lower than that of the control seedlings. The dry weight and the cotyledon area of MF exposed seedlings were also significantly lower than those of the control seedlings (Yano et al., 2004).

A MF of around 4 mT had beneficial effects, regardless of the direction of magnetic field, on the growth promotion and enhancement of CO_2 uptake of potato plantlets *in vitro*. However, the direction of magnetic field at the MF tested had no effects on the growth and CO_2 exchange rate (Iimoto et al., 1998).

A permanent magnetic field induces significant changes in bean leaf fluorescence spectra and temperature. The fluorescence intensity ratio (FIR) and change of leaf temperature ΔT increase with the increase of magnetic field intensity. The increase of ΔT due to magnetic fields is explained in bean with a simple ion velocity model. Reasonable agreement between calculated ΔT, based on the model, and measured ΔT was obtained (Jovanic and Sarvan, 2004).

The contents of maize photosynthetic pigments and total carbohydrates declined by 13% and 18%, respectively, in 4 h exposure treatments to increased MF compared to unexposed control (Kumar et al., 2016). Furthermore, the activity of starch-hydrolyzing enzymes α- and β-amylases increased by similar to 92% and 94%, respectively, at an exposure duration of 4 h, over that in the control. In response to 4 h exposure treatment, the activity of sucrolytic enzymes acid invertases and alkaline invertases increased by 88% and 266%, whereas the specific activities of phosphohydrolytic enzymes (acid phosphatases and alkaline phosphatases) showed initial increase and then declined at >2 h exposure duration. The results of this study indicate MF inhibited seedling growth of *Z. mays* by interfering with starch and sucrose metabolism (Kumar et al., 2016).

The effects of enhanced MF on growth and Chl *a* fluorescence of *Lemna minor* plants were investigated under controlled conditions in extreme geomagnetic environments of 150 mT. The strong static magnetic field seems to have the potential to increase initial Chl *a* fluorescence and energy dissipation in *Lemna minor* plants (Jan et al., 2015).

3.3.7 Effects of High MF on Lipid Composition

In radish seedlings grown in lowlight and darkness in an extremely low frequency (ELF) magnetic field characterized by 50 Hz frequency and approximate to 500 µT flux density, MF exposure increased the production of polar lipids by threefold specifically, glycolipids content increased fourfold, and phospholipids content rose 2.5 times, compared to seeds. MF stimulated lipid synthesis in chloroplast, mitochondrial, and other cell membranes (Novitskii et al., 2014). Furthermore, among fatty acids, MF exerted the strongest effect on the content of erucic acid: it increased in the light and in darkness approximately by 25% and decreased in the light by 13%. Therefore, MF behaved as a correction factor affecting lipid metabolism on the background of light and temperature action (Novitskaya et al., 2010).

Plasma membranes of seeds of tomato plants were purified, extracted, and applied to a silicon substrate in a buffer suspension and their molecular structure was studied using X-ray diffraction. While MFs had no observable effect on protein structure, enhanced lipid order was observed, leading to an increase in the gel components and a decrease in the fluid component of the lipids (Poinapen et al., 2013b).

A field experiment on cardoon seeds (*Cynara cardunculus* L.) was carried out during two successive seasons to study the effect of electromagnetic fields (EMF) on cardoon growth and its palmitic acid content. A 75 mT (millitesla) MF was used on cardoon seeds (*Cynara cardunculus* L.) during two successive seasons to study the effect of MF on plant growth and palmitic acid content. The EMF had significant effects on the palmitic acid (C16:0) content in producing seeds and the maximum value of palmitic acid content was 11.83% compared to a control value of 9.30%. These results suggest that MF treatments of cardoon seeds might have the potential to enhance the cardoon plant growth and the palmitic acid content (Sharaf-Eldin, 2016).

3.3.8 Other Effects of High MF on Plants

MF-induced DNA damage and methylation was studied in wheat calli by using random amplified polymorphic DNA and coupled restriction enzyme digestion-random amplification techniques. When calli were exposed to 7 mT static MF for 24, 48, 72, 96, or 120 h of incubation, the highest change in polymorphism rate was obtained after 120 h in both 7- and 14-day-old calli. Moreover, increase in MF duration caused DNA hypermethylation in both 7- and 14-day-old calli. The highest methylation level with a value of 25.1% was found in 7-day-old calli exposed to MF for 120 h (Aydin et al., 2016).

The effectiveness of magnetopriming was assessed for alleviation of salt-induced adverse effects on soybean growth. Soybean seeds were pretreated with static MF of 200 mT for 1h to evaluate the effect of magnetopriming on growth, carbon and nitrogen metabolism, and yield of soybean plants under different salinity levels (0, 25, and 50 mM NaCl). MF pretreatment significantly increased the number of root nodules, nodules, fresh weight, biomass accumulation, and photosynthetic performance under both nonsaline and saline conditions as compared to untreated seeds. Furthermore, nitrate reductase activity, PIABS, photosynthetic pigments, and net rate of photosynthesis were also higher in plants that emerged from MF pretreated seeds as compared to untreated seeds. MF pretreatment also increased leghemoglobin content and hemechrome content in root nodules, indicating that pre-sowing exposure of seeds to MF enhanced carbon and nitrogen metabolism, improved the yield of soybeans and alleviated salinity stress (Baghel et al., 2016).

Inflorescences from *Tradescantia* clones subjected to high MF showed pink mutations in stamen hair cells were observed (Baum and Nauman, 1984), whereas pollen grains of papaya (*Carica papaya*) exposed to MF germinated faster and produced longer pollen tubes than the controls (Alexander and Ganeshan, 1990).

In kiwifruit (*Actinidia deliciosa*), MF treatment partially removed the inhibitory effect caused by the lack of Ca^{2+} in the pollen culture medium, inducing a release of internal Ca^{2+} stored in the secretory vesicles of pollen plasma membrane (Betti et al., 2011).

Short day strawberry (*Fragaria vesca*) plants treated with MF strengths of 0.096, 0.192, and 0.384 Tesla (T) in heated greenhouse conditions showed increased fruit yield per plant (208.50 and 246.07 g, respectively) and fruit number per plant (25.9 and 27.6, respectively), but higher MF strengths than 0.096 T reduced fruit yield and fruit number. Increasing MF strength from control to 0.384 T also increased contents of N, K, Ca, Mg, Cu, Fe, Mn, Na, and Zn, but reduced P and S contents (Esitken and Turan, 2004).

The effects of pre-sowing magnetic treatments on growth and yield of tomato increased significantly (P < 0.05) the mean fruit weight, the fruit yield per plant, the fruit yield per area, and the equatorial diameter of fruits in comparison with the controls. Total dry matter was also significantly higher for plants from magnetically treated seeds than controls (De Souza et al., 2006).

In the presence of a static MF, the rhythmic leaflet movements of the plant *Desmodium gyrans* tended to slowdown. Leaflets moving up and down in a MF of approximately 50 mT flux density increased the period by about 10% due to a slower motion in the "up" position. Since, during this position, a rapid change of the extracellular potentials of the pulvinus occurs, it was proposed that the effects could be mediated via the electric processes in the pulvinus tissue (Sharma et al., 2000).

Electric process implies ion flux variations. The influence of a high-gradient MF on spatial distribution of ion fluxes along the roots, cytoplasmic streaming, and the processes of plant cell growth connected with intracellular mass and charge transfer was demonstrated (Kondrachuk and Belyavskaya, 2001).

In tomato, a significant delay in the appearance of first symptoms of geminivirus and early blight and a reduced infection rate of early blight were observed in the plants from exposed seeds to increased MFs (De Souza et al., 2006).

Single suspension-cultured plant cells of the Madagascar rosy periwinkle (*Catharanthus roseus*) and their protoplasts were anchored to a glass plate and exposed to a MF of 302 ± 8 mT for several hours. Analysis suggested that exposure to the magnetic field roughly tripled Young's modulus of the newly synthesized cell wall without any lag (Haneda et al., 2006).

In vitro tissue cultures of *Paulownia tomentosa* and *Paulownia fortunei* exposed to a magnetic flow density of 2.9–4.8 mT and 1 m s^{-1} flow rate for a period of 0, 2.2, 6.6, and 19.8 s showed increased regeneration capability of *Paulownia* cultures and a shortening of the regeneration time. When the cultures were exposed to a MF with strength of 2.9–4.8 mT for 19.8 s, the regenerated *P. tomentosa* and *P. fortunei* plants dominated the control plants (Yaycili and Alikamanoglu, 2005).

Increase in MF conditions may also affect secondary plant metabolism. The growth of suspension cultures of *Taxus chinensis* var. *mairei* and Taxol production were promoted both by a sinusoidal alternating current magnetic field (50 Hz, 3.5 mT) and by a direct current magnetic field (3.5 mT). Taxol production increased rapidly from the fourth day with the direct current MF but most slowly with the alternating current MF. The maximal yield of Taxol was 490 μg l^{-1} with the direct current MF and 425 μg l^{-1} with the alternating current MF after 8 days of culture, which were, respectively, 1.4-fold and 1.2-fold of that without exposure to a MF (Shang et al., 2004).

The biological impact of MF strengths up to 30 T on transgenic Arabidopsis plants engineered with a stress response gene consisting of the alcohol dehydrogenase (Adh) gene promoter driving the β-glucuronidase (GUS) gene reporter. Field strengths in excess of about 15 T induce expression of the Adh/GUS transgene in the roots and leaves. From the microarray analyses that surveyed 8,000 genes, 114 genes were differentially expressed to a degree greater than 2.5-fold over the control. The data suggest that MF in excess of 15 T have far-reaching effect on the genome. The widespread induction of stress-related genes and transcription factors, and a depression of genes associated with cell wall metabolism, are prominent examples. The roles of magnetic field orientation of macromolecules and magnetophoretic effects are possible factors that contribute to the mounting of this response (Paul et al., 2006).

The influence of high MF was also studied on the growth and biomass composition of *Spirulina* sp. and *Chlorella fusca* cultivated in vertical tubular photobioreactors. MFs of

30 and 60 mT for 1 h d⁻¹ stimulated *Spirulina* growth, leading to higher biomass concentration by comparison with the control culture. Increase in productivity, protein and carbo-
hydrate contents were also observed by showing that MF may also influence the growth of
Spirulina sp. (Deamici et al., 2016a,b).

3.4 Possible Mechanisms of Magnetoreception

For a number of years, laboratory studies on the biological effects of MF have demonstrated that MFs can produce or alter a wide range of phenomena. Explaining the diversity
of the reported effects is a central problem. In recent years, the following types of physical
processes or models underlying hypothetically primary mechanisms of the interaction of
MF responses in biological systems have been proposed: (a) classical and quantum oscillator models; (b) cyclotron resonance model; (c) interference of quantum states of bound
ions and electrons; (d) coherent quantum excitations; (e) biological effects of torsion fields
accompanying MF; (f) biologically active metastable states of liquid water; (g) free-radical
reactions and other "spin" mechanisms; (h) parametric resonance model; (i) stochastic
resonance as an amplifier mechanism in magnetobiology and other random processes; (j)
phase transitions in biophysical systems displaying liquid crystal ordering; (k) bifurcation
behavior of solutions of nonlinear chemical kinetics equations; (l) radio-technical models,
in which biological structures and tissues are portrayed as equivalent electric circuits; and
(m) macroscopic charged vortices in cytoplasm. Although mechanisms combining these
concepts and models cannot be excluded (Belyavskaya, 2004), a critical survey is needed
(see also Chapter 7 in *BBA*).

Observation of resonance effects at specific frequencies, combined with new theoretical considerations and calculations, indicates that birds use a radical pair with special
properties that is optimally designed as a receptor in a biological compass. This radical
pair design might be realized by cryptochrome photoreceptors if paired with molecular
oxygen as a reaction partner (Ritz et al., 2009; Ritz et al., 2010). Therefore, several considerations have suggested that cryptochromes are likely to be the primary sensory molecules of the light-dependent magnetodetection mechanism, which has been suggested
to be radical pair based (Liedvogel and Mouritsen, 2010). The molecular mechanism that
leads to formation of a stabilized, magnetic field–sensitive radical pair has despite various theoretical and experimental efforts not been unambiguously identified yet. By using
a quantum mechanical molecular dynamics approach, it was possible to follow the time
evolution of the electron transfer in an unbiased fashion and to reveal the molecular driving force that ensures fast electron transfer in cryptochrome guaranteeing formation of a
persistent radical pair suitable for magnetoreception (Ludemann et al., 2015).

In plants, cryptochromes control different aspects of growth and development (Wang
et al., 2014; Liu et al., 2016); i.e., involvement in de-etiolation responses such as inhibition
of hypocotyl growth (Ahmad and Cashmore, 1993; Lin, 2002), anthocyanin accumulation
(Ahmad et al., 1995), leaf and cotyledon expansion (Cashmore et al., 1999; Lin, 2002), transitions to flowering (El-Assal et al., 2003), or regulation of blue-light-regulated genes (Jiao
et al., 2003). In Arabidopsis, cryptochromes are encoded by two similar genes, *cry1* and
cry2. CRY2 protein levels in seedlings decrease rapidly upon illumination by blue light,
presumably as a result of protein degradation of the light-activated form of the receptor
(Ahmad et al., 2007). Like photolyases, plant cryptochromes undergo a light-dependent

electron transfer reaction, known as photoactivation, that leads to photoreduction of the flavin cofactor, FAD (Giovani et al., 2003).

Particular attention has been paid to the potential role of cryptochrome as a plant magnetosensor (Ahmad and Cashmore, 1993; Ang et al., 1998; Chattopadhyay et al., 1998; Mockler et al., 1999; Lin, 2002; El-Assal et al., 2003; Giovani et al., 2003; Jiao et al., 2003; Zeugner et al., 2005; Ahmad et al., 2007; Bouly et al., 2007; Kleine et al., 2007; Solov'yov et al., 2008; Harris et al., 2009; Liedvogel and Mouritsen, 2010; Ritz et al., 2010; Solov'yov and Schulten, 2012; Wan et al., 2015; Wan et al., 2016; Wang et al., 2016; Xu et al., 2017a,b).

Experiments on Arabidopsis have suggested that magnetic intensity affects cryptochrome-dependent growth responses (Ahmad et al., 2007). But, as discussed above, these reported cryptochrome-mediated magnetic field effects on plant growth could not be replicated in an independent study (Harris et al., 2009). These findings would be very important, if they turn out to exist and be independently replicable, since even though magnetic responses do not seem biologically relevant for the plant, they would show in principle that biological tissue is sensitive to the magnetic field responses that are linked to cryptochrome-dependent signaling pathways. They could thus confirm the ability of cryptochrome to mediate magnetic field responses (Liedvogel and Mouritsen, 2010).

The claimed magnetosensitive responses can best be explained by the radical pair model, as Arabidopsis cryptochromes form radical pairs after photoexcitation (Giovani et al., 2003; Zeugner et al., 2005; Bouly et al., 2007) and these experiments might reflect common physical properties of photoexcited cryptochromes in both plants and animals.

The radical-pair mechanism is currently the only physically plausible mechanism by which magnetic interactions that are orders of magnitude weaker than the average thermal energy, $k_B T$, can affect chemical reactions. The kinetics and quantum yields of photo-induced flavin-tryptophan radical pairs in cryptochrome are indeed magnetically sensitive and cryptochrome is a good candidate as a chemical magnetoreceptor. Cryptochromes have also attracted attention as potential mediators of biological effects of extremely low frequency (ELF) electromagnetic fields and possess properties required to respond to Earth-strength (approximately 50 μT) fields at physiological temperatures (Maeda et al., 2012).

Recently, a combination of quantum biology and molecular dynamics simulations on plant cryptochrome has demonstrated that after photoexcitation a radical pair forms, becomes stabilized through proton transfer, and decays back to the protein's resting state on time scales allowing the protein, in principle, to act as a radical pair-based magnetic sensor (Solov'yov and Schulten, 2012 and references therein; Maffei, 2014; Occhipinti et al., 2014). Furthermore, the elimination of the local geomagnetic field weakens the inhibition of Arabidopsis hypocotyl growth by white light, and delays flowering time. The expression changes of three Arabidopsis cryptochrome-signaling-related genes (*PHYB*, *CO*, and *FT*) suggest that the effects of a near-null magnetic field are cryptochrome-related, which may be revealed by a modification of the active state of cryptochrome and the subsequent signaling cascade plant cryptochrome has been suggested to act as a magnetoreceptor (Xu et al., 2012).

3.5 Conclusion and Perspectives

Revealing the relationships between MF and plant responses is becoming more and more important as new evidence reveals the ability of plants to perceive and respond quickly to varying MF by altering their gene expression and phenotype. The recent implications of MF reversal with plant evolution (Occhipinti et al., 2014; Bertea et al., 2015) open new horizons not only in plant science but also to the whole biosphere, from the simplest organisms to human beings.

Magnetotactic bacteria are a diverse group of microorganisms with the ability to orient and migrate along geomagnetic field lines (Yan et al., 2012); the avian magnetic compass has been well characterized in behavioral tests (Ritz et al., 2009); magnetic alignment, which constitutes the simplest directional response to the GMF, has been demonstrated in diverse animals including insects, amphibians, fish, and mammals (Begall et al., 2013); concerns of possible biological effects of environmental electromagnetic fields on the basis of the energy required to rotate the small crystals of biogenic magnetite that have been discovered in various human tissues have been discussed (Kobayashi and Kirschvink, 1995). The overall picture is thus a general effect of GMF on life forms.

Life evolved on Earth along changes in the GMF life history. Any other environment lacking a GMF is expected to generate reactions in living organisms. These concerns become urgent questions in light of planned long-term flights to other planets (Belyavskaya, 2004). Understanding GMF effects on life will provide the fundamental background necessary to understand evolution of life forms in our planet and will help us to develop scientific recommendations for design of life-support systems and their biotic components for future space exploration.

References

Abe, K., N. Fujii, I. Mogi, M. Motokawa, and H. Takahashi. 1997. Effect of a high magnetic field on plant. *Biol Sci Space* 11: 240–247.

Ahmad, M., and A.R. Cashmore. 1993. Hy4 gene of *A. thaliana* encodes a protein with characteristics of a blue-light photoreceptor. *Nature* 366: 162–166.

Ahmad, M., P. Galland, T. Ritz, R. Wiltschko, and W. Wiltschko. 2007. Magnetic intensity affects cryptochrome-dependent responses in *Arabidopsis thaliana*. *Planta* 225: 615–624.

Ahmad, M., C.T. Lin, and A.R. Cashmore. 1995. Mutations throughout an arabidopsis blue-light photoreceptor impair blue-light-responsive anthocyanin accumulation and inhibition of hypocotyl elongation. *Plant J* 8: 653–658.

Aksenov, S.I., A.A. Bulychev, T.Y. Grunina, and V.B. Turovetskii. 2000. Effect of low-frequency magnetic field on esterase activity and pH changes near the wheat germ during imbibition of seeds. *Biofizika* 45: 737–745.

Aleman, E.I., A. Mbogholi, Y.F. Boix, J. Gonzalez-Ohnedo, and A. Chalfun. 2014. Effects of EMFs on some biological parameters in coffee plants (*Coffea arabica* L.) obtained by in vitro propagation. *Polish J Environ Stud* 23: 95–101.

Alexander, M.P., and S. Ganeshan. 1990. Electromagnetic field-induced in vitro pollen germination and tube growth. *Current Sci* 59: 276–277.

Anand, A., S. Nagarajan, A. Verma, D. Joshi, P. Pathak, and J. Bhardwaj. 2012. Pre-treatment of seeds with static magnetic field ameliorates soil water stress in seedlings of maize (*Zea mays* L.). *Indian J Biochem Biophys* 49: 63–70.

Ang, L.H., S. Chattopadhyay, N. Wei, et al., 1998. Molecular interaction between COP1 and HY5 defines a regulatory switch for light control of Arabidopsis development. *Mol Cell* 1: 213–222.

Aydin, M., M.S. Taspinar, Z.E. Cakmak, R. Dumlupinar, and G. Agar. 2016. Static magnetic field induced epigenetic changes in wheat callus. *Bioelectromagnetics* 37: 504–511.

Baby, S.M., G.K. Narayanaswamy, and A. Anand. 2011. Superoxide radical production and performance index of Photosystem II in leaves from magnetoprimed soybean seeds. *Plant Sign Behav* 6: 1635–1637.

Baghel, L., S. Kataria, and K.N. Guruprasad. 2016. Static magnetic field treatment of seeds improves carbon and nitrogen metabolism under salinity stress in soybean. *Bioelectromagnetics* 37: 455–470.

Baum, J.W., and C.H. Nauman. 1984. Influence of strong magnetic fields on genetic endpoints in *Tradescantia tetrads* and stamen hairs. *Environ Mutagen* 6: 49–58.

Begall, S., E. Pascal Malkemper, J. Cerveny, P. Nemec, and H. Burda. 2013. Magnetic alignment in mammals and other animals. *Mammal Biol* 78: 10–20.

Belov, K.P., and N.G. Bochkarev. 1983. *Magnetism on the Earth and in Space.* Moskow: Nauka.

Belyavskaya, N.A. 2001. Ultrastructure and calcium balance in meristem cells of pea roots exposed to extremely low magnetic fields. *Adv Space Res* 28: 645–650.

Belyavskaya, N.A. 2004. Biological effects due to weak magnetic field on plants. *Adv Space Res* 34: 1566–1574.

Bertea, C.M., R. Narayana, C. Agliassa, C.T. Rodgers, and M.E. Maffei. 2015. Geomagnetic field (GMF) and plant evolution: investigating the effects of GMF reversal on *Arabidospis thaliana* development and gene expression. *J Visual Exp* 105: e53286.

Betti, L., G. Trebbi, F. Fregola, et al., 2011. Weak static and extremely low frequency magnetic fields affect in vitro pollen germination. *Sci World J* 11: 875–890.

Bhardwaj, J., A. Anand, and S. Nagarajan. 2012. Biochemical and biophysical changes associated with magnetopriming in germinating cucumber seeds. *Plant Physiol Biochem* 57: 67–73.

Bhardwaj, J., A. Anand, V.K. Pandita, and S. Nagarajan. 2016. Pulsed magnetic field improves seed quality of aged green pea seeds by homeostasis of free radical content. *J Food Sci Technol* 53: 3969–3977.

Bilalis, D.J., N. Katsenios, A. Efthimiadou, and A. Karkanis. 2012. Pulsed electromagnetic field: an organic compatible method to promote plant growth and yield in two corn types. *Electromagn Biol Med* 31: 333–343.

Bittl, R., and S. Weber. 2005. Transient radical pairs studied by time-resolved EPR. *Biochim Biophys Acta-Bioenerg* 1707: 117–126.

Boe, A.A., and D.K. Salunkhe. 1963. Effects of Magnetic Fields on Tomato Ripening. *Nature* 199: 91–92.

Bogatina, N.I., B.I. Verkin, and V.A. Kordyum. 1978. Effect of permanent magnetic fields with different intensities on the wheat growth rate. *Dokl Akad Nauk Ukr SSR, Ser B* 4: 352–356.

Bouly, J.P., E. Schleicher, M. Onisio-Sese, et al., 2007. Cryptochrome blue light photoreceptors are activated through interconversion of flavin redox states. *J Biol Chem* 282: 9383–9391.

Cakmak, T., Z.E. Cakmak, R. Dumlupinar, and T. Tekinay. 2012. Analysis of apoplastic and symplastic antioxidant system in shallot leaves: Impacts of weak static electric and magnetic field. *J Plant Physiol* 169: 1066–1073.

Cakmak, T., R. Dumlupinar, and S. Erdal. 2010. Acceleration of germination and early growth of wheat and bean seedlings grown under various magnetic field and osmotic conditions. *Bioelectromagnetics* 31: 120–129.

Carbonell, M.V., M. Florez, E. Martinez, R. Maqueda, and J. Amaya. 2011. Study of stationary magnetic fields on initial growth of pea (*Pisum sativum* L.) seeds. *Seed Sci Technol* 39: 673–679.

Cashmore, A.R., J.A. Jarillo, Y.J. Wu, and D.M. Liu. 1999. Cryptochromes: Blue light receptors for plants and animals. *Science* 284: 760–765.

Chattopadhyay, S., L.H. Ang, P. Puente, X.W. Deng, and N. Wei. 1998. Arabidopsis bZIP protein HY5 directly interacts with light-responsive promoters in mediating light control of gene expression. *Plant Cell* 10: 673–683.

Chen, Y.P., R. Li, and J.M. He. 2011. Magnetic field can alleviate toxicological effect induced by cadmium in mungbean seedlings. *Ecotoxicology* 20: 760–769.

De Souza, A., D. Garcia, L. Sueiro, F. Gilart, E. Porras, and L. Licea. 2006. Pre-sowing magnetic treatments of tomato seeds increase the growth and yield of plants. *Bioelectromagnetics* 27: 247–257.

De Souza, A., L. Sueiro, D. Garcia, and E. Porras. 2010. Extremely low frequency non-uniform magnetic fields improve tomato seed germination and early seedling growth. *Seed Sci Technol* 38: 61–72.

Deamici, K.M., B.B. Cardias, J.A. Vieira Costa, and L.O. Santos. 2016a. Static magnetic fields in culture of Chlorella fusca: Bioeffects on growth and biomass composition. *Process Biochemistry* 51: 912–916.

Deamici, K.M., J.A. Costa, and L.O. Santos. 2016b. Magnetic fields as triggers of microalga growth: evaluation of its effect on Spirulina sp. *Bioresour Technol* 220: 62–67.

El-Assal, S.E.D., C. Alonso-Blanco, A.J.M. Peeters, C. Wagemaker, J.L. Weller, and M. Koornneef. 2003. The role of cryptochrome 2 in flowering in Arabidopsis. *Plant Physiol* 133: 1504–1516.

Esitken, A., and M. Turan. 2004. Alternating magnetic field effects on yield and plant nutrient element composition of strawberry (*Fragaria x ananassa* cv. Camarosa). *Acta Agric Scand Sect B-Soil Plant Sci* 54: 135–139.

Firn, R.D., and J. Digby. 1997. Solving the puzzle of gravitropism—Has a lost piece been found? *Planta* 203: S159–S163.

Fischer, G., M. Tausz, M. Kock, and D. Grill. 2004. Effects of weak 162/3 Hz magnetic fields on growth parameters of young sunflower and wheat seedlings. *Bioelectromagnetics* 25: 638–641.

Florez, M., M.V. Carbonell, and E. Martinez. 2004. Early sprouting and first stages of growth of rice seeds exposed to a magnetic field. *Electromagn Biol Med* 23: 157–166.

Florez, M., M.V. Carbonell, and E. Martinez. 2007. Exposure of maize seeds to stationary magnetic fields: Effects on germination and early growth. *Environ Exper Bot* 59: 68–75.

Galland, P., and A. Pazur. 2005. Magnetoreception in plants. *J Plant Res* 118: 371–389.

Giovani, B., M. Byrdin, M. Ahmad, and K. Brettel. 2003. Light-induced electron transfer in a cryptochrome blue-light photoreceptor. *Nature Struct Biol* 10: 489–490.

Haghighat, N., P. Abdolmaleki, F. Ghanati, M. Behmanesh, and A. Payez. 2014. Modification of catalase and MAPK in *Vicia faba* cultivated in soil with high natural radioactivity and treated with a static magnetic field. *J Plant Physiol* 171: 99–103.

Haneda, T., Y. Fujimura, and M. Iino. 2006. Magnetic field exposure stiffens regenerating plant protoplast cell walls. *Bioelectromagnetics* 27: 98–104.

Harris, S.R., K.B. Henbest, K. Maeda, et al., 2009. Effect of magnetic fields on cryptochrome-dependent responses in *Arabidopsis thaliana*. *J Royal Soc Interf* 6: 1193–1205.

Hasenstein, K.H., S. John, P. Scherp, D. Povinelli, and S. Mopper. 2013. Analysis of Magnetic Gradients to Study Gravitropism. *Am J Bot* 100: 249–255.

Hasenstein, K.H., and O.A. Kuznetsov. 1999. The response of lazy-2 tomato seedlings to curvature-inducing magnetic gradients is modulated by light. *Planta* 208: 59–65.

Herranz, R., A.I. Manzano, J.J.W.A. van Loon, P.C.M. Christianen, and F.J. Medina. 2013. Proteomic signature of arabidopsis cell cultures exposed to magnetically induced hyper- and microgravity environments. *Astrobiology* 13: 217–224.

Iimoto, M., K. Watanabe, and K. Fujiwara. 1998. Effects of magnetic flux density and direction of the magnetic field on growth and CO_2 exchange rate of potato plantlets in vitro. *Acta Hortic* 440: 606–610.

Iqbal, M., D. Muhammad, U.H. Zia, Y. Jamil, and M. Ahmad. 2012. Effect of pre-sowing magnetic field treatment to garden pea (*Pisum sativum* L.) seed on germination and seedling growth. *Pakistan J Bot* 44: 1851–1856.

Izmaylov, A.F., J.C. Tully, and M.J. Frisch. 2009. Relativistic interactions in the radical pair model of magnetic field sense in CRY-1 protein of *Arabidopsis thaliana*. *J Phys Chem A* 113: 12276–12284.

Jan, L., D. Fefer, K. Kosmelj, A. Gaberscik, and I. Jerman. 2015. Geomagnetic and strong staticmagnetic field effects on growth and chlorophylla fluorescencein lemna minor. *Bioelectromagnetics* 36: 190–203.

Javed, N., M. Ashraf, N.A. Akram, and F. Al-Qurainy. 2011. Alleviation of adverse effects of drought stress on growth and some potential physiological attributes in maize (*Zea mays* L.) by seed electromagnetic treatment. *Photochem Photobiol* 87: 1354–1362.

Jiao, Y., H. Yang, L. Ma, et al., 2003. A genome-wide analysis of blue-light regulation of Arabidopsis transcription factor gene expression during seedling development. *Plant Physiol* 133: 1480–1493.

Jouni, F.J., P. Abdolmaleki, and F. Ghanati. 2012. Oxidative stress in broad bean (*Vicia faba* L.) induced by static magnetic field under natural radioactivity. *Mut Res -Gen Toxicol Environ Mutag* 741: 116–121.

Jovanic, B.R., and M.Z. Sarvan. 2004. Permanent magnetic field and plant leaf temperature. *Electromagn Biol Med* 23: 1–5.

Kleine, T., P. Kindgren, C. Benedict, L. Hendrickson, and A. Strand. 2007. Genome-wide gene expression analysis reveals a critical role for CRYPTOCHROME1 in the response of arabidopsis to high irradiance. *Plant Physiol* 144: 1391–1406.

Kobayashi, A., and J.L. Kirschvink. 1995. Magnetoreception and electromagnetic field effects: Sensory perception of the geomagnetic field in animals and humans. *Adv Chem Ser* 250: 367–394.

Kobayashi, M., N. Soda, T. Miyo, and Y. Ueda. 2004. Effects of combined DC and AC magnetic fields on germination of hornwort seeds. *Bioelectromagnetics* 25: 552–559.

Kondrachuk, A., and N. Belyavskaya. 2001. The influence of the HGMF on mass-charge transfer in gravisensing cells. *J Gravit Physiol* 8: 37–38.

Kordyum, E.L., N.I. Bogatina, Y.M. Kalinina, and N.V. Sheykina. 2005. A weak combined magnetic field changes root gravitropism. *Adv Space Res* 36: 1229–1236.

Krylov, A., and G.A. Tarakonova. 1960. Plant physiology. *Fiziol Rost* 7: 156.

Kumar, A., H.P. Singh, D.R. Batish, S. Kaur, and R.K. Kohli. 2016. EMF radiations (1800 MHz)-inhibited early seedling growth of maize (Zea mays) involves alterations in starch and sucrose metabolism. *Protoplasma* 253: 1043–1049.

Kumar, M., B. Singh, S. Ahuja, A. Dahuja, and A. Anand. 2015. Gamma radiation and magnetic field mediated delay in effect of accelerated ageing of soybean. *J Food Sci Technol* 52: 4785–4796.

Kuznetsov, O.A., and K.H. Hasenstein. 1996. Intracellular magnetophoresis of amyloplasts and induction of root curvature. *Planta* 198: 87–94.

Kuznetsov, O.A., and K.H. Hasenstein. 1997. Magnetophoretic induction of curvature in coleoptiles and hypocotyls. *J Exper Bot* 48: 1951–1957.

Kuznetsov, O.A., J. Schwuchow, F.D. Sack, and K.H. Hasenstein. 1999. Curvature induced by amyloplast magnetophoresis in protonemata of the moss *Ceratodon purpureus*. *Plant Physiol* 119: 645–650.

Lebedev, S.I., P.I. Baranskiy, L.G. Litvinenko, and L.T. Shiyan. 1977. Barley growth in superweak magnetic field. *Electr Treat Mat* 3: 71–73.

Li, A. 2000. Effect of gradient magnetic field on growth of stem pearls of *Dioscorea opposita* during seedling stage. *Zhongg Zhong Zazhi* 25: 341–343.

Liedvogel, M., and H. Mouritsen. 2010. Cryptochromes-a potential magnetoreceptor: what do we know and what do we want to know? *J Royal Soc Interf* 7: S147–S162.

Lin, C.T. 2002. Blue light receptors and signal transduction. *Plant Cell* 14: S207–S225.

Liu, B.B., Z.H. Yang, A. Gomez, B. Liu, C.T. Lin, and Y. Oka. 2016. Signaling mechanisms of plant cryptochromes in Arabidopsis thaliana. *J Plant Res* 129: 137–148.

Ludemann, G., I.A. Solov'yov, T. Kubar, and M. Elstner. 2015. Solvent driving force ensures fast formation of a persistent and well-separated radical pair in plant cryptochrome. *J Am Chem Soc* 137: 1147–1156.

Maeda, K., A.J. Robinson, K.B. Henbest, et al., 2012. Magnetically sensitive light-induced reactions in cryptochrome are consistent with its proposed role as a magnetoreceptor. *Proc Natl Acad Sci USA* 109: 4774–4779.

Maffei, M.E. 2014. Magnetic field effects on plant growth, development, and evolution. *Front Plant Sci* 5.

Mahajan, T.S., and O.P. Pandey. 2014. Magnetic-time model at off-season germination. *Int Agrophys* 28: 57–62.

Manzano, A.I., O.J. Larkin, C.E. Dijkstra, et al., 2013. Meristematic cell proliferation and ribosome biogenesis are decoupled in diamagnetically levitated Arabidopsis seedlings. *Bmc Plant Biol* 13.

Martinez, E., M.V. Carbonell, and J.M. Amaya. 2000. A static magnetic field of 125 mT stimulates the initial growth stages of barley (*Hordeum vulgare* L.). *Electro Magnetobiol* 19: 271–277.

Minorsky, P.V. 2007. Do geomagnetic variations affect plant function? *J Atm Solar-Terrestr Phys* 69: 1770–1774.

Mockler, T.C., H.W. Guo, H.Y. Yang, H. Duong, and C.T. Lin. 1999. Antagonistic actions of Arabidopsis cryptochromes and phytochrome B in the regulation of floral induction. *Development* 126: 2073–2082.

Nanushyan, E.R., and V.V. Murashov. 2001. Plant meristem cell response to stress factors of the geomagnetic field (GMF) fluctuations. In *Plant under Environmental Stress*, pp. 204–205. Moscow: Friendship University of Russia.

Naz, A., Y. Jamil, Z. ul Haq, et al., 2012. Enhancement in the germination, growth and yield of Okra (*Abelmoschus esculentus*) using pre-sowing magnetic treatment of seeds. *Indian J Biochem Biophysi* 49: 211–214.

Nedukha, O., E. Kordyum, N. Bogatina, M. Sobol, T. Vorobyeva, and Y. Ovcharenko. 2007. The influence of combined magnetic field on the fusion of plant protoplasts. *J Gravit Physiol* 14: 117–118.

Negishi, Y., A. Hashimoto, M. Tsushima, C. Dobrota, M. Yamashita, and T. Nakamura. 1999. Growth of pea epicotyl in low magnetic field implication for space research. *Adv Space Res* 23: 2029–2032.

Novitskaya, G.V., D. Molokanov, T. Kocheshkova, and Yu.I. Novitskii. 2010. Effect of weak constant magnetic field on the composition and content of lipids in radish seedlings at various temperatures. *Russ J Plant Physiol* 57: 52–61.

Novitskii, Y., G. Novitskaya, and Y. Serdyukov. 2016. Effect of weak permanent magnetic field on lipid composition and content in perilla leaves. *Bioelectromagnetics* 37: 108–115.

Novitskii, Y.I., G.V. Novitskaya, and Y.A. Serdyukov. 2014. Lipid utilization in radish seedlings as affected by weak horizontal extremely low frequency magnetic field. *Bioelectromagnetics* 35: 91–99.

Occhipinti, A., A. De Santis, and M.E. Maffei. 2014. Magnetoreception: an unavoidable step for plant evolution? *Trends Plant Sci* 19: 1–4.

Paul, A.L., R.J. Ferl, and M.W. Meisel. 2006. High magnetic field induced changes of gene expression in arabidopsis. *Biomagn Res Technol* 4: 7.

Payez, A., F. Ghanati, M. Behmanesh, P. Abdolmaleki, A. Hajnorouzi, and E. Rajabbeigi. 2013. Increase of seed germination, growth and membrane integrity of wheat seedlings by exposure to static and a 10-KHz electromagnetic field. *Electromagn Biol Med* 32: 417–429.

Phirke, P.S., A.B. Kubde, and S.P. Umbarkar. 1996. The influence of magnetic field on plant growth. *Seed Sci Technol* 24: 375–392.

Poinapen, D., D.C.W. Brown, and G.K. Beeharry. 2013a. Seed orientation and magnetic field strength have more influence on tomato seed performance than relative humidity and duration of exposure to non-uniform static magnetic fields. *J Plant Physiol* 170: 1251–1258.

Poinapen, D., L. Toppozini, H. Dies, D.C.W. Brown, and M.C. Rheinstadter. 2013b. Static magnetic fields enhance lipid order in native plant plasma membrane. *Soft Matter* 9: 6804–6813.

Polovinkina, E., E. Kal'yasova, Yu.V. Sinitsina, and A. Veselov. 2011. Effect of weak pulse magnetic fields on lipid peroxidation and activities of antioxidant complex components in pea chloroplasts. *Russ J Plant Physiol* 58: 1069–1073.

Qamili, E., A. De Santis, A. Isac, M. Mandea, B. Duka, and A. Simonyan. 2013. Geomagnetic jerks as chaotic fluctuations of the Earth's magnetic field. *Geochem Geophys Geosys* 14: 839–850.

Radhakrishnan, R., and B.D.R. Kumari. 2012. Pulsed magnetic field: A contemporary approach offers to enhance plant growth and yield of soybean. *Plant Physiol Biochem* 51: 139–144.

Radhakrishnan, R., and B.D.R. Kumari. 2013. Influence of pulsed magnetic field on soybean (*Glycine max* L.) seed germination, seedling growth and soil microbial population. *Indian J Biochem Biophys* 50: 312–317.

Rajabbeigi, E., F. Ghanati, P. Abdolmaleki, and A. Payez. 2013. Antioxidant capacity of parsley cells (*Petroselinum crispum* L.) in relation to iron-induced ferritin levels and static magnetic field. *Electromagn Biol Med* 32: 430–441.

Rakosy-Tican, L., C.M. Aurori, and V.V. Morariu. 2005. Influence of near null magnetic field on in vitro growth of potato and wild Solanum species. *Bioelectromagnetics* 26: 548–557.

Regoli, F., S. Gorbi, N. Marchella, S. Tedesco, and G. Principato. 2005. Pro-oxidant effects of extremely low frequency electromagnetic fields in the land snail *Helix aspesa*. *Free Radic Biol Med* 39: 1620–1628.

Ritz, T., R. Wiltschko, P.J. Hore, et al., 2009. Magnetic Compass of Birds Is Based on a Molecule with Optimal Directional Sensitivity. *Biophys J* 96: 3451–3457.

Ritz, T., T. Yoshii, C. Helfrich-Foester, and M. Ahmad. 2010. Cryptochrome: A photoreceptor with the properties of a magnetoreceptor? *Commun Integr Biol* 3: 24–27.

Rochalska, M. 2005. Influence of frequent magnetic field on chlorophyll content in leaves of sugar beet plants. *Nukleonika* 50: S25–S28.

Rochalska, M. 2008. The influence of low frequency magnetic field upon cultivable plant physiology. *Nukleonika* 53: S17–S20.

Rochalska, M., and A. Orzeszko-Rywka. 2005. Magnetic field treatment improves seed performance. *Seed Sci Technol* 33: 669–674.

Sakhnini, L. 2007. Influence of Ca^{2+} in biological stimulating effects of AC magnetic fields on germination of bean seeds. *J Magnet Magn Mater* 310: E1032–E1034.

Serdyukov, Y.A., and Y.I. Novitskii. 2013. Impact of weak permanent magnetic field on antioxidant enzyme activities in radish seedlings. *Russ J Plant Physiol* 60: 69–76.

Shang, G.M., J.C. Wu, and Y.J. Yuan. 2004. Improved cell growth and Taxol production of suspension-cultured *Taxus chinensis* var. *mairei* in alternating and direct current magnetic fields. *Biotechnol Lett* 26: 875–878.

Sharaf-Eldin, M.A. 2016. The effects of electromagnetic treatments on the growth and palmitic acid content of *Cynara cardunculus*. *J Anim Plant Sci* 26: 1081–1086.

Sharma, V.K., W. Engelmann, and A. Johnsson. 2000. Effects of static magnetic field on the ultradian lateral leaflet movement rhythm in *Desmodium gyrans*. *Z Naturforsc C-J Biosci* 55: 638–642.

Shine, M., and K. Guruprasad. 2012. Impact of pre-sowing magnetic field exposure of seeds to stationary magnetic field on growth, reactive oxygen species and photosynthesis of maize under field conditions. *Acta Physiol Plant* 34: 255–265.

Shine, M., K. Guruprasad, and A. Anand. 2011. Enhancement of germination, growth, and photosynthesis in soybean by pre-treatment of seeds with magnetic field. *Bioelectromagnetics* 32: 474–484.

Shine, M., K. Guruprasad, and A. Anand. 2012. Effect of stationary magnetic field strengths of 150 and 200 mT on reactive oxygen species production in soybean. *Bioelectromagnetics* 33: 428–437.

Solov'yov, I.A., D.E. Chandler, and K. Schulten. 2008. Exploring the possibilities for radical pair effects in cryptochrome. *Plant Sign Behav* 3: 676–677.

Solov'yov, I.A., and K. Schulten. 2012. Reaction kinetics and mechanism of magnetic field effects in cryptochrome. *J Phys Chem B* 116: 1089–1099.

Stange, B.C., R.E. Rowland, B.I. Rapley, and J.V. Podd. 2002. ELF magnetic fields increase amino acid uptake into Vicia faba L. roots and alter ion movement across the plasma membrane. *Bioelectromagnetics* 23: 347–354.

Teixeira da Silva, J.A., and J. Dobranszki. 2015. How do magnetic fields affect plants in vitro? *In Vitro Cell Dev Biol-Plant* 51: 233–240.

Teixeira da Silva, J.A., and J. Dobranszki. 2016. Magnetic fields: how is plant growth and development impacted? *Protoplasma* 253: 231–248.

Turker, M., C. Temirci, P. Battal, and M.E. Erez. 2007. The effects of an artificial and static magnetic field on plant growth, chlorophyll and phytohormone levels in maize and sunflower plants. *Phyton-Ann Rei Botan* 46: 271–284.

Vanderstraeten, J., and H. Burda. 2012. Does magnetoreception mediate biological effects of power-frequency magnetic fields? *Sci Tot Environ* 417: 299–304.

Vashisth, A., and D.K. Joshi. 2017. Growth Characteristics of Maize Seeds Exposed to Magnetic Field. *Bioelectromagnetics* 38: 151–157.

Vashisth, A., and S. Nagarajan. 2008. Exposure of seeds to static magnetic field enhances germination and early growth characteristics in chickpea (*Cicer arietinum* L.). *Bioelectromagnetics* 29: 571–578.

Vashisth, A., and S. Nagarajan. 2010. Effect on germination and early growth characteristics in sunflower (*Helianthus annuus*) seeds exposed to static magnetic field. *J Plant Physiol* 167: 149–156.

Volpe, P. 2003. Interactions of zero-frequency and oscillating magnetic fields with biostructures and biosystems. *Photochem Photobiol Sci* 2: 637–648.

Voznyak, V.M., I.B. Ganago, A.A. Moskalenko, and E.I. Elfimov. 1980. Magnetic field-induced fluorescence changes in chlorophyll-proteins enriched with P-700. *Biochim Biophys Acta* 592: 364–368.

Wan, G.-J., W.-J. Wang, J.-J. Xu, et al., 2015. Cryptochromes and hormone signal transduction under near-zero magnetic fields: new clues to magnetic field effects in a rice planthopper. *Plos One* 10: e0132966.

Wan, G.-J., R. Yuan, W.-J. Wang, et al., 2016. Reduced geomagnetic field may affect positive phototaxis and flight capacity of a migratory rice planthopper. *Anim Behav* 121: 107–116.

Wang, W.X., H.L. Lian, L.D. Zhang, et al., 2016. Transcriptome analyses reveal the involvement of both c and n termini of cryptochrome 1 in its regulation of phytohormone-responsive gene expression in arabidopsis. *Front Plant Sci* 7: 294

Wang, X., Q. Wang, P. Nguyen, and C.T. Lin. 2014. Cryptochrome-mediated light responses in plants. In Machida, Y., C. Lin and F. Tamanoi (Eds.) *Enzymes*, Vol. 35: Signaling Pathways in Plants, pp. 167–189. San Diego: Elsevier Academic Press Inc.

Weise, S.E., O.A. Kuznetsov, K.H. Hasenstein, and J.Z. Kiss. 2000. Curvature in Arabidopsis inflorescence stems is limited to the region of amyloplast displacement. *Plant Cell Physiol* 41: 702–709.

Xia, L., and J. Guo. 2000. Effect of magnetic field on peroxidase activation and isozyme in Leymus chinensis. *Ying Yong Sheng Tai Xue Bao* 11: 699–702.

Xu, C., Y. Li, Y. Yu, Y. Zhang, and S. Wei. 2015. Suppression of Arabidopsis flowering by near-null magnetic field is affected by light. *Bioelectromagnetics* 36: 476–479.

Xu, C., Y. Lv, C. Chen, Y. Zhang, and S. Wei. 2014. Blue light-dependent phosphorylations of cryptochromes are affected by magnetic fields in *Arabidopsis*. *Adv Space Res* 53: 1118–1124.

Xu, C., Y. Yu, Y. Zhang, Y. Li, and S. Wei. 2017a. Gibberellins are involved in effect of near-null magnetic field on Arabidopsis flowering. *Bioelectromagnetics* 38: 1–10.

Xu, C.X., S.F. Wei, Y. Lu, Y.X. Zhang, C.F. Chen, and T. Song. 2013. Removal of the local geomagnetic field affects reproductive growth in Arabidopsis. *Bioelectromagnetics* 34: 437–442.

Xu, C.X., X. Yin, Y. Lv, C.Z. Wu, Y.X. Zhang, and T. Song. 2012. A near-null magnetic field affects cryptochrome-related hypocotyl growth and flowering in Arabidopsis. *Adv Space Res* 49: 834–840.

Xu, J., W. Pan, Y. Zhang, et al., 2017b. Behavioral evidence for a magnetic sense in the oriental armyworm, Mythimna separata. *Biology Open* 6: 340–347.

Yamashita, M., K. Tomita-Yokotani, H. Hashimoto, M. Takai, M. Tsushima, and T. Nakamura. 2004. Experimental concept for examination of biological effects of magnetic field concealed by gravity. *Adv Space Res* 34: 1575–1578.

Yan, L., S. Zhang, P. Chen, H. Liu, H. Yin, and H. Li. 2012. Magnetotactic bacteria, magnetosomes and their application. *Microbiol Res* 167: 507–519.

Yano, A., Y. Ohashi, T. Hirasaki, and K. Fuliwara. 2004. Effects of a 60 Hz magnetic field on photosynthetic CO_2 uptake and early growth of radish seedlings. *Bioelectromagnetics* 25: 572–581.

Yao, W., and Y. Shen. 2015. Effect of magnetic treatment on seed germination of loblolly pine (Pinus taeda L.). *Scandinavian Journal of Forest Research* 30: 639–642.

Yaycili, O., and S. Alikamanoglu. 2005. The effect of magnetic field on *Paulownia* tissue cultures. *Plant Cell Tiss Organ Cult* 83: 109–114.

Zeugner, A., M. Byrdin, J.P. Bouly, et al., 2005. Light-induced electron transfer in Arabidopsis cryptochrome-1 correlates with in vivo function. *J Biol Chem* 280: 19437–19440.

4

Evaluation of the Toxicity and Potential Oncogenicity of Extremely Low Frequency Magnetic Fields in Laboratory Animal Models

David L. McCormick
IIT Research Institute

CONTENTS

4.1 Introduction

Over the past four decades, the possible relationship between exposure to power frequency (50 and 60 Hz) electromagnetic fields (EMFs) and adverse human health outcomes has received significant attention in both the scientific community and the general population. Based on widely circulated accounts in the popular press [1], and on mass media reports of the results of selected epidemiologic investigations [2,3], a public perception developed in the 1980s and 1990s that human exposure to EMF may be associated with a range of adverse health effects, including reproductive dysfunction, developmental abnormalities, and cancer. The results of a number of epidemiologic studies published at that time provided limited support for the hypothesis that EMF exposure may be associated with an increased risk of neoplasia in several organ sites in humans. Among these sites, the hematopoietic system, breast, and brain were identified most commonly as possibly sensitive targets for EMF action (reviewed in [4]).

Although data from a number of more recent epidemiology studies continue to provide suggestive evidence of the potential oncogenicity of EMF in these sites [*c.f.*, 5–7], many other well-designed epidemiology studies and meta-analyses have failed to identify increased cancer risks in populations receiving either environmental or occupational exposure to EMF [*c.f.*, 8–10]. On this basis, it must be concluded that the total body of epidemiologic data linking EMF exposure and cancer risk is inconclusive.

Since 1990, well over one hundred epidemiology studies designed to investigate the possible association between occupational or residential exposure to magnetic fields and cancer risk have been published (reviewed in [11,12]). The methods used in these more recent studies are often substantially improved in comparison to methods used in earlier investigations; specific areas of improvement include the use of larger sample sizes and better exposure assessment. However, despite these improvements in epidemiologic methods, EMF cancer epidemiology studies continue to generate both positive and negative results. When considered together, the results of these studies are insufficient to either support or refute the hypothesis that exposure to EMF is a significant risk factor for human cancer.

In situations where epidemiology does not support the conclusive identification and quantitation of the potential risks associated with exposure to an environmental agent, laboratory studies conducted in appropriate experimental model systems increase in importance. Well-designed and controlled animal studies permit evaluation of biological effects *in vivo* under tightly controlled exposure and environmental conditions, and in the absence of potential confounding variables. In consideration of the conflicting results of EMF epidemiology studies, and difficulties associated with exposure assessment in such studies, animal studies may provide the best opportunity to identify effects of EMF exposure that could translate into human health hazards.

A large body of research addressing the potential toxicity and oncogenicity of EMF in animal model systems has been published. This review provides a brief review and analysis of this literature. For the purposes of the review, published toxicology and carcinogenesis bioassays of EMF in animal model systems are divided into five sections.

- In Section 4.2, studies designed to investigate the general and organ-specific toxicity of exposure to power frequency EMF are summarized. These studies include both general toxicity bioassays that have been conducted using standard rodent model systems, and specialized toxicology studies that are designed to identify possible specific toxic effects such as developmental toxicity (teratology), reproductive toxicity, or immunotoxicity.

- In Section 4.3, investigations into the possible oncogenicity of EMF as a single agent are reviewed. The most comprehensive studies reviewed in this section are chronic oncogenicity bioassays that are performed in rodents using standardized toxicity testing protocols. The designs of these studies include evaluations of the risk of oncogenesis in essentially all major organ systems; the experimental designs have been developed to satisfy the safety assessment requirements of regulatory agencies such as the US Environmental Protection Agency and the US Food and Drug Administration. Over several decades, an extensive database has developed that supports the utility of the chronic oncogenicity bioassay in rodents as a predictor of oncogenicity in humans.

- In Section 4.4, studies designed to evaluate the activity of EMF exposure as a cocarcinogen or tumor promoter will be reviewed. These studies involve simultaneous or sequential exposures to EMF in combination with another agent in order to identify possible activity as a tumor initiator, tumor promoter, or co-carcinogen in specific organ sites. Most such studies have been conducted using animal models that were designed primarily for use as research tools to study site-specific carcinogenesis. As a result, the utility of these assays as predictors of human oncogenicity is less completely understood than are the results of the 2-year bioassay.

- Section 4.5 encompasses a discussion of studies in which the potential oncogenicity of EMF exposure has been evaluated using genetically modified (transgenic or gene knockout) animals. Via insertion of cancer-associated genes (oncogenes) or deletion of tumor suppressor genes from the germ line, transgenic and knockout animal strains have been developed that demonstrate a genetic predisposition to neoplasia. The use of these models to evaluate the potential oncogenicity of EMF exposure may identify biological effects that occur in sensitive subpopulations, but which may not occur in the general population. Given the relative novelty of these genetically engineered animal models and the often very limited background database for their use in hazard identification, little information exists on which their utility as predictors of human oncogenicity can be evaluated.

- Section 4.6 is a brief review of potential biological mechanisms through which EMF exposure has been proposed to induce or stimulate carcinogenesis. An exhaustive compilation and discussion of the literature related to all possibly relevant biological activities of EMF is well beyond the scope of this review. For this reason, this section is focused specifically on the effects of EMF exposure on biochemical and molecular markers that may be mechanistically linked to the process of neoplastic development, with specific emphasis on studies performed in whole animal model systems.

4.2 Animal Toxicity Bioassays of EMF

4.2.1 General Toxicology Bioassays of EMF

Although many thousands of humans have received occupational exposure to EMF for extended periods, no documented case reports of generalized human toxicity resulting from EMF exposure have been published in the peer-reviewed literature. On this basis, it is generally agreed that acute, subchronic, or chronic exposure to EMF is not a significant risk factor for systemic or generalized toxicity in humans. Because certain occupational environments contain "high field" areas in which EMF flux densities often exceed residential EMF levels by factors of tens to hundreds, it is logical to expect that populations working in such "high field" environments would be the primary groups in which EMF toxicities would be observed. Because no case reports of EMF-associated generalized toxicity or malaise in any exposed worker has been published, it is logical to conclude that EMF exposure is not a significant risk factor for the induction of such generalized toxicity.

The lack of systemic toxicity of EMF exposure in humans is clearly supported by the results of acute and subchronic bioassays conducted in animal model systems. In these studies, rats and/or mice have been exposed to EMF at levels ranging from low milliGauss/microTesla (mG/µT) up to as much as 20 G (equivalent to 2000 µT). Bioassays conducted in different laboratories have studied the effects of both linearly polarized and circularly polarized EMFs.

Although the experimental endpoints evaluated in these bioassays vary by study, most include evaluations of the possible effects of EMF exposure on survival, overall health as monitored by clinical and physical observations, body weight, food consumption, hematology, clinical chemistry, and histopathologic evaluation of tissues. Although occasional instances of statistically significant differences in EMF-exposed animals from sham-exposed controls have been observed in one or more endpoints, no reproducible pattern of EMF toxicity has been identified in any bioassay with known predictability for human responses (*c.f.,* [13–15]); other studies reviewed in [4]. The lack of hematologic toxicity of EMF identified in these animal studies is consistent with the data from an experimental exposure study conducted in humans [16].

Although long-term studies have generally been focused on the possible activity of EMF as a carcinogen or tumor promoter, many of the chronic EMF exposure studies (discussed in succeeding sections of this review) also included evaluations of toxicological endpoints such as body weight, clinical and physical observations, and hematology. As was the case with the acute and subchronic exposure studies, studies involving chronic EMF exposures have failed to identify any evidence of systemic toxicity (see, for example, [17–19]).

Summarizing the available data, no evidence of generalized toxicity associated with EMF exposure has been identified in epidemiology studies of human populations receiving occupational exposure, or in experimental exposure studies in either animals or humans. On this basis, it can be concluded that the risks of generalized or systemic toxicity resulting from acute, subchronic, or chronic exposure to EMF are very small.

4.2.2 Developmental and Reproductive Toxicity Studies of EMF

Investigations into the possible developmental and reproductive toxicity of EMF were stimulated by early reports of teratogenesis in chick embryos exposed to high EMF flux densities (reviewed in [20]). Although the processes of prenatal development in chickens differ substantially from those in humans, the induction of terata in early chick embryos has been interpreted by some investigators to support the hypothesis that EMF is a teratogen. By contrast, however, teratologists who use animal models to develop human hazard assessments for chemical and physical agents have questioned the value of the chick embryo model for human hazard identification. In consideration of both the positive and negative results of studies designed to examine the effects of EMF exposure on chick embryo development, and the unknown ability of studies in chickens and other avian species to predict human developmental toxicity, data from developmental toxicity studies of EMF in chickens are considered to offer relatively little insight into human hazard assessment [20].

It should be noted, however, that the early teratology data generated in chicken models were extended by reports of small increases in the incidence of birth defects and spontaneous abortions in women who used electric blankets and electric water bed heaters during pregnancy (reviewed in [4]). These early findings were hypothesis generating, but were limited in that they were retrospective studies that included no measurements of EMF exposure. Furthermore, the design of these studies essentially precluded the separation of possible EMF effects from thermal effects that could result from the use of an electric blanket or bed heater.

Since the publication of these early findings, a large number of epidemiology studies have been performed to investigate the hypothesis that EMF exposure is a risk factor for teratogenesis. These studies have examined the incidence of birth defects, growth retardation, and premature delivery, among other endpoints, in the offspring of women who used electric blankets or electric bed heaters during pregnancy. Other studies have examined rates of these abnormalities in pregnant women with different levels of residential EMF exposure and in pregnant women with different measured or imputed levels of occupational EMF exposure. In general, although occasional EMF-associated differences have been reported, the results of these studies failed to confirm the hypothesis that EMF exposure during pregnancy is a significant risk to the developing fetus (reviewed in [4]). In most studies, no statistically significant relationships have been found between EMF exposure and the risk of birth defects or other developmental abnormalities. The source of the EMF exposure (use of an electric blanket or bed heater, overall higher level of residential EMF, or occupational EMF exposure) was inconsequential with respect to possible effects on the risk of teratogenesis.

Supporting these epidemiologic data are the negative results of more than a dozen teratology studies in which pregnant rodents were exposed to EMF flux densities of up to 20 G (2000 µT; *c.f.*, [21–25]; others reviewed in [20]). It is important to note that the rodent models, study designs, and periods of exposure used in several EMF developmental toxicity studies have been used for many years to evaluate the possible teratogenicity of pharmaceuticals and environmental chemicals; these models have been validated extensively, and have been shown to be generally predictive of human responses. The results of these EMF teratology studies, which have been conducted by several different teams of investigators in several different countries, have been uniformly negative.

When the negative results generated in these experimental evaluations of EMF teratogenesis are considered together with the negative results of most epidemiology studies, the overwhelming majority of available teratology data do not support the hypothesis that exposure to power frequency EMF during pregnancy constitutes an important hazard to the developing fetus. Interestingly, Mevissen and colleagues [26] found no significant adverse effects of fetal exposure to 50 Hz EMF in rats, but reported a significant reduction in fetal survival in rats receiving gestational exposure to 30 mT static EMFs. Similarly, Saito and colleagues reported the induction of terata by exposure of pregnant mice to an extremely high static EMF (400 mT, which is 8,000 times the earth's static EMF [27]). These results suggest that very high static EMFs may have development effects that are not induced by exposure to power frequency EMF.

As is the case with developmental toxicity (teratology) studies of EMF, no compelling body of evidence from animal studies implicates EMF as a significant risk for either male or female fertility. The total number of relevant studies is small, and includes assessments of the potential reproductive toxicity of both power frequency electric and magnetic fields ([28,29]; other studies reviewed in [30]). However, the results of these studies, which have commonly involved exposure of several generations of rodents to EMF, have failed to identify any decreases in fertility in either male or female animals receiving such exposures.

4.2.3 Immunotoxicity Studies of EMF

Evaluation of the possible effects of EMF exposure on immune function is important to support our understanding of the possible role of EMF in carcinogenesis and as a modifier of host resistance to infection. Any reproducible downregulation of immune function in EMF-exposed animals could have important consequences in terms of the host's ability to resist infectious disease challenge and/or to provide effective immune surveillance against neoplastic cells.

Over several decades, a database has developed in which immunotoxic effects observed in rodent models have been linked to similar effects in humans. On this basis, the results of immune function studies in established rodent models appear to provide the best experimental tool to predict possible effects in humans. Studies have been reported in which the effects of EMF on immune-related parameters have been evaluated in non-rodent species such as sheep [31]; however, the utility of these species as predictors of human responses in unknown. For this reason, the most relevant data set for the possible effects of EMF exposure on immune function is that which has been generated in rodents.

In the rodent studies, a battery of immune function assays (lymphoid organ weight, lymphoid organ cellularity, lymphoid organ histology, B- and T-cell-mediated immune responses, NK cell function, lymphocyte subset analysis, host resistance assays) were evaluated in mice and/or rats exposed to magnetic field flux densities of up to 20 G for periods ranging from 4 weeks to 3 months. The results of studies performed in two different laboratories demonstrated that EMF-exposed animals demonstrated no deficits in lymphoid organ weights, lymphoid organ cellularity, or lymphoid organ histology; similarly, no deficits in T-cell function or B-cell function were identified, and lymphocyte subset analysis did not reveal any effects of EMF exposure [32,33]. Interestingly, however, a statistically significant suppression of NK cell function was seen in two studies performed in female mice; this alteration was not seen in male mice of the same strain, nor in either sex of rats evaluated in a parallel study [32,34].

Although the authors conclude that this suppression of NK cell function is real [34], it appears to have little or no biological significance. The primary role of NK cells appears to be in immune surveillance against cancer cells. However, completely negative results were obtained in a 2-year carcinogenesis bioassay of EMF performed in the same strain of mice that demonstrated the reduction in NK cell function [19]. Because the deficit in NK cell function was not associated with an increase in cancer risk, it is concluded that either (a) the quantitative reduction (approximately 30%) in NK cell function induced by EMF is too small to be biologically significant, or (b) other arms of the host immune system were able to perform required immune surveillance in these animals.

4.3 Assessment of the Possible Oncogenic Activity of EMF Exposure using Chronic Exposure Studies in Rodents

4.3.1 Design of Chronic Exposure Studies

Several teams of investigators have published the results of studies that are designed to investigate the possible carcinogenic activity of chronic exposure to EMF alone (as opposed to EMF exposure in combination with simultaneous or sequential exposure to other agents). These studies have generally been conducted using a standardized study design that is commonly referred to as the "Chronic Oncogenicity Bioassay in Rodents." This study design has been used widely as the basis to evaluate the potential carcinogenicity of new drugs, agricultural chemicals, occupational chemicals, and a wide range of environmental agents, and is considered to be a useful predictor of human oncogenicity. The International Agency for Research on Cancer (IARC) and United States National Toxicology Program (NTP) have both performed analyses demonstrating the utility of the rodent chronic bioassay as a predictor of predict human carcinogenicity. As a result, it is generally accepted among toxicologists that the chronic rodent bioassay currently provides the best available experimental approach to identify agents that may be carcinogenic in humans.

In the chronic rodent oncogenicity bioassay, groups of rats or mice are exposed to the test agent for a period than encompasses the majority of their normal life span (2 years in most studies; some studies in mice are conducted for 18 months). The bioassay includes a standard series of in-life toxicology observations and evaluations; however, its key experimental endpoint is histopathology.

Histopathologic evaluations performed at the conclusion of chronic rodent bioassays generally include classification of all gross lesions identified at necropsy, and examination of 45–50 tissues from each animal in the high-dose and control groups. In addition to the complete histopathologic evaluations of high-dose and control animals, histopathology is generally performed on gross lesions and identified target tissues in animals in the middle- and low-dose groups.

A significant strength of the use of the chronic rodent bioassay to identify potentially carcinogenic agents is the ability to compare tumor incidence patterns of exposed groups to both contemporaneous controls (i.e., the control group from that specific study), as well as to tumor incidence patterns in historical control animals. Historical control databases for tumor incidence are commonly maintained both within conducting laboratories and by animal suppliers. The historical control database is particularly large for studies conducted for the NTP. Because all rats and mice used in NTP chronic oncogenicity studies are bred in the same animal colonies, the NTP database includes the results of tumor incidence data generated during histopathologic evaluations of many thousands of control animals.

4.3.2 Results of Chronic Rodent Oncogenicity Bioassays

4.3.2.1 IIT Research Institute (USA) Chronic Oncogenicity Bioassays in Rats and Mice

The largest and most comprehensive evaluations of the potential carcinogenicity of EMF exposure in rodents were conducted at IIT Research Institute (IITRI), under the sponsorship of the NTP. The quality and comprehensive nature of these studies was specifically highlighted in a commentary written by the Director of the Food and Drug Administration's National Center for Toxicological Research; this commentary was published in *Toxicologic Pathology* [35].

In this evaluation program, parallel studies were conducted in F344 rats [18] and in B6C3F1 mice [19]. In each study, groups of 100 animals per sex were exposed for 18.5 hours per day for 2 years to pure, linearly polarized 60 Hz EMFs. It is useful to note that this group size is twice that commonly used in chronic rodent bioassays; this increase in group size confers increased statistical power to the experimental design, and thereby increases its ability to identify weak effects. Experimental groups included animals receiving continuous exposure to field strengths of 20 mG (equivalent to 2 μT), 2 G (200 μT), or 10 G (1000 μT), or intermittent exposures (1 hour on/1 hour off) to 10 G (1000 μT). Parallel sham control groups were housed within an identical exposure array, but were exposed to ambient EMFs only.

The design of these studies included continuous monitoring of EMF strength and waveform throughout the 2-year exposure period. At termination, all animals received a complete necropsy, and complete histopathologic evaluations were performed on all gross lesions collected from all study animals, in addition to approximately 50 tissues per animal in all study groups.

The results from these studies provided no evidence of increased cancer incidence in any of the putative target tissues (hematopoietic system, brain, breast) for EMF oncogenicity, and do not support the hypothesis that EMF is a significant risk factor for human neoplasia in any site.

- The results of the study conducted in B6C3F1 mice demonstrated no increases from sham control in the incidence of neoplasia in any tissue. When compared to sham controls, the only statistically significant differences in tumor incidence in groups exposed to EMF were:
  - a statistically significant decrease in the incidence of malignant lymphoma in female mice exposed intermittently to 10 G EMF,
  - significant decreases in the incidence of lung tumors in both sexes of mice exposed to EMF at 20 mG or 2 G (but not at 10 G).
- The results of the oncogenicity study conducted in F344 rats also failed to provide evidence to support the hypothesis that EMF is a significant risk factor for human cancer. Similar to the results of the study in mice, no significant increases in the incidence of neoplasia in the hematopoietic system, breast, or brain were seen in any study group. Significant differences from control tumor incidences included:
  - a statistically significant decrease in the incidence of leukemia in male rats exposed intermittently to 10 G EMF,
  - a statistically significant decrease in the incidence of preputial gland carcinomas in male rats exposed to 2 G (but not to 10 G) EMF,
  - a statistically significant decrease in the incidence of trichoepitheliomas of the skin in male rats exposed continuously to 10 G EMF,
  - a statistically significant decrease in the incidence of adrenal cortical adenomas in female rats exposed intermittently to 10 G EMF,
  - a statistically significant increase in incidence of thyroid C-cell tumors in male rats exposed to EMF at field strengths of 20 mG or 2 G (but not at 10 G).

When considered together, the results of these studies provide no evidence that EMF exposure is a significant risk factor for human cancer. No increases in the incidence of neoplasia in the brain, breast, or hematopoietic system were observed in either sex of either species in any group receiving chronic EMF exposure. Similarly, although a number of statistically significant differences from control tumor incidence were observed in the two studies, seven of the nine differences were reductions, rather than increases in tumor incidence.

4.3.2.2 Institut Armand Frappier (Canada) Chronic Oncogenicity Bioassay in Rats

Scientists at the Institut Armand Frappier (IAF) in Laval, Quebec conducted a chronic bioassay in which F344 rats were exposed to pure, linearly polarized 60 Hz EMFs for 20 hours per day for 2 years [33]. Although group sizes used in the IAF study were smaller than those used in the chronic rat oncogenicity study conducted at IITRI, the experimental designs of the two rat oncogenicity bioassays were generally comparable. Two factors did distinguish the experimental design of the IAF study:

- EMF exposures were initiated 2 days prior to animal birth, rather than in young adult animals,
- study participants were "blinded" to the identify of study groups until after study completion.

The most common approach to the conduct of rodent oncogenicity bioassays is to begin exposure to the test agent when animals are young adults (6–8 weeks old), and to identify the exposure status of each experimental group so that all study participants are aware of group identities. Because the IAF study included exposures during the perinatal and juvenile periods, its design addresses the possibly enhanced sensitivity of younger animals to EMF effects. Furthermore, the conduct of the bioassay using a "blinded" design precludes any possible influence of investigator bias on study results.

The design of this study included 50 rats per sex per group. Experimental groups included cage controls, sham controls, and groups exposed to EMF at field strengths of 20 mG (2 μT), 200 mG (20 μT), 2 G (200 μT), and 20 G (2000 μT). Toxicologic endpoints included a standard battery of in-life evaluations and histopathologic evaluation of gross lesions and approximately 50 tissues per animal.

Similar to the data generated in the IITRI/NTP studies, the results of the IAF study failed to support an association between EMF exposure and increased risk of neoplasia in the brain, breast, hematopoietic system, or any other tissue examined. The study authors summarize their data by stating that "no statistically significant, consistent, positive dose-related trends with the number of tumor-bearing animals per study group could be attributed to EMF exposure." Although not statistically significant at the 5% level of confidence, total tumor incidence in all groups exposed to magnetic fields was decreased in comparison to tumor incidences observed in the cage control and sham control groups.

In the IAF study, the incidences of brain tumors (astrocytomas, gliomas, etc.), malignant mammary tumors (adenocarcinomas), and leukemias were low in all groups, and demonstrated no pattern of differences between control groups and groups exposed to EMF. Benign mammary tumors (fibroadenomas) were common in all groups, and were present in similar incidences, regardless of EMF exposure. The most common tumor identified in the study was a benign pituitary tumor (adenoma); although differences did not always attain statistical significance, the incidences of pituitary adenomas in all groups exposed to EMF were decreased from those seen in both the sham control group and the cage control group. *In toto*, the results of the IAF study are comparable to those from the IITRI study, and extend these results to include EMF exposures that were initiated during the perinatal period.

4.3.2.3 *Mitsubishi Kasei Institute (Japan) Chronic Oncogenicity Bioassay in Rats*

Scientists at the Mitsubishi Kasei Institute (MKI) of Toxicological and Environmental Sciences, Ibaraki, Japan conducted a 2-year bioassay in F344 rats to evaluate the potential oncogenicity of chronic exposure to linearly polarized, 50 Hz EMF [36]. The 50 Hz sine wave is the primary component of power frequency EMF associated with the generation and distribution of electricity in Europe and Asia. In this study, groups of 48 rats per sex were exposed for > 21 hours per day for 2 years to 50 Hz EMF at field strengths of 5 G (500 μT) or 50 G (5000 μT); an identically sized control group received sham exposure for the same period. At study termination, all animals received a complete necropsy. Complete histopathologic evaluations were performed on all gross lesions, and approximately 45 additional tissues per animal from all animals in all study groups.

Survival was comparable in all study groups, and differential white blood cell counts performed after 52, 78, and 104 weeks of exposures failed to identify any effects of EMF exposure. Consistent with the results of studies conducted at IITRI and IAF, the MKI study found no increased risk of neoplasia in animals receiving chronic exposure to EMF. The MKI team reported that EMF exposure had no effect on animal survival in either sex, and had no effect on the total incidence or number of neoplasms. Within a sex, incidences of leukemia, brain tumors, and mammary tumors in groups exposed to EMF were comparable to those of sex-matched sham controls.

The only statistically significant histopathologic findings from the study were an increase in the incidence of a benign lesion (fibroma) in the subcutis of male rats exposed to 50 G EMF, and a decrease in the total incidence of invasive neoplasms in male rats in the 5 G EMF group. Although the increased incidence of fibromas in male rats exposed to 50 G EMF was statistically significant when compared to concurrent male sham controls, lesion incidence was comparable to that observed in historical controls in the laboratory. On this basis, the authors concluded that this increase in fibroma incidence in rats exposed to 50 G EMF was not biologically significant. Similarly, because no differences in the incidence of metastatic neoplasms were seen in the study, the observed decrease in the incidence of invasive malignancy appears to be without biological significance.

4.3.2.4 Ramazzini Institute (Italy) Chronic Multi-Agent Bioassays in Rats

Scientists at the Ramazzini Institute (Italy) have recently published two papers reporting the results of chronic bioassays in which rats were exposed to 50 Hz EMF in combination with other agents [37,38]. In addition to expanding the database of studies in which the carcinogenicity of EMF (as a single agent) has been evaluated, these studies were designed to identify possible interactions between EMF and either formaldehyde or γ radiation in the induction of malignant lesions.

In one study [37], groups of male and female rats received chronic exposure to EMF (1 mT; 10 G) alone; formaldehyde alone (50 mg/liter, in drinking water); EMF + formaldehyde; or no exposure (control). Group sizes were unusually large for chronic bioassays: the control group (no exposure) included 500+ rats per sex, while exposed groups included 200+ rats per sex. Large group sizes commonly increase the statistical power of a study. It should be noted, however, that the design of these studies was unusual, in that animals were permitted to live until their natural death rather than being euthanized after 2 years of exposure. The authors propose that this study design (large group sizes and extended study duration) maximizes the opportunity to identify carcinogenic effects; however, the design has been criticized based on the high incidences of age-related malignancies expected in all groups as a result of the extended period of observation. In addition, the extended duration of the in-life period in this study makes comparisons with the results of 2-year bioassays impossible; this eliminates the possible use of historical control data from other chronic bioassays in the analysis of study results.

The authors reported no increases in cancer incidence in rats receiving chronic exposure to either EMF alone or to formaldehyde alone; the observed lack of carcinogenic activity of EMF (as a single agent) in this study confirms and extends the results of previous chronic bioassays of EMF in rodents [18,19,33,36]. By contrast to the lack of carcinogenicity of EMF alone or formaldehyde alone, the authors did report statistically significant increases in the incidences of total malignant tumors, C-cell carcinomas of the thyroid, and lymphomas/leukemias in male rats exposed to EMF + formaldehyde. These changes were not seen in female rats. The authors propose that EMF and formaldehyde interact synergistically in the induction of these malignant lesions; however, whether any interaction is synergistic, additive, or potentiating cannot be determined on the basis of the study data.

In the second study [38], groups of pregnant female rats either received no EMF exposure (controls) or were exposed to EMF (20 μT [200 mG] or 1 mT [10 G]) beginning on gestation day 12. EMF exposure (20 µT or 1 mT) was continuous throughout gestation and after pups were born. Pups were assorted into four treatment groups: single exposure to γ radiation (0.1 Gray; Gy) at 6 weeks of age + chronic exposure to EMF (20 µT); single exposure to γ radiation + chronic exposure to EMF (1 mT); single exposure to γ radiation only (no EMF exposure); and no treatment. EMF exposure in 20 µT and 1 mT groups was continued until termination of the study. As in the formaldehyde study, group sizes were large: the control group (no exposure; this appears to be the same control group used in the formaldehyde study), included 500+ rats per sex, and exposed groups included 100+ rats per sex. As in the formaldehyde study, animals were permitted to live until their natural death rather than being euthanized after 2 years of exposure. Although significant increases in cancer incidence were seen in exposed groups in comparison to untreated controls, no clear evidence of EMF effects on carcinogenesis was presented.

4.3.2.5 Overview of Chronic Rodent Oncogenicity Studies

Although minor differences can be identified, the overall experimental designs used in the bioassays performed at IITRI (USA), IAF (Canada), and MKI (Japan) were very similar; all study designs conform with harmonized regulatory requirements for chronic oncogenicity testing in rodents. The results of the four studies conducted in these three laboratories are also in close agreement. In all studies, chronic exposure to power frequency EMF had no effect on the incidence of neoplasia in any of the three putative targets for EMF action (brain, breast, and hematopoietic system). Furthermore, chronic exposure to EMF did not induce any pattern of biologically significant increases in cancer incidence in other tissues. The very close comparability of the results of four chronic rodent oncogenicity bioassays conducted independently in three laboratories strengthens the conclusion that exposure to EMFs does not induce cancer in rodents. On the basis of the demonstrated predictive nature of the rodent 2-year bioassay, these findings do not support the hypothesis that EMF exposure is a significant risk factor in the etiology of human neoplasia.

4.3.3 Results of Site-Specific Oncogenicity Bioassays in Rodents

4.3.3.1 University of California at Los Angeles (USA) Lymphoma/Brain Tumor Bioassay in Mice

A chronic murine bioassay was conducted at the University of California at Los Angeles (UCLA)/Veterans Administration Hospital to evaluate the potential interaction between EMF and ionizing radiation in the induction of hematopoietic neoplasia in mice [39]. Although the primary focus of this study was the interaction between EMF and ionizing radiation, the study design did include several experimental groups that were exposed to EMF alone. Neoplastic responses in EMF-exposed and sham control groups that received no exposure to ionizing radiation are suitable for use in assessing the potential oncogenicity of exposure to EMF.

In this study, one group of 380 female C57BL/6 mice was exposed to circularly polarized 60 Hz EMF at a field strength of 14.2 G (1.42 mT) for up to 852 days. The incidence of hematopoietic neoplasia in these EMF-exposed mice was compared with that observed in a negative (untreated) control group consisting of 380 female C57BL/6 mice, and in a sham control group consisting of 190 female C57BL/6 mice. In addition to the investigation of EMF effects on hematopoietic neoplasia, a *post hoc* histopathologic analysis of brain tissues from this study was performed to investigate the possible activity of EMF as a causative agent for primary brain tumors [39].

Chronic exposure to EMF had no statistically significant effects on animal survival or on the incidence or latency of hematopoietic malignancy in this study [39]. At study termination, the final incidence of lymphoma in mice exposed to circularly polarized EMF was 36.8%, as compared to a lymphoma incidence of 34.7% in sham controls. The incidence of histiocytic sarcomas was 23.7% in mice receiving EMF exposure versus 22.1% in sham controls, yielding a total incidence of hematopoietic neoplasia of 56.3% in sham controls versus a total incidence of 59.2% in the group exposed to circularly polarized EMF. Relative risks for various types of hematopoietic neoplasia in the EMF group ranged from 0.94 to 1.03; all 95% confidence intervals included 1.00, and none differed from sham control at the 5% level of significance.

Consistent with the results for hematopoietic neoplasia, histopathologic evaluation of brains from this study provided no support for the hypothesis that EMF exposure is a significant risk factor for brain tumor induction. In this study, brains from a total of 950 nonirradiated mice were evaluated (total of control and EMF-exposed groups that received no exposure to ionizing radiation); only 2 benign brain tumors were identified [40]. Because the incidence of brain cancer in the negative control group, sham control group, and the EMF-exposed group were all below 0.25%, these data provide no evidence that exposure to circularly polarized EMF is oncogenic in the brain of C57BL/6 mice.

Although lack of proximity to power transmission and distribution lines ensures that most humans are not exposed to circularly polarized EMF, the possible carcinogenicity of circularly polarized fields has received only very limited study. The primary strengths of this study are that it evaluated the potential oncogenicity of a previously unstudied exposure metric (circularly polarized rather than linearly polarized EMF), and used very large experimental groups. The large group sizes used in the study greatly increase its statistical power, and therefore improve its ability to identify effects of modest magnitude.

It must be noted, however, that the study design was quite limited in that it included histopathologic evaluations of only the hematopoietic/lymphoid system and brain. As such, while the study data provide no support for the hypothesis that EMF exposure is causally associated with the induction of neoplasia in the hematopoietic system and brain, the lack of systematic evaluation of other tissues precludes any conclusions about possible influences on neoplasia in other sites.

4.3.3.2 Technical University of Nova Scotia (Canada) Lymphoma Bioassay in Mice

Using a unique study design in which three consecutive generations of CFW mice were exposed to extremely high flux densities (250 G [25 mT] of 60 Hz EMF, [41]), data were presented that suggested an increased incidence of malignant lymphoma in the second and third generations of exposed animals. The strength of this study lies in its innovative design involving exposure of multiple generations, and its examination of flux densities that greatly exceed those that have been used in other studies. In consideration of the exposure regimen used in this study, it can be argued that this investigation provided the maximum likelihood of identifying a positive oncogenic activity of EMF. Indeed, this study is the only report in the peer-reviewed literature in which long-term EMF exposure in otherwise untreated animals has been associated with an increased incidence of malignancy.

Although the results of this study were clearly a novel finding, it must be noted that the experimental design and interpretation of this study has been strongly criticized for several reasons [42,43]. These reasons include:

- Group sizes are small and variable, and the number of observed malignant lesions is very small.

- Exposure assessment, environmental control, and control of possible confounding of study results by the heat and vibration generated by the EMF exposure system present serious questions as to the validity of results. Indeed, noise and vibration associated with ventilation equipment needed to dissipate the heat generated by the EMF generation and exposure system, as well as temperature control for exposed animals, were very different than those used for control animals; control animals were housed in a different room, and were not exposed to these environmental factors.

- The onset of lymphoma in mice is age-related, yet the study design included large discrepancies between the ages of EMF-exposed mice and the control groups to which they were compared.

- Peer review of photomicrographs indicates that some lesions identified by the investigators as neoplasms may, in fact, represent hyperplastic rather than malignant lesions.

4.4 Assessment of the Possible Co-Carcinogenic or Tumor Promoting Activity of EMF Exposure using Multistage Rodent Models

It is generally accepted that exposure to power frequency EMF does not induce mutations or other genetic damage that is identifiable using standard genetic toxicology model systems [44–46]. Because EMF is apparently not genotoxic, it is logical to conclude that any oncogenic effects of exposure are mediated through co-carcinogenic or tumor promotion/progression mechanisms. To address this possibility, a relatively large number of *in vivo* studies have been conducted to identify possible co-carcinogenic or tumor promoting effects of EMF in various target tissues. The design of these studies involves simultaneous or sequential exposure to EMF in combination with another agent, and generally focuses on neoplastic development in a specific organ. It should be noted, however, that most multistage tumorigenesis studies of EMF have been conducted using animal models that were designed as research tools to study site-specific carcinogenesis. As a result, the utility of these assays as predictors of human oncogenicity is less completely understood than are the results of the chronic oncogenicity bioassay.

The design of most multistage tumorigenesis studies is based on the initiation-promotion paradigm that was originally developed in mouse skin. In the initiation-promotion model in mouse skin, mice are exposed to a single sub-threshold dose of a genotoxic agent (e.g., benzo[*a*]pyrene or 7,12-dimethylbenz[*a*]anthracene), followed by repetitive administration of a nongenotoxic agent (e.g., 12-*O*-tetradecanoylphorbol-13-acetate). Over the past 50 years, this paradigm has been extended to include tumor induction models in more than a dozen organ sites, several of which have been used in EMF studies. Most multistage evaluations of the potential oncogenicity of EMF have been performed in animal models for neoplastic development in the breast, brain, skin, liver, and hematopoietic system.

In view of the relative large literature related to possible tumor promotion by EMF, analysis, and discussion of all possibly relevant multistage oncogenicity evaluations is beyond the scope of the present review. For this reason, discussion in this section is limited to a brief review of the studies that have been conducted in organ systems that have been suggested by epidemiology data as possible targets for EMF oncogenicity (brain, breast, and hematopoietic system).

4.4.1 Design of Multistage Oncogenicity Studies

The design of multistage oncogenicity studies is site-specific: the selection of animal species and strain, carcinogen exposure regimen, observation period, and endpoint analyses vary by animal model system. As a general rule, animals are exposed to one or a few doses of a genotoxic agent (the initiator), which is then followed by subchronic or chronic exposure to EMF (the putative promoter). Many, but not all, multistage studies that are designed to evaluate the activity of EMF as a promoter include a positive control group that is exposed to the same dose of initiating agent, followed by exposure to an agent with known promoting activity.

In consideration of their site specificity, multistage tumorigenesis studies are often conducted in a single sex, and employ group sizes that are smaller than those used in chronic rodent bioassays. The species and strain of animals used in these organ-specific tumorigenesis studies is selected on the basis of previous literature demonstrating appropriate sensitivity to neoplastic development in the organ site of interest. Under optimal conditions, the carcinogen dosing regimen (initiating regimen) is selected to be a threshold dose that will induce a low incidence (<10%) of neoplasia in otherwise untreated animals; unfortunately, the value of a several multistage tumorigenicity evaluations of EMF is undermined by inappropriate selection of initiator doses. The period of observation and type of endpoint observations are also model-specific; optimal study design in these areas is based on previous studies using the same model system.

4.4.2 Multistage Oncogenicity Studies in the Brain

The peer-reviewed literature contains two reports of experimental studies in which the activity of 60 Hz EMF as a promoter of brain tumor induction has been evaluated. These reports include an evaluation of the activity of EMF as a promoter of neurogenic tumors induced in F344 rats by transplacental exposure to *N*-ethyl-*N*-nitrosourea [47], and a study to evaluate the activity of EMF as a promoter of brain tumors induced in C57BL/6 mice by ionizing radiation [40]. Neither study demonstrated any significant activity of EMF as a promoter of brain tumor induction.

4.4.2.1 Institut Armand Frappier (Canada) Brain Tumor Promotion Study in Rats

Mandeville and colleagues [47] have reported a study to evaluate the influence of EMF exposure on the induction of brain and spinal tumors by transplacental exposure to the nitrosamide, *N*-ethyl-*N*-nitrosourea (ENU). The transplacental ENU model in rats has been used widely in studies of neurogenic carcinogenesis, and is considered to be an appropriate model system for such evaluations.

In this study, groups of 50 pregnant female F344 rats received a single intraperitoneal dose of 5 mg ENU per kg body weight on day 18 of gestation. The F1 generation was exposed to EMF beginning on day 20 of gestation and continuing until study termination;

flux densities (20 mG [2 μT], 200 mG [20 μT], 2 G [200 μT], and 20 G [2000 μT]) and environmental conditions in the laboratory were identical to those used in the chronic oncogenicity bioassay conducted at IAF.

EMF exposure had no effect on animal survival in the study and had no influence on the incidence of neurogenic tumors. The results of this study do not support the hypothesis that EMF is a potent promoter of neural tumorigenesis.

4.4.2.2 University of California at Los Angeles (USA) Brain Tumor Promotion Study in Mice

A chronic murine bioassay was conducted at the University of California at Los Angeles (UCLA)/Veterans Administration Hospital to evaluate the potential interaction between EMF and ionizing radiation in the induction of hematopoietic neoplasia in mice [39]. As an adjunct to this study, the possible activity of EMF as a promoter of brain tumor induction was evaluated via histopathologic evaluation of brains from mice exposed to graded doses of ionizing radiation followed by exposure to either ambient EMFs (sham controls) or circularly polarized EMF (14.2 G [1.4 mT]) for up to 852 days [40].

When compared to matched sham controls, EMF exposure had no statistically significant effect on animal survival in any group. Total brain tumor incidence in the study was <0.5% (a total of 7 brain tumors in 1707 irradiated mice), and no evidence of increased brain tumor incidence was observed in any group exposed to EMF. These data provide no evidence that exposure to circularly polarized EMF has tumor promoting activity in the brain of C57BL/6 mice.

In spite of its large group sizes, one issue in the interpretation of the results of this study is its sensitivity and ability to identify any neurocarcinogenic effects of EMF exposure. The small number of brain cancers seen in all experimental groups could be interpreted as evidence that the mouse brain is relatively insensitive to neural tumor induction. Alternatively, however, the low incidence of brain cancers observed in otherwise unexposed animals could suggest that brain cancer incidence in study animals is at a response "threshold," and that exposure to any agent that stimulates cancer induction should increase brain cancer response. Regardless of the strength of the finding, the data from the present study provide no support for the hypothesis that EMF exposure is a significant risk factor for cancer induction in the brain.

4.4.3 Multistage Oncogenicity Studies in the Mammary Gland

The carcinogen-induced mammary adenocarcinoma in female rats is an organ-specific cancer model that is highly suitable for use as a test system in which to identify and quantitate EMF bioeffects. Epidemiologic evidence suggests that the breast may be a sensitive target tissue for the biological activity of EMF, and a well-defined and extensively studied multistage model system has been established that is suitable for the identification of possible mammary gland carcinogens and tumor promoters [48]. Numerous studies have been conducted to investigate the possible activity of EMF as a promoter of carcinogenesis in the rat mammary gland, and considerable controversy has developed concerning whether EMF exposure does indeed stimulate neoplastic development in this model system.

The general design of studies to evaluate the possible activity of EMF as a promoter of tumor induction in the rat mammary gland involves administration of one to four doses of a chemical carcinogen (7,12-dimethylbenz[*a*]anthracene [DMBA] or *N*-methyl-*N*-nitrosourea [MNU]) to young adult rats, followed by whole body exposure to exposure to either EMF or sham fields. Tumor development is monitored by palpation at regular intervals throughout the in-life period; at study termination, tumors are excised and evaluated histopathologically to confirm their malignant phenotype.

Several critical factors must be considered in the evaluating of the quality of studies reporting evaluations of the potential oncogenicity of EMF in the rat mammary gland.

- It is essential that study designs include histopathological evaluation of induced tumors. Absent such histologic confirmation, it impossible to demonstrate that masses palpated during in-life observations are indeed malignant, and do not represent either benign tumors (adenomas or fibroadenomas) or nonmalignant lesions (e.g., mammary cysts).

- Dose selection for the chemical carcinogen is also a critical factor. In order to demonstrate promotional activity, the dose of carcinogen that is administered to test animals must induce a relatively low incidence of lesions, thereby providing a baseline cancer incidence against which a statistically significant increase in incidence can be achieved. If the cancer incidence induced by the carcinogen dose is too high, demonstration of promotional activity will be impossible.

- The mammary tumor response to the carcinogen must fall within accepted incidence and multiplicity ranges; these ranges have been established over more than 30 years through the work of many independent researchers. It is critical to note that this model has been used for several decades in studies of hormonal carcinogenesis and in efficacy evaluations of cancer chemopreventive agents. As such, dose-response parameters for mammary tumor induction are well established. In instances where reported dose-response relationships fall outside of the established dose-response parameters, it becomes impossible to exclude technical deficiencies in study conduct.

4.4.3.1 Oncology Research Center (Georgia) Mammary Tumor Promotion Studies in Rats

In 1991, Beniashvili and colleagues [49] published the first report of the enhancement of rat mammary carcinogenesis by EMF exposure, and later published a confirming study [50]. In this work, exposure of rats to either static or 50 Hz EMFs alone did not induce mammary cancer. However, exposure of rats to static or 50 Hz EMF following administration of chemical carcinogen (MNU) increased the incidence and reduced the latency of mammary tumors in comparison to controls exposed to MNU only. Tumor incidence was higher in animals exposed to MNU + 50 Hz EMF than to either MNU + static fields or MNU only. The authors interpret these findings to suggest that EMF is not oncogenic by itself, but may present a cancer hazard for both humans and animals.

The value of the data from these papers is compromised by the lack of information regarding the exposure system used, and limited detail regarding experimental methods. However, these data were clearly suggestive and stimulated the conduct of a number of similar studies in other laboratories.

4.4.3.2 Hannover School of Veterinary Medicine (Germany) Mammary Tumor Promotion Studies in Rats

The largest number of studies investigating the influence of EMF on rat mammary carcinogenesis has been published by Loscher and colleagues from the School of Veterinary

Medicine at Hannover in the Federal Republic of Germany [51–58]. In these studies, rats were exposed to DMBA followed by exposure to 50 Hz EMF or sham fields for periods ranging from 13 to 27 weeks.

The initial study from this group [57] reported an increase in mammary tumor incidence in rats exposed to 50 Hz EMF at a flux density of 1 G (100 μT). However, no histopathologic evaluations were performed in this study, and tumor size measurements were based on estimates performed via palpation. In a follow-up study conducted at lower doses that are more relevant to residential environments, Loscher et al. [51] reported that exposure to a 50 Hz EMF gradient of field strengths ranging from 3 to 10 mG (0.3 to 1.0 μT) reduced nocturnal melatonin levels, but had no effect on mammary carcinogenesis. In this study, EMF exposure for 13 weeks had no effect on mammary cancer incidence, mammary tumor size, or the incidence of preneoplastic lesions. The data from these studies were interpreted to suggest that exposure to EMF at high flux densities stimulates mammary tumor induction in rats, but that such effects do not occur as a result of exposure to EMF at low field strengths (such as those encountered in residential environments).

In a subsequent study, Loscher and Mevissen [52] reported a linear increase in mammary tumor incidence at 13 weeks in rats receiving DMBA and exposed to 50 Hz EMF at field strengths of 100 mG, 500 mG, and 1 G (10, 50, and 100 μT). Confirming these data, the same group of investigators reported that exposure to 500 mG (50 μT) EMF increased both the number and growth rate of mammary tumors [53], and the total incidence of mammary tumors [58]. By contrast, however, another confirming study [54] published the same year as the initial investigation of this series reported no increase in mammary tumor incidence, number, or size in rats exposed to 50 Hz EMF at 100 mG (10 μT). A fourth confirming study conducted for 26 weeks [55] found a much smaller increase from sham control in the incidence of mammary tumors in groups exposed to the 500 mG EMF; although the authors state statistical significance for the finding, the reported difference appears to be within the intrinsic variability of the DMBA mammary cancer system.

4.4.3.3 Battelle-Pacific Northwest Laboratories (USA) Mammary Tumor Promotion Studies in Rats

A series of studies supported by the NTP and conducted at Battelle-Pacific Northwest Laboratories (PNL) was designed to replicate and extend the mammary carcinogenesis studies reported by Loscher and colleagues. In these studies, groups of 100 female rats received sham EMF exposure or were exposed to either 50 or 60 Hz EMF at field strengths of 1 or 5 G (100 or 500 μT).

The initial study conducted was a 13-week bioassay that was designed to replicate the findings of Loscher et al. [57] and Loscher and Mevissen [52]. The results of this replication study demonstrated no differences from DMBA-treated sham controls in mammary cancer incidence, mammary cancer number, or mammary cancer size in DMBA-treated rats that were exposed to either 50 or 60 Hz EMF [59]. Therefore, the replication study conducted at PNL failed to confirm the findings of the Hannover group.

The second study conducted at PNL used the same exposure metrics, and was designed to replicate the results of the 26-week mammary cancer bioassays reported by Loscher and colleagues. Similar to the results of the 13-week study conducted at PNL, the results of the 26-week study demonstrated no significant increases in mammary cancer incidence in any group exposed to EMF. Furthermore, statistically significant decreases in the total number of mammary cancers were seen in groups exposed to 50 or 60 Hz EMF field strengths of 1 G [11].

Investigators at PNL and in Hannover have collaborated in the attempt to identify reasons underlying the inability of PNL investigators to reproduce the results reported by Loscher and colleagues [58]. The Hannover group has attributed the inability of the PNL group to reproduce their findings to differences in EMF responsiveness of different substrains of Sprague-Dawley rats [60].

4.4.3.4 National Institute for Working Life (Sweden) Mammary Tumor Promotion Studies in Rats

One study has been published by investigators from the National Institute for Working Life in Sweden in which the possible promoting activity of 50 Hz EMF was evaluated in the DMBA rat mammary carcinogenesis model system [61]. In this study, groups of female rats were exposed to DMBA followed by exposure to a transient-producing EMF at flux densities of 2.5 or 5 G (250 or 500 μT) for 25 weeks. No statistically significant differences from sham control were observed in mammary tumor incidence, mammary tumor number, total tumor weight, or tumor volume in either group exposed to EMF. The results of this study do not support the hypothesis that EMF exposure is an important risk factor for breast cancer.

4.4.4 Multistage Oncogenicity Studies in the Hematopoietic System

Two studies have been reported in which the activity of EMF as an inducer of lymphoma in standard (nontransgenic) animals has been evaluated. Several additional studies using genetically modified animals (transgenic and knockout strains) have also been published; the results of these studies are summarized in Section 4.5.

4.4.4.1 Zhejiang Medical University (China) Lymphoma Promotion Study in Mice

Shen and colleagues [62] presented the results of a study designed to evaluate the possible activity of a 1 mT 50 Hz EMF in the promotion of lymphoma induction in newborn mice treated with DMBA. In this study, 320 newborn mice received a single injection of carcinogen within 24 hours of birth; sham exposure (155 mice) or EMF exposure (165 mice) was initiated at 2 weeks of age, and was continued until study termination at 16 weeks. The incidence of lymphoma was histologically confirmed.

At the termination of the study, lymphoma incidence was 22% in sham controls, and 24% in the group receiving EMF exposure, demonstrating that EMF exposure had no promoting activity under the conditions of this study. However, the incidence of metastatic infiltration into the liver was higher in EMF-exposed mice than in controls; the significance of this finding, if any, is unclear.

4.4.4.2 University of California at Los Angeles (USA) Lymphoma Promotion Study in Mice

A chronic murine bioassay was conducted at the University of California at Los Angeles (UCLA)/Veterans Administration Hospital to evaluate the potential interaction between EMF and ionizing radiation in the induction of hematopoietic neoplasia in mice [39]. In this study, groups of mice were exposed to graded doses of ionizing radiation followed by exposure to either ambient EMFs (sham controls) or circularly polarized EMF (14.2 G [1.4 mT]) for up to 852 days. Details of the design of this study were provided in Section 4.3.

When compared to matched sham controls, EMF exposure had no statistically significant effect on animal survival in any group, and did not increase the incidence of lymphoma in any group. In fact, the only statistically significant difference from matched sham controls was a reduction in lymphoma risk in mice exposed to EMF after exposure to an ionizing radiation dose of 5.1 Gray. Extending the results of the complete carcinogenesis component of this study, the results of the lymphoma promotion cohorts of the study provide no evidence that exposure to circularly polarized EMF promotes the induction of lymphoma in C57BL/6 mice.

4.4.4.3 Overview of Multistage Oncogenicity Studies

Overall, the peer-reviewed literature provides little compelling evidence that exposure to EMF has co-carcinogenic or tumor-promoting activity in any organ site in experimental animals. Although the results of epidemiology studies have identified the brain, breast, and hematopoietic system as possible targets of EMF action, no consistent pattern of EMF effects has been seen in any of these sites in experimental carcinogenesis models. Similarly, carcinogenesis studies conducted in animal model systems have not identified any other organ as a potential target of EMF oncogenicity.

Studies conducted in animal models for lymphoma and brain cancer provide no evidence of tumor promoting or co-carcinogenic activity associated with exposure to EMF. The observed lack of activity in the promotion of hematopoietic neoplasia in multistage model systems is supported by similar results from studies conducted in transgenic and knockout models of lymphoma induction.

Several reports of tumor promoting activity in the rat mammary gland have been presented in the peer-reviewed literature. However, these reports come from only two laboratories, and tumor-promoting activity was identified on the basis of different endpoints in different studies. More importantly, however, independent efforts to replicate these studies in other laboratories have failed. On this basis, the body of evidence supporting tumor-promoting activity for EMF in the rat mammary gland must be considered to be weak, at best.

Although not reviewed in detail in this chapter, similar negative results have been obtained in experimental studies conducted in animal models for neoplasia of the skin and liver. Although one report of skin tumor promotion by EMF has been presented [63], subsequent studies conducted in several laboratories have failed to identify either any tumor-promoting effects of EMF in mouse skin [64–67] or any effects of EMF exposure on biomarkers of tumor promotion in the skin [68]. Studies designed to determine the effects of EMF exposure on the induction of altered liver foci (a preneoplastic lesion in rat liver) also fail to provide clear evidence of tumor promotion by EMF [69, 70].

4.5 Assessment of the Possible Oncogenic Activity of EMF Exposure using Genetically Modified (Transgenic and Gene Knockout) Rodent Models

Insights into the molecular mechanisms of carcinogenesis provide the scientific basis for the development and use of genetically modified animals to study cancer induction and the application of these models in hazard identification and toxicity evaluation. The use of genetically modified animals in safety assessment is an emerging technology that lacks the long historical precedent of the 2-year bioassay and other standardized approaches to toxicity testing. However, understanding of the utility of these model systems and their value in safety assessment is evolving rapidly, and their use in toxicology is expanding. In this regard, it should be noted that oncogenicity studies in two genetically modified models, the p53 knockout mouse and the *ras*H2 mouse, are accepted by the FDA as suitable models for preclinical assessments of potential carcinogenicity.

The science supporting the use of genetically modified models in safety assessment stems from initial observations that the incidence of malignancy is increased and/or its latency is decreased in animal strains into whose germ line a tumor-associated gene (oncogene) has been inserted. Subsequent work demonstrated similar changes in patterns of neoplasia in animal strains from whose germ line a tumor-suppressor gene has been deleted. On this basis, transgenic animals (into whose germ line a tumor-associated gene has been inserted) and knockout animals (from whose genome a tumor-suppressor gene has been deleted) demonstrate a genetic predisposition to neoplasia; this predisposition may be exploited as an approach to the use of animal models whose sensitivity to oncogenesis is increased.

These models have several desirable attributes that support their use in the study of EMF effects. First, oncogenicity studies in transgenic or knockout models involve evaluations of biological activity in animals in which exposure to a test agent is superimposed upon a genetic predisposition to disease. Such evaluations may identify oncogenic effects that occur in sensitive subpopulations, and rarely or not at all in the general population. As a result, genetically modified models may demonstrate sensitivity to EMF effects that is substantially greater than that of standard animal strains. Second, transgenic or knockout animals provide experimental models that may be considered as analogous to co-carcinogenesis and initiation-promotion models; tumorigenesis in some transgenic and knockout model systems does not require exposure to a chemical carcinogen. Finally, the conduct of parallel assessments of the possible oncogenicity of EMF in animals with different genetic alterations can generate information regarding (a) the generality of any observed effects and (b) possible molecular mechanisms underlying such effects.

Because genetically modified animals have a less extensive history of use in safety assessment than do standard-bred rodents, many fewer studies are available on which the utility of these models to predict human oncogenicity can be evaluated. When considered alone, oncogenicity assessments in genetically modified animals may be of limited value in predicting human responses. However, when considered in combination with studies performed using standardized model systems, the increased sensitivity of transgenic and knockout models to disease processes may support the identification of low-dose effects and effects in sensitive subpopulations.

4.5.1 Design of Oncogenicity Studies in Genetically Modified Animals

The design of oncogenicity studies in transgenic and knockout animals generally parallel the designs used for oncogenicity bioassays in standard strains of rodents. However, these bioassays differ from the design of chronic oncogenicity bioassays in duration, group size, and experimental endpoints. Primary differences from the 2-year bioassay are as follows:

- The duration of oncogenicity studies in genetically modified animals varies by animal strain. The primary determinant of study duration is the kinetics of spontaneous oncogenesis in the animal model being used in the bioassay. Most commonly, oncogenicity assessments are designed for completion using an in-life period of

6 months; however, the in-life period in certain models can be extended to include much longer periods of exposure. For example, the protocol developed by the NTP for oncogenicity bioassays in heterozygous p53 knockout mice involves 26 weeks of agent exposure; this protocol is now used widely in safety assessments of novel drugs and natural products being submitted for FDA approval. By contrast, studies in PIM transgenic mice (as cited below) have ranged in duration from 6 months to 18 months.

- Group size in these studies rarely exceeds 30 per sex per group, versus 50–100 in standard oncogenicity bioassays. A group size of 25 per sex per group is routinely required by the FDA for studies in the p53 knockout mouse.

- In most cases, studies in genetically modified animals are designed to examine effects of a test agent on neoplastic development in a specific site, and histopathologic evaluations are limited to that site. In EMF studies, the primary focus has been on the possible influence of EMF exposure on the incidence of lymphoma. As such, histopathologic evaluation of tissues in these studies has been limited to lymphoid organs.

4.5.2 Results of Oncogenicity Studies in Genetically Modified Animals

4.5.2.1 IITRI (USA) Lymphoma Bioassays in PIM Transgenic and Heterozygous p53 Knockout Mice

As part of a larger program supported by the NTP and the United States National Institute of Environmental Health Sciences (NIEHS), scientists at IITRI conducted 6-month studies to determine the influence of EMF exposure on lymphoma induction in PIM transgenic mice and heterozygous p53 knockout mice [71]. Both genetically modified mouse strains were used as models for lymphoma: the PIM mouse receives a single dose of carcinogen (*N*-ethyl-*N*-nitrosourea) prior to EMF exposure and is considered to be a "high incidence" lymphoma model over a 6-month observation period. The heterozygous p53 knockout mouse receives no carcinogen exposure and is a "low incidence" lymphoma model system over this same observation period.

4.5.2.1.1 Results of IITRI (USA) Lymphoma Bioassay in PIM Transgenic Mice

The PIM transgenic mouse carries the *pim*-1 oncogene [72] and is a rapid model for the study of lymphoma. We have previously demonstrated that this model system is useful for studies of the modulation of lymphoma promotion by cancer chemopreventive agents [73]. However, there is little data to correlate neoplastic responses in other organs in the PIM mouse model with responses to chemicals in 2-year bioassays for oncogenicity. As such, the PIM mouse must be considered to be at an early stage of development for use in the identification of agents that may stimulate the induction of leukemia/lymphoma.

EMF exposure metrics used in the PIM mouse oncogenicity bioassay [71] were identical to those used in the chronic animal bioassays of EMF that were conducted at IITRI. Groups of 30 mice per sex received a single intraperitoneal dose of 25 mg ENU and were then were exposed for 18.5 hours per day for 23 weeks to pure, linearly polarized 60 Hz EMFs. Experimental groups included animals receiving continuous exposure to field strengths of 20 mG (2 μT), 2 G (200 μT), or 10 G (1000 μT), or intermittent exposures (1 hour on/1 hour off) to 10 G (1000 μT). Parallel sham control groups were housed within an identical exposure array, but were exposed to ambient EMFs only. At the conclusion of the exposures, animals underwent a limited gross necropsy focused on the lymphoid system, and histopathologic evaluations were performed on the spleen, thymus, mandibular lymph node, liver, kidney, and lung.

When compared to sham controls, exposure to 60 Hz EMF did not increase the incidence of lymphoma in any experimental group. In fact, the only statistically significant difference from sham control was a significant decrease in the incidence of lymphoma in male mice exposed continuously to EMF (23% incidence, versus 49% incidence in sham controls; $p=0.041$ via Fisher's exact test). On this basis, the results of this study do not support the hypothesis that exposure to EMF is a significant risk factor for hematopoietic neoplasia.

4.5.2.1.2 Results of IITRI (USA) Lymphoma Bioassay in p53 Knockout Mice

As a result of deletion of one allele of the p53 tumor-suppressor gene, heterozygous p53 knockout mice are highly sensitive to spontaneous neoplasia in several sites, as well as to the induction of neoplasia by carcinogens. By 18 months of age, approximately 50% of otherwise untreated heterozygous p53 knockout mice will develop malignant lesions, with particular predisposition to tumors of the bone and hematopoietic system [74]. Carcinogen exposure greatly accelerates neoplastic development in this model; in this context p53 knockout mice were used as a model system for the study of EMF effects on lymphoma induction.

In this study, groups of 30 mice per sex were exposed for 18.5 hours per day for 23 weeks to either pure, linearly polarized 60 Hz EMF at 10 G (1000 µT), or to sham fields. At the conclusion of the exposures, animals underwent a limited gross necropsy focused on the lymphoid system, and histopathologic evaluations were performed on the spleen, thymus, mandibular lymph node, liver, kidney, and lung.

Consistent with the results of the lymphoma bioassay in PIM mice, exposure to 60 Hz EMF at a flux density of 10 G had no effect on lymphoma induction in heterozygous p53 knockout mice. Lymphoma incidence in both sexes in the sham control group was 3% (1/30). By comparison, lymphoma incidence in male mice in the 10 G group was 0% (0/30), while female mice exposed to 10 G had a 7% incidence of lymphoma (2/30). Although this study was of limited statistical power, it provides no evidence to support the hypothesis that EMF exposure is a risk factor for lymphoma induction.

4.5.2.2 Walter and Eliza Hall Institute of Medical Research (Australia) Lymphoma Bioassay in PIM Transgenic Mice

A very large lymphoma induction study using the PIM mouse model was conducted at the Walter and Eliza Hall Institute of Medical Research in Melbourne, Australia [75]. In this study, groups of approximately 100 female PIM mice were continuously exposed for 18 months to linearly polarized 50 Hz EMF at flux densities of 10 mG (1 µT), 1 G (100 µT), or 10 G (1000 µT), or intermittently exposed (15 minutes on/15 minutes off) to 10 G (1000 µT) for the same period. In contrast to the design of the PIM mouse study conducted at IITRI, EMF and sham-exposed mice in the present study received no carcinogen.

Although the study designs were very different, the conclusions drawn from the results of this study were quite similar to those of the PIM mouse study conducted at IITRI. When compared to sham controls, no statistically significant increase in the incidence or latency of lymphoma was seen in any group of mice exposed to EMF: in comparison to a lymphoma incidence of 29% in the sham control group, the incidence of lymphoma in groups exposed to EMF ranged from 26% to 35% ($p > 0.05$ for all comparisons). By contrast, mice exposed to a positive control material (*N*-ethyl-*N*-nitrosourea) demonstrated a lymphoma incidence of 60% at 9 months.

4.5.2.3 Overview of Oncogenicity Studies in Genetically Modified Animals

Although the total number of completed oncogenicity evaluations of EMF in genetically modified animals is small, the goals and results of these studies are both very consistent. The peer-reviewed literature contains reports of three studies in which the influence of EMF exposure on lymphoma induction has been assessed using genetically modified animals. The three studies were conducted using vastly different experimental models and designs (carcinogen-treated PIM mouse, noncarcinogen PIM mouse, and noncarcinogen-treated p53 knockout mouse). Furthermore, the three models used demonstrated large differences in the incidence of lymphoma in sham control groups. However, the results of all three studies were very comparable: in all studies, exposure to EMF was not associated with a significant increase in any experimental group.

The relatively recent development of genetically modified animals precludes a long history of their use in safety assessment. As a result, data are insufficient to support a broad assessment of the predictive nature of these models for human oncogenesis. However, the results of oncogenicity evaluations of EMF exposure that have been conducted in standard animal strains and in genetically modified animal models are quite comparable. On this basis, the results of EMF lymphoma studies in the PIM transgenic and p53 knockout model systems can be considered to confirm and extend the results obtained in 2-year bioassays of EMF.

4.6 Proposed Mechanisms of EMF Action in Oncogenesis

A number of mechanisms have been proposed though which exposure to EMF may induce or stimulate neoplastic development; these possible mechanisms include a wide range of effects at the molecular, cellular, and organismal level. An exhaustive presentation and evaluation of the literature relevant to possible mechanisms of EMF action is beyond the scope of this review. However, a brief discussion of the more commonly proposed mechanisms for EMF action is relevant to an evaluation of exposure to EMF as a risk factor for cancer and other diseases. Detailed reviews of possible mechanisms of EMF action have been presented in the assessment of EMF health effects prepared by the U.S. National Institute of Environmental Health Sciences [4] and in the International Agency for Research on Cancer evaluation of the potential carcinogenicity of EMF [11].

Review of the published scientific literature provides no clear support for any specific mechanism of EMF action in carcinogenesis. Furthermore, no reproducible body of scientific evidence exists to link EMF exposure to alterations in any biological endpoint that is mechanistically related to neoplastic development in any tissue.

Most hypothesized mechanisms of EMF action in carcinogenesis can be grouped into five types of effects:

- Genetic toxicity (DNA damage, clastogenesis, or mutagenesis),
- Alterations in gene expression,
- Biochemical changes associated with regulation of cell proliferation,
- Alterations in immune function,
- Alterations in melatonin levels or action.

These general classifications are necessarily arbitrary, and were developed to simplify the purposes of this review. It is clear that several of these mechanisms overlap, and that all possible mechanisms of EMF action are not included in these five groups. However, these groups do encompass the vast majority of mechanisms proposed for EMF bioeffects, and include mechanisms that have received the most extensive study in order to identify possible linkages between EMF exposure and carcinogenesis.

4.6.1 Genetic Toxicology Studies of EMF Exposure

The scientific literature includes over 100 reports of studies that were conducted to determine if exposure to EMF induces clastogenesis, mutagenesis, or other types of DNA damage. Many of these studies were conducted using standard experimental model systems (Ames test, micronucleus test) that are widely used in safety assessments of new drugs, industrial and agricultural chemicals, environmental contaminants, and other agents. As such, the predictive nature of several of the assay systems used to study the genetic toxicology of EMF is well known.

The authors of a comprehensive review of the genetic toxicology literature related to EMF concluded that "the preponderance of evidence suggests that ELF electric or magnetic fields do not have genotoxic potential" [44]. Several investigators have presented study data that indicate positive mutagenic or clastogenic activity of EMF exposure; however, an independent scientific review of these studies suggests that none of these results satisfies basic quality criteria for data reproducibility, consistency, and completeness. By contrast, a number of well-designed, complete, reproducible, and apparently well-conducted studies have failed to demonstrate any genotoxic effects of EMF [44].

It is generally agreed by investigators in the field that ELF magnetic fields do not possess sufficient energy to damage DNA via direct interaction (reviewed in [4]). Although it is possible that power frequency EMF could damage DNA through an indirect mechanism (i.e., via generation of free radicals), the vast majority of well-designed genetic toxicology studies conducted in models with demonstrated predictiveness for DNA damaging activity have failed to identify any significant mutagenic or clastogenic effects of EMF exposure. As such, it is the consensus among toxicologists that exposure to power frequency EMF presents little to no risk of genetic toxicity. On this basis, the induction of DNA damage by EMF exposure appears unlikely to provide a mechanism for cancer induction.

4.6.2 Alterations in Gene Expression

The possible influence of EMF exposure on the expression of cancer-related genes was for many years a highly controversial area of research in bioelectromagnetics. Several groups reported increases in the expression of one or more proto-oncogenes (generally c-*myc* or c-*fos*) in cell cultures exposed to 60 Hz EMF [76–78]. However, replication studies conducted by many other groups did not confirm these findings [79–83]. Other, more broadly based screening efforts to identify cancer-related genes that are up- or downregulated by EMF exposure have generally yielded negative results [84,85]. On this basis, the robustness of the reports of altered expression of these cancer-associated genes, as well as the generality of those findings, must be questioned.

Given the huge universe of genetic targets in the mammalian cell and the common use of microarray and other genome-wide screening technologies to identify effects of exogenous agents on gene expression, it is logical to expect that exposure to 50 and 60 Hz EMF will be found to alter the expression of numerous genes. Indeed, a substantial number of recent publications have reported that exposure to 50 or 60 Hz EMF modifies the expression of genetic and/or epigenetic targets and their associated molecular signaling pathways [*c.f.*, 86–88]. It is important to note, however, that a finding of enhanced expression of an oncogene or any other gene is not, by itself, sufficient evidence to suggest physiologic or pathophysiologic activity. Because many cellular pathways exhibit biological redundancy, alterations in one pathway may be compensated for by an antagonistic change in another pathway. For this reason, although findings of altered gene expression may be considered as generally suggestive of a biologically important effect of EMF exposure, demonstration of upregulation or downregulation of some effector function is necessary to establish the biological relevance of the observed alteration in gene expression. Lacking the demonstration of a physiological/pathophysiological effect, an isolated finding of altered gene expression cannot be construed to be biologically significant. Restated with emphasis on the process of carcinogenesis, a finding of altered expression of an oncogene or a tumor suppressor gene as a result of EMF exposure can by no means be equated with any activity of EMF as a carcinogen or tumor promoter.

4.6.3 Biochemical Changes Associated with Regulation of Cell Proliferation

Changes in the expression or activity of enzymes and protein products involved in cell proliferation, cell-cycle regulation, and apoptosis would be expected if EMF exposure is significantly associated with either complete carcinogenesis or tumor promotion. For example, several reports of EMF-associated alterations in the activity of ornithine decarboxylase, the rate-limiting step in polyamine biosynthesis, have been presented in the literature [89,90]. However, other investigators have either failed to confirm these findings in replication studies [91], or have found no effects of EMF on ornithine decarboxylase activity in other *in vitro* or *in vivo* model systems [92,93]. A similar lack of consistency has been found in studies of biochemical endpoints such as induction of heat shock proteins [94–98].

Clearly, a single finding of an alteration in a specific biochemical parameter is insufficient to support its alteration as a general mechanism for EMF activity. As discussed above with regard to possible alterations in gene expression, an isolated finding of changes in enzyme activity or other pathway in cells that are exposed to EMF can be considered to be no more than suggestive of a possible adverse outcome. Linkage of these biochemical or cell-based effects to the physiological or pathophysiological effect is essential to demonstrate their biological significance.

4.6.4 Alterations in Immune Function

Downregulation of the host immune response by EMF is a tempting hypothesis through which EMF exposure could be associated with risk of carcinogenesis; however, this hypothesis is supported by very little experimental evidence. In fact, several studies conducted in standard rodent models for immunotoxicology testing have failed to demonstrate any significant adverse effects of EMF exposure on either cell-mediated or humoral immune responses [33,99].

The only exception to these negative studies is an apparently reproducible suppression of NK cell function that was seen in B6C3F1 female mice in two studies [32,34]. Interestingly, this suppression was not observed in male B6C3F1 mice, or male and female F344 rats used in these same studies. Furthermore, the reduction in NK cell function does not appear to result in a functional deficit, since negative results were obtained in a 2-year carcinogenesis bioassay of EMF in the same animal species and sex (female B6C3F1 mouse) in which the NK cell functional deficits were observed [19]. On this basis, although the deficit in NK cell function was statistically significant, it appears to be without biological significance in terms of host resistance to neoplasia.

As such, although the hypothesis that EMF exposure may stimulate tumorigenesis through an indirect mechanism involving suppression of host immunity may be intellectually appealing, it is unsupported by any credible body of experimental evidence.

4.6.5 Alterations in Melatonin Levels or Action

The "melatonin hypothesis" was for many years perhaps the most widely accepted potential mechanism for the biological effects of EMF exposure. A simplified version of this hypothesis states that EMF effects are mediated through alterations in the function of the pineal gland; these changes in pineal function are then responsible for alterations in patterns of melatonin synthesis, kinetics, or action [100]. Ultimately, reductions in melatonin synthesis may have a number of potential adverse effects on the host, including reduced activity as an endogenous free radical scavenger, and influences on the hypothalamic-pituitary-gonadal axis [101].

A considerable body of evidence to support the melatonin hypothesis was generated in studies performed during the 1980s and early 1990s (reviewed in [102,103]). In these studies, reductions in circulating melatonin levels and/or time shifts in the circadian rhythm of melatonin biosynthesis were reported in both experimental animals and in humans. However, several investigators who had previously reported significant effects of EMF exposure on pineal function were later unable to replicate their own data [104–107]; replication failures were most commonly attributed to the use of new, more sophisticated EMF exposure and monitoring equipment in replication studies. Later papers from other laboratories (reviewed in [108,109]) have failed to demonstrate any consistent pattern of effects of EMF exposure on melatonin synthesis or kinetics in humans or in rodent model systems.

One notable exception to this trend is a series of studies that have been conducted using the Siberian hamster as a model system; EMF effects on melatonin secretion in this species appear to be a generally reproducible finding [110,111]. However, this animal demonstrates a seasonal circadian rhythm that is considerably different from that seen in either humans or rodent species that are commonly used for safety assessments; as such, a relationship between this finding and possible human health effects is difficult to establish.

Concomitant with the weakening of the data set relating EMF exposure to alterations in pineal function, the melatonin hypothesis has been revised to suggest that EMF influences on melatonin may be affected through alteration in melatonin effects at the level of the target cell, rather than through effects on its synthesis or secretion. The database supporting this hypothesis is very limited, and is considered insufficient to provide strong support for this potential mechanism of EMF action.

4.7 Summary and Conclusions

Over the past 30 years, a large number of well-designed and carefully conducted studies have been performed to evaluate the toxicity and possible oncogenicity of power frequency [50/60 Hz] magnetic fields (EMFs) in experimental animals. The results of acute, subchronic, and chronic toxicity and oncogenicity studies conducted using standardized toxicology bioassay protocols in rodent models provide little support for the hypothesis that exposure to power frequency EMFs is a significant risk factor for human disease. Although positive results have been reported in a small number of animal studies, essentially all of those results either (a) have not been replicated in in other laboratories or (b) were generated using nontraditional experimental models whose value as predictors of human responses is largely or completely unknown.

Perhaps most importantly, the results of chronic toxicity and oncogenicity bioassays in rodents provide no compelling evidence of either significant chronic toxicity or oncogenicity of EMF in any organ. Similarly, the results of multistage oncogenicity studies in site-specific animal models for skin cancer, brain cancer, and hematopoietic neoplasia provide no evidence that EMF acts as a co-carcinogen or tumor promoter in these organ sites. Studies performed using genetically modified (transgenic and gene knockout) animals also demonstrate no activity of EMF as promoter of hematopoietic neoplasia in genetically sensitive subpopulations.

The only experimental evidence of tumor promotion or enhancement by EMF comes from studies in which EMF exposure has been combined with administration of a chemical carcinogen or ionizing radiation. Two long-term studies were recently reported in which increased incidences of neoplasia were seen in rats exposed to EMF in combination with formaldehyde or γ radiation; the relevance of these studies for human hazard identification and EMF risk assessment is currently unclear. Most other positive studies were performed in the rat mammary gland; however, reports of enhancement of mammary carcinogenesis by EMF come from only two laboratories, and attempts at independent replication of these results have failed. The limited nature of the positive mammary cancer data is further suggested by the negative results of mammary tumor promotion studies conducted by other investigators. The experimental literature also fails to provide significant data to support any of several proposed mechanisms for EMF as a carcinogen or tumor promoter.

Some adverse effects of EMF exposure have been reported in studies designed to investigate its possible developmental toxicity (induction of birth defects; teratogenicity) and immunotoxicity. However, adverse effects of EMF on fetal development have been reported only in studies performed using nonstandard models; evaluations of the possible developmental and reproductive toxicity of EMF in animal models that are commonly used for hazard assessment have been uniformly negative. Although immunotoxicity bioassays of EMF have generated both positive and negative results, any reductions in specific immune parameters resulting from EMF exposure have not been linked to any functional deficit in immunity.

Clearly, the safety of human exposure to EMF (or any other chemical or physical agent) cannot be conclusively determined on the basis of studies in animal models alone. Interspecies extrapolation of results, and requirements for extrapolation of high-dose exposure data in animals to low-dose exposures in humans both require the acceptance of mechanistic assumptions that may ultimately prove to be inaccurate. For this reason, the most effective hazard assessments are based on the integration of results from appropriate animal test systems with available data from studies of exposed human populations.

In the case of EMF hazard assessment, evaluation of data from specific toxicologic endpoints that have been examined both in experimental models and in epidemiology studies demonstrates that the results of animal studies agree quite closely with data from studies in human populations. This relationship suggests that, where appropriate comparative data exist, the results of well-designed studies in appropriate animal model systems are largely predictive of human responses to EMF.

Ultimately, the key issue in EMF hazard assessment is whether animal data can be used to predict human risk for cancer and other disease processes for which the epidemiologic data are inconsistent or unavailable. On the basis of the close agreement between animal and human data in both general toxicology and organ site-specific toxicity studies, and the negative results of the overwhelming majority of oncogenicity evaluations of EMF in animal model systems, it is concluded that exposure to EMF is unlikely to be a significant risk factor for human oncogenesis.

References

1. Brodeur, P., *The Great Power-Line Cover-Up*, New York: Little, Brown, and Company, 1993.
2. Wertheimer, N. and Leeper, E., Electrical wiring configurations and childhood cancer, *Am. J. Epidemiol.*, 190, 273–284, 1979.
3. Savitz, D., Wachtel, H., Barnes, F.A., John, E.M., and Tvrdik, J.G., Case-control study of childhood cancer and exposure to 60-Hz magnetic fields, *Am. J. Epidemiol.*, 128, 21–38, 1998.
4. Portier, C.J., and Wolfe, M.S. (Eds.), *Assessment of Health Effects from Exposure to Power-Line Frequency Electric and Magnetic Fields*, NIEHS Working Group Report. NIH Publication No. 98–3981, Research Triangle Park, NC, pp. 85–208, 1998.
5. Zhao, L., Liu, X., Wang, C., Yan, K., Lin, X., Li, S., Bao, H., and Liu, X., Magnetic fields exposure and childhood leukemia risk: a meta-analysis based on 11,699 cases and 13,194 controls, *Leuk. Res.*, 38, 269–274, 2014.
6. Koeman, T., van den Brandt, P.A., Slottje, P., Schouten, L.J., Goldbohm, R.A., Kromhout, H., and Vermeulen, R., Occupational extremely low-frequency field exposure and selected cancer outcomes in a prospective Dutch cohort, *Cancer Causes Control*, 25, 203–214, 2014.
7. Kheifets, L., Crespi, C.M., Hooper, C., Amoon, A.T., and Vergara, X.P., Residential magnetic fields exposure and childhood leukemia: a population-based case-control study in California, *Cancer Causes Control*, 28, 1117–1123, 2017.
8. Johansen, C., Raaschou Nielsen, O., Olsen, J.H., and Schüz, H., Risk for leukaemia and brain and breast cancer among Danish utility workers: a second follow-up, *Occup. Environ. Med.*, 64, 782–784, 2007.
9. Li, W., Ray, R.M., Thomas, D.B., Yost, M., Davis, S., Breslow, N., Gao, D.L., Fitzgibbons, E.D., Camp, J.E., Wong, E., Wernli, K.J., and Checkoway, H., Occupational exposure to magnetic fields and breast cancer among women textile workers in Shanghai, China, *Am. J. Epidemiol.*, 178, 1038–1045, 2013.
10. Repacholi, M.H., Lerchl, A., Röösli, M., Sienkiewicz, Z., Auvinen, A., Breckenkamp, J., D'Inzeo, G., Elliott, P., Frei, P., Heinrich, S., Lagroye, I., Lahkola, A., McCormick, D.L., Thomas, S., and Vecchia, P., Systematic review of wireless phone use and brain cancer and other head tumors, *Bioelectromagnetics*, 33, 187–206, 2012.
11. International Agency for Research on Cancer, *IARC Monographs on the Evaluation of Carcinogenic Risks to Humans*, Non-ionizing radiation, Part 1: Static and extremely low-frequency (ELF) electric and magnetic fields, Vol. 80, IARC Press, Lyon, 2002.
12. Schüz, J., and Erdmann, F., Environmental exposure and risk of childhood leukemia, *Arch. Med. Res.*, 47, 607–614, 2016.
13. Margonato, V., Veicsteinas, A., Conti, R., Nicolini, P., and Cerretelli, P., Biologic effects of prolonged exposure to ELF electromagnetic fields in rats: I. 50 Hz electric fields, *Bioelectromagnetics*, 14, 479–493, 1993.
14. Margonato, V., Nicolini, P., Conti, R., Zecca, L., Veicsteinas, A., and Cerretelli, P., Biologic effects of prolonged exposure to ELF electromagnetic fields in rats: II. 50 Hz magnetic fields, *Bioelectromagnetics*, 16, 343–355, 1995.

15. Boorman, G.A., Gauger, J.R., Johnson, T.R., Tomlinson, M.J., Findlay, J.C., Travlos, G.S., and McCormick, D.L., Eight-week toxicity study of 60 Hz magnetic fields in F344 rats and B6C3F1 mice, *Fundam. Appl. Toxicol.*, 35, 55–63, 1997.
16. Selmaoui, B., Bogdan, A., Auzeby, A., Lambrozo, J., and Touitou, Y., Acute exposure to 50 Hz magnetic field does not alter hematologic or immunologic functions in healthy young men: a circadian study, *Bioelectromagnetics*, 17, 364–372, 1996.
17. Boorman, G.A., Anderson, L.E., Morris, J.E., Sasser, L.B., Mann, P.C., Grumbein, S.L., Hailey, J.R., McNally, A., Sills, R.C., and Haseman, J.K., Effect of 26-week magnetic field exposures in a DMBA initiation-promotion mammary gland model in Sprague-Dawley rats, *Carcinogenesis*, 20, 899–904, 1999.
18. Boorman, G.A., McCormick, D.L., Findlay, J.C., Hailey, J.R., Gauger, J.R., Johnson, T.R., Kovatch, R.M., Sills, R.C., and Haseman, J.K., Chronic toxicity/oncogenicity evaluation of 60 Hz (power frequency) magnetic fields in F344/N rats, *Toxicol. Pathol.*, 27, 267–278, 1999.
19. McCormick, D.L., Boorman, G.A., Findlay, J.C., Hailey, J.R., Johnson, T.R., Gauger, J.R., Pletcher, J.M., Sills, R.C., and Haseman, J.K., Chronic toxicity/oncogenicity evaluation of 60 Hz (power frequency) magnetic fields in B6C3F1 mice, *Toxicol. Pathol.*, 27, 279–285, 1999.
20. Brent, R.L., Reproductive and teratologic effects of low-frequency electromagnetic fields: a review of *in vivo* and *in vitro* studies using animal models, *Teratology*, 59, 261–286, 1999.
21. Ryan, B.M., Mallett, E. Jr., Johnson, T.R., Gauger, J.R., and McCormick, D.L., Developmental toxicity study of 60 Hz (power frequency) magnetic fields in rats, *Teratology*, 54, 73–83, 1996.
22. Ryan, B.M., Polen, M., Gauger, J.R., Mallett, E., Jr, Kearns, M.B., Bryan, T.L., and McCormick, D.L., Evaluation of the developmental toxicity of 60 Hz magnetic fields and harmonic frequencies in Sprague-Dawley rats, *Radiat. Res.*, 153, 637–641, 2000.
23. Rommereim, D.N., Rommereim, R.L., Miller, D.L., Buschbom, R.L., and Anderson, L.E., Developmental toxicology evaluation of 60-Hz horizontal magnetic fields in rats, *Appl. Occup. Environ. Hyg.*, 11, 307–312, 1996.
24. Negishi, T., Imai, S., Itabashi, M., Nishimura, I., and Sasano, T., Studies of 50 Hz circularly polarized magnetic fields of up to 350 microT on reproduction and embryo-fetal development in rats: exposure during organogenesis or during preimplantation, *Bioelectromagnetics*, 23, 369–389, 2002.
25. Chung, M.K., Kim, J.C., Myung, S.H., and Lee, D.I., Developmental toxicity evaluation of ELF magnetic fields in Sprague-Dawley rats, *Bioelectromagnetics*, 24, 231–240, 2003.
26. Mevissen, M., Buntenkotter, S., and Loscher, W., Effects of static and time-varying (50-Hz) magnetic fields on reproduction and fetal development in rats, *Teratology*, 50, 229–237, 1994.
27. Saito, K., Suzuki, H., and Suzuki, K., Teratogenic effects of static magnetic fields on mouse fetuses, *Reprod. Toxicol.*, 22, 118–124, 2006.
28. Rommereim, D.N., Rommereim, R.L., Miller, D.L., Buschbom, R.L., and Anderson, L.E., Developmental toxicology evaluation of 60-Hz horizontal magnetic fields in rats, *Appl. Occup. Environ. Hyg.*, 11, 307–312, 1996.
29. Ryan, B.M., Symanski, R.R., Pomeranz, L.E., Johnson, T.R., Gauger, J.R., and McCormick, D.L., Multigeneration reproductive toxicity assessment of 60-Hz magnetic fields using a continuous breeding protocol in rats, *Teratology*, 59, 156–162, 1999.
30. Chernoff, N., Rogers, J.M., and Kavet, R., A review of the literature on potential reproductive and developmental toxicity of electric and magnetic fields, *Toxicology*, 74, 91–126, 1992.
31. Hefeneider, S.H., McCoy, S.L., Hausman, F.A., Christensen, H.L., Takahashi, D., Perrin, N., Bracken, T.D., Shin, K.Y., and Hall, A.S., Long-term effects of 60-Hz electric vs. magnetic fields on IL-1 and IL-2 activity in sheep, *Bioelectromagnetics*, 22, 170–177, 2001.
32. House, R.V., Ratajczak, H.V., Gauger, J.R., Johnson, T.R., Thomas, P.T., and McCormick, D.L., Immune function and host defense in rodents exposed to 60-Hz magnetic fields, *Fundam. Appl. Toxicol.*, 34, 228–239, 1996.
33. Mandeville, R., Franco, E., Sidrac-Ghali, S., Paris-Nadon, L., Rocheleau, N. Mercier, G., Desy, M., and Gaboury, L., Evaluation of the potential carcinogenicity of 60 Hz linear sinusoidal continuous-wave magnetic fields in Fischer F344 rats, *FASEB J.*, 11, 1127–1136, 1997.

34. House, R.V. and McCormick, D.L., Modulation of natural killer cell function after exposure to 60 Hz magnetic fields: confirmation of the effect in mature B6C3F1 mice, *Radiat. Res.*, 153, 722–724, 2000.

35. Schwetz, B., Commentary: Rodent carcinogenicity studies on magnetic fields, *Toxicol. Pathol.*, 27, 286, 1999.

36. Yasui, M., Kikuchi, T., Ogawa, M., Otaka, Y., Tsuchitani, M., and Iwata, H., Carcinogenicity test of 50 Hz sinusoidal magnetic fields in rats, *Bioelectromagnetics*, 18, 531–540, 1997.

37. Soffriti, M., Tibaldi, E., Padovani, M., Hoel, D.G., Giuliani, L., Bua, L., Lauriolo, M., Falcioni, L., Manservigi, M., Manservisi, F., and Belpoggi, F., Synergism between sinusoidal-50 Hz magnetic field and formaldehyde in triggering carcinogenic effects in male Sprague-Dawley rats, *Am. J. Ind. Med.*, 59, 509–521, 2016.

38. Soffriti, M., Tibaldi, E., Padovani, M., Hoel, D.G., Giuliani, L., Bua, L., Lauriolo, M., Falcioni, L., Manservigi, M., Manservisi, F., Panzacchi, S., and Belpoggi, F., Life-span exposure to sinusoidal-50 Hz magnetic field and acute low-dose γ radiation induce carcinogenic effects in Sprague-Dawley rats, *Int. J. Radiat. Biol.*, 92, 202–214, 2016.

39. Babbitt, J.T., Kharazi, A.I., Taylor, J.M., Bonds, C.B., Mirell, S.G., Frumkin, E., Zhuang, D., and Hahn, T.J., Hematopoietic neoplasia in C57BL/6 mice exposed to split-dose ionizing radiation and circularly polarized 60 Hz magnetic fields, *Carcinogenesis*, 21, 1379–1389, 2000.

40. Kharazi, A.I., Babbitt, J.T., and Hahn, T.J., Primary brain tumor incidence in mice exposed to split-dose ionizing radiation and circularly polarized 60 Hz magnetic fields, *Cancer Lett.*, 147, 149–156, 1999.

41. Fam, W.Z. and Mikhail, E.L., Lymphoma induced in mice chronically exposed to very strong low-frequency electromagnetic field, *Cancer Lett.*, 105, 257–269, 1996.

42. Boorman, G.A., McCormick, D.L., Ward, J.M., Haseman, J.K., and Sills, R.C., Magnetic fields and mammary cancer in rodents: a critical review and evaluation of published literature, *Radiat. Res.*, 153, 617–626, 2000.

43. Boorman, G.A., Rafferty, C.N., Ward, J.M., and Sills, R.C., Leukemia and lymphoma incidence in rodents exposed to low-frequency magnetic fields, *Radiat. Res.*, 153, 627–636, 2000.

44. McCann, J., Dietrich, F., and Rafferty, C., The genotoxic potential of electric and magnetic fields: An update, *Mutat. Res.*, 411, 45–86, 1998.

45. Stronati, L., Testa, A., Villani, P., Marino, C., Lovislo, G.A., Conti, D., Russo, F., Fresegna, A.M., and Cordelli, E., Absence of genotoxicity in human blood cells exposed to 50 Hz magnetic fields as assessed by comet assay, chromosome aberration, micronucleus, and sister chromatid exchange analyses, *Bioelectromagnetics*, 25, 41–48. 2004.

46. Verschaeve, L., Anthonissen, R., Grudniewska, M., Wudarski, J., Gevaert, L., and Maes, A., Genotoxicity investigation of ELF-magnetic fields in Salmonella typhimurium with the sensitive SOS-based VITOTOX test, *Bioelectromagnetics*, 32, 580–584, 2011.

47. Mandeville, R., Franco, E., Sidrac-Ghali, S., Paris-Nadon, L., Rocheleau, N., Mercier, G., Desy, M., Devaux, C., and Gaboury, L., Evaluation of the potential promoting effect of 60 Hz magnetic fields on N-ethyl-N-nitrosourea induced neurogenic tumors in female F344 rats, *Bioelectromagnetics*, 21, 84–93, 2000.

48. McCormick, D.L. and Moon, R.C., Vitamin A deficiency and cancer, In Bauernfeind, J.C. (Ed.) *Vitamin A Deficiency and Its Control*, Academic Press, New York, 1985, pp. 245–284.

49. Beniashvili, D.S., Bilanishvili, V.G., and Menabde, M.Z., Low-frequency electromagnetic radiation enhances the induction of rat mammary tumors by nitrosomethyl urea, *Cancer Lett.*, 61, 75–79, 1991.

50. Anisimov, V.N., Zhukova, O.V., Beniashvili, D.S., Menabde, M.Z., and Gupta, D., Effect of light/dark regimen and electromagnetic fields on mammary carcinogenesis in female rats, *Biofizika*, 41, 807–814, 1996.

51. Loscher, W., Wahnschaffe, U., Mevissen, M., Lerchl, A., and Stamm, A., Effects of weak alternating magnetic fields on nocturnal melatonin production and mammary carcinogenesis in rats, *Oncology*, 51, 288–295, 1994.

52. Loscher, W. and Mevissen, M., Linear relationship between flux density and tumor co-promoting effect of prolonged magnetic field exposure in a breast cancer model, *Cancer Lett.*, 96, 175–180, 1995.

53. Mevissen, M., Lerchl, A., and Loscher, W., Study on pineal function and DMBA-induced breast cancer formation in rats during exposure to a 100-mG, 50 Hz magnetic field, *J. Toxicol. Environ. Health*, 48, 169–185, 1996.

54. Mevissen, M., Lerchl, A., Szamel, M., and Loscher, W., Exposure of DMBA-treated female rats in a 50-Hz, 50 microTesla magnetic field: effects on mammary tumor growth, melatonin levels, and T lymphocyte activation, *Carcinogenesis*, 17, 903–910, 1996.

55. Thun-Battersby, S. Mevissen, M., and Loscher, W., Exposure of Sprague-Dawley rats to a 50-Hertz, 100-microTesla magnetic field for 27 weeks facilitates mammary tumorigenesis in the 7, 12-dimethylbenz[a]-anthracene model of breast cancer, *Cancer Res.*, 59, 3627–3633, 1999.

56. Fedrowitz, M., Kamino, K., and Loscher, W., Significant differences in the effects of magnetic field exposure on 7,12-dimethylbenz(a)anthracene-induced mammary carcinogenesis in two substrains of Sprague-Dawley rats, *Cancer Res.*, 64, 243–251, 2004.

57. Loscher, W., Mevissen, M., Lehmacher, W., and Stamm, A., Tumor promotion in a breast cancer model by exposure to a weak alternating magnetic field, *Cancer Lett.*, 71, 75–81, 1993.

58. Mevissen, M., Haussler, M., Lerchl, A., and Loscher, W., Acceleration of mammary tumorigenesis by exposure of 7, 12-dimethylbenz[a]anthracene-treated female rats in a 50-Hz, 100-microT magnetic field: replication study, *J. Toxicol. Environ. Health*, 53, 401–418, 1998.

59. Anderson, L.E., Boorman, G.A., Morris, J.E., Sassar, L.B., Mann, P.C., Grumbein, S.L., Hailey, J.R., McNally, A., Sills, R.C., and Haseman, J.K., Effect of 13-week magnetic field exposures on DMBA-initiated mammary gland carcinomas in female Sprague-Dawley rats, *Carcinogenesis*, 20, 1615–1620, 1999.

60. Anderson, L.E., Morris, J.E., Sasser, L.B., and Loscher, W., Effects of 50- or 60-hertz, 100 microT magnetic field exposure in the DMBA mammary cancer model in Sprague-Dawley rats: possible explanations for different results from two laboratories, *Environ. Health Perspect.*, 108, 797–802, 2000.

61. Ekstrom, T., Mild, K.H., and Holmberg, B., Mammary tumours in Sprague-Dawley rats after initiation with DMBA followed by exposure to 50 Hz electromagnetic fields in a promotional scheme, *Cancer Lett.*, 123, 107–111, 1998.

62. Shen, Y.H., Shao, B.J., Chiang, H., Fu, Y.D., and Yu, M., The effects of 50 Hz magnetic field exposure on dimethylbenz(alpha)anthracene induced thymic lymphoma/leukemia in mice, *Bioelectromagnetics*, 18, 360–364, 1997.

63. Stuchly, M.A., McLean, J.R., Burnett, R., Goddard, M., Lecuyer, D.W., and Mitchel, R.E., Modification of tumor promotion in the mouse skin by exposure to an alternating magnetic field, *Cancer Lett.*, 65, 1–7, 1992.

64. McLean, J.R., Thansandote, A., McNamee, J.P., Tryphonas, L., Lecuyer, D., and Gajda, G., A 60 Hz magnetic field does not affect the incidence of squamous cell carcinomas in SENCAR mice, *Bioelectromagnetics*, 24, 75–81, 2003.

65. Sasser, L.B., Anderson, L.E., Morris, J.E., Miller, D.L., Walborg, E.F., Jr., Kavet, R., Johnston, D.A., and DiGiovanni, J., Lack of a co-promoting effect of a 60 Hz magnetic field on skin tumorigenesis in SENCAR mice, *Carcinogenesis*, 19, 1617–1621, 1999.

66. McLean, J.R., Thansandote, A., Lecuyer, D., and Goddard, M., The effect of 60-Hz magnetic fields on co-promotion of chemically induced skin tumors on SENCAR mice: a discussion of three studies, *Environ. Health Perspect.*, 105, 94–96, 1997.

67. Rannug, A., Ekström, T., Mild, K.H., Holmberg, B., Gimenez-Conti, I., and Slaga, T.J., A study on skin tumour formation in mice with 50 Hz magnetic field exposure. *Carcinogenesis*, 14, 573–578, 1993.

68. DiGiovanni, J., Johnston, D.A., Rupp, T., Sasser, L.B., Anderson, L.E., Morris, J.E., Miller, D.L., Kavet, R., and Walborg, E.F., Jr., Lack of effect of a 60 Hz magnetic field on biomarkers of tumor promotion in the skin of SENCAR mice, *Carcinogenesis*, 20, 685–689, 1999.

69. Rannug, A., Holmberg, B., and Mild, K.H., A rat liver foci promotion study with 50-Hz magnetic fields, *Environ. Res.*, 62, 223–229, 1993.
70. Rannug, A., Holmberg, B., Ekström, T., and Mild, K.H., Rat liver foci study on coexposure with 50 Hz magnetic fields and known carcinogens, *Bioelectromagnetics*, 14, 17–27, 1993.
71. McCormick, D.L., Ryan, B.M., Findlay, J.C., Gauger, J.R., Johnson, T.R., Morrissey, R.L., and Boorman, G.A., Exposure to 60 Hz magnetic fields and risk of lymphoma in PIM transgenic and TSG-p53 (p53 knockout) mice, *Carcinogenesis*, 19, 1649–1653, 1998.
72. Breuer, M.L., Slebos, R., Verbeek, S., van Lohuizen, M., Wientjens, E., and Berns, A., Very high frequency of lymphoma induction by a chemical carcinogen in *pim*-1 transgenic mice, *Nature*, 340, 61–63, 1989.
73. McCormick, D.L., Johnson, W.D., Rao, K.V.N., Bowman-Gram, T.A., Steele, V.E., Lubet, R.A., and Kelloff, G.J., Comparative activity of N-(4-hydroxyphenyl)-all-*trans*-retinamide and αdifluoromethyl-ornithine as inhibitors of lymphoma induction in PIM transgenic mice, *Carcinogenesis*, 17, 2513–2517, 1996.
74. Donehower, L.A., Harvey, M., Slagle, B.L., McArthur, M.J., Montgomery, C.A., Jr., Butel, J.S., and Bradley, A., Mice deficient for p53 are developmentally normal but susceptible to spontaneous tumours, *Nature*, 356, 215–221, 1992.
75. Harris, A.W., Basten, A., Gebski, V., Noonan, D., Finnie, J., Bath, M.L., Bangay, M.J., and Repacholi, M.H., A test of lymphoma induction by long-term exposure of E mu-Pim1 transgenic mice to 50 Hz magnetic fields, *Radiat. Res.*, 149, 300–307, 1998.
76. Wei, L.X., Goodman, R., and Henderson, A., Changes in levels of c-myc and histone H2B following exposure of cells to low-frequency sinusoidal electromagnetic fields: evidence for a window effect, *Bioelectromagnetics*, 11, 269–272, 1990.
77. Phillips, J.L., Effects of electromagnetic field exposure on gene transcription. *J. Cell Biochem.*, 51, 381–386, 1993.
78. Karabakhtsian, R., Broude, N., Shalts, N., Kochlatyi, S., Goodman, R., and Henderson, A.S., Calcium is necessary in the cell response to EM fields, *FEBS Lett.*, 349, 1–6, 1994.
79. Saffer, J.D., and Thurston, S.J., Short exposures to 60 Hz magnetic fields do not alter MYC expression in HL60 or Daudi cells, *Radiat. Res.*, 144, 18–25, 1995.
80. Lacy-Hulbert, A., Wilkins, R.C., Hesketh, T.R., and Metcalfe, J.C., No effect of 60 Hz electromagnetic fields on MYC or beta-actin expression in human leukemic cells, *Radiat. Res.*, 144, 9–17, 1995.
81. Owen, R.D., MYC mRNA abundance is unchanged in subcultures of HL60 cells exposed to power-line frequency magnetic fields, *Radiat. Res.*, 150, 23–30, 1998.
82. Jahreis, G.P., Johnson, P.G., Zhao, Y.L., and Hui, S.W., Absence of 60-Hz, 0.1-mT magnetic field-induced changes in oncogene transcription rates or levels in CEM-CM3 cells, *Biochim. Biophys. Acta*, 1443, 334–342, 1998.
83. Yomori, H., Yasunaga, K., Takahashi, C., Tanaka, A., Takashima, S., and Sekijima, M., Elliptically polarized magnetic fields do not alter immediate early response genes expression levels in human glioblastoma cells, *Bioelectromagnetics*, 23, 89–96, 2002.
84. Loberg, L.I., Gauger, J.R., Buthod, J.L., Engdahl, W.R., and McCormick, D.L., Gene expression in human breast epithelial cells exposed to 60 Hz magnetic fields, *Carcinogenesis*, 20, 1633–1636, 1999.
85. Balcer-Kubiczek, E.K., Harrison, G.H., Davis, C.C., Haas, M.L., and Koffman, B.H., Expression analysis of human HL60 cells exposed to 60 Hz square- or sine-wave magnetic fields, *Radiat. Res.*, 153, 670–678, 2000.
86. Chen, G., Lu, D., Chiang, H., Leszczynski, D., and Xu, Z., Using model organism Saccharomyces cerevisiae to evaluate the effects of ELF-MF and RF-EMF exposure on global gene expression, *Bioelectromagnetics*, 33, 550–560, 2012.
87. Lee, H.C., Hong, M.N., Jung, S.H., Kim, B.C., Suh, Y.J., Ko, Y.G., Lee, Y.S., Lee, B.Y., Cho, Y.Go, Myung, S.H., and Lee, J.S., Effect of extremely low frequency magnetic fields on cell proliferation and gene expression, *Bioelectromagnetics*, 36, 506–516, 2015.

88. Parham, F., Portier, C.J., Chang, X., and Mevissen, M., The use of signal-transduction and metabolic pathways to predict human disease targets from electric and magnetic fields using *in vitro* data in human cell lines, *Front. Public Health*, 4, 193, 2016. DOI:10.3389/fpubh.2016.00193, 2016.

89. Byus, C.V., Pieper, S.E., and Adey, W.R., The effects of low-energy 60-Hz environmental electromagnetic fields upon the growth-related enzyme ornithine decarboxylase, *Carcinogenesis*, 8, 1385–1389, 1987.

90. Mullins, J.M., Penafiel, L.M., Juutilainen, J., and Litovitz, T.A., Dose-response of electromagnetic field-enhanced ornithine decarboxylase activity, *Bioelectrochem. Bioenerg.*, 48, 193–199, 1999.

91. Cress, L.W., Owen, R.D., and Desta, A.B., Ornithine decarboxylase activity in L929 cells following exposure to 60 Hz magnetic fields, *Carcinogenesis*, 20, 1025–1030, 1999.

92. Kumlin, T., Alhonen, L., Jänne, J., Lang, S., Kosma, V.M., and Juutilainen, J., Epidermal ornithine decarboxylase and polyamines in mice exposed to 50 Hz magnetic fields and UV radiation, *Bioelectromagnetics*, 19, 388–391, 1998.

93. McDonald, L.J., Loberg, L.I., Savage, R.E., Jr., Zhu, H., Lotz, W.G., Mandeville, R., Owen, R.D., Cress, L.W., Desta, A.B., Gauger, J.R., and McCormick, D.L., Ornithine decarboxylase activity in tissues from rats exposed to 60 Hz magnetic fields including harmonic and transient field characteristics, *Toxicol. Mechanisms and Methods*, 13, 31–38, 2003.

94. Lin, H., Head, M., Blank, M., Han, L., Jin, M., and Goodman, R., Myc-mediated transactivation of HSP70 expression following exposure to magnetic fields, *J. Cell Biochem.*, 69, 181–188, 1998.

95. Malagoli, D., Lusvardi, M., Gobba, F., and Ottaviani, E., 50 Hz magnetic fields activate mussel immunocyte p38 MAP kinase and induce HSP70 and 90, *Comp. Biochem. Physiol. C Toxicol. Pharmacol.*, 137, 75–79, 2004.

96. Kang, K.I., Bouhouche, I., Fortin, D., Baulieu, E.E., and Catelli, M.G., Luciferase activity and synthesis of Hsp70 and Hsp90 are insensitive to 50Hz electromagnetic fields, *Life Sci.*, 63, 489–497, 1998.

97. Morehouse, C.A., and Owen, R.D., Exposure to low-frequency electromagnetic fields does not alter HSP70 expression or HSF-HSE binding in HL60 cells, *Radiat. Res.*, 153, 658–662, 2000.

98. Mariucci, G., Vilarini, M., Moretti, M., Taha, E., Conte, C., Minelli, A., Aristei, C., and Ambrosini, M.V., Brain DNA damage and 70-kDa heat shock protein expression in CD1 mice exposed to extremely low frequency magnetic fields, *Int. J. Radiat. Biol.*, 86, 701–701, 2010.

99. Thun-Battersby, S., Westermann, J., and Löscher, W., Lymphocyte subset analyses in blood, spleen and lymph nodes of female Sprague-Dawley rats after short or prolonged exposure to a 50 Hz 100-microT magnetic field, *Radiat. Res.*, 152, 436–443, 1999.

100. Stevens, R.G., and Davis, S., The melatonin hypothesis: Electric power and breast cancer, *Environ. Health Perspect.*, 104(Suppl 1), 135–140, 1996.

101. Reiter, R.J., Tan, D.X., Manchester, L.C., Lopez-Burillo, S., Sainz, R.M., and Mayo, J.C., Melatonin: Detoxification of oxygen and nitrogen-based toxic reactants, *Adv. Exp. Med. Biol.*, 527, 539–548, 2003.

102. Reiter, R.J., Alterations of the circadian melatonin rhythm by the electromagnetic spectrum: A study in environmental toxicology, *Regul. Toxicol. Pharmacol.*, 15, 226–244, 1992.

103. Brainard, G.C., Kavet, R., and Kheifets, L.I., The relationship between electromagnetic field and light exposures to melatonin and breast cancer risk: a review of the relevant literature, *J. Pineal. Res.*, 26, 65–100, 1999.

104. Graham, C., Cook, M.R., Riffle, D.W., Gerkovich, M.M., and Cohen, H.D., Nocturnal melatonin levels in human volunteers exposed to intermittent 60 Hz magnetic fields, *Bioelectromagnetics*, 17, 263–273, 1996.

105. Graham, C., Cook, M.R., Sastre, A., Riffle, D.W., and Gerkovich, M.M., Multi-night exposure to 60 Hz magnetic fields: effects on melatonin and its enzymatic metabolite, *J. Pineal. Res.*, 28, 1–8, 2000.

106. Graham, C., Cook, M.R, Gerkovich, M.M, and Sastre, A., Examination of the melatonin hypothesis in women exposed at night to EMF or bright light, *Environ. Health Perspect.*, 109, 501–507, 2001.

107. Löscher, W., Mevissen, M., and Lerchl, A., Exposure of female rats to a 100-microT 50 Hz magnetic field does not induce consistent changes in nocturnal levels of melatonin, *Radiat. Res.*, 150, 557–567, 1998.
108. Lewczuk, B., Redlarski, G., Zak, A., Ziólkowska, N., Przybylska-Gornowicz, B., and Krawczuk, M., Influence of electric, magnetic, and electromagnetic fields on the circadian system: current stage of knowledge, *Biomed. Res. Int.*, 2014, 169459, 2014. DOI:10.1155/2014/169459, 2014.
109. Touitou, Y., and Selmaoui, B., The effects of extremely low-frequency magnetic fields on melatonin and cortisol, two marker rhythms of the circadian system, *Dialogues Clin. Neurosci.*, 14, 381–390, 2012.
110. Yellon, S.M., Acute 60 Hz magnetic field exposure effects on the melatonin rhythm in the pineal gland and circulation of the adult Djungarian hamster, *J. Pineal. Res.*, 16, 136–144, 1994.
111. Brendel, H., Niehaus, M., and Lerchl, A., Direct suppressive effects of weak magnetic fields (50 Hz and 16 2/3 Hz) on melatonin synthesis in the pineal gland of Djungarian hamsters (Phodopus sungorus), *J. Pineal. Res.*, 29, 228–233, 2000.

5

Evaluation of the Potential Oncogenicity of Radiofrequency Fields in Experimental Animal Models

David L. McCormick

IIT Research Institute

CONTENTS

5.1 Introduction 148
    5.1.1 Possible Health Effects of Radiofrequency Radiation from Mobile Telephones and Other Wireless Communications Devices 148
    5.1.2 Strategies to Identify Possible Health Effects of Radiofrequency Radiation from Mobile Telephones and Other Wireless Communications Devices 149
    5.1.3 Investigative Studies of RFR Exposure in Laboratory Animal Models 151
5.2 Assessment of the Possible Oncogenic Activity of RFR using the Rodent 2-Year Bioassay 152
    5.2.1 Design of the Rodent 2-Year Oncogenicity Bioassay 152
    5.2.2 Results of 2-Year Rodent Oncogenicity Bioassays of RFR 152
        5.2.2.1 IIT Research Institute (USA) Chronic Bioassays of GSM- and CDMA-Modulated 900 MHz RFR in Sprague-Dawley Rats 153
        5.2.2.2 University of Washington (USA) Chronic Bioassay of 2450 MHz Microwaves in Sprague-Dawley Rats 155
        5.2.2.3 University of Tübingen (Germany) Chronic Bioassays of Pulsed 900 MHz GSM RFR in Sprague-Dawley Rats 155
        5.2.2.4 Washington University in St. Louis (USA) Chronic Bioassays of FDMA and CDMA RFR in F344 Rats 156
        5.2.2.5 Battelle (USA) Chronic Bioassay of 1.6 GHz RFR in F344 Rats 156
        5.2.2.6 RCC, Ltd. (Switzerland) Chronic Bioassay of GSM and DCS RFR in Han Wistar Rats 157
        5.2.2.7 IIT Research Institute (USA) Chronic Bioassays of GSM- and CDMA-Modulated 1900 MHz RFR in B6C3F1 Mice 157
        5.2.2.8 Fraunhofer (Germany) Chronic Bioassay of GSM and DCS RFR in B6C3F1 Mice 158
        5.2.2.9 Overview of Chronic Rodent Oncogenicity Studies 159
5.3 Assessment of the Possible Oncogenic Activity of RFR Using Tumor-Prone Rodent Models 160
    5.3.1 Results of Oncogenicity Bioassays of RFR in Genetically Engineered Tumor-Prone Rodent Models 161
        5.3.1.1 Oncogenicity Studies in the Eμ-*pim*-1 transgenic mouse 161

5.1 Introduction

5.1.1 Possible Health Effects of Radiofrequency Radiation from Mobile Telephones and Other Wireless Communications Devices

Wireless communications devices are ubiquitous components of the modern lifestyle in both industrialized countries and less developed areas of the world. Although mobile telephones and other wireless devices now seem essential for everyday life, their history of use is relatively short. In 1983, the Motorola DynaTAC 8000X was the first mobile phone approved by the Federal Communications Commission for use in the United States [1]. Growth in mobile phone usage since that time has been extraordinary: whereas the number of U.S. cell phone subscriptions in 1990 was equal to only 2% of the American population [2], the number of U.S. cell phone subscriptions in 2017 [3] approaches 75% of the American population.

Calendar year 2017 data from the Global System For Mobile Communications (GSM) Association, an industry trade group, indicates that more than 2/3 of the world's population currently has access to a mobile communications device, and more than five billion subscriptions to wireless services are now active [4]. Primarily as a result of the continuing rapid growth in wireless device use in India and other parts of Asia, the GSM Association predicts that the number of wireless subscriptions worldwide will reach 5.7 billion by 2020 [4].

Because wireless devices communicate through the use of radiofrequency radiation (RFR), a consequence of the nearly universal use of cellular telephones and other wireless devices is that billions of people worldwide receive daily exposure to RFR. Over the past two decades, a substantial number of laboratory and epidemiology studies have been performed to investigate whether exposure to RFR may lead to adverse health outcomes.

Both positive and negative findings have been reported from studies in laboratory animals and in humans [reviewed in 5–7], but no consistent pattern of RFR health effects has been identified. As a result, no scientific consensus has emerged concerning the possible risks of human exposure to RFR. However, in consideration of the extremely large number of people who are regularly exposed to RFR, even a small increase in the risk of cancer or other disease that may result from the use of cellular telephones or other wireless communications devices could have important public health implications.

A substantial body of literature published over more than 50 years clearly demonstrates that exposure to microwaves or RFR at high field strengths (power levels that are substantially higher than those emitted by wireless communications devices) can induce tissue heating. As a consequence of this tissue heating, exposure to high levels of RFR (as generated by radar equipment, diathermy machines, unshielded microwave devices, and other equipment) may induce temperature-dependent changes in several tissues. Adverse health effects of tissue heating by RFR in animal models includes induction of cataracts [8,9,10] and adverse reproductive outcomes [11,12].

Although the use of mobile phones results in the local deposition of RF energy in the brain and other tissues in the head [13,14,15], flux densities of RF fields generated by wireless communications devices are well below the levels that will induce measurable tissue heating. For this reason, identification of possible adverse effects of exposure to nonthermal levels of RFR has become the central focus of health effects research related to the use of wireless communications devices. The key question to be resolved in RFR health effects research is "does exposure to RFR generated by cellular telephones and other wireless devices induce nonthermal effects that will induce or exacerbate disease?"

5.1.2 Strategies to Identify Possible Health Effects of Radiofrequency Radiation from Mobile Telephones and Other Wireless Communications Devices

It has become increasingly clear that a comprehensive evaluation of the possible health risks of human exposure to RFR should be based on a "weight of the evidence" approach that integrates data from (a) epidemiology studies in human populations; (b) hazard identification studies in predictive animal models; and (c) mechanistic studies in relevant *in vivo* and *in vitro* test systems [16]. At the present time, neither epidemiology alone, experimental bioassays alone, nor mechanistic studies alone are sufficiently informative to support a broad assessment of RFR health effects.

Although epidemiology offers the obvious advantage of examining health effects in humans receiving "real world" exposures, RFR epidemiology has several important limitations. In addition to the strengths and limitations of all epidemiology studies [17], key issues in RFR epidemiology include:

- the unknown duration of RFR exposure that is required to induce an adverse health effect. Because broad public use of wireless communications devices has a relatively brief history [2], the duration of human exposure to RFR may be too short for epidemiology to identify chronic toxicities or other adverse effects (including some malignancies) with long latent periods. For this reason, definitive epidemiology data for the possible relationship between RFR exposure and some cancers may not be generated for 20 years or more. In consideration of this possibility, important unanswered questions include: (a) what duration of RFR exposure is necessary to induce an adverse health effect, and (b) when should monitoring of exposed populations be initiated to identify such effects?

- challenges in the quantitation of actual RFR exposures for users of mobile telephones and other wireless communications devices. Although a number of approaches to exposure assessment have been used in RFR epidemiology studies [18,19,20], accurate assessment of human exposure to RFR generated by mobile telephones remains a major challenge. Clearly, reliable quantitation of RFR exposure is essential to support epidemiologic findings of adverse health effects [18].

- the need for adverse health outcomes to have occurred prior to hazard identification, thus delaying the possible identification of a true human hazard for years, if not decades. This is considered to be perhaps the most important limitation of RFR epidemiology. Given the potentially long latency of RFR-induced health effects, identification of such effects through epidemiology alone may require years (or decades) of exposure. Should epidemiology identify significant adverse health effects of RFR exposure, billions of people will have already been exposed to RFR for extended periods and will therefore be at risk of those health effects. Given the truly massive population exposure to RFR from wireless devices, avoidance of a potentially major public health crisis mandates that risks be identified more quickly than can be accomplished through epidemiology alone.

Studies in predictive animal models may identify potential human health hazards years (or decades) earlier than can epidemiology. This shorter time required to identify possible health hazards of RFR increases in importance when those hazards may include neoplasms with long latent periods. Importantly, a large body of evidence has developed to support the predictive power of well-designed animal bioassays, particularly the 2-year oncogenicity bioassay in rodents, to identify human carcinogens [reviewed in 21,22]. Well-designed and conducted animal bioassays also offer the opportunity to evaluate possible health effects under tightly controlled exposure conditions that support the characterization of dose-response (or exposure-response) relationships, and reduce or eliminate factors that could confound or otherwise impact results. That said, however, the need to extrapolate animal bioassay data from rodents to humans, and the common requirement to extrapolate effects of high-dose exposures in rodents to possible effects of much lower exposure levels in humans greatly complicate the interpretation of animal bioassay data [23].

Data from mechanistic studies performed using *in vivo* or *in vitro* model systems may identify cellular, biochemical, or molecular mechanisms that underlie effects of RFR identified in epidemiology studies or animal bioassays. It should be noted, however, that identification of a mechanism of action is not essential to identify an agent as being hazardous or possibly hazardous to humans. Furthermore, although demonstration of specific cellular, biochemical, or molecular effects of RFR that may be relevant to the induction of cancer or other diseases is clearly relevant to hazard identification, such data are not, in themselves, sufficient to identify a hazard. Because most critical physiological processes are regulated by redundant mechanisms, identification of an effect on a single mechanism may or may not be biologically significant for the organism. For this reason, findings of effects on disease-related mechanisms are most often considered to be secondary data that can be used to understand, support, and interpret the results of epidemiology studies or animal bioassays. Without evidence of a hazard identified by epidemiology studies or bioassays in experimental animal models, mechanistic data alone cannot be interpreted as definitive evidence that a health hazard exists.

Based on the complementary strengths and limitations of epidemiology studies and animal bioassays, and the secondary role played by mechanistic data in hazard identification, it is clear that integration of data from all three types of investigations provides the most comprehensive approach to identifying possible health hazards that may result from human exposure to RFR. In situations where the epidemiology data are incomplete, inconclusive, or conflicting, the importance of animal bioassays increases. In this chapter, the results of animal bioassays of RFR are reviewed and interpreted in the context of developing a comprehensive assessment of the possible health effects of RFR exposure.

5.1.3 Investigative Studies of RFR Exposure in Laboratory Animal Models

The scientific literature contains a substantial body of research addressing the toxicity and potential oncogenicity of RFR in animal models. For the purposes of this review, toxicology and carcinogenesis bioassays of RFR in animal models are summarized in three sections of this chapter.

- In Section 5.2, chronic studies to investigate the possible oncogenicity of RFR in standard-bred animal models are reviewed. The most comprehensive studies included in this section are 2-year oncogenicity bioassays performed in rodents. Over several decades, a substantial database has developed that supports the value of the 2-year oncogenicity bioassay in rodents in predicting carcinogenic activity in humans [reviewed in 21]. The design of these studies involves observation of relatively large groups of animals over the majority of their normal lifespan. These studies also include microscopic evaluation of a large list of tissues from all study animals, and therefore support an evaluation of the risk of oncogenesis in all major organs. In most cases, studies are designed to comply with the safety assessment requirements of organizations such as the United States Food and Drug Administration (FDA; the regulatory body responsible for the oversight of the safety of cellular telephones and other wireless communications devices in the United States); the United States Environmental Protection Agency (EPA); and/or the International Council for Harmonisation (ICH, an international organization focused on standardizing safety testing protocols used around the world).

- In Section 5.3, studies designed to evaluate the potential carcinogenic activity of RFR in tumor-prone mice will be reviewed. Studies discussed in this section include those performed using (a) animals that have been genetically engineered by insertion of an oncogene or deletion of a tumor suppressor gene, resulting in increased sensitivity to neoplastic development, and (b) animal strains that have been selectively bred to increase sensitivity to neoplastic development in specific tissues. In addition to supplementing data from 2-year oncogenicity bioassays, these models may identify carcinogenic effects of RFR that occur in sensitive subpopulations. It is important to note, however, that most tumor-prone animals lack a long history of use in hazard identification; as such, their value in predicting human responses has generally not been established.

- In Section 5.4, studies are reviewed in which exposure to RFR is combined with simultaneous or sequential exposure to other chemical or physical agents to characterize the possible activity of RFR as a tumor initiator, a tumor promoter, or a co-carcinogen in one or more organs. These multistage carcinogenesis bioassays are most commonly performed using animal models that have been designed for use as research tools to study organ-specific carcinogenesis. As is the case with tumor-prone animals, the value of data from multistage carcinogenesis bioassays in predicting human cancer responses to exogenous agents has not been established.

5.2 Assessment of the Possible Oncogenic Activity of RFR using the Rodent 2-Year Bioassay

5.2.1 Design of the Rodent 2-Year Oncogenicity Bioassay

The chronic (2-year) rodent oncogenicity bioassay is considered to be the "gold standard" protocol for the experimental assessment of carcinogenic activity. Two-year bioassays in rodents have been demonstrated to be useful predictors of human carcinogenic responses [21]; data from these bioassays are accepted by American and international regulatory agencies as providing the most comprehensive and most predictive experimental approach to assess agent carcinogenicity.

In a well-designed chronic rodent bioassay, elements of the study protocol (e.g., group sizes, exposure levels) are designed to maximize the likelihood of identifying an increase in cancer incidence following long-term exposure to agents with carcinogenic activity. The design of these studies was discussed in detail in the chapter in this volume entitled "Evaluation of the Toxicity and Potential Oncogenicity of ELF Magnetic Fields in Experimental Animal Model Systems," and will not be repeated here. Briefly, however, exposures begin either *in utero* or when mice or rats are young adults, and continue for 2 years. The 2-year exposure period encompasses the majority of the normal lifespan of these species, and thereby maximizes the probability of identifying an oncogenic effect. Group sizes (≥50 animals per sex per group) are larger than are used in other toxicology bioassays, and are often increased to as many as 100 (or more) animals per sex per group to increase statistical power. Study designs generally include complete histopathologic evaluation of approximately 45 tissues from each study animal, thereby permitting the assessment of oncogenicity in all major organs in the body.

These studies are most often conducted using a standardized study design that is referred to as the "Chronic Oncogenicity Bioassay in Rodents." This study design has been used widely as the basis to evaluate the potential carcinogenicity of new drugs, agricultural chemicals, occupational chemicals, and a wide range of environmental agents, and is considered to be a useful predictor of human oncogenicity [21]. The International Agency for Research on Cancer (IARC) and United States National Toxicology Program (NTP) have both performed analyses demonstrating the utility of the rodent chronic bioassay as a predictor of predict human carcinogenicity. As a result, it is generally accepted among toxicologists that the chronic rodent bioassay currently provides the best available experimental approach to identify agents that may be carcinogenic in humans.

5.2.2 Results of 2-Year Rodent Oncogenicity Bioassays of RFR

Two-year bioassays of RFR and microwaves of a similar frequency have been performed in three strains of rats (Sprague-Dawley, Fischer [F344], Wistar) and in one strain of mice (B6C3F1).

It is important to note that these studies were performed using several different RFR exposure metrics and delivery systems; study protocols also include substantial differences in the duration of daily exposure. Several chronic bioassays of RFR were performed using "head only" or "head first" exposures, in which restrained rodents are exposed using a "Ferris wheel" type of exposure system. This type of exposure system directs RFR to the head of the animal, and in this manner simulates the regional deposition of RF energy that humans may receive from a mobile telephone. On this basis, use of a "head-only" exposure system may provide an advantage in terms of the specific parts of the body in which RFR is deposited. However, the need to restrain animals during exposures performed using these systems limits the duration of daily RFR exposure to several hours, and may also induce restraint stress.

By contrast, other chronic bioassays of RFR were performed using systems that expose unrestrained animals in their home cages. This type of exposure system permits animals to be exposed to RFR for much longer periods each day, and may thereby increase the likelihood of identifying carcinogenic effects of RFR (if such effects exist). Exposure in these studies is whole-body, and as such, does not recapitulate the spatial deposition of RFR seen in users of mobile telephones. However, exposure of unrestrained animals in their home cages allows much longer daily exposures than can be performed using a "head-only" system, and also removes the possible confounder of restraint stress.

5.2.2.1 IIT Research Institute (USA) Chronic Bioassays of GSM- and CDMA-Modulated 900 MHz RFR in Sprague-Dawley Rats

The largest chronic oncogenicity bioassay of RFR in rats was performed at IIT Research Institute under contract to the NTP. Although complete results from this study have not been published, peer review of selected neoplastic lesions has been completed, and the NTP has presented a summary of tumor incidence data from selected tissues [24] in this study. The data presented in [24] have also been presented and discussed at a recent international scientific meeting [25].

The RFR exposure system used in the study was based on a reverberation chamber concept; details of the exposure system design and associated animal dosimetry have been published [26,27]. Seven groups of Sprague-Dawley rats (100/sex/group) received chronic whole body exposure to 900 MHz RFR at specific absorption rates (SARs) of 0 (sham control), 1.5, 3.0, or 6.0 W/kg. Data from a preliminary study demonstrated that an SAR of 6.0 W/kg is the maximum RFR exposure level to which rats can be exposed without increasing mean body temperature by more than 1°C. On this basis, all three exposure levels used in this study were defined as being "nonthermal."

The study design included 3 groups of rats exposed to 900 MHz RFR with Global System for Mobile Communications (GSM) modulation; 3 groups of rats exposed to 900 MHz RFR with Code Division Multiple Access (CDMA) modulation; and a sham control group that was housed in an identical reverberation chamber but received no exposure to RFR. Rats were exposed to RFR for 18.5 hours per day, 7 days per week, using a schedule of 10 minutes on/10 minutes off. To maintain constant exposure levels (SARs) over time, the intensity of RFR signals was adjusted on a regular schedule throughout the exposure period to reflect changes in mean body weight in each group. RFR signal intensity and environmental conditions (temperature, humidity, airflows, light cycle) in each chamber were monitored continuously throughout the 2+-year exposure period.

RFR exposures in all groups were initiated *in utero* (on gestation day 6), and were continued through gestation, parturition, the neonatal and juvenile periods, and for 2 years after weaning. An interim necropsy of 10 rats per sex per group was performed at 13 weeks after weaning; remaining animals in each group were exposed until the time of their death or for a minimum of 104 weeks after weaning. A comprehensive microscopic examination of tissues from all animals in all groups was performed. Additional details of the study design have been presented [24].

The results of this study demonstrated that chronic exposure to 900 MHz RFR with either GSM or CDMA modulations at SARs of up to 6 W/kg induced no gross clinical evidence of toxicity in any study animal. RFR exposure had no biologically significant effects on group mean body weight or body weight gain, and had no effect on hematology parameters evaluated after 13 weeks of exposure. Surprisingly, however, all groups of male rats exposed to RFR demonstrated statistically significant increases in survival when compared to male rats in the sham control group; by contrast, survival in female rats exposed to RFR was not significantly different from that in female sham controls. The increased survival in RFR-exposed male rats was attributed by the Study Pathologist to be the result of reduced nephropathy; nephropathy is a common age-related change in rats, and is responsible for a substantial fraction of mortality in 2-year studies in this species.

When compared to female sham controls, one or more groups of female rats receiving chronic exposure to RFR demonstrated statistically significant reductions in (a) the total incidence of primary neoplasms; (b) the total incidence of malignant neoplasms; (c) the total incidence of benign neoplasms; and (d) total incidences of neoplasms in the liver, mammary gland, or pituitary gland. A trend towards increased incidence of thyroid C-cell carcinomas with increasing exposure was seen in female rats exposed to GSM RFR; however, no statistically significant differences from sham control were seen in the incidences of proliferative brain lesions or Schwann cell lesions in female rats exposed to RFR. In consideration of the reductions in the total incidences of malignant and benign tumors in RFR-exposed female rats, and the lower incidences of neoplasms in several specific organ sites in these animals, these data do not support the hypothesis that chronic exposure to nonthermal levels of RFR is carcinogenic in female rats.

The situation in male rats was quite different. Male rats exposed to CDMA-modulated RFR demonstrated a statistically significant trend towards increased incidences of proliferative brain lesions (malignant glioma + glial cell hyperplasia [a preneoplastic lesion]) with increasing RFR exposure. Whereas 0/90 male rats in the sham control group demonstrated proliferative brain lesions, the incidences of proliferative brain lesions in male rats exposed to CDMA-modulated RFR at the low, mid, and high levels were 2/90, 0/90, and 5/90, respectively ($p < 0.05$ for dose-dependent trend). Similarly, incidences of proliferative brain lesions in male rats exposed to GSM-modulated RFR at the low, mid, and high levels were 5/90, 6/90, and 3/90, respectively.

Male rats exposed to either GSM- or CDMA-modulated RFR also demonstrated statistically significant, dose-dependent trends towards increased incidences of proliferative Schwann cell lesions of the heart. Whereas no proliferative Schwann cell lesions were identified in male sham controls (0/90 rats), 7/90 male rats exposed to GSM-modulated RFR at 6 W/kg and 9/90 male rats exposed to CDMA-modulated RFR at 6 W/kg demonstrated proliferative Schwann cell lesions; lower incidences of Schwann cell lesions were seen in male rats exposed to RFR at 1.5 or 3 W/kg.

As mentioned previously, all groups of male rats exposed to RFR demonstrated significantly greater survival than did male rats receiving sham exposure; the improved survival in RFR-exposed male rats was attributed to decreased nephropathy. In consideration of the greater survival of male rats exposed to RFR, the increased incidences of brain and

Schwann cell lesions in these animals could be the result of increased longevity. Clearly, possible effects of survival cannot be excluded. However, statistical analyses performed by the NTP did include age adjustments [24], suggesting that the increased incidences of neoplastic and preneoplastic lesions in the brain and heart of male rats exposed to RFR were an effect of exposure and were not due solely to improved survival.

5.2.2.2 University of Washington (USA) Chronic Bioassay of 2450 MHz Microwaves in Sprague-Dawley Rats

Although not designed specifically to examine the effects of long-term exposure to RFR, an early study performed at the University of Washington did evaluate the effects of chronic exposure to 2450 MHz microwaves in male rats [28]. The 2450 MHz signal frequency used in this study is close to frequencies used in some wireless communications devices systems.

Beginning at 8 weeks of age, male Sprague-Dawley rats (100/group) received either sham exposure or exposure to 2450 MHz pulsed microwaves for 21.5 hours per day, 7 days per week, for 25 months. The microwave signal used was 800 pps with a 10 μs pulse width; because exposure levels were not adjusted during the in-life period to account for changes in animal body weight, SAR values in the study ranged from approximately 0.4 W/kg in young rats to approximately 0.15 W/kg in older rats at their peak body weights. Based on a maximum SAR of 0.4 W/kg and a daily exposure period of 21.5 hours, the maximum daily exposure received by rats in this study is <20% of that received in the IIT Research Institute/NTP study described above.

Male rats exposed to 2450 MHz microwaves for 2 years demonstrated mortality patterns and mean body weights that were comparable to those of sham controls. Microwave exposure was not associated with statistically significant increases in the incidence of any benign or malignant tumor in any organ. Although rats exposed to microwaves did demonstrate a higher total incidence of malignant lesions than did sham controls, this increase resulted from pooling of nonsignificant increases in the incidence of malignant lesions in several sites. On this basis, this increase is not seen as being biologically significant.

5.2.2.3 University of Tübingen (Germany) Chronic Bioassays of Pulsed 900 MHz GSM RFR in Sprague-Dawley Rats

A team of scientists at the University of Tübingen performed four small studies in female Sprague-Dawley rats to evaluate the possible oncogenicity of low-dose exposure to pulsed 900 MHz RFR with GSM modulation [29]. In all studies, rats received either sham exposure or exposure to 217 Hz pulsed 900 MHz RFR with GSM modulation for 23 hours per day, 7 days per week, for up to 37 months. RFR exposure levels used in these studies were substantially lower than those used in other chronic bioassays performed in Sprague-Dawley rats: whole body SARs measured during the in-life periods of these studies ranged from 15 to 130 mW/kg; these exposures compare with the peak SAR of 400 mW/kg used in the University of Washington study and constant SARs of 1.5, 3, and 6 W/kg used in the IIT Research Institute/NTP study.

In addition to the use of low RFR exposure levels, the four studies have several important design weaknesses that diminish their value for use in hazard identification. Because the four studies were performed separately over a period of approximately 11 years, their results cannot reasonably be pooled. In addition, group sizes in each study were much smaller than are commonly used in 2-year bioassays: the first two studies each included only 12 rats per group, while the third and fourth studies each included only 30 rats per group. Finally, detailed microscopic evaluation of tissues was performed in only one of the four studies reported in this publication.

When compared to cancer incidences observed in animals in the sham control group, no significant increases in cancer incidence were identified in any tissue in rats receiving long-term exposure to RF. On this basis, the results of these studies do not support the hypothesis that RF exposure is a significant risk factor for carcinogenesis in rats. However, the substantial design weaknesses in these studies greatly limit their value for hazard identification. On the basis of these design flaws (most notably small group sizes and inadequate microscopic evaluations), the results of these studies must be considered to be inconclusive.

5.2.2.4 Washington University in St. Louis (USA) Chronic Bioassays of FDMA and CDMA RFR in F344 Rats

La Regina and colleagues from Washington University in St. Louis performed a 2-year study to determine the effects of exposure to Frequency Division Multiple Access (FDMA) RFR or Code Division Multiple Access (CDMA) RFR signals in F344 (Fischer) rats. Beginning at age 6 weeks, groups of 80 rats per sex received sham exposure (control) or were exposed to 835.62 MHz FDMA or 847.74 MHz CDMA for 4 hours per day, 5 days per week for 24 months. The nominal time-averaged SAR in the brain was 1.3 ± 0.5 W/kg in groups exposed to each RFR signal. RFR or sham exposure was initiated when rats were 6 weeks old; animals were restrained during their daily periods of RFR or sham exposure.

Survival and body weights in RFR-exposed groups were comparable to those of sex-matched sham controls. Comparisons of tumor incidences in exposed groups versus sham controls failed to identify any statistically significant differences in the incidences of any tumor in any organ site. The authors concluded that chronic exposure to 835.62 MHz FDMA or 847.7 MHz CDMA for up to 4 hours per day, 5 days per week for 2 years had no significant effect on tumor incidence in either sex of F344 rats.

5.2.2.5 Battelle (USA) Chronic Bioassay of 1.6 GHz RFR in F344 Rats

Scientists at Battelle-Pacific Northwest Laboratories performed a chronic bioassay in F344 rats to identify possible adverse effects of long-term exposure to a 1.6 GHz (1600 MHz) RFR signal; this signal was used in the Iridium satellite-based network for wireless communication. In this study, three groups of 36 timed-pregnant rats received sham exposure or whole body exposure to a far-field Iridium signal that resulted in an SAR of 0.16 W/kg in the brain of the fetus. Far-field RFR or sham exposures were initiated at gestation day 19, and were continued through parturition and the neonatal and early juvenile periods (until weaning at approximately 23 days after parturition). Rats were not restrained during these exposures. Beginning at 36 days after parturition, pups from RFR-exposed dams were assorted into groups of 90 F_1 rats per sex and received "head-first" exposure to a near-field Iridium signal at levels selected to induce SARs of 0.16 or 1.6 W/kg in the brain. A sham control group of 90 F_1 pups born to dams that received sham exposure only was exposed to sham fields beginning at age 36 days. F_1 rats in all groups were restrained and exposed for 2 hours per day, 5 days per week until they reached 2 years of age. In addition, a (non-exposed) shelf control group of equal size was included in the study design.

Exposure of pregnant dams to the Iridium signal had no effect on the number of live pups per litter, pup survival, or pup body weight. When compared to F_1 rats in the sham control group, F_1 rats receiving chronic exposure to the Iridium signal demonstrated no statistically significant differences in survival, clinical signs, or tumor incidence in any site. It was concluded that the results of this study do not support the hypothesis that exposure to the 1.6 GHz Iridium signal induces significant adverse health effects (including cancer) in either sex of F344 rats.

5.2.2.6 RCC, Ltd. (Switzerland) Chronic Bioassay of GSM and DCS RFR in Han Wistar Rats

Smith et al. [32] performed a very large study to evaluate the chronic toxicity and possible oncogenicity of a 902 MHz GSM RFR signal and a 1747 MHz digital communication system (DCS) RFR signal in rats. Beginning at approximately 6 weeks of age, groups of 65 Han Wistar rats per sex were exposed for 2 hours per day, 5 days per week at nominal SARs of 0 (sham control), 0.44, 1.33, or 4.0 W/kg. Rats were restrained during daily RFR exposure. Fifteen rats per sex per group were euthanized at 52 weeks for an interim necropsy; remaining animals in each group were exposed until their natural death or the terminal necropsy after 104 weeks of exposure. The study design also included a cage control group that was not restrained or exposed to RFR.

Toxicological endpoints evaluated during the in-life portion of the study included survival, clinical signs, body weight, food consumption, ophthalmoscopy, and clinical pathology; rats were also palpated regularly throughout the study to identify gross lesions in the mammary gland and other tissues. Terminal and postmortem evaluations included organ weights, gross pathology at necropsy, and microscopic evaluation of tissues.

The authors did not identify any adverse effects of chronic exposure to either GSM or DCS RFR. Sham control and RFR-exposed rats demonstrated comparable survival, mean body weights, mean individual organ weights, and numbers and types of both neoplastic and non-neoplastic lesions. When compared to the sham control group, RFR-exposed groups did not demonstrate statistically significant differences in the total incidences of primary tumors; the total incidences of malignant tumors; the total incidences of benign tumors; median tumor latency or multiplicity (for organs such as the mammary gland in which multiple tumors may be identified and the latency determined); or the number of rats with metastatic lesions. The authors concluded that the results of this study do not support the hypotheses that chronic exposure to either a 902 MHz GSM RFR signal or a 1747 MHz DCS RFR signal induces significant adverse health effects in either sex of Han Wistar rats.

5.2.2.7 IIT Research Institute (USA) Chronic Bioassays of GSM- and CDMA-Modulated 1900 MHz RFR in B6C3F1 Mice

The largest chronic oncogenicity bioassay of RFR in mice was performed at IIT Research Institute (USA) simultaneously with the rat study discussed in Section 5.2.2.1. This study was also supported by the NTP.

As discussed in Section 5.2.2.1, the RFR exposure system used in the study was based on a reverberation chamber concept [26,27]. Seven groups of B6C3F1 mice (105/sex/group) received chronic whole body exposure to 1900 MHz RFR at SARs of 0 (sham control), 2.5, 5.0, or 10.0 W/kg. Data from a preliminary study demonstrated that mice can be exposed to 1900 MHz RFR at an SAR of 10.0 W/kg without increasing mean body temperature by more than 1°C. On this basis, all three exposure levels used in this study were defined as being "nonthermal."

The study included 3 groups of mice exposed to 1900 MHz RFR with GSM modulation, 3 groups of mice exposed to 1900 MHz RFR with CDMA modulation, and a sham control group that was housed in an identical reverberation chamber but received no RFR exposure. RFR exposures were 18.5 hours per day, 7 days per week, using a schedule of 10 minutes on/10 minutes off. To maintain constant exposure levels (SARs) over time, the intensity of RFR signals was adjusted on a regular schedule throughout the exposure period to reflect changes in group mean body weights. RFR signal intensity and environmental conditions (temperature, humidity, airflows, light cycle) in each chamber were monitored continuously throughout the 2-year exposure period.

RFR exposures were initiated when mice were 5–6 weeks of age. An interim necropsy of 15 mice per sex per group was performed after 13 weeks of RFR or sham exposure; remaining mice in each group were exposed until the time of their death or for 104 weeks. All mice received a complete necropsy, followed by a comprehensive microscopic examination of tissues.

The results of this study demonstrated that chronic exposure of mice to 1900 MHz RFR with either GSM or CDMA modulations at SARs of up to 10 W/kg for 2 years induced no gross clinical evidence of toxicity. RFR exposure had no adverse effects on survival; in fact, survival in eleven of the twelve groups of RFR-exposed mice exceeded survival in sex-matched sham controls. Clinical and physical observations were also generally unremarkable. Although transient differences in group mean body weight were identified sporadically during the study, these differences were not considered to be biologically significant.

Histopathologic evaluation of tissues failed to provide clear evidence of chronic toxicity or carcinogenicity in either male or female mice receiving chronic exposure to GSM or CDMA RFR. The incidences of non-neoplastic lesions in all RFR-exposed groups were comparable to incidences of those lesions in mice in the sham control groups. As such, comparisons of patterns of non-neoplastic lesions in RFR- and sham-exposed mice did not identify any target organs for the chronic toxicity of RFR exposure.

When compared to sex-matched sham controls, no statistically significant differences in the incidences of total neoplasms, total malignant neoplasms, or total metastatic neoplasms were seen in any group of male or female mice exposed to GSM- or CDMA-modulated RFR. Female mice in the 10 W/kg GSM group demonstrated a significant decrease in the total incidence of malignant+benign neoplasms, and male mice in the 5 W/kg GSM group and male mice in the 2.5 W/kg CDMA group demonstrated statistically significant increases in the total incidence of benign neoplasms. Because these increases were not seen in male mice exposed to RFR at higher field strengths, the biological significance of these findings appears to be limited.

When compared to male and female sham controls, statistically significant differences (increases or decreases) in the incidences of several benign and malignant neoplasms were identified in one or more groups of mice exposed to GSM or CDMA RFR. In all cases, tumor incidences in RFR-exposed mice that differed significantly from those in sex-matched sham controls were all either within or very close to incidence ranges reported for NTP historical controls. On the basis of the lack of any clear pattern of dose-related neoplastic or non-neoplastic lesions in mice exposed to RFR in this study, it was concluded that these study data provide little to no evidence to support the hypothesis that chronic exposure to GSM or CDMA RFR at SARs of up to 10 W/kg is carcinogenic or induces chronic toxicity in B6C3F1 mice.

5.2.2.8 Fraunhofer (Germany) Chronic Bioassay of GSM and DCS RFR in B6C3F1 Mice

In a companion bioassay to the rat study discussed in Section 5.2.2.6, Tillmann and colleagues [33] evaluated the chronic toxicity and possible oncogenicity of a 902 MHz GSM

RFR signal and a 1747 MHz DCS RFR signal in B6C3F1 mice. Beginning at 8–9 weeks of age, groups of 50 mice per sex were exposed to RFR or sham signals for 2 hours per day, 5 days per week at nominal SARs of 0 (sham control), 0.44, 1.33, or 4.0 W/kg. Mice were restrained during the daily period of RFR exposure. All mice were exposed until their death or for 104 weeks; the design also included a cage control group that was not restrained or exposed.

When compared to sex-matched sham controls, no statistically significant increases in tumor incidence were seen in any group exposed to RFR for 2 years; furthermore, tumor incidences in all study groups were within ranges reported for historical controls. The data were interpreted by the authors as providing no support for the hypothesis that chronic exposure to either GSM- or DCS-modulated RFR increases the incidence of any benign or malignant tumor in B6C3F1 mice.

5.2.2.9 Overview of Chronic Rodent Oncogenicity Studies

Eight two-year toxicity/oncogenicity bioassays of cell phone RFR (five in rats, two in mice) or pulsed microwaves (one in rats) have been performed. The results of seven of the eight studies are interpreted as negative. In these studies, chronic exposure of rats or mice to RFR was not associated with any pattern of statistically significant, exposure-related increases in the incidences of (a) total tumors, (b) total malignant tumors, (c) total benign tumors, or (d) tumor incidences in any individual organ site. In the oncogenicity study with pulsed microwaves [28], an increased incidence of total malignant tumors (all sites) was seen. However, this finding is considered to be of limited biological significance, since it resulted from pooling of nonsignificant changes in tumor incidence in several organs.

It is important to note that in several of the studies whose results are interpreted as negative, statistically significant increases or decreases in the incidences of benign or malignant tumors were seen in one or more organ sites in animals exposed to RFR. Obviously, a finding of decreased tumor incidence in groups exposed to RFR does not suggest risk. In all cases where increases in tumor incidence were seen in RFR-exposed groups, these increases were not dose-related and were within or very close to historical incidences seen in control animals of the same species and strain. Absent any pattern of statistically significant, dose-related increases in the incidence of specific tumors, these differences are interpreted indicative of biological variability within the model system, and the overall study data are interpreted as negative.

It should be noted, however, that several of the 2-year oncogenicity studies appear to have less than optimal sensitivity to identify possible carcinogenic effects of RFR exposure. This limited sensitivity results from two issues in study design:

- The SARs used in several studies [28–30] were relatively low (whole body or brain SARs ranging from 0.015 to 0.4 W/kg). In two carcinogenicity studies in Sprague-Dawley rats [28,29], the highest levels of RFR exposure (0.4 and 0.13 W/kg) were more than an order of magnitude below exposure levels that induced no elevations in body temperature or clinical evidence of toxicity in other studies performed in rats [24,32]. Ideally, carcinogen identification studies should be designed to maximize the likelihood of identifying a carcinogenic effect. Studies using RFR exposures that are well below the threshold for thermal effects appear unlikely to have achieved this goal.

- Several studies [31–33] were performed using RFR exposure systems that required animal restraint during exposures. In addition to the possible confounding of study data by induction of restraint stress, the duration of RFR exposure using these systems was limited to either 2 or 4 hours per day. In addition to these short daily exposures not maximizing the likelihood of identifying a carcinogenic effect, many human users of wireless communications devices use their devices for more than 2 hours per day. As a result, studies whose designs included only short daily exposures to RFR do not appear to have maximum sensitivity for hazard identification.

By contrast to the negative results of other bioassays, the largest 2-year oncogenicity study performed in rats (the IIT Research Institute/NTP bioassay of GSM and CDMA RFR in Sprague-Dawley rats) appears to have generated positive results: statistically significant, dose-related increases in the incidences of proliferative brain lesions (gliomas and glial cell hyperplasias) and proliferative Schwann cell lesions (Schwannomas and Schwann cell hyperplasias) of the heart were seen in male rats exposed to RFR. These increases were not seen in female rats exposed to RFR at the same SARs and were not seen in either male or female mice in a companion study performed in the same laboratory. It is important to note that gliomas and Schwann cell tumors of the acoustic nerve (acoustic neuromas) have been identified in epidemiology studies performed by one group as tumors whose incidence may be increased in users of wireless communications devices [34,35].

Although these data suggest a possible hazard of chronic exposure to RFR, the observed increases in the incidence of these preneoplastic and neoplastic lesions in male rats (only) may have been secondary to statistically significant increases in survival in male rats in RFR-exposed groups. Increased survival in male rats exposed to RFR was the apparent result of reduced nephropathy, a common age-related change in rats that is the apparent cause of death in a large fraction of rats in 2-year bioassays. The mechanism underlying reduced nephropathy in male rats exposed to RFR is unknown.

Increased incidences of proliferative glial cell lesions in the brain and proliferative Schwann cell lesions in the heart were seen only in male rats exposed to RFR; similarly, significant increases in survival versus sex-matched sham controls were seen only in male rats exposed to RFR. By contrast, female rats, female mice, and male mice exposed to RFR had survival patterns that were comparable to those of sex- and species-matched sham controls, and did not demonstrate significant, dose-related incidences in the incidence of proliferative glial cell lesions or Schwann cell lesions.

Although the increased incidences of brain and Schwann cell lesions in male rats in this study persisted when data were adjusted for mortality [24], increased longevity cannot conclusively be excluded as a possible factor underlying the observed differences in response. Cancer is an age-related disease in both rodents and humans; the possibility that significantly increased longevity in male rats exposed to RFR is at least partially responsible for the observed increases in preneoplastic and neoplastic lesions glial cell and Schwann cell lesions cannot be ruled out.

5.3 Assessment of the Possible Oncogenic Activity of RFR Using Tumor-Prone Rodent Models

Many animal strains and models have been developed that demonstrate increased sensitivity to neoplastic development in specific organs. In recent years, the overwhelming majority of new tumor-prone animal models have been generated through genetic engineering, either by deletion of a tumor suppressor or other regulatory gene or by insertion of an oncogene into the germ line. In this regard, however, many valuable tumor-prone animal models that are still in use were developed using traditional selective breeding strategies over multiple generations. Both types of models have been used in hazard identification studies with RFR.

In most cases, tumor-prone animal models were developed primarily for use in mechanistic studies and/or efficacy studies of novel therapeutics. As a result, most tumor-prone animal models have only a very limited history of use in hazard identification. For this reason, the ability of these models to predict human responses to potential carcinogens is generally unknown, and these models have not been validated for use in hazard identification.

Although the predictive value of many tumor-prone models has not been studied extensively, the conduct of hazard identification studies using such models may (at least theoretically) increase the ability of a test battery to identify agents with weak or equivocal carcinogenic activity. The value of these models may also increase when the primary focus is on evaluations of potential carcinogenic activity in specific organs. In addition, studies in tumor-prone animal models may be useful in the identification of chemical or physical agents that induce cancer only in sensitive subpopulations; such populations include individuals who have either (a) concomitant or past exposure to potentially carcinogenic agents and/or (b) an underlying genetic predisposition to neoplasia.

The designs of carcinogenicity studies in tumor-prone models are commonly model-specific. Study durations and endpoint evaluations in these studies have often been developed based on use of a model in mechanistic or drug efficacy studies, rather than with the goal of providing a systematic framework for hazard identification. For this reason, endpoints that may be considered critical for hazard identification (e.g., comprehensive microscopic evaluation of tissues) are often not performed, potentially reducing the value of hazard identification data generated in those studies.

5.3.1 Results of Oncogenicity Bioassays of RFR in Genetically Engineered Tumor-Prone Rodent Models

5.3.1.1 Oncogenicity Studies in the Eµ-pim-1 transgenic mouse

Three studies have been reported in which the effects of chronic exposure to RFR on the induction of lymphoma were evaluated in the heterozygous Eµ-*pim*-1 transgenic mouse. Neoplastic development in the Eµ-*pim*-1 mouse is driven by the *pim*-1 oncogene, a highly conserved serine/threonine kinase that is present in both mice and humans [36]. Aging but otherwise untreated *pim*-1 mice develop lymphomas in high incidence [37]; the kinetics of lymphoma development in this model can be greatly accelerated by administration of a single dose of a chemical carcinogen such as N-ethyl-N-nitrosourea [ENU; 38]. The Eµ-*pim*-1 transgenic mouse has been used previously to evaluate the possible effects of exposure to 60 Hz magnetic fields on lymphoma induction [39].

5.3.1.1.1 Royal Adelaide Hospital (Australia) Chronic Bioassay of Pulsed 900 MHz RFR in Eµ-pim-1 Mice

The first study of RFR action in the Eµ-*pim*-1 mouse model was reported by Repacholi and colleagues in 1997 [40]. In this study, heterozygous female Eµ-*pim*-1 mice received either sham exposure (100 mice) or twice daily exposure for 30 minutes (101 mice) to a pulsed 900 MHz RF field (pulse repeat frequency of 217 Hz, pulse width of 0.6 msec). Mean SARs in exposed mice ranged from 0.13 to 1.4 W/kg. RFR or sham exposures began when mice were 6–8 weeks of age, and continued for up to 18 months.

The authors reported that mice receiving chronic exposure to RFR demonstrated a 2.4-fold increase in the risk of lymphoma versus sham controls (p = 0.006). Most neoplasms were diagnosed as follicular lymphomas.

Although this study provides an apparently clear result, it suffers from several important weaknesses in design. Perhaps the most important weakness is the lack of systematic microscopic evaluation of lymphoid tissues from study animals. At study termination, mice that were identified as "healthy" on the basis of clinical observations were counted as survivors and were not evaluated further. These animals were not necropsied, and no microscopic evaluations were performed on tissues from "healthy" surviving animals. On this basis, it is considered highly likely that lymphoma incidence in this study was under-reported; microscopic neoplasms that had not yet resulted in clinical signs of illness were almost certainly present in at least some apparently healthy mice, yet were not identified. This underreporting may have had a substantive impact on study data.

5.3.1.1.2 *Institute of Veterinary and Medical Science (Australia) Chronic Bioassay of GSM-Modulated 898.4 MHz RFR in Eμ-pim-1 Mice*

A second, much larger study using both Eμ-*pim*-1 transgenic mice and wild-type control mice was performed by Utteridge and colleagues [41] to confirm and extend the results of Repacholi et al. [40]. Although the exposure metric used in the Utteridge study was not identical to that used in the Repacholi study, both the exposure metric and the designs of *in vivo* elements of the two studies were similar.

In this study, groups of 120 heterozygous female Eμ-*pim*-1 mice and 120 wild-type female mice received either sham exposure or exposure to GSM-modulated 898.4 MHz RFR at SARs of 0.25, 1.0, 2.0, or 4.0 W/kg. Mice were exposed to RFR or sham fields for 1 hour per day, 5 days per week, for up to 104 weeks. RFR and sham exposures were performed using a "Ferris wheel" type of exposure system that required animal restraint during exposures. To control for possible effects of restraint stress, an unrestrained negative control group (shelf control group) was also included in the study design.

This study has several important advantages over the study reported by Repacholi et al. [40]. The inclusion of multiple RFR exposure groups (including two groups exposed to higher SARs than in the Repacholi study) increases the potential sensitivity of the bioassay, and also permits the characterization of dose-response relationships for any enhancement or promotion of lymphoma induction by RFR. More importantly, this study included microscopic evaluations of tissues from all study animals; the inclusion of histopathology addresses one of the key weaknesses of the study performed by Repacholi et al.

As expected on the basis of their genetic predisposition to neoplasia, survival in Eμ-*pim*-1 mice (both sham control and RFR-exposed groups) was significantly reduced in comparison to survival in comparably treated wild type mice. More importantly for the purposes of the study, comparisons of survival and group mean body weight in both wild-type and Eμ-*pim*-1 transgenic mice failed to identify statistically significant differences between sham controls and strain-matched RFR-exposed groups. In Eμ-*pim*-1 mice, the incidence of lymphoma in sham controls was comparable to incidences seen in all groups exposed to RFR exposure.

The authors interpreted the results of this study as negative and were unable to confirm the positive result reported by Repacholi and colleagues [40].

5.3.1.1.3 Istituto di Ricerche Biomediche LCG-RBM (Italy) Chronic Bioassay of Pulsed 900 MHz RFR in Eμ-pim-1 Mice

A third chronic study to determine the effects of RFR exposure on lymphoma induction in the Eμ-*pim*-1 transgenic mouse was reported by Oberto and colleagues [42]. The authors described this study as a replication and extension of the study reported by Repacholi et al. [40]. The RFR exposure metric used in this study was essentially identical to that used by Repacholi, but the study design was expanded to include three RFR exposure levels and both sexes of transgenic mice.

Groups of Eμ-*pim*-1 transgenic mice (50/sex/group) were exposed to a pulsed 900 MHz RFR signal (pulse repeat frequency of 217 Hz, pulse width of 0.577 ms) at whole body SARs of 0 (sham control), 0.5, 1.4, or 4.0 W/kg. Mice received sham or RFR exposure twice daily for 30 minutes per exposure, 7 days per week for up to 18 months. Mice were restrained during exposures; to control for possible restraint stress, groups of unexposed and unrestrained (cage control) mice were also included in the study design.

Male mice exposed to RFR at all SARs demonstrated decreased survival in comparison to male sham controls. Female mice in the lowest RFR group (0.5 W/kg) also demonstrated decreased survival versus female sham controls. RFR exposure had no effect on body weight in either sex at any exposure level.

In both sexes, the incidence of lymphoma in Eμ-*pim*-1 transgenic mice was comparable in the sham control group and in all groups exposed to RFR. On this basis, the results of this study did not confirm the earlier findings of Repacholi et al. [40] and were comparable to the results reported by Utteridge et al. [41].

It should be noted that male mice (but not female mice) exposed to RFR at SARs of 0.5 or 4.0 W/kg demonstrated increased incidences of benign tumors of the Harderian gland; the increased incidence of Harderian gland tumors resulted in a significant increase in the total incidence of benign tumors seen in male mice exposed to RFR. However, because the murine Harderian gland has no human equivalent [43], this finding is considered to have little or no relevance to human hazard identification.

5.3.1.1.4 Summary of Chronic Bioassays of RFR in Eμ-pim-1 Mice

Three studies have been reported in which the influence of chronic exposure to RFR on the incidence of lymphoma in Eμ-*pim*-1 transgenic mice was investigated. In the earliest study [40], a significant increase in the incidence of lymphoma was reported in the group of female Eμ-*pim*-1 transgenic mice exposed to RFR (SAR range, 0.13–1.4 W/kg). By contrast, two later studies using the same animal model and a very similar RFR signal found no effects of exposure to RFR on lymphoma incidence. The second study performed in female Eμ-*pim*-1 transgenic mice [41] included four RFR exposure levels (SARs of 0.25, 1.0, 2.0, and 4.0 W/kg). The third study was performed in both male and female Eμ-*pim*-1 transgenic mice [42], and included three RFR exposure levels (SARs of 0.5, 1.4, and 4.0 W/kg).

The designs of the two later studies [41,42] appear to be superior to that of the first study [40]. Both later studies included multiple RFR exposure groups, including groups with SARs that were higher than those used in the first study. In addition, both later studies included microscopic evaluation of lymphoid tissues of all animals, while no systematic microscopic evaluations were performed in the study in which an effect of RFR was reported [40].

On the basis of the failure to replicate an initial positive finding in two later studies whose designs were superior, the overall data set for possible induction or enhancement of lymphomas in Eμ-*pim*-1 transgenic mice by RFR is interpreted to be negative.

5.3.1.2 Italian National Agency for New Technologies, Energy and Sustainable Economic Development (ENEA; Italy) Bioassay of 900 MHz RFR in Ptc1⁺/⁻ Knockout Mice

One study has been reported in which the effect of exposure to a 900 MHz GSM signal on the induction of brain tumors in neonatal wild type and heterozygous Patched1 knockout (Ptc1$^{+/-}$) mice was determined [44]. In this study, wild-type and Ptc1$^{+/-}$ mice (22–36/sex/group) received sham exposure or exposure to a 900 MHz GSM signal from postnatal day (PND) 2 to PND 6; the schedule for RFR exposures was selected based on the sensitivity of the neonatal Ptc1$^{+/-}$ mouse to brain tumor induction by ionizing radiation. Mice were exposed twice daily for 30 minutes per exposure period at an SAR of 4.0 W/kg. Mice were monitored for survival and tumor development throughout their lifespans.

RFR exposure had no effect on survival in either wild type or Ptc1$^{+/-}$ mice. No significant differences in the incidence of brain tumors or other malignancies were identified in comparisons of sham-exposed and RFR-exposed groups. The authors concluded that a short-term exposure to RFR during the neonatal period had no tumorigenic activity in the Ptc1$^{+/-}$ mouse. It must be noted, however, that the period of RFR exposure in this study was extremely short, and may be insufficient to detect effects of nonionizing radiation.

5.3.2 Results of Oncogenicity Bioassays of RFR in Other Tumor-Prone Rodent Models

5.3.2.1 Oncogenicity Bioassays in AKR Mice

Three studies designed to evaluate the effect of RFR on the induction of leukemia/lymphoma in the AKR mouse have been reported. The AKR mouse carries the murine leukemia virus, and has been used in studies of the induction and biology of leukemia and lymphoma for over 50 years. As a result of its viral status, otherwise untreated AKR mice develop leukemia and lymphoma in high incidence as they age. On this basis, this mouse provides a sensitive model for use in studies of the mechanisms of leukemogenesis and lymphomagenesis. The AKR mouse has also been used widely to identify chemical and physical agents that stimulate or enhance leukemia/lymphoma induction, and has been used as a model system to identify novel agents with preventive or therapeutic activity against lymphoid neoplasia.

5.3.2.1.1 International University Bremen (Germany) Chronic Bioassay of 900 MHz RFR in AKR/J Mice

Groups of 160 female AKR/J mice received sham exposure or were exposed to a 900 MHz, GSM-like RF signal (mean whole body SAR of 0.4 W/kg) for 24 hours per day, 7 days per week, for approximately 40 weeks [45]. Mice were group-housed (6–7 mice per cage) and were exposed while unrestrained in their home cages. After completion of the exposure period, all animals were necropsied, and microscopic evaluations were performed on primary sites of lymphoma development and infiltration.

Survival rates in sham control and RFR-exposed mice were similar: median survival time was 183 days in the sham control group and 190 days in the RFR-exposed group. Mean body weight in the RFR group was significantly greater than mean body weight in the sham control group. Essentially all mortality in the study was the result of lymphoblastic lymphomas; no significant difference was seen in the incidence of lymphoma in sham controls versus RFR-exposed mice. The results of this study are interpreted as negative.

5.3.2.1.2 Jacobs University Bremen (Germany) Chronic
Bioassay of UTMS RFR in AKR/J Mice

A parallel study to that described in Section 5.3.2.1.1 [45] was performed by the same group to evaluate the possible oncogenicity of a UTMS RFR signal in AKR/J mice [46]. In this study, groups of 160 female AKR/J mice received sham exposure or were exposed to a generic UTMS signal (mean whole body SAR of 0.4 W/kg) for 24 hours per day, 7 days per week, until mice reached approximately 43 weeks of age. Mice were group-housed (6–7 mice per cage) and were exposed unrestrained in their home cages. An additional group of 30 female mice was used as a cage control group. After the exposure period was completed, all mice were necropsied, and microscopic evaluations were performed to characterize lymphoma histology and sites of metastatic infiltration.

No statistically significant differences in survival time, mean body weight, or disease severity were seen in comparisons of sham control and RFR-exposed groups. The authors interpreted these data as confirming their previous results in this model with 900 MHz RFR, and concluded that chronic exposure to UTMS RFR at an SAR of 0.4 W/kg had no adverse effects on the health of AKR/J mice.

5.3.2.1.3 Ewha University (Korea) Chronic Bioassay of Combined
CDMA and WCDMA RFR in AKR/J Mice

In the third study examining the effects of RFR on lymphomagenesis in AKR mice [47], groups of 40 AKR/J mice per sex were either sham-exposed or exposed to a combined RFR signal that contained both a CDMA component (848.5 MHz, 2 W/kg) and a WCDMA component (1950 MHz, 2 W/kg). Mice received sham or RFR exposure for 45 minutes per day, 5 days per week, for up to 42 weeks. At study termination, mice were necropsied and lymphoid tissues were evaluated microscopically.

When compared to sex-matched sham controls, RFR-exposed mice demonstrated no statistically significant differences in median survival time, group mean body weight, or incidence of lymphoma. On this basis, the authors interpreted the results of the study as negative. It should be noted, however, that lymphoma incidence in all groups (both RFR-exposed and sham-exposed) was ≥75%, and thus provided limited sensitivity to identify an agent that may increase lymphoma incidence.

5.3.2.1.4 Summary of Chronic Bioassays of RFR in AKR Mice

Three studies have been reported in which the influence of chronic exposure to RFR on the incidence of lymphoma in AKR mice was investigated. Although the sensitivity to detect a positive effect is questionable in one study, none of the three studies identified any significant increases in lymphoma incidence or decrease in lymphoma-associated survival in AKR mice exposed to RFR. On the basis of these three negative findings, the data for possible induction or enhancement of lymphomas by RFR exposure in AKR mice are interpreted to be negative.

5.3.2.2 Oncogenicity Bioassays in C3H Mice

C3H mice develop a high incidence of mammary tumors as they age and are also susceptible to mammary tumor induction by administration of hormones and other exogenous agents [48]. The C3H mouse has been used widely as a model system to study mechanisms of carcinogenesis in the mammary gland, and may also serve as a sensitive model to identify possible effects of RFR on breast cancer induction in sensitive subpopulations.

5.3.2.2.1 Georgia Institute of Technology (USA) Chronic
Bioassay of 435 MHz RFR in C3H Mice

To determine if long-term exposure to RFR increases mammary tumor incidence and/or decreases mammary tumor latency in C3H mice, Toler and colleagues [49] exposed groups of 200 female C3H/HeJ mice to sham fields or horizontally polarized 435 MHz pulsed RFR (1.0 kHz pulse rate; 1.0 μsec pulse width) for 22 hours per day, 7 days per week, for 21 months. At the end of the exposure period, all animals underwent a gross necropsy, and mammary tumors were evaluated microscopically.

The authors reported that in comparison to sham controls, RFR had no statistically significant effects on survival, group mean body weight, mammary tumor incidence, mammary tumor latency, or mammary tumor growth rate. The results of this study were interpreted as negative.

5.3.2.2.2 Trinity University (USA) Chronic Bioassays of
2450 MHz Microwaves in C3H Mice

Frei and colleagues performed two studies to evaluate the effects of exposure to 2450 MHz microwaves on mammary tumorigenesis in C3H mice. In the first study [50], groups of 100 female C3H mice were exposed to circularly polarized 2450 MHz microwaves or sham-exposed for 20 hours per day, 7 days per week, for 18 months. The mean whole body SAR in the RFR-exposed group was 0.3 W/kg. No significant differences between sham controls and microwave-exposed mice were observed in survival, group mean body weight, mammary tumor incidence (52% in sham controls versus 44% in exposed mice), mean tumor latency (62 weeks in sham controls versus 64 weeks in exposed mice), or rate of mammary tumor growth. Histopathologic evaluation of tissues also failed to identify and differences in the numbers of malignant, metastatic, or benign mammary tumor in the two groups.

The second study [51] was performed using an almost identical experimental design, except that animals were exposed to 2450 MHz microwaves at a higher SAR (1.0 W/kg). Again, the authors reported no statistically significant effects of microwave exposure on animal survival, group mean body weight, mammary tumor incidence (30% in sham controls versus 38% in exposed mice), mammary tumor latency (62 weeks in sham controls versus 63 weeks in exposed mice), or mammary tumor growth. No significant differences in the numbers of malignant, metastatic, or benign mammary tumor in the two groups were identified in microscopic examinations.

Both studies conducted by Frei and colleagues were interpreted as negative.

5.3.2.2.3 Air Force Research Laboratory (USA) Chronic Bioassay
of Ultra-Wideband Pulses in C3H Mice

In a study performed by the same team of investigators as the Frei studies [50,51], groups of 100 female C3H/HeJ mice received either sham exposure or exposure to ultra-wide band (UWB) electromagnetic pulses with a rise time of 176 psec, a fall time of 3.5 nsec, a pulse width of 1.9 nsec, a repetition rate of 1 kHz, and a peak electric field of 40 kV/m [52]. Mice were exposed for 2 minutes per week for 12 weeks, and were observed for an additional 64 weeks.

The authors reported no statistically significant differences between sham-exposed and UWB-exposed groups in survival, incidence of palpable mammary tumors, median tumor latency, or tumor growth rate. Microscopic evaluations also failed to identify significant differences in the incidence or number of mammary gland neoplasms in the sham control versus and UWB-exposed groups.

5.3.2.2.4 *Summary of Chronic Bioassays of RFR in C3H Mice*

Four studies have been reported in which various electromagnetic signals (435 MHz, 2450 Hz UWB) were evaluated for effects on mammary tumor induction in female C3H mice. In each of these studies, no statistically significant differences in mammary tumor incidence, mammary tumor multiplicity, or mammary tumor latency were identified in comparisons of sham control and exposed groups. On the basis of these four findings, the database for the possible enhancement of mammary tumorigenesis in C3H mice by RFR and similar electromagnetic signals mice is completely negative.

5.3.3 Overview of Oncogenicity Bioassays of RFR in Tumor-Prone Mouse Models

Four tumor-prone mouse models have been used to identify possible effects of RFR exposure on neoplastic development. Three of these models were investigated in at least three studies each; some studies were designed as replication studies.

The results of three studies performed to determine the possible effects of chronic exposure to RFR on the induction of leukemia/lymphoma in AKR mice were completely negative. Similarly, the results of four studies to identify possible effects on mammary tumor induction in C3H mice were completely negative. None of these studies provides support for the hypothesis that exposure to RFR induces or enhances tumorigenesis in tumor-prone animals or in sensitive subpopulations.

One study was performed to examine the influence of short-term (neonatal) exposure to RFR on the induction of brain tumors in the heterozygous Ptc1$^{+/-}$ knockout mouse. Although the results of this study were negative, the very short duration of RFR exposure used in this study may have been insufficient to support an adequate assessment of RFR activity. The results of this study are considered to be inconclusive.

By contrast to the uniformly negative results of three studies in the AKR mouse model for leukemia/lymphoma, four studies in the C3H mouse model for breast cancer, and one study in heterozygous Ptc1$^{+/-}$ knockout mouse model for brain cancer, a somewhat less clear pattern emerges from three studies performed in the Eμ-*pim*-1 transgenic mouse model of lymphoma. In the first study performed in the Eμ-*pim*-1 transgenic mouse, the authors reported a statistically significant increase in lymphoma incidence in female mice exposed to RFR. However, the design of this study had several important weaknesses, and its results were not confirmed in two subsequent studies with stronger experimental designs. Because the designs of the two later studies were superior to that of the first study, it is concluded that the overall data set from studies in the Eμ-*pim*-1 transgenic mouse provides no substantive evidence that RFR exposure enhances the induction of lymphomas in this model.

Overall, it is concluded that studies in tumor-prone animals do not provide significant evidence that chronic exposure to RFR stimulates tumorigenesis in any tumor site evaluated.

5.4 Assessment of the Possible Co-Carcinogenic or Tumor-Promoting Activity of RFR in Multistage Rodent Models

Numerous *in vivo* studies have been conducted to identify possible co-carcinogenic or tumor-promoting effects of RFR in specific target organs; the designs of these studies were discussed in detail in Chapter 4 in this volume entitled "Evaluation of the Toxicity and

Potential Oncogenicity of ELF Magnetic Fields in Experimental Animal Model Systems." Briefly, co-carcinogenesis and tumor promotion studies involve simultaneous or sequential exposure to RFR in combination with exposure to a known carcinogen or other chemical or physical agent. Co-carcinogenic or tumor-promoting activity is operationally defined as a statistically significant increase in the incidence or multiplicity of tumors in groups exposed to the chemical or physical agent+RFR in comparison to a control group receiving the chemical or physical agent+sham exposure. Additional details concerning the design of individual co-carcinogenesis and tumor promotion studies with RFR are presented in the International Agency for Research on Cancer (IARC) Monograph on RFR [5].

As was the case with tumor-prone animal models, co-carcinogenesis and multistage (initiation-promotion) tumor models were ordinarily designed as research tools to study carcinogenesis in specific organ sites. In addition, some of these models have been used widely to evaluate the efficacy of novel agents under investigation for activity in cancer chemoprevention. However, because these models were not specifically developed for use in hazard identification, their value in predicting oncogenicity in humans has not been evaluated systematically.

In consideration of the large number of studies in which the possible co-carcinogenic or tumor-promoting activity of RFR has been examined, and the uncertain value of these studies in predicting human responses, analysis and discussion of all possibly relevant co-carcinogenesis and tumor promotion studies of RFR is beyond the scope of the present review. Many studies of RFR action have been performed using well-established multistage carcinogenesis models and can be used to support reasonable assessments of the possible co-carcinogenic or tumor-promoting activity of RFR; these models are discussed in this section.

By contrast, however, other studies of RFR action were performed in animal models with no history of use, and for which there are little or no data to support the biological relevance of the test system. In addition, the protocols used in some studies had important design weaknesses (e.g., small group sizes, poor dosimetry, inadequate tumor assessments) that greatly reduce their value for hazard assessment. These studies are not discussed.

5.4.1 Initiation-Promotion and Co-Carcinogenesis Studies of RFR in Brain Tumor Models

Because RF energy in users of mobile telephones is deposited primarily in the brain [13–15], the possible activity of RFR as a promoter of neoplastic development in the brain is a central focus of hazard identification studies. The rationale for studies of RFR as a possible causal agent for brain cancer is also supported by several epidemiology studies in which increased incidences of glioma were reported in users of mobile telephones (reviewed in [7]).

Six *in vivo* studies [53–58; Table 5.1] have been performed to evaluate the possible activity of RFR as a promoter of brain tumor induction in rats. Although the specific protocols used in different studies demonstrated some differences, all six studies were performed using the same experimental model. In this model, rats receive transplacental exposure to the chemical carcinogen, ENU, and develop brain and spinal cord tumors in low incidence as a result of this *in utero* exposure. Studies listed in Table 5.1 were performed to determine whether post-natal exposure to RFR enhances the incidence of neurogenic tumors induced by ENU; the activity of several different RFR metrics was examined.

The results of these studies were uniformly negative: no evidence of brain tumor promotion by RFR was identified in any study. On this basis, it is concluded that the data set from multistage (initiation-promotion) studies of brain carcinogenesis using the rat ENU model

TABLE 5.1

Initiation-Promotion and Co-Carcinogenesis Studies of RFR in Brain Tumor Models

Species	RFR Exposure Metric	SAR (W/kg)	Other Agent[a]	Endpoint	Results	Reference
Rat	836 MHz NDAC	1.1–1.6	ENU	Brain and CNS tumors	Negative	[53]
Rat	836.55 MHz	1.1–1.6	ENU	Brain and CNS tumors	Negative	[54]
Rat	860 MHz TDMA	1.0	ENU	Brain and CNS tumors	Negative	[55]
Rat	860 MHz CWRF	1.0	ENU	Brain and CNS tumors	Negative	[55]
Rat	1.439 GHz TDMA	0.67, 2.0	ENU	Brain and CNS tumors	Negative	[56]
Rat	860 MHz TDMA	1.0	ENU	Brain and CNS tumors	Negative	[57]
Rat	1.95 GHz W-CDMA	0.67, 2.0	ENU	Brain and CNS tumors	Negative	[58]

[a] ENU, *N*-ethyl-*N*-nitrosourea.

provides no support for the hypothesis that RFR has co-carcinogenic or tumor-promoting activity in the brain.

5.4.2 Initiation-Promotion Studies of RFR in Mammary Tumor Models

Five studies have been reported in which the possible activity of RFR as a promoter of mammary carcinogenesis in the rat was evaluated [59–62; Table 5.2]. All five studies were performed using the rat mammary cancer model induced by 7,12-dimethylbenz[a anthracene

TABLE 5.2

Initiation-Promotion and Co-Carcinogenesis Studies of RFR in Mammary Tumor Models

Species	RFR Exposure Metric	SAR (W/kg)	Other Agent[a]	Endpoint	Results/Conclusions	Reference
Rat	Pulsed 900 MHz GSM	0.015–0.130	DMBA	Mammary cancer	Negative	[59]
Rat	900 MHz GSM	1.4, 2.2, 3.5	DMBA	Mammary cancer	No difference in tumor incidence or tumor number; decreased latency at 1.4 and 2.2 W/kg, not at 3.5	[60]
Rat	900 MHz GSM	0.1, 0.7, 1.4	DMBA	Mammary cancer	Decreased tumor number at 1.4 W/kg	[60]
Rat	900 MHz GSM	0.44, 1.33, 4.0	DMBA	Mammary cancer	Negative	[61]
Rat	902 MHz GSM	0.4, 1.3, 4.0	DMBA	Mammary cancer	All differences between groups were incidental findings	[62]

[a] DMBA, 7,12-dimethylbenz[a]anthracene.

[DMBA; 63]. The rat DMBA model has been used widely to study mechanisms of mammary carcinogenesis and the effects of hormones on mammary cancer induction; these studies have contributed greatly to our understanding of the etiology of human breast cancer. The rat DMBA model has also been widely used as a preclinical model to characterize the activity of novel agents being developed for breast cancer chemoprevention. Our understanding of the biology, hormone dependence, pathogenesis, and regulation of carcinogenesis in the rat DMBA mammary cancer model is extensive; this model also demonstrates many similarities to the biology of human breast cancer.

The results of all five studies of RFR action in the DMBA rat mammary cancer model were interpreted as negative by the study authors: no evidence of RFR activity as a mammary tumor promoter was identified in any study. On this basis of these data, it is concluded that the multistage mammary carcinogenesis studies performed in the well-studied DMBA model provide no support for the hypothesis that RFR has tumor-promoting activity in the rat mammary gland.

5.4.3 Initiation-Promotion and Co-Carcinogenesis Studies of RFR in Skin Tumor Models

Although no substantive body of evidence exists to suggest that the skin is a target for RFR carcinogenesis, studies in the initiation-promotion model in mouse skin have been critical to our understanding of carcinogenesis and cancer biology. For this reason, studies to identify the possible tumor-promoting activity of RFR in mouse skin are relevant to an overall assessment of its activity.

Most tumorigenesis studies in mouse skin are performed using a well-established model in which tumor initiation is achieved by topical application of a single dose of DMBA or other genotoxic agent to the back of a mouse, and tumor promotion is achieved by repeated (usually twice weekly) topical administration of a nongenotoxic tumor promoter (most commonly, 12-*O*-tetradecanoylphorbol-13-acetate (TPA)) to the same site. The DMBA/TPA regimen induces benign skin tumors (papillomas) in high incidence with a relatively short latency. This model has been used widely to identify agents that act as tumor promoters or inhibitors of tumor promotion.

Six studies have been reported in four publications which the activity of RFR as a promoter of DMBA-initiated skin tumors has been assessed [64–67; Table 5.3]; a wide range

TABLE 5.3

Initiation-Promotion and Co-Carcinogenesis Studies of RFR in Skin Tumor Models

Species	RFR Exposure Metric	SAR (W/kg)	Other Agent[a]	Endpoint	Results	Reference
Mouse	1.49 GHz TDMA	2.0	DMBA	Skin Papillomas	Negative	[64]
Mouse	849 MHz CDMA	0.4	DMBA	Skin Papillomas	Negative	[65]
Mouse	1.763 GHz CDMA	0.4	DMBA	Skin Papillomas	Negative	[65]
Mouse	112 MHz AM	0.75	DMBA	Skin Papillomas	Negative	[66]
Mouse	2.45 GHZ	0.1	DMBA	Skin Papillomas	Negative	[66]
Mouse	94 GHZ MMW	1.0	DMBA	Skin Papillomas	Negative	[67]
Rat	900 MHz GSM	0.075,0.27	B(a)P	Skin Sarcoma	Negative	[68]

[a] DMBA, 7,12-dimethylbenz[a]anthracene; B[a]P, benzo[a]pyrene.

of RFR metrics was evaluated in these studies. In each study, mice were initiated with a single dose of DMBA and subsequently received sham or RFR exposure; in most studies, a positive control group was exposed to a single dose of DMBA followed by repeat-dose exposure to TPA.

The results of all studies of RFR action in the mouse skin initiation-promotion model were negative: when compared to DMBA-treated sham controls, no increases in the number of skin tumors were seen in mice exposed to DMBA+RFR in any study. It is concluded that the results of initiation-promotion studies in mouse skin provide no evidence that exposure to RFR has activity as a tumor promoter.

A similar result was seen in a rat sarcoma model in which animals were exposed to the polycyclic aromatic hydrocarbon, benzo[a]pyrene, by injection [68]. The incidence of sarcomas in RFR-exposed rats in this study did not differ from the incidence seen in sham controls.

5.4.4 Initiation-Promotion Studies of RFR in Models of Preneoplasia in the Liver

Two studies were performed by one group of investigators to determine the effects of RFR exposure on the induction of preneoplastic lesions in rat liver [69,70; Table 5.4]. The endpoint in these studies, liver foci that stain for the placental form of glutathione S-transferase (GST-P), is accepted as a precursor to liver cancer in the rat [71]. On this basis, this assay has been used widely to identify agents with tumor-promoting activity.

In these studies, rats were exposed to a genotoxic chemical carcinogen (diethylnitrosamine) followed by a partial hepatectomy. This regimen stimulates cell proliferation, which is followed by development of hepatic foci; GST-P positive foci can be characterized in terms of their incidence, multiplicity, and/or size. In longer term studies in which hepatocellular carcinomas develop, the number and size of GST-P positive hepatic foci are strongly correlated with liver cancer response [71].

The results of both assays of RFR in the GST-P liver assay were negative: in both studies, the number of GST-P positive foci in RFR-exposed rats was comparable to those in sham controls. These studies provide no evidence to support the hypothesis that RFR has tumor-promoting activity in the liver.

5.4.5 Initiation-Promotion and Co-Carcinogenesis Studies of RFR in Tumor Models in Other Sites

Three studies have been reported in which the possible tumor-promoting or co-carcinogenic activity of RFR in other sites has been evaluated (Table 5.5).

TABLE 5.4

Initiation-Promotion and Co-Carcinogenesis Studies of RFR in Models of Preneoplasia in Liver

Species	RFR Exposure Metric	SAR (W/kg)	Other Agent(s)[a]	Endpoint	Results	Reference
Rat	929.2 MHz TDMA	1.7–2.0	DEN+partial hepatectomy	GST-P positive foci	Negative	[69]
Rat	1.439 GHz TDMA	0.937–1.91	DEN+partial hepatectomy	GST-P positive foci	Negative	[70]

[a] DEN, diethylnitrosamine.

TABLE 5.5

Initiation-Promotion and Co-Carcinogenesis Studies of RFR in Tumor Models in Other Sites

Species	RFR Exposure Metric	SAR (W/kg)	Other Agent(s)[a]	Endpoint	Results	Reference
Mouse	2.45 GHz	10–12	DMH	Colon cancer incidence	Negative	[72]
Mouse	1.966 GHz UMTS	0.62–5.76	ENU	Lung and liver tumor incidence	Increased incidence of lung and liver tumors	[73]
Mouse	1.966 GHz UMTS	0.04, 0.4, 2.0	ENU	Cancer incidence in multiple sites	Increased incidence of lymphoma, lung, and liver tumors	[74]

[a] DMH, dimethylhydrazine; ENU, *N*-ethyl-*N*-nitrosourea.

In one study [72], the potential activity of 2.45 GHz microwaves in the promotion of colon carcinogenesis was evaluated in mice exposed to a known colon carcinogen, dimethyl-hydrazine (DMH). The incidence of colon cancer was comparable in DMH-treated mice receiving either sham exposure or microwave exposure. The results of this study provided no evidence of promoting activity for the 2.45 GHz microwave signal.

Two studies have been reported in which the possible promoting activity of a 1.966 GHz UMTS RFR signal was evaluated in mice receiving transplacental exposure to ENU [73,74]. The first study (Tillmann et al. [73]) appears to have been a failed attempt to transfer the well-studied rat transplacental ENU brain cancer model to mice. In this study, B6C3F1 mice received transplacental exposure to ENU, followed by post-natal exposure to RFR or sham fields. Transplacental exposure to ENU failed to induce brain or other neurogenic tumors in mice. Perhaps surprisingly, however, mice receiving transplacental exposure to ENU followed by post-natal exposure to RFR demonstrated increased incidences of lung and liver tumors when compared to the incidences of lung and liver tumors seen in mice receiving transplacental exposure to ENU followed by sham exposure.

This finding was replicated by Lerchl et al. [74], who reported that when compared to mice receiving transplacental exposure to ENU followed by post-natal sham exposure, mice receiving transplacental exposure to ENU and post-natal exposure to RFR demonstrated increased incidences of lymphoma, lung tumors, and liver tumors.

The transplacental ENU mouse model used in these studies has not been used in other hazard assessment studies, and no other studies in this model have been reported in the literature. As a result, neither the biology of cancer induction in this model nor its value as a predictor of human responses has been characterized. However, increased incidences of tumors in two sites (lung and liver) were seen in both studies in mice exposed to ENU+RFR when compared to ENU-treated sham controls. The apparent replication of a positive finding is unique among RFR carcinogenesis studies.

5.4.6 Overview of Multistage Oncogenicity Studies

The scientific literature provides little evidence to support the hypothesis that exposure to RFR has co-carcinogenic or tumor-promoting activity in animal models. Numerous studies in well-studied multistage carcinogenesis models have been published; all studies have had negative results. Seven studies have been reported in the transplacental ENU brain cancer model in rats; the results of all seven studies were negative [53–58]. Similarly, the negative results obtained in all five studies in the DMBA mammary cancer model in rats [59–62], all seven studies in the initiation-promotion model in mouse skin [64–68], both studies in the GST-P focus model in rat liver [69–70], and one study in the DMH colon cancer model in mice [72] provide no evidence that RFR is active as a co-carcinogen or tumor promoter. A total of 22 studies have been performed in well-studied multistage carcinogenesis models; all 22 studies generated negative results for RFR as a co-carcinogen or tumor promoter.

That said, however, a possibly important finding is the apparent enhancement of lung and liver tumors (and possibly lymphomas) by RFR in mice receiving transplacental exposure to ENU. This model has no history of use for other purposes, its biology has not been studied in any detail, and its relevance to human hazard identification is unknown. However, the finding of an apparent tumor-promoting activity of RFR, which has now been reported by two laboratories, merits further investigation.

5.5 Conclusion

Eight two-year toxicity/oncogenicity bioassays in rodents have been performed to evaluate the carcinogenicity of RFR or pulsed microwaves; seven of the eight studies were negative [25,28–33]. The 2-year bioassay is considered by toxicologists to be the "gold standard" for hazard identification in animal models, and a strong correlation has been demonstrated between the results of 2-year bioassays and carcinogenicity in humans [21]. On this basis, studies performed using this design carry substantially more weight in an overall evaluation of carcinogenicity than do studies in tumor-prone animals or initiation-promotion/co-carcinogenesis studies.

Although one positive result was reported in lymphoma studies in the Eμ-*pim*-1 transgenic mouse [40], the results of two subsequent studies in the same animal model using apparently superior designs were both negative [41,42]. Three studies in the AKR mouse leukemia/lymphoma model were negative [45–47], as were four studies in the C3H mouse mammary tumor model [49–52] and one study in the heterozygous Ptc1$^{+/-}$ knockout mouse brain cancer model [44]. Because the only reported positive finding in a tumor-prone mouse model was not replicated in two later studies, these data are interpreted as providing no evidence that RFR is carcinogenic in tumor-prone mouse models.

Similarly, none of the 22 studies performed in multistage and initiation-promotion models for cancer of the brain [53–58], breast [59–62], skin [64–68], liver [69,70], or colon [72] demonstrated significant activity for RFR as a tumor promoter or co-carcinogen. The results of these studies, all of which were performed in established multistage rodent models of carcinogenesis, do not support the hypothesis that RFR has tumor-promoting or co-carcinogenic activity in these organs.

Although the vast majority of studies performed in animal models to identify possible carcinogenic effects of RFR exposure have generated negative results, three studies do provide what may be interpreted as positive signals.

As discussed above, the results of 7 of the 8 two-year oncogenicity bioassays of RFR are interpreted as negative. However, the largest 2-year bioassay of RFR in rats [IIT Research Institute/NTP; 24,25] demonstrated statistically significant increases in the incidences of proliferative glial cell lesions (gliomas, glial cell hyperplasias) in the brain of male rats and proliferative Schwann cell lesions (Schwannomas, Schwann cell hyperplasias) in the heart of male rats. Both gliomas and Schwann cell tumors (acoustic neuromas) have been identified in several epidemiology studies as possible sites of RFR oncogenicity in humans [reviewed in 5,7].

The exposure system used in the IIT Research Institute/NTP study permitted exposure of rats to higher but nonthermal levels of RFR (SARS up to 6.0 W/kg) than had been used in prior studies. Furthermore, the use of an exposure system that did not involve animal restraint permitted animals to be exposed to RFR for much longer periods each day. On these bases, it can logically be proposed that the greater daily duration and intensity of nonthermal RFR exposures increased the sensitivity of this bioassay to detect carcinogenic effects versus that of other 2-year studies.

That said, however, the findings of increased incidences of proliferative lesions in the brain and heart may be associated with the improved survival seen in male rats in this study. All groups of male rats in the IIT Research Institute/NTP study demonstrated significant increases in survival in comparison to male sham controls; male rats also demonstrated increased incidences of proliferative lesions in the brain and heart. By contrast, female rats, male mice, and female mice demonstrated neither increased survival nor increased incidences of these lesions. Although the data from this study were mortality-adjusted during statistical analyses, the differential survival in these animals, and its possible effect on tumorigenesis, cannot be ignored. The differential survival in male rats demonstrating these lesions greatly complicates interpretation of study data.

The apparent enhancement of lung and liver tumorigenesis (and possibly lymphomagenesis) by RFR in mice receiving transplacental exposure to ENU [73,74] is another signal that may suggest possible positive carcinogenic activity of RFR. A significant strength of these data is the fact that the finding has been replicated independently. However, the model system used in these studies has not been used to evaluate the carcinogenicity of other agents, and its biology and relevance to human hazard identification are unknown. That said, this finding clearly merits further investigation.

Neither epidemiology alone nor animal studies alone currently provide a comprehensive assessment of the possible carcinogenicity of human exposure to RFR. For this reason, it is proposed that adequate assessments of the possible carcinogenicity of RFR should be based on a "weight of the evidence" approach in which epidemiology data, experimental data, and mechanistic data are integrated and considered together. No conclusive evidence of RFR carcinogenicity has been demonstrated in either epidemiology or experimental studies. However, the positive signals from three animal studies suggest that reasonable attempts to minimize exposure to RFR may be prudent.

References

1. Uswitch. History of mobile phones and the first mobile phone. www.uswitch.com/mobiles/guides/history-of-mobile-phones/. Accessed October 31, 2017.
2. Infoplease. Cell phone subscribers in the U.S., 1985 to 2010. www.infoplease.com/science-health/cellphone-use/cell-phone-subscribers-us-1985-2010. Accessed October 31, 2017.
3. Statista. Number of cell phone users in the United States from spring 2008 to spring 2017. www.statista.com/statistics/231612/number-of-cell-phone-users-usa/. Accessed October 31, 2017.
4. GSMA. Number of global mobile subscribers to surpass five billion this year, finds new GSMA study. www.gsma.com/newsroom/press-release/number-of-global-mobile-subscribers-to-surpass-five-billion-this-year/. Accessed October 31, 2017.

5. International Agency for Research on Cancer. Non-ionizing radiation, Part 2: Radiofrequency electromagnetic fields. *IARC Monogr Eval Carcinog Risks Hum*, 102, 1–460, 2013.

6. Repacholi, M.H., Lerchl, A., Röösli, M., Sienkiewicz, Z., Auvinen, A., Breckenkamp, J., D'Inzeo, G., Elliott, P., Frei, P., Heinrich, S., Lagroye, I., Lahkola, A., McCormick, D.L., Thomas, S., and Vecchia, P. Systematic review of wireless phone use and brain cancer and other head tumors. *Bioelectromagnetics*, 33, 187–206, 2012.

7. Carlberg, M., and Hardell, L. Evaluation of mobile phone and cordless phone use and glioma risk using the Bradford Hill viewpoints from 1965 on association or causation. *Biomed Res Int*, 2017, 9218486, 2017, DOI:10.1155/2017/9218486.

8. Hirsch, S.E., Appleton, B., Fine, B.S., and Brown, P.V. Effects of repeated microwave irradiations to the albino rabbit eye. *Invest Ophthalmol Vis Sci*, 16, 315–319, 1977.

9. Kramar, P., Harris, C., Emery, A.F., and Guy, A.W. Acute microwave irradiation and cataract formation in rabbits and monkeys. *J Microw Power*, 13, 239–249, 1978.

10. Elder, J.A. Ocular effects of radiofrequency energy. *Bioelectromagnetics*, (Suppl. 6), S148–S161, 2003.

11. Berman, E., Carter, H.B., and House, D. Tests of mutagenesis and reproduction in male rats exposed to 2,450-MHz (CW) microwaves. *Bioelectromagnetics*, 1, 65–76, 1980.

12. Heynick, L.N., and Merritt, J.H. Radiofrequency fields and teratogenesis. *Bioelectromagnetics*, (Suppl. 6), S174–S186, 2003.

13. Christ, A., and Kuster, N. Differences in RF energy absorption in the heads of adults and children. *Bioelectromagnetics*, (Suppl. 7), S31–S44, 2005.

14. Cardis, E., Deltour, I., Mann, S., Moissonnier, M., Taki, M., Varsier, N., Wake, K., and Wiart, J. Distribution of RF energy emitted by mobile phones in anatomical structures of the brain. *Phys Med Biol*, 53, 2771–2783, 2008.

15. Varsier, N., Wake, K., Taki, M., and Watanabe, S. Influence of use conditions and mobile phone categories on the distribution of specific absorption rate in different anatomical parts in the brain. *IEEE Trans Microwave Theory Tech*, 57, 899–904, 2009.

16. McCormick, D.L. Integration of experimental and epidemiologic data into a "Weight of the Evidence" evaluation of possible risks of exposure to radiofrequency fields generated by wireless telephones. *Proc XIII Inte. Cong Toxicol*, W6-1, 2013.

17. McCormick, D.L. Animal studies in carcinogen identification: the example of power frequency (50/60 Hz) magnetic fields. In: Obe, G., Jandrig, B., Marchant, G., Schütz, H., and Wiedemann, P. (Eds.) *Cancer Risk Evaluation: Methods and Trends*. Wiley-VCH, Berlin, pp. 125–136, 2011.

18. Neubauer, G., Cecil, S., Giczi, W., Petric, B., Preiner, P., Frölich, J., and Röösli, M. The association between exposure determined by radiofrequency personal exposimeters and human exposure: a simulation study. *Bioelectromagnetics*, 31, 535–545, 2010.

19. Goedhart, G., Kromhout, H., Wiart, J., and Vermeulen, R. Validating self-reported mobile phone use in adults using a newly developed smartphone application. *Occup Environ Med*, 72, 812–818, 2015.

20. Choi, K.H., Ha, M., Burm, E., Ha, E.H., Park, H., Kim, Y., Lee, A.K., Kwon, J.H., Choi, H.D., and Kim, N. Multiple assessment methods of prenatal exposure to radio frequency radiation from telecommunication in the Mothers and Children's Environmental Health (MOCEH) study. *Int J Occup Med Environ Health*, 29, 959–972, 2016.

21. Huff, J. Value, validity, and historical development of carcinogenesis studies for predicting and confirming carcinogenic risks to humans. In: Kitchin, K.T. (Ed.) *Carcinogenicity Testing, Predicting, and Interpreting Chemical Effects*. Marcel Dekker, New York, pp. 21–123, 1999.

22. McCormick, D.L. Preclinical evaluation of carcinogenicity using standard-bred and genetically engineered rodent models. In: A.S. Faqi (Ed.) *A Comprehensive Guide to Toxicology in Nonclinical Drug Development*, 2nd Edition. Elsevier, New York, pp. 274–292, 2017.

23. Cohen, S.M. Human carcinogenic risk evaluation: an alternative approach to the two-year rodent bioassay. *Toxicol Sci*, 80, 225–229, 2004.

24. Wyde, M., Cesta, M., Blystone, C., Elmore, S., Foster, P., Hooth, M., Kissling, G., Malarkey, D., Sills, R., Stout, M., Walker, N., Witt, K., Wolfe, M., and Bucher, J. Report of partial findings from the National Toxicology Program carcinogenesis studies of cell phone

radiofrequency radiation in Hsd: Sprague Dawley® SD rats (whole body exposure). www.biorxiv.org/ content/early/2016/06/23/055699, 2016. Accessed November 15, 2017.

25. McCormick, D. Two-year oncogenicity evaluations of cell phone radiofrequency radiation in Sprague-Dawley rats and B6C3F1 mice. *Toxicol Lett*, 280S, S31, 2017.

26. Capstick, M.H., Kuehn, S., Berdinas-Torres, V., Gong, Y., Wilson, P.F., Ladbury, J.M., Koepke, G., McCormick, D.L., Gauger, J., Melnick, R.L., and Kuster, N. A radio frequency radiation exposure system for rodents based on reverberation chambers. *IEEE Trans on Electromagn Compat*, 59, 1041–1052, 2017.

27. Gong, Y., Capstick, M.H., Kuehn, S., Wilson, P.F., Ladbury, J.M., Koepke, G., McCormick, D.L., Melnick, R.L., and Kuster, N. Life-time dosimetric assessment for mice and rats exposed in reverberation chambers for the two-year NTP cancer bioassay study on cell phone radiation. *IEEE Trans on Electromagn Compat*, 59, 1798–1808, 2017.

28. Chou, C.K., Guy, A.W., Kunz, L.L., Johnson, R.B., Crowley, J.J., and Krupp, J.H. Long-term, low level microwave irradiation of rats. *Bioelectromagnetics*, 13, 469–496, 1992.

29. Bartsch, H., Küpper, H., Scheurlen, U., Deerberg, F., Seebald, E., Dietz, K., Mecke, D., Probst, H., Stehle, T., and Bartsch, C. Effect of chronic exposure to a GSM-like signal (mobile phone) on survival of female Sprague-Dawley rats: modulatory effects by month of birth and possibly stage of the solar cycle. *Neuro Endocrinol Let*, 31, 457–473, 2010.

30. La Regina, M., Moros, E.G., Pickard, W.F., Straube, W.L., Baty, J., and Roti Roti, J. The effect of chronic exposure to 835.62 MHz FDMA or 847.74 MHz CDMA radiofrequency radiation on the incidence of spontaneous tumors in rats. *Radiat Res*, 160, 143–151, 2003.

31. Anderson, L.E., Sheen, D.M., Wilson, B.W., Grumbein, S.L., Creim, J.A., and Sasser, L.B. Two-year chronic bioassay study of rats exposed to a 1.6 GHz radiofrequency signal. *Radiat Res*, 162, 201–210, 2004.

32. Smith, P., Kuster, N., Ebert, S., and Chevalier, H.J. GSM and DCS wireless communication signals: combined chronic toxicity/carcinogenicity study in the Wistar rat. *Radiat Res*, 168, 480–492, 2007.

33. Tillmann, T., Ernst, H., Ebert, S., Kuster, N., Behnke, W., Rittinghausen, S., and Dasenbrock, C. Carcinogenicity study of GSM and DCS wireless communication signals in B6C3F1 mice. *Bioelectromagnetics*, 28, 173–187, 2007.

34. Hardell, L., Carlberg, M., and Hansson Mild, K. Use of mobile phones and cordless phones is associated with increased risk for glioma and acoustic neuroma. *Pathophysiology*, 20, 85–110, 2013.

35. Hardell, L., and Carlberg, M. Using the Hill viewpoints from 1965 for evaluating strengths of evidence of the risk for brain tumors associated with use of mobile and cordless phones. *Res Environ Health*, 28, 97–102, 2013.

36. Nawijn, M.C., Alendar, A., and Berns, A. For better or for worse: The role of Pim oncogenes in tumorigenesis. *Nat Rev Cancer*, 11, 23–34, 2011.

37. Van Lohuizen, M., Verbeek, S., Krimpenfort, P., Domen, J., Saris, C., Radaszkiewicz, T., and Berns, A. Predisposition to lymphomagenesis in pim-1 transgenic mice: cooperation with c-myc and N-myc in murine leukemia virus-induced tumors. *Cell*, 56, 673–682, 1989.

38. Breuer, M.L. Slebos, R., Verbeek, S., van Lohuizen, M., Wientjens, E., and Berns, A., Very high frequency of lymphoma induction by a chemical carcinogen in pim-1 transgenic mice. *Nature*, 340, 61–63, 1989.

39. McCormick, D.L., Ryan, B.M., Findlay, J.C., Gauger, J.R., Johnson, T.R., Morrissey, R.L., and Boorman, G.A., Exposure to 60 Hz magnetic fields and risk of lymphoma in PIM transgenic and TSG-p53 (p53 knockout) mice, *Carcinogenesis*, 19, 1649–1653, 1998.

40. Repacholi, M.H., Basten, A., Gebski, V., Noonan, D., Finnie, J., and Harris, A.W. Lymphomas in E mu-Pim1 transgenic mice exposed to pulsed 900 MHZ electromagnetic fields. *Radiat Res*, 147, 631–640, 1997.

41. Utteridge, T.D., Gebski, V., Finnie, J.W., Vernon-Roberts, B., and Kuckel, T.R. Long-term exposure of E-mu-Pim1 transgenic mice to 898.4 MHz microwaves does not increase lymphoma incidence. *Radiat Res*, 158, 357–364, 2002.

42. Oberto, G., Rolfo, K., Yu, P., Carbonatto, M., Peano, S., Kuster, N., Ebert, S., and Tofani, S. Carcinogenicity study of 217 Hz pulsed 900 MHz electromagnetic fields in Pim1 transgenic mice. *Radiat Res*, 168, 316–326, 2007.

43. Albert, D.M., Frayer, W.C., Black, H.E., Massicotte, S.J., Sang, D.N., and Soque, J. The Harderian gland: its tumors and its relevance to humans. *Trans Amer Opththalmol Soc*, 84, 312–341, 1986.

44. Saran, A., Pazzaglia, S., Mancuso, M., Rebessi, S., DiMajo, V., Tanori, M., Lovisolo, G.A., Pinto, R., and Marino, C. Effects of exposure of newborn patched1 heterozygous mice to GSM, 900 MHz. *Radiat Res*, 168, 733–740, 2007.

45. Sommer, A.M., Streckert, J.M., Bitz, A.K., Hansen, V.W., and Lerchl, A. No effects of GSM-modulated 900 MHz electromagnetic fields on survival rate and spontaneous development of lymphoma in female AKR/J mice. *BMC Cancer*, 4, 77, 2007.

46. Sommer, A.M., Bitz, A.K., Streckert, J., Hansen, V.W., and Lerchl, A. Lymphoma development in mice chronically exposed to UMTS-modulated radiofrequency electromagnetic fields. *Radiat Res*, 168, 72–80, 2007.

47. Lee, H.J., Jin, Y.B., Lee, J.-S., Choi, S.Y., Kim, T.-H., Pack, J.-K., Choi, H.D., Kim, N., and Lee, Y.-S. Lymphoma development of simultaneously combined exposure to two radiofrequency signals in AKR/J mice. *Bioelectromagnetics*, 32, 485–492, 2011.

48. Medina, D. Of mice and women: A short history of mouse mammary cancer research with an emphasis on the paradigms inspired by the transplantation method. *Cold Spring Harb Perspect Biol*, 2(20), a004523, 2010.

49. Toler, J.C., Shelton, W.W., Frei, M.R., Merritt, J.H., and Stedham, M.A. Long-term, low-level exposure of mice prone to mammary tumors to 435 MHz radiofrequency radiation. *Radiat Res*, 148, 227–234, 1997.

50. Frei, M.R., Berger, R.E., Dusch, S.J., Guel, V., Jauchem, J.R., Merritt, J.H., and Stedham, M.A. Chronic exposure of cancer-prone mice to low-level 2450 MHz radiofrequency radiation. *Bioelectromagnetics*, 19, 20–31, 1998.

51. Frei, M.R., Jauchem, J.R., Dusch, S.J., Merritt, J.H., Berger, R.E., and Stedham, M.A. Chronic, low-level (1.0 W/kg) exposure of mice prone to mammary cancer to 2450 MHz microwaves. *Radiat Res*, 150, 568–576, 1998.

52. Jauchem, J.R., Ryan, K.L., Frei, M.R., Dusch, S.J., Lehnert, H.M., and Kovatch, R.M. Repeated exposure of C3H/HeJ mice to ultra-wideband electromagnetic pulses: Lack of effects on mammary tumors. *Radiat Res*, 155, 369–377, 2001.

53. Adey, W.R., Byus, C.V., Cain, C.D., Higgins, R.J., Jones, R.A., Kean, C.J., Kuster, N., MacMurray, A., Stagg, R.B., Zimmerman, G., Phillips, J.L., and Haggren, W. Spontaneous and nitrosourea-induced primary tumors of the central nervous system in Fischer 344 rats chronically exposed to 836 MHz modulated microwaves. *Radiat Res*, 152, 293–302, 1999.

54. Adey, W.R., Byus, C.V., Cain, C.D., Higgins, R.J., Jones, R.A., Kean, C.J., Kuster, N., MacMurray, A., Stagg, R.B., and Zimmerman, G. Spontaneous and nitrosourea-induced primary tumors of the central nervous system in Fischer 344 rats exposed to frequency-modulated microwave fields. *Cancer Res*, 60, 1857–1863, 2000.

55. Zook, B.C., and Simmens, S.J. The effects of 860 MHz radiofrequency radiation on the induction or promotion of brain tumors and other neoplasms in rats. *Radiat Res*, 155, 572–583, 2001.

56. Shirai, T., Kawabe, M., Ichihara, T., Fujiwara, O., Taki, M., Watanabe, S., Wake, K., Yamanaka, Y., Imaida, K., Asamoto, M., and Tamano, S. Chronic exposure to a 1.439 GHz electromagnetic field used for cellular phones does not promote N-ethylnitrosourea induced central nervous system tumors in F344 rats. *Bioelectromagnetics*, 26, 59–68, 2005.

57. Zook, B.C., and Simmens, S.J. The effects of pulsed 860 MHz radiofrequency radiation on the promotion of neurogenic tumors in rats. *Radiat Res*, 165, 608–615, 2006.

58. Shirai, T., Ichihara, T., Wake, K., Watanabe, S., Yamanaka, Y., Kawabe, M., Taki, M., Fujiwara, O., Wang, J., Takahashi, S., and Tamano, S. Lack of promoting effects of chronic exposure to 1.95-GHz W-CDMA signals for IMT-2000 cellular system on development of N-ethylnitrosourea-induced central nervous system tumors in F344 rats. *Bioelectromagnetics*, 28, 562–572, 2007.

59. Bartsch, H., Bartsch, C., Seebald, E., Deerberg, F., Dietz, K., Vollrath, L., and Mecke, D. Chronic exposure to a GSM-like signal (mobile phone) does not stimulate the development of DMBA-induced mammary tumors in rats: results of three consecutive studies. *Radiat Res*, 157, 183–190, 2002.

60. Anane, R., Dulou, P.E., Taxile, M., Geffard, M., Crespeau, F.L., and Veyret, B. Effects of GSM-900 microwaves on DMBA-induced mammary gland tumors in female Sprague-Dawley rats. *Radiat Res*, 160, 492–497, 2003.

61. Yu, D., Shen, Y., Kuster, N., Fu, Y., and Chiang, H. Effects of 900 MHz GSM wireless communication signals on DMBA-induced mammary tumors in rats. *Radiat Res*, 165, 174–180, 2006.

62. Hruby, R., Neubauer, G., Kuster, N., and Frauscher, M. Study on potential effects of "902-MHz GSM-type Wireless Communication Signals" on DMBA-induced mammary tumours in Sprague-Dawley rats. *Mutat Res*, 649, 34–44, 2008.

63. McCormick, D.L., and Moon, R.C. Tumorigenesis of the rat mammary gland. In: H.A. Milman and E.K. Weisburger (Eds.) *Handbook of Carcinogen Testing*. Noyes Publications, Park Ridge, NJ, pp. 215–229, 1985.

64. Imaida, K., Kuzutani, K., Wang, J., Fujiwara, O., Ogiso, T., Kato, K., and Shirai, T. Lack of promotion of 7,12-dimethylbenz[a]anthracene-initiated mouse skin carcinogenesis by 1.5 GHz electromagnetic near fields. *Carcinogenesis*, 22, 1837–1841, 2001.

65. Huang, T.Q., Lee, J.S., Kim, T.H., Pack, J.K., Jang, J.J., and Seo, J.S. Effect of radiofrequency radiation exposure on mouse skin tumorigenesis initiated by 7,12-dimethybenz[alpha]anthracene. *Int J Radiat Biol*, 81, 861–867, 2005.

66. Paulraj, R., and Behari, J. Effects of low level microwave radiation on carcinogenesis in Swiss Albino mice. *Mol Cell Biochem*, 348, 191–197, 2011.

67. Mason, P.A., Walters, T.J., DiGiovanni, J., Beason, C.W., Jauchem, J.R., Dick, E.J., Jr., Mahajan, K., Dusch, S.J., Shields, B.A., Merritt, J.H., Murphy, M.R., and Ryan, K.L. Lack of effect of 94 GHz radio frequency radiation exposure in an animal model of skin carcinogenesis. *Carcinogenesis*, 22, 1701–1708, 2001.

68. Chagnaud, J.L., Moreau, J.M., and Veyret, B. No effect of short-term exposure to GSM-modulated low-power microwaves on benzo(a)pyrene-induced tumours in rat. *Int J Radiat Biol*, 75, 1251–1256, 1999.

69. Imaida, K., Taki, M., Watanabe, S., Kamimura, Y., Ito, T., Yamaguchi, T., Ito, N., and Shirai, T. The 1.5 GHz electromagnetic near-field used for cellular phones does not promote rat liver carcinogenesis in a medium-term liver bioassay. *Jpn J Cancer Res*, 89, 995–1002, 1998.

70. Imaida, K., Taki, M., Yamaguchi, T., Ito, T., Watanabe, S., Wake, K., Aimoto, A., Kamimura, Y., Ito, N., and Shirai, T. Lack of promoting effects of the electromagnetic near-field used for cellular phones (929.2 MHz) on rat liver carcinogenesis in a medium-term liver bioassay. *Carcinogenesis*, 19, 311–314, 1998.

71. Tsuda, H., Fukushima, S., Wanibuchi, H., Morimura, K., Nakae, D., Imaida, K., Tatematsu, M., Hirose, M., Wakabayashi, K., and Moore, M.A. Value of GST-P positive preneoplastic hepatic foci in dose-response studies of hepatocarcinogenesis: Evidence for practical thresholds with both genotoxic and nongenotoxic carcinogens. A review of recent work. *Toxicol Pathol*, 31, 80–86, 2003.

72. Wu, R.Y., Chiang, H., Shao, B.J., Li, N.G., and Fu, Y.D. Effects of 2.45-GHz microwave radiation and phorbol ester 12-O-tetradecanoylphorbol-13-acetate on dimethylhydrazine-induced colon cancer in mice. *Bioelectromagnetics*, 15, 531–538, 1994.

73. Tillmann, T., Ernst, H., Streckert, J., Zhou, Y., Taugner, F., Hansen, V., and Dasenbrock, C. Indication of cocarcinogenic potential of chronic UMTS-modulated radiofrequency exposure in an ethylnitrosourea mouse model. *Int J Radiat Biol*, 86, 529–541, 2010.

74. Lerchl, A., Klose, M., Grote, K., Wilhelm, A.F., Spathmann, O., Fiedler, T., Streckert, J., Hansen, V., and Clemens, M. Tumor promotion by exposure to radiofrequency electromagnetic fields below exposure limits for humans. *Biochem Biophys Res Commun*, 459, 585–590, 2015.

6

Biological Effects of Millimeter and Submillimeter Waves

Stanislav I. Alekseev
Russian Academy of Sciences

Marvin C. Ziskin
Temple University School of Medicine

CONTENTS

6.1 Biological Effects of Millimeter Waves

6.1.1 Introduction

Millimeter (mm) waves comprise the region of electromagnetic spectrum between 30 and 300 GHz (wavelength (λ) = 1–10 mm in free space). However, in common practice, mm wave studies of biological effects cover the frequency range between 30 and 100 GHz. Submillimeter waves or terahertz radiation spectrum (1 THz = 10^{12} Hz) is typically defined as 100–10,000 GHz or 0.1–10 THz, i.e., GHz and THz radiations are between the radiofrequencies and the far infrared radiations.

Humans are increasingly exposed to mm and THz waves from many different sources, such as wireless telecommunication devices (Kallfass et al., 2011), airport security scanners (Sheen et al., 2001), automotive collision avoidance systems (Nicolson et al., 2008), and nonlethal crowd control weaponry (Chen et al., 2012). In addition, mm waves have been used as a therapeutic modality in medical devices (Rojavin and Ziskin, 1998). Newly developed 5G mobile communication systems will significantly add to this exposure. The increasing utilization of mm wave and THz technologies creates considerable interest in the potential effects of mm waves and THz radiation on biological systems. Research on the mm wave and THz biological effects is especially important for establishment of accurate safety standards.

Pakhomov et al. (1998) presented a comprehensive review of biological effects of mm waves at different organization levels of organisms. This review covered about 50 papers published in peer reviewed Western sources and more than 300 papers published in the Former Soviet Union before the year 1997. Remarkable progress in bioelectromagnetics research has been achieved in the past two decades. In the present review, we provide the updated results of studies of biological effects of mm waves published since 1997 in the peer reviewed sources, except for a few essential citations of earlier publications. We review the studies of THz biological effects in Part II of this chapter. All of the publications reviewed are listed in the References located at the end of this chapter.

It should be noted that some of the early results were confirmed in independent recent studies. However, most effects of low-intensity mm wave irradiation are still waiting for their replication. There have been systematic studies of mm wave effects on nervous and immune systems as well as on gene expression, cell proliferation, and artificial lipid membranes.

The present review is focused on experimental findings of mm wave effects on subcellular and cellular levels, effects on cellular proliferation and gene expression, effects on excitable tissues, involvement of nervous and immune systems in mm wave effects, physiologic effects of high power mm waves, effects of mm waves on eyes, and skin heating. The review also includes the theoretical analysis of mechanisms of mm wave action on biological objects and typical artifacts encountered when conducting experiments with mm waves.

6.1.2 Basic Characteristics of mm Wave Radiation

6.1.2.1 Propagation of mm Waves in Free Space and Lossy Dielectric

The plane periodic mm waves traveling in free space in the z direction can be expressed as follows (Olver, 1992):

$$E = E_0 e^{j(\omega t - \beta_0 z)} \tag{6.1}$$

where E is the electric field (V/m), E_0 is amplitude factor (V/m), ω is angular frequency, equal to $2\pi f$, f is frequency (Hz), β_0 is the propagation constant (m^{-1}), $\beta_0 = 2\pi/\lambda_0$, λ_0 is the wavelength in free space (m), and $j = (-1)^{1/2}$.

In a lossy dielectric, Equation (6.1) is transformed to the following form:

$$E = E_0 e^{j\omega t - \gamma z} \tag{6.2}$$

where γ is the complex propagation factor expressed as:

$$\gamma = \alpha + j\beta \tag{6.3}$$

The attenuation coefficient α (m^{-1}) is given by:

$$\alpha = \omega \sqrt{\frac{\mu \varepsilon'}{2} \left[\left(1 + \left(\frac{\varepsilon''}{\varepsilon'} \right)^2 \right)^{1/2} - 1 \right]} \tag{6.4}$$

The propagation coefficient β is given by:

$$\beta = \omega \sqrt{\frac{\mu \varepsilon'}{2} \left[\left(1 + \left(\frac{\varepsilon''}{\varepsilon'} \right)^2 \right)^{1/2} + 1 \right]} \tag{6.5}$$

The wavelength in a lossy dielectric is less than that in free space and can be found as:

$$\lambda = \frac{2\pi}{\beta} \tag{6.6}$$

The attenuation coefficient α is also known as absorption coefficient of medium at the angular frequency ω. Its inverse is called the depth of penetration of mm waves, $\delta = 1/\alpha$.

δ equals the distance into a medium at which the amplitude of the E field drops to $1/e$ of the initial value. The power penetration depth L is expressed as $L = \delta/2 = 1/2\alpha$.

The power density (PD) for a plane-polarized field can be written as follows (Ramo et al., 1993; IEEE C95.1, 2005):

$$PD = \frac{E^2}{\eta} = \eta \cdot H^2 \qquad (6.7)$$

where η is the wave impedance (Ω):

$$\eta = \sqrt{\frac{\mu}{\varepsilon'[1 - j(\varepsilon''/\varepsilon')]}} \qquad (6.8)$$

$\eta = 377\ \Omega$ in free space.

The amplitude reflection coefficient R of mm waves having parallel polarization, i.e., the E-field is parallel to the surface of incidence, is given by

$$R = \frac{\eta_2 - \eta_1}{\eta_2 + \eta_1} \qquad (6.9)$$

where η_1 and η_2 are the wave impedances of medium 1 and 2, respectively. The transmission coefficient T is defined as

$$T = \frac{E_2}{E_1} = \frac{2\eta_2}{\eta_2 + \eta_1} \qquad (6.10)$$

The energy absorbed by biological material is characterized by the specific absorption rate (SAR, W/kg) that is given by

$$\text{SAR} = \frac{\sigma \cdot E^2}{2\rho} \qquad (6.11)$$

where σ is the conductivity (S/m), ρ is mass density (kg/m^3), and E is the electric field strength (V/m).

In biological experiments, objects are exposed to mm waves in the far field or near field of antennas. The far field typically begins at a distance $l = 2D/\lambda$, where D is the longest dimension of the radiating structure, and λ is the wavelength in air. Rectangular horn antennas frequently used in biological experiments have the longest dimension of 2 cm (Alekseev and Ziskin, 2003). The far field distance at 42.25 GHz for this antenna is 11.3 cm. Actually, the far field is a term describing the plane wave exposure field. In far field exposure, the interaction or "coupling" between the antenna and object is absent. Irradiation at a distance less than l is termed near field exposure. The near field exposure especially in the reactive region of antenna is characterized by the strong interaction between the radiation source and object depending on the shape and size of the source and the geometrical and electrical properties of the object.

6.1.2.2 E-field Strength and PD Measurements

The mm wave E-field distribution is measured with E-field probes. As the size of the commercially available E-field probes is relatively large (1–10 mm), their use in the near field of an antenna is limited. Moreover, in the reactive or radiating near field region where reactive fields or standing waves exist, the PD distribution is too complicated. In this case, numerical calculation of the E-field and PD distribution using the finite-difference time domain method (FDTD) (Zhadobov et al., 2017) or other numerical methods such as the finite element method (FEM), finite difference, and Monte Carlo are preferable (Wang and Wu, 2007). For measurement of the E-field strength at frequencies between 40 and 52 GHz, Pakhomov et al. (1997) successfully used a Narda miniature flat crystal detector with a custom made holder for the detector allowing precise movements in any direction over the irradiated area.

Mapping of the PD distribution can be performed using a calibrated receiving antenna such as a horn antenna or open-ended waveguide connected to a power meter. More detailed mapping of the PD distribution is achieved by using an open-ended waveguide due to small size of its aperture (Walters et al., 2000).

Most of the laboratory studies of bioeffects of mm waves have been performed in exposures where the biological structure is placed close to a small antenna. Thus, the object is exposed in the near field of the narrow irradiating mm wave beam. In this case, the SAR and PD values can best be obtained by measuring the initial temperature rise rate on the object surface as described in Section 6.1.4.2.

6.1.2.3 Calibration of Measuring Devices

Calibration methods are addressed in IEEE C95.3 (2002). Three basic methods of calibration of microwave survey devices are used: free-space standard field method, guided wave method, and transfer probe method. For mm wave devices, only a free-space standard method is suitable for accurate calibration in the frequency range above 1 GHz. Standard gain horn antennas are commonly used to establish accurate electromagnetic field intensities. The PD in the far field can be calculated from

$$PD = \frac{P_r \cdot G}{4\pi \cdot r^2} \tag{6.12}$$

where PD is the power density (W/m²), G is the isotropic gain of the antenna, P_r is the radiated power (W), r is a distance from the horn antenna aperture to the on-axis field point (m). Gain is defined as $G = E_{antenna} \cdot D$, where $E_{antenna}$ is efficiency and D is directivity of antenna. For common open-ended waveguide apertures with a two-to-one aspect ratio, i.e., $a/b = 2$, the far-field gain is approximated by the following equation (Kanda and Orr, 1987):

$$G = 21.6 \, fa \tag{6.13}$$

where f is frequency (GHz) and a is the width (m) (larger dimension) of the waveguide aperture. For calculation of on-axis gain of the horn antenna, the equations given by Larsen (1978) can be used:

$$G(dB) = 10Log(AB) + 10.08 - R_H(dB) - R_E(dB) \tag{6.14}$$

where A is the wavelength normalized width of the horn aperture, B is the wavelength normalized height of the horn aperture, R_H is the gain reduction factor due to the H-plane flair of the horn, and R_E is the gain reduction factor due to the E-plane flair of the horn. The gain reduction factors are given by

$$R_H(\text{dB}) = 0.01\alpha(1 + 10.19\alpha + 0.51\alpha^2 - 0.097\alpha^3)$$ (6.15)

$$R_E(\text{dB}) = 0.1\beta^2(2.31 + 0.053\beta)$$ (6.16)

$$\alpha = A^2(1/L_H + 1/r)$$ (6.17)

$$\beta = B^2(1/L_E + 1/r)$$ (6.18)

where L_H and L_E are the wavelength normalized values of the slant lengths and r is the wavelength normalized distance from the aperture of the horn to the on-axis field point.

6.1.2.4 Generation of mm Waves

Millimeter wave generators use different sources of oscillators. Vacuum tube based sources include backward wave oscillators (BWO), orotrons (high-power BWO), magnetrons, gyrotrons, gyro-klystrons, and gyro-traveling wave tubes (gyro-TWT). Solid-state sources include widely used Gunn diodes and impact ionization avalanche transit-time (IMPATT) diodes. Magnetrons, gyrotrons, gyro-klystrons, and gyro-TWT are used in high output power generators. Pulse magnetrons operate in the frequency range up to 220 GHz with peak power of 30 kW. Gyrotrons depending on cooling conditions can generate power at fixed frequencies up to 20 kW. Gyro-klystrons operate at fixed frequencies with output power up to 340 kW. Gyro-TWT can generate peak power up to 180 kW. The low output generators commonly used in biological experiments have oscillators such as BWO, Gunn diodes, and IMPATT diodes. These sources of mm waves cover the frequency range of 30–178 GHz at maximum output power up to 400 mW. Generators based on BWO operate at frequencies from 36 to 178 GHz with output powers up to 80 mW. BWO are the most wide-banded sources with electronic control of frequency. Cavity stabilized Gunn oscillators generate from 40 to 140 GHz with maximum CW power at lower frequencies up to 200 mW, which drops at higher frequencies to 30 mW. CW IMPATT diodes are used for oscillators and amplifiers. They operate in the frequency range of 30–140 GHz with output power up to 400 mW. IMPATT diodes are used in noise generators. Some generators use frequency synthesizers. A frequency synthesizer is an electronic circuit for generating any of a range of frequencies from a single fixed oscillator. A frequency synthesizer uses the techniques of frequency multiplication, frequency division, direct digital synthesis, and frequency mixing (photomixing) to generate new frequencies, which have the same stability and accuracy as the master oscillator. Commercially available synthesizers cover the frequency ranges from 36 to 1250 GHz and 0.45 to 2.85 THz.

6.1.3 Permittivity of Biological Material

6.1.3.1 Electric and Magnetic Properties of Biological Material

The response of biological material (skin, tissue, cells) to mm wave exposure depends on its electric and magnetic properties at the exposure frequency. Magnetic properties of material are described by complex permeability μ:

$$\mu = \mu' - j\mu''$$ (6.19)

In biological non-ferromagnetic materials, magnetic response is very weak, and the permeability differs very little from the permeability of free space (μ_0), i.e., $\mu \approx \mu_0 = 4\pi \cdot 10^{-7}\,\text{H/m}$.

The electric properties of material are characterized by the frequency-dependent complex permittivity:

$$\varepsilon^* = \varepsilon' - j\varepsilon'' \tag{6.20}$$

where ε' is the relative dielectric constant and ε'' is the relative loss factor of the material. The total conductivity σ is related to ε'' by

$$\varepsilon'' = \frac{\sigma}{\omega \cdot \varepsilon_0} \tag{6.21}$$

The permittivity of free space is given by $\varepsilon_0 = 8.85 \cdot 10^{-12}\,\text{F/m}$. The total conductivity σ includes a contribution from the frequency independent ionic conductivity and is associated with the frequency-dependent dielectric loss of material. The loss tangent is a measure of how "lossy" or energy absorbing a material is. It is defined as

$$\tan\delta = \frac{\varepsilon''}{\varepsilon'} \tag{6.22}$$

Two relaxation functions are often used to fit dielectric data, the Debye, and Cole–Cole equations. The Cole–Cole equation is given by

$$\varepsilon^* = \varepsilon_\infty + \frac{\Delta\varepsilon}{(1 + j\omega\tau)^{1-\alpha}} + \frac{\sigma_i}{j\omega\varepsilon_0} \tag{6.23}$$

where ε_∞ is the optical permittivity, $\Delta\varepsilon = \varepsilon_s - \varepsilon_\infty$ is the magnitude of the dispersion of material, ε_s is the permittivity at $\omega\tau \ll 1$, $\omega = 2\pi f$, ω is an angular frequency, f is the frequency (Hz), τ is the relaxation time (s), σ_i is the ionic conductivity (S/m), and α is the distribution parameter. At $\alpha = 0$, Equation 6.23 transforms to the well-known Debye equation.

According to Foster and Schwan (1986), the loss factor can be expressed as follows:

$$\varepsilon'' = \frac{\Delta\varepsilon \cdot \omega\tau}{1 + (\omega\tau)^2} + \frac{\sigma_i}{\omega\varepsilon_0} \tag{6.24}$$

The total conductivity is proportional to the loss factor ε'' (Equation 6.21): $\sigma = \omega\varepsilon_0\varepsilon''$. The contribution of ionic conductivity decreases with increasing frequency. At mm wave frequencies, the total conductivity is defined mainly by the dielectric loss of material.

The dielectric spectrum of biological tissue is characterized by major relaxation regions such as α, β, and γ dispersions at low, medium, and high frequencies, respectively. Some minor relaxation regions such as δ dispersion may also contribute to the dielectric spectrum of tissue (Schwan, 1977; Foster and Schwan, 1986). The relaxation frequency of the γ dispersion in skin is about 22 GHz at 37°C (Gabriel et al., 1996), i.e., the γ dispersion is exhibited in the mm-wave frequency range.

The complex refractive index of a material is defined as

$$n^* = n' - j \cdot n'' = \sqrt{\varepsilon^*} \tag{6.25}$$

6.1.3.2 Permittivity of Skin

In biological tissue (skin), water is a main absorber of mm waves. The photon energy of mm waves, $h\nu$, ranges from 0.12 to 1.24 meV, where h is Planck's constant and ν is frequency. The energy of electron removal from an atom or molecule is typically 12 eV. Unlike ionizing radiation, the photon energy of mm waves is not enough to disrupt molecular bonds. Therefore, mm waves are regarded as nonionizing radiation. The energy of molecular vibration is in the range of 0.01–0.1 eV. The energy of thermal motion, kT, at room temperature is about 0.025 eV, where k is a Boltzmann constant and T is temperature. Hence, the photon energy of mm waves is even lower than the energy of thermal motion. Only the energy of orientation motion of the molecular dipoles (10^{-3}–10^{-4} eV) is lower than the photon energy of mm waves. Thus, mm waves can interact with molecules that have rotational degree of freedom such as water molecules. This type of interaction raises the thermal energy of water molecules, i.e. produces heating of water.

With the exception of the stratum corneum (SC) layer, skin consists of about 70% of water. Some of the water molecules interact with soluble tissue components and form a hydration shell. This motionally restricted water is called "bound" water. The remaining water molecules are free in motion and compose the "free" water of tissue. Dispersion of "bound" water and dispersion of tissue components such as proteins and lipids occur at lower microwave frequencies (Schwan, 1965; Grant, 1982; Smith and Foster, 1985; Mashimo et al., 1987). The "free" water relaxation region is characterized by the γ dispersion that is well described by the Debye equation.

At higher frequencies (>100 GHz), Buchner et al. (1999) and Ellison (2007) found an additional minor relaxation region in the dielectric spectrum of water. There is only a small difference between the permittivity dispersion curves calculated using the Debye equation with either one or two relaxation frequencies at mm waves. However, at THz frequencies, the second relaxation region brings in a significant contribution to permittivity. The main absorber of mm waves in biological tissues including skin is "free" water. Permittivity of pure water at 298 K is shown in Figure 6.1.

In most cases, skin permittivity is derived using the direct reflection measurements (Hwang et al., 2003; Alekseev and Ziskin, 2007), time domain reflectometry (Mashimo et al., 1987; Naito et al., 1997), and a quasi-optical method (Alabaster, 2003). Direct mm wave

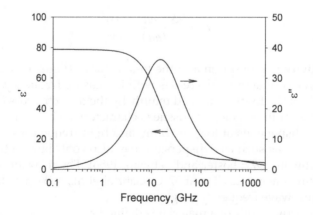

FIGURE 6.1
Permittivity of pure water calculated using the double Debye equation (Equation 6.32) with parameters from the paper by Pickwell et al. (2004a).

TABLE 6.1

Skin Permittivity at 60 GHz Obtained by Different Methods

Reference	e^*	$T(°C)$	Method	Sample Type
Gabriel et al. (1996)	$7.98-j10.90$	37	E	*In vivo*
Gandhi and Riazi (1986)	$8.89-j13.15$	37	E	*In vitro*
Hwang et al. (2014)	$8.05-j4.13$	24–26	M	*In vivo*
Alabaster (2003)	$9.90-j9.0$	23	M	*In vitro*
Alabaster (2003)	$13.2-j10.3$	37	E	*In vitro*
Alekseev and Ziskin (2007)	$8.12-j11.4$	32.6	M	*In vivo*
Zhadobov et al. (2008)	$9.38-j12.49$	30	T	-

E, extrapolation; *M*, direct measurement; and *T*, theoretical value.

measurements often require sophisticated equipment, such as mm wave vector network analyzers. The permittivity data obtained for a homogeneous model of skin at 60 GHz is given in Table 6.1 (Zhadobov et al., 2011).

Obtained data shows that in 10–100 GHz range the relative permittivity of skin decreases with increasing frequency while conductivity of skin increases with the increase of frequency.

6.1.4 Interaction of mm Waves With Skin

6.1.4.1 Skin Organization

The human skin consists of three individual layers: the epidermis, dermis, and hypodermis. The epidermis, the outermost layer of skin, is about 0.1 mm thick but on the palms of the hands it can be 0.7 mm thick or more (Bloom and Fawcett, 1968; Odland, 1971; El Gammal et al., 1999; Welzel et al., 2004). The majority of cells in the epidermis are keratinocytes. The surface layer of the epidermis is called the SC. The SC is made up of flattened dead keratinocytes, which have lost their internal structure. The thickness of the SC in the forearm skin is about 0.012–0.018 mm (Kligman, 1964; Rajadhyaksha et al., 1999; Huzaira et al., 2001; Caspers et al., 2003; Sandby-Moller et al., 2003). The rest of the epidermis (without the SC) consisting of live cells is called the viable epidermis. The dermis is organized into a papillary (outer) and a reticular (inner) region. The distinction between the two layers is based mostly on their differences in connective tissue. Literature data of the dermis thickness depend on location and on the methods used for thickness measurements, and vary from 1.0 to 2.0 mm (Meema et al., 1964; Black, 1969; Shuster et al., 1975; Dykes and Marks, 1977; Fornage and Deshayes, 1986; Branchet et al., 1990; Gniadecka and Quistorff, 1996). The hypodermis is composed mainly of fat cells and connects the dermis to underlying tissues and muscle.

6.1.4.2 Depth of Penetration of mm Waves into Skin

To evaluate the biological effect of mm waves, it is important to know the PD distribution within the skin, which can be defined based on the knowledge of the penetration depth of radiation and reflection of mm waves from the skin.

Two models were developed to describe the interaction of mm waves with skin: one-layer (or homogeneous) and multilayer skin models. Multilayer models consist of the SC, the viable epidermis and dermis, and the fat layer (Alekseev and Ziskin, 2007). The power reflection coefficient for the homogeneous skin model in terms of refractive indices and at normal incidence of mm waves is expressed as

$$R = \left| \frac{n_1 - n_2}{n_1 + n_2} \right|^2 \tag{6.26}$$

where n_1 and n_2 are refractive indices of medium 1 and 2, respectively. If medium 1 is air, as commonly used in experiments, $n_1 = 1$. The power reflection coefficient decreases from 0.43 to 0.18 as the frequency increases from 30 to 100 GHz (Alekseev et al., 2008).

The amplitude penetration depth (m) is expressed as $\delta = c/\omega n''$, where c is the velocity of light (10^8 m/s), ω is an angular frequency (Hz), and n'' is the imaginary part of the refractive index of medium. The frequency dependence of penetration depth is presented in Figure 6.2. As can be seen, the penetration depth decreases with increasing the frequency.

As the wavelengths of mm waves are small in comparison with the size of human body, the geometrical optics concepts can be applied for calculations of interaction of mm waves with skin. That is, mm waves can be considered as rays. The skin can be presented as a flat semi-infinite surface exposed to plane mm waves. To characterize mm wave exposure intensity, the safety standards FCC (1996), ICNIRP (1998), and IEEE (2005) recommend using PD. The PD distribution in lossy homogeneous material is given by the Beer-Lambert law:

$$PD(z) = PD_0 \cdot e^{-2z/\delta} \tag{6.27}$$

where δ is the amplitude penetration depth (m) and PD_0 is the incident PD (W/m²). More than 90% of mm wave energy is absorbed within the epidermis and dermis. The rest of mm wave energy is absorbed in the subcutaneous tissue.

In the reactive near field of a radiating antenna, it is not an easy task to derive accurate values of PD. Therefore, an application of the SAR commonly used at lower frequencies for characterization of absorbed energy is reasonable at mm wave frequencies also. Moreover, SAR is used for calculations of skin heating. SAR at a depth of z of the homogeneous skin model is given by (Gandhi and Riazi, 1986).

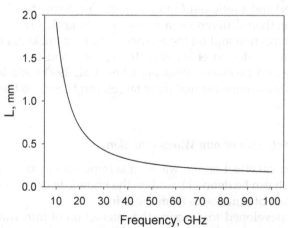

FIGURE 6.2 Power penetration depth in the human skin. The penetration depth is calculated using permittivity data from Alekseev and Ziskin (2007).

$$\text{SAR}(z) = \frac{2 \cdot (1 - R)}{\rho \cdot \delta} \cdot \text{PD}_0 \cdot e^{-2z/\delta} \tag{6.28}$$

where R is the power reflection coefficient, ρ is the mass density (kg/m^3), and other symbols are the same as in Equation 6.27. The SAR increases rapidly with increasing frequency due to decreasing the power reflection coefficient and penetration depth. If PD_0 is not known, SAR can be estimated by measuring the initial temperature rise rate in tissue:

$$\text{SAR} = C \frac{dT}{dt} \Big|_{t=0} \tag{6.29}$$

where C is the specific heat capacity (J/kg/$°$C). However, the thermal noise obscuring the initial phase of the heating kinetics reduces the accuracy in SAR determination. The most reliable way to determine SAR is by fitting of a thermal model to the experimental heating kinetics and then to calculate SAR from the model (Alekseev and Ziskin, 2003; Chahat et al., 2012; Zhadobov et al., 2017).

Millimeter waves penetrate deep enough into the skin to affect skin structures located in the epidermis and dermis. Main targets for the mm wave effect in the epidermis are the keratinocytes, melanocytes, and Langerhans cells as well as the Merkel cells located at the dermal-epidermal junction (Bloom and Fawcett, 1968; Holbrook and Wolff, 1993; Mehregan et al., 1995). In the papillary dermis, the mm wave PD is still high. The papillary dermis contains free nerve endings, the most widespread and important sensory receptors. Some free nerve endings extend into the epidermis. Another type of sensory receptor, the Meissner corpuscle, is also located in the papillary dermis. Monocytes and macrophages, as well as mast cells, are commonly present in this region.

The microcirculatory beds in skin include arterioles, precapillary sphincters, arterial and venous capillaries, postcapillary venules, and collecting venules (Rhodin, 1967, 1968). At the junction between the papillary and reticular dermis, terminal arterioles form a horizontal subpapillary plexus giving rise to the capillary loops extending into the papillary dermis. Venous capillaries drain into venules that lie above and below the arteriolar subpapillary plexus. Thus, a large amount of blood vessels and ultimately blood cells are exposed to mm waves at a relatively high PD. Thus, most skin structures present in the epidermis and dermis could be primary targets for the mm wave action in human skin.

Most theoretical calculations of the PD and SAR distributions in skin were performed using Equations 6.27 and 6.28 for a homogeneous skin model. The skin structures such as blood vessels and appendages (hair, sweat ducts, and sebaceous glands) with electrical properties different from the average electrical properties of skin tissue cause either selective absorption of mm wave energy or local distortion of the mm wave field in their vicinity (Alekseev and Ziskin, 2001, 2009a). In the blood vessels located in the human and murine dermis and oriented parallel to the E-field, the SAR could exceed the average SAR in the surrounding dermis by ~40% (Alekseev and Ziskin, 2009a). In murine skin, SAR in blood vessels normally traversing the fat layer achieved its maximal value at the parallel orientation of the E-field to the vessel axis. At 42 GHz exposure, the maximal SAR in small blood vessels could be more than 30 times greater than that in the skin (Alekseev and Ziskin, 2011). Analysis of mm wave absorption by blood vessels did not reveal strong frequency dependence of this effect. In evaluating the threshold intensities of biological effects in skin, it is important to take into account the heterogeneous structure of the exposed region. The greater the difference between the electrical properties of skin structures (blood vessels, hair, sweat pores, etc.) and skin, the greater is the distortion of the

E-field distribution near these structures. Selective absorption of mm-wave energy by small cutaneous blood vessels could hardly result in excessive temperature elevation due to the effective heat dissipation by blood flow and heat conduction to the surrounding tissue. However, the increased E-field strength in the close vicinity of innervated skin appendages and blood vessels could result in a neural effect.

6.1.4.3 Heating of Skin

Absorption of mm wave energy of any intensity will produce a temperature elevation. If the intensity is sufficiently high, the temperature elevation in tissue will be significant. A modification in function or structure of a biological structure by a large temperature elevation is called a thermal bioeffect. However, thermoregulatory systems of mammals are capable of keeping integral body temperature at nearly the same level even when exposed to an intensity as high as 10 mW/cm². Bioeffects occurring at low exposure intensities producing a temperature rise ≤0.1°C are accepted as nonthermal (Betsky, 1993). This occurs at intensities less than 10 mW/cm². Any effect of electromagnetic energy absorption not associated with the production of heat or a measurable temperature rise is classified as nonthermal (IEEE C95-3, 2002).

As the skin heating is important for understanding the mechanisms of mm wave action and development of safety standards, human skin heating has been studied extensively and the results of these experimental studies are widely present in literature (Walters et al., 2000, 2004; Nelson et al., 2003; Alekseev and Ziskin, 2003; Alekseev et al., 2005). In experiments, skin is exposed with antennas forming Gaussian beams on the skin surface of different size (between 4.8 and 40 mm in diameter) (Alekseev and Ziskin, 2003; Walters et al., 2000, 2004). It is shown that the temperature elevation depends on the location of the exposed site on a body, the beam size, and blood flow rate (Walters et al., 2004; Alekseev et al., 2005). Different thermal models are used for predictions of temperature distributions in skin exposed to mm waves (Nelson et al., 2000, 2003; Alekseev et al., 2005; Stewart et al., 2006; Kanezaki et al., 2008, 2010; Foster et al., 2010, 2016; Shafirstein and Moros, 2011; Zilberty et al., 2013, 2014; Morimoto et al., 2017). Most of them are based on the Pennes bio-heat transfer equation (BHTE) (Pennes, 1948) that accounts for the blood flow effect. One and two-dimensional BHTE applied to homogeneous skin have been frequently used, primarily due to their relative simplicity and accuracy in predictions of temperature fields in tissue regions without large (>1 mm) blood vessels. Two-dimensional BHTE is typically applied for modeling radially symmetric beam (Gaussian beam) exposure in the near-field of an antenna (Alekseev et al., 2005). The one-dimensional BHTE is given by (Foster et al., 1978)

$$\rho C \cdot \frac{\partial T}{\partial t} = k \cdot \frac{\partial^2 T}{\partial z^2} - V_s \cdot T + \text{SAR}(z) \cdot \rho \qquad (6.30)$$

where $T = T_t - T_b$, T_t is tissue temperature (°C), T_b is arterial blood temperature (°C), k is the coefficient of tissue heat conduction (W/m · °C), $V_s = f_b \cdot \rho_b \cdot C_b$, f_b is the specific blood flow rate (mL/s/mL), ρ_b (kg/m³) and C_b (J/kg · °C) are the density and specific heat of blood, respectively, SAR (z) is the SAR distribution in tissue, ρ is the density of tissue (kg/m³), C is the specific heat of tissue (J/kg/°C), and z is distance from tissue surface in the direction of the beam axis (m). In the equation, a term accounting for metabolic heat production is neglected because its contribution to heat production in resting man is relatively low (Hardy, 1982; Nelson et al., 2000), and would not change much during mm-wave exposure.

The irradiating beam size plays a significant role in mm wave heating. The broader the beam, the higher is the surface temperature elevation and the deeper is the heat penetration into tissue (Alekseev et al., 2005).

The BHTE accurately predicts skin heating only at low blood perfusion rates. Blood perfusion produces a cooling effect and reduces the temperature elevation in skin. "Effective conductivity" models have been introduced by Crezee and Lagendijk (1990), Ducharme and Tikuisis (1991), Crezee et al. (1994), and Kolios et al. (1996). To fit the experimental data, the blood flow dependent effective thermal conductivity, k_{eff}, is applied to account for the thermal response in the areas of body (finger) with relatively high blood flow (Alekseev et al., 2005; Alekseev and Ziskin, 2009b).

Three or four layer thermal models are much closer to the real structure of skin and underlying tissue (Stolwijk and Hardy, 1977; Emery and Sekins, 1982; Xu and Werner, 1997; Kanezaki et al., 2008, 2010). They include dermal, fat, and muscle blood flows. As the multilayer models reflect physiological conditions of different tissue layers, they are more adequate for describing thermal events in the skin. In modeling skin heating with mm waves, Alekseev and Ziskin (2009b) used a four-layer model consisting of the epidermis, dermis, fat, and muscle layers (Figure 6.3). At skin blood flow rate typical for abdomen and the fat thickness of 2 mm, the temperature elevation on skin surface at the incident PD of 10 mW/cm^2 and frequency of 42 GHz was about 1.2°C. When applying a one-layer model with the same blood flow rate, the temperature elevation was about 2 times smaller. The fat layer plays a role of thermal insulator. With increasing the thickness of the fat layer, the temperature elevation in skin exposed to mm waves is also increased. The areas of skin with low blood flow and thick fat have the maximum temperature elevation. Heat diffuses deep into tissue reaching the fat and muscle layers. Kanezaki et al. (2010) obtained similar results with a model consisting of the skin, fat, and muscle layers. The temperature elevation decreases when skin is exposed to a narrow Gaussian-type beam. Experimentally measured temperature elevation of skin surface exposed to 1.06 cm beam was only 0.5°C at the peak PD of 10 W/cm^2 (Alekseev et al., 2005).

Thus, exposure of skin to 10 mW/cm^2 definitely can produce thermal effect on cells and structures located not only in the skin but also in the fat and muscle layers.

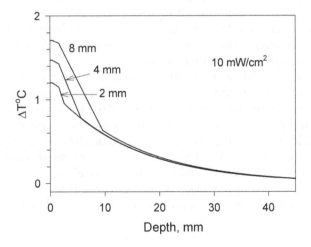

FIGURE 6.3
Temperature increment distributions within tissue calculated for different thicknesses of the fat layer (2, 4, and 8 mm) in a four-layer model. Blood flows in skin, fat and muscle layers were 1.4×10^{-3}, 0.43×10^{-5}, and 5.33×10^{-4} mL/s/mL, respectively.

6.1.5 Millimeter Wave Effects on Eyes

The eyes, located on the surface of the body like skin, are directly exposed to mm wave irradiation. Exposure to high-intensity mm waves can produce adverse effects in the eye. The eye is especially vulnerable to thermal damage because there is no blood flow to internal structures such as the lens. Within the anterior chamber of the eye, heat dissipates only via conduction through the sclera and convection from the surface of the cornea. Overheating of the eyes causes corneal burns and cataracts. Whether the exposure is accidental or occurs in military applications, it is important to determine the thresholds for damage in order to establish appropriate safety standards.

Kues et al. (1999) studied the ocular effects of 60 GHz mm waves at an intensity of 10 mW/cm². Nonhuman primates and rabbits were exposed once for 8 h, and for 4 h per day during 5 consecutive days. The authors did not find any ocular changes at microscopic examination and diagnostic procedures that could be attributed to mm wave exposure. Thus, the low intensity mm wave exposure does not result in any detectable ocular damage.

However, mm wave exposures at high intensities produce adverse effects on eyes. Rosenthal et al. (1976) reported the results of the study of the mm wave effects on rabbit eyes exposed to 35 and 107 GHz at 50 mW/cm² for 15–80 min. These exposures induced both epithelial damage and stromal edema in the cornea. The immediate stromal damage produced by 107 GHz exposure recovered by the next day.

Chalfin et al. (2002) investigated the effects of pulsed 35 and 94 GHz exposure on the anterior segment of the nonhuman primate eye at the exposure intensities of 2 and 8 W/cm². The corneal temperature elevation at 94 GHz exposure was 35°C. The authors detected distinct lesions, involving only superficial layers of the cornea. The corneal damage caused by 35 GHz exposure at 2 W/cm² for 1.5–5 s was reversible within 24 h. The mean threshold fluence required to produce a corneal lesion was 7.5 J/cm² at 35 GHz and 5 J/cm² at 94 GHz.

The effect of high-intensity 60 GHz exposure on the rabbit eye was studied by Kojima et al. (2009). Exposure for 6 min at the intensity of 1,898 mW/cm² led to an elevation of the corneal surface temperature to 54.2°C accompanied with corneal edema and epithelial cell loss. Anterior uveitis also occurred resulting in acute miosis, an increase in flares, and iris vasodilatation. Heat generated by mm wave exposure could apparently penetrate below the surface of the eye inducing the observed thermal effects. The effects of mm waves were dependent on the intensity and duration of exposure.

Different numerical models were developed to describe the temperature distribution in rabbit, nonhuman primate, and human eyes following mm wave exposure (Scott, 1988; Foster et al., 2003; Papaioannou and Samara, 2011; Karampatzakis and Theodoros, 2010, 2013). For example, Foster et al. (2003) modeled the empirical temperature data obtained by Chalfin et al. (2002). The results of calculations using one-dimensional heat conduction equation were in agreement with experimental data. The thresholds for damage to the cornea corresponded to temperature elevation by about 20°C at both irradiation frequencies 35 and 94 GHz. The authors concluded that the simple heat conduction equation could be used for predictions of thermal damage thresholds to the cornea.

The experimental results show that low-intensity (10 mW/cm²) mm wave irradiation does not produce any harmful effect on eyes. However, the high-intensity mm wave exposure results in adverse effects on eye. The ocular damage is induced by the thermal effect of mm waves and depends on the frequency, intensity, and duration of exposure.

6.1.6 Millimeter Wave Effects on Subcellular and Cellular Levels

6.1.6.1 Effects on Membrane Level

6.1.6.1.1 Artificial Lipid Membranes

Cellular membrane is believed to be one of the main targets of mm wave action. This belief is substantiated by the theoretical works by Frölich (1968, 1970, 1972, 1978) suggesting that microwaves are capable of producing coherent longitudinal electrical oscillations in lipid membranes. Artificial lipid membranes are simple and convenient models for the study of mm wave effects on ion transport, phase transition, hydration, membrane surface charge, lipid peroxidation, and other processes.

Many studies were carried out on models of cellular membranes such as liposomes and bilayer lipid membranes (Alekseev and Ziskin, 1995; Logani and Ziskin, 1996, 1998; Ramundo-Orlando et al., 2009; Di Donato et al., 2012; Beneduci et al., 2012, 2013, 2014; Albini et al., 2014). Di Donato et al. (2012) found the increase of permeability of cationic liposomes loaded with carbonic anhydrase and exposed to 53.37 GHz with an intensity as low as 0.1 mW/cm². In a number of papers, the effects of mm waves on giant phospholipid vesicles were reported (Ramundo-Orlando et al., 2009; Albini et al., 2014). Giant liposomes dispersed in 0.2 M sucrose solution were exposed from the top of a chamber to 53.37 GHz mm waves at 0.1 mW/cm². Direct optical observations in real time allowed authors to discover induced diffusion of fluorescent dye di-8-ANEPPS into the bilayer membrane (BLM), elongation of vesicles, increased attraction between vesicles, and their vectorial movement. It was concluded that the observed effects cannot be attributed to local heating. However, the effect of convection, induced in the liquid medium by mm wave exposure, on the properties of lipid vesicles could not be excluded. Beneduci et al. (2013) reported the effect of mm waves on phosphatidylcholine vesicles using deuterium nuclear magnetic resonance (²H-NMR) spectroscopy. Multilamellar vesicles were exposed to 53.57–78.33 GHz frequency range at 0.0035–0.010 mW/cm² with a Teflon antenna inserted into the NMR probe. Exposure at temperatures close to the phase transition of the membrane produced a transition of the membrane from the fluid to the gel phase. During phase transitions, the significant structural changes occur in the membrane, and the membrane becomes sensitive to external physical influences. The authors interpreted the results as a hydrogen-dependent reduction of the water ordering around the phosphatidylcholine headgroups (Beneduci et al., 2014).

Liposomes were used to study the effect of mm waves on lipid peroxidation in the presence and absence of melanin, a pigment produced in the epidermis by melanocytes (Logani and Ziskin, 1996). Liposomes were exposed to 53.6, 61.2, and 78.2 GHz at incident power densities of 10, 1.0, and 500 mW/cm², respectively. The authors did not find an enhancement of the formation of lipid peroxides compared to unexposed samples. Direct exposure of melanin also did not exhibit an increased formation of superoxide or hydrogen peroxide.

Zhadobov et al. (2006) investigated the effect of mm waves on superficial pressure and microdomain distribution in phospholipid monolayers. Microdomains reflect functional specialization of the different membrane regions and play an important role in membrane interaction processes. Exposure at 60 GHz and PD of 0.9 mW/cm² for 5 h resulted in increase of lateral pressure. Low-power mm wave exposure did not induce significant transformations in the phospholipid domain organization in model membranes.

Direct measurements of the conductance and capacitance of lipid BLMs exposed to mm waves in the range of 54–76 GHz did not reveal any of the effects found in the experiments with giant liposomes, which could affect the electrical properties of BLM (Alekseev and Ziskin, 1995). A waveguide isolated from the solution by thin Teflon film was placed at specific distances d (d ≥ 0 mm) from the BLM formed on a tip of plastic pipette. The pipette was located in the center of a chamber. Such an experimental setup excluded artifacts caused by the evaporation of water on the surface of solution when exposed from the top of a chamber, or influence of the bottom material and its size when exposed from the bottom of a chamber. Some membranes were modified by gramicidin A, amphotericin B, or tetraphenylboron anions, which increased the conductance of BLM. Gramicidin A and amphotericin B form ionic channels in a membrane, and model the ionic channels in excitable cells. Tetraphenylboron is a lipid soluble ion. BLM was exposed to continuous wave (CW) and pulsed wave (PW) mm waves at repetition rates ranging from 1 to 100 pulses per second (pps) and PW at 1000 pps. In the 54–76 GHz range at 1 GHz steps, no resonance-like effects on capacitance and conductance of modified membranes were detected. All changes in membrane capacitance and conductance were independent on the modulation employed, and were equivalent to heating by ~1.1°C with an SAR of 2 kW/kg. These results clearly demonstrate that coherent oscillations in BLM are not excited in the frequency range of 54–76 GHz.

Thus, some results obtained in experiments with artificial lipid membranes are inconsistent with the thermal effect of mm waves. However, the mechanisms underlying these effects are not clear. It is obvious that more studies with better control of the exposure conditions are required to evaluate the validity of these results.

6.1.6.1.2 Cellular Membranes

The results of early studies of mm wave effects on ionic channels of cellular membranes are described in details in the review by Pakhomov et al. (1998). Most of the studies reported the positive effects of nonthermal low-intensity mm waves on Ca^{++}-activated K^+ channels (Geletyuk et al., 1995; Fesenko et al., 1995), and chloride and calcium channels (Kataev et al., 1993). Here, we describe the results of two studies of mm wave action on K^+ and Ca^{++} currents in snail neurons (Alekseev and Ziskin, 1999) and voltage-gated sodium and potassium channels expressed by *Xenopus laevis* oocytes (Shapiro et al., 2013).

Alekseev and Ziskin (1999) investigated the effects of mm waves 60.22–62.22 and 75 GHz on A-type K^+ currents, and the effects of 61.22 GHz on Ca^{++} currents of Lymnaea neurons. In a study of the frequency-dependent effects of irradiation on the peak amplitude and inactivation components of A-currents, the frequency was changed at 0.1 GHz intervals within the 60.22–62.22 GHz range. A neuron attached to a polythene pipette was exposed with a waveguide opening covered with thin Teflon film and placed into solution close to the neuron. The SAR was in the range of 0–2400 W/kg. This type of setup allowed authors to record ionic currents during exposure without artifacts. Millimeter wave exposure increased the peak amplitudes, activation and inactivation rates of both ionic currents. These changes were independent of frequency and resulted from the temperature rise produced by the irradiation. No additional effects of irradiation on A-type K^+ currents other than thermal were found when tested at the phase transition temperature. Millimeter waves had no effect on the steady-state activation and inactivation curves, suggesting that the membrane surface charge and binding of calcium ions to the membrane in the area of channel locations did not change. The absence of resonance-like frequency-dependent effects of mm waves on BLM (Alekseev and Ziskin, 1995) and cellular membrane does not support Frölich's theory. However, it is not excluded that the resonance-like effects may occur in a different frequency range.

In the recent article by Shapiro et al. (2013), the results of study of 60 GHz exposure effects on the voltage-gated sodium and potassium channels in oocytes were presented. The irradiation power was delivered to oocytes through an open-ended waveguide from the bottom of a recording chamber. The power densities at the top and bottom of oocytes were 1–33 and 18–60 mW/cm^2, respectively. Oocyte sat on the bottom of a chamber on a 0.25 mm quartz coverslip. This setup excluded most of artifacts in recording ionic currents except those arising from convection currents resulting from the elevated temperature (Zhadobov et al., 2017). The observed changes in the kinetics and activity levels of voltage-gated potassium and sodium channels were consistent with a thermal mechanism. The authors suggested that mm wave exposure produced significant thermally mediated effects on excitable cells via basic thermodynamic mechanisms.

Thus, the more recent studies do not confirm the nonthermal effects of mm waves on electrical events in cell membranes.

6.1.6.2 Effects on Gene Expression

Gene expression is a process by which information from a gene is used to synthesize a functional gene product. These products are often proteins. Disturbances in gene expression if they are accompanied with DNA damage may result in serious medical conditions including cancer. That is why the studies of mm wave effects on gene expression and DNA damage, genotoxic effects, are very important and attract the efforts of the scientific community.

Vijayalaxmi et al. (2004) investigated the genotoxic potential of mm wave radiation on mice exposed to 42.2 GHz at the incident PD of 31.5 mW/cm^2. The radiation was applied locally to the nasal region of mice for 30 min/day for 3 consecutive days. The extent of genotoxicity was assessed from the incidence of micronuclei in polychromatic erythrocytes of peripheral blood and bone marrow cells collected 24 h after treatment. The results indicated that there was no evidence for the induction of genotoxicity in the peripheral blood and bone marrow cells of mice exposed to mm waves.

The influence of 60 GHz mm wave exposure at an intensity of 0.54 mW/cm^2 on a set of stress-sensitive gene expression of molecular chaperones, clusterin, and Hsp70, in a human brain cell line was investigated in experiments with long exposure durations up to 33 h (Zhadobov et al., 2007). The results demonstrated the absence of significant modifications in gene transcription, mRNA, and protein amount for the evaluated stress-sensitive genes. The authors concluded that low-power 60 GHz radiation does not modify stress-sensitive gene expression of chaperon proteins.

The effects of mm waves on endoplasmic reticulum stress sensor gene expression were reported in a number of papers (Nicolaz et al., 2009a,b; Le Quement et al., 2014). Exposure at a frequency of 60 GHz (or 8 frequencies within the 59–61 GHz range) with different intensities up to 20 mW/cm^2 did not change the gene expression.

Soubere Mahamoud et al. (2016) analyzed modifications of the whole genome of a human keratinocyte model exposed to 60.4 GHz at the incident PD of 20 mW/cm^2 for 3 h. No keratinocyte transcriptome modifications were observed. The effects of mm waves on cell metabolism were tested by co-treating mm wave exposed cells with a glycolysis inhibitor, 2-deoxyglucose. Whole genome expression was evaluated along with the ATP content. In this case, the treatment did not alter the keratinocyte ATP content, but it slightly altered the transcriptome, which indicated the capacity of mm waves to interfere with the bioenergetic stress response.

The effect of mm waves on neuronal differentiation was studied using a neuron-like cell line (PC 12) (Haas et al., 2016a). PC12 cell monolayers were exposed to 60.4 GHz for 24 h at the incident PD of 10 mW/cm^2. The PC 12 neurite outgrowth and cytoskeleton protein expression were assessed. No changes in protein expression were found. A slight increase in neurite outgrowth was related to the thermal effect of mm wave exposure. The same authors used a PC 12 subclone Neuroscreen-1 cell line to investigate the effects of mm waves on the expression of receptors of the Transient Receptor Potential cation channel subfamily TRPV1 and purinergic receptor P2X (Haas et al., 2016b). Exposure to 60.4 GHz with the incident PD of 10 mW/cm^2 revealed no effect on protein expression of Hsp70, TRPV1, TRPV2, and P2X3.

To test the genotoxic effect of mm waves at frequency of 60 GHz and intensity of 1.0 mW/cm^2, Koyama et al. (2016a) used human corneal and lens epithelial cells. Exposure for 24 h did not reveal any genotoxic effect of mm waves in human eye cells.

Changes in gene expression were discovered in rat skin following exposure to 35 GHz at 75 mW/cm^2 resulting in overheating of the skin up to 42°C–43°C (Millenbaugh et al., 2008). Microscopic findings observed in the dermis of rats included aggregation of neutrophils in vessels, degeneration of stromal cells, and breakdown of collagen. Changes were detected in 56 genes at 6 h exposure and 58 genes at 24 h exposure. Genes associated with regulation of transcription, protein folding, oxidative stress, immune response, and tissue matrix turnover were affected at both times. The obtained results indicate that prolonged exposure to high-intensity mm waves causes thermally related stress and injury in skin while triggering repair processes involving inflammation and tissue matrix recovery.

In another paper, the effect of high-intensity mm waves on biological activity of soluble factors in the plasma of exposed rats was reported (Sypniewska et al., 2010). Rats were exposed to 35 GHz at 75 mW/cm^2 until core temperature reached 41.0°C. NR8383 rat microphages were incubated with 10% plasma of exposed rats. Plasma from exposed rats increased the expression of 11 proteins and level of 3-nitrotyrosine, a marker of macrophage stimulation, in seven proteins. The altered proteins are associated with inflammation, oxidative stress, and energy metabolism.

Thus, no genotoxic effect was found in cells exposed to mm waves at intensities up to 75 mW/cm^2. Most studies show the absence of the effects of mm waves on gene expression at exposure intensities $\leq$20 mW/cm^2. Changes in gene expression occur at much higher exposure intensities causing significant temperature elevations in skin.

6.1.6.3 Effects on Cellular Proliferation

The antitumor effects of mm waves are studied using animal models and in experiments on a cellular level *in vitro*.

The murine experimental model of B16 F10 melanoma was used to evaluate the ability of mm waves to influence tumor growth (Radzievsky et al., 2004a). The nasal area of mice was exposed to 61.22 GHz with the average incident PD of 13.3 mW/cm^2 for 15 min a day during 5 consecutive days. The temperature elevation at the tip of the nose was 1.05°C. The mm wave treatment induced suppression of the subcutaneous tumor growth. Moreover, endogenous opioids were involved in this effect.

One of the major side effects of cyclophosphamide (CPA), a commonly used anti-cancer drug, is that it can enhance tumor metastasis due to suppression of natural killer (NK) cell activity. Logani et al. (2006) studied the ability of mm waves to inhibit tumor metastasis enhanced by CPA. Tumor metastasis was evaluated in mice that were injected through a tail vein with melanoma cells. Animals were exposed at the nasal area to 42.2 GHz with an incident PD of 36.5 mW/cm^2 and SAR = 730 W/kg for a 30-min exposure that caused a maximum temperature rise of 1.5°C. CPA caused a marked enhancement of tumor colonies in lungs, which was significantly reduced when CPA-treated animals were irradiated with mm waves. Millimeter wave exposure increased NK cell activity suppressed by CPA, suggesting that a reduction in tumor metastasis by mm waves is mediated through activation of NK cells.

Antiproliferative effect of low-intensity mm waves on a cellular level *in vitro* was described by a group of authors with Beneduci (Chidichimo et al., 2002; Beneduci et al., 2005a,b; 2007; Beneduci, 2009). Using a noise generator in the frequency range of 53.57–78.33 GHz or monochromatic frequencies in the range of 52–78 GHz with output powers of generator less than 1 mW, the authors were able to observe the effective inhibition of melanoma cell growth. Similar results were obtained under the same exposure conditions in a study of the antiproliferative effect of mm waves on human erythromyeloid leukemia cells in culture (Beneduci et al., 2007). The power densities used in these experiments were too low to cause a thermal effect. The proposed explanation of the possible mechanisms of mm wave action underlying the antiproliferative effect is yet to be proved.

Li et al. (2012, 2014) reported on the different effects of mm waves on chondrocyte proliferation. Chondrocytes produce and maintain the cartilaginous matrix, which protects the ends of long bones at the joints. Chondrocytes were isolated from the rat knee. The second generation of chondrocytes was exposed to mm waves (7.0–10.0 mm) from the top of the Petri dish at an intensity of 4 mW/cm². Millimeter wave irradiation caused progression of the cell cycle of chondrocytes *in vitro* thus promoting chondrocyte proliferation. The actual intensity of mm waves at the cell layer located on the bottom of the Petri dish is much lower than the incident PD due to the strong absorption of mm waves by the liquid medium. However, a thermal mechanism of the mm wave action is not ruled out due to convective stirring of bulk culture medium above the heated medium on the surface.

Escherichia coli bacterial cell viability and metabolic activity was used to evaluate the mm wave effect on cell proliferation (Cohen et al., 2010). Cell suspension was exposed to 99 GHz at 0.2 mW/cm². One-hour exposure produced no effect on *E. coli* viability and colony characteristics. Exposure for 19 h caused a slight proliferation but did not influence the metabolic activity of cells. The authors concluded that the slight proliferation (fivefold) following 19 h exposure was not biologically significant.

Thus, mm wave irradiation of cell cultures and in animals has an anticancer effect. However, the proliferative effect of mm waves on other cells is controversial in spite of the comparable exposure intensities. The indirect effect of mm waves in animals seems to be mediated through the nervous system and subsequently involving secretion of endogenous opioids.

6.1.6.4 Resonance Effects

Knowing the temperature responses of biological objects, the thermal effects of mm waves are well predictable. Therefore, investigation of mm wave specific effects (not related to heating) requires exposures with intensities that would be incapable of significant temperature elevation. Consequently, many if not most publications available in peer reviewed literature sources are devoted to the study of mm wave effects at low intensities ≤10 mW/cm².

Some early studies had discovered sharp resonance-like frequency-dependent effects (Gründler et al., 1977, 1992; Gründler and Keilmann, 1983, 1989; Belyaev et al., 1994, 1996; Gapeev et al., 1996). Gründler and coauthors found that the growth rate of the yeast *Saccharomyces cerevisiae* was strongly dependent on exposure frequency in the very narrow range 41.8–42.0 GHz. The effect of about the same magnitude was observed in the wide range of exposure intensities from 5 pW/cm^2 to 10 mW/cm^2. However, careful attempts to reproduce these results by other authors were not successful (Furia et al., 1986; Gos et al., 1997).

Belyaev et al. (1993a,b, 1994, 1996) reported that mm wave exposure at intensities as low as 10^{-19} W/cm^2 produced the frequency-dependent changes in the genome conformational state of *E. coli* cells with resonance peaks at 51.76 and 41.34 GHz. The dependence of resonance frequencies on the length of haploid genome allowed authors to suggest the involvement of the chromosomal DNA in the resonance interaction of mm waves with cells. These results were obtained using an anomalous viscosity time-dependent technique. However, this method is not common for this type of study and its interpretation is questionable (Pakhomov et al., 1998).

Gapeyev et al. (1996) found the frequency-dependent inhibition of the production of oxygen active forms by neutrophils opsonized by zymozan. This effect was observed only in the near field of an antenna in the narrow frequency range 41.5–42.7 GHz at 2.5 mW/cm^2. Exposure in the far field of the antenna resulted in elimination of the frequency dependence of the effect. This result indicates that the frequency-dependent effect may be caused by the "geometrical" resonances appearing in the near field of the antenna (Betsky, 1993; Khizhnyak and Ziskin, 1994).

It should be noted that the resonance frequencies mentioned in the above studies lay in the same frequency range of 41–43 GHz. The interest to the possible resonance effects of mm waves has remained a constant subject of debates (Shneider and Pekker, 2013, 2014). However, independent thorough replications of the above claimed resonance effects are necessary before the resonance mechanism can be accepted as a biological action of mm waves.

However, there has been a recent finding of an interesting resonant effect. Feldman et al. (2008) have proposed that sweat ducts in Human skin act as helical antennas in the mm and submillimeter wave range. Within the 95–110 GHz frequency range, there is an enhanced absorption due to a resonance with the sweat ducts twisted into a helical coil and filled with sweat, a high water containing fluid. This enhanced absorption could lead to a highly localized temperature increase that would rapidly diffuse. Any bioeffect resulting from this effect would be from the temperature elevation if the incident intensities were sufficiently great.

6.1.6.5 Cellular Effects

Keratinocytes are the most numerous cells of the epidermis. The effect of mm waves on human keratinocytes was studied in experiments *in vitro* at exposures to 61.22 and 42.25 GHz with intensities 29 mW/cm^2 (SAR = 770 W/kg) and 1.67 W/cm^2, respectively (Szabo et al., 2003). The viability of keratinocytes, the productions of heat shock protein (Hsp70) and chemokines, including RANTES and IP-10, were analyzed. In addition, the intercellular gap junctional communication in keratinocyte monolayers was investigated. At low-intensity exposure (29 mW/cm^2) no significant changes in keratinocyte viability and in constitutive RANTES and inducible IP-10 production were found. No alterations in Hsp70 production and the gap junctional intercellular communication were observed. Exposure at intensity of 1.67 W/cm^2 induced cellular damage and heat stress reaction. The maximal temperature at the end of 30-min exposure reached 45.2°C. The authors stressed that exposure at low intensity (29 mW/cm^2) provided no evidence of skin inflammation or keratinocyte damage.

The same authors studied the effect of mm wave exposure to 61.22 GHz with SAR of 770 W/kg on proliferation, adhesion, chemotaxis, and interleukin-1beta (IL-1beta) production in human keratinocytes (Szabo et al., 2001). Exposure duration was 15–30 min. Exposure did not produce any effect on spontaneous proliferation, adhesion, chemotaxis except for a modest, but statistically significant increase in the intracellular level of IL-1beta. It seems that mm waves can cause activation of basal keratinocytes resulting in an elevated level of IL-1beta production.

The absence of the effect of mm wave exposures to 30.16 GHz with intensities of 1.0 and 3.5 mW/cm^2 on gap junction intercellular communication in human keratinocytes was confirmed by Chen et al. (2004).

The effect of 94 GHz exposure on skeletal muscle contraction was studied by Chatterjee et al. (2013). Electric field magnitude in excess of 2.6 kV/m was able to cause a reproducible decrease in force production of skeletal muscle in the absence of measurable changes in temperature. The authors measured temperature only in the fluid forcibly circulated around the excised muscle. As calculated by Wu et al. (2015), the electric field in excess of 2.6 kV/m would result in an SARρ level in muscle well in excess of 1000 kW/m^3, which would definitely result in muscle heating.

A new mechanism of mm wave action on cellular level was discovered by Szabo et al. (2006). Exposure of the human keratinocytes and murine melanoma cells to 42.25 GHz at the incident PD of 1.23 W/cm^2 induced reversible externalization of phosphatidylserine (PS) molecules without detectable membrane damage. The negatively charged PS molecules are normally localized within the internal leaflets of the phospholipid bilayer of plasma membranes in live cells. Their surface expression, that is, rotation of the negatively charged pole of the PS molecule from the inner surface of the cell membrane to the outer surface is called externalization. The externally exposed portion of the molecule apparently possesses active sites upon which ligands and other molecules can attach and activate biological processes. Externalization is an early event of programmed cell death allowing recognition of apoptotic cells by phagocytes (Fadok et al., 1992; Martin et al., 1995). Jurkat cells exposed to much lower intensity of 34.5 mW/cm^2 also showed reversible PS externalization. The authors could not exclude the effect of enhanced convection in liquid medium produced by local heating of sample by 3.5°C as the possible mechanism of mm wave action. The involvement of nonthermal mechanisms in the effect cannot be ruled out either, but there is not enough data to develop a specific model.

Thus, low-intensity mm wave exposure did not reveal changes in functioning of cellular systems. The effects induced by high-power irradiation had most probably a thermal origin. The data on PS externalization show a new potential of mm wave action on cellular membranes and needs further verification in independent studies.

6.1.7 Millimeter Wave Effects on Excitable Tissues

A great number of early studies, mostly in the former Soviet Union, were carried out exploring the effects of low-intensity (≤10 mW/cm^2) mm waves on conduction of the compound action potential (CAP) in isolated nerves. Several positive effects were reported in the literature (Pakhomov et al., 1998). Pakhomov et al. (1997) investigated the effects of mm waves (CW, 40–52 GHz, 0.24–3.0 mW/cm^2) on the CAP conduction in an isolated frog sciatic nerve preparation, and found none of the reported positive effects on CAP conduction. The low-rate electrical stimulation of the nerve mm wave exposure for 10–60 min at 0.24–1.5 mW/cm^2, either at various constant frequencies or with a stepwise frequency change (0.1 or 0.01 GHz/min), did not cause any detectable changes in CAP conduction or nerve refractoriness. The changes in CAP observed at higher intensities of 2–3 mW/cm^2 were both qualitatively and quantitatively similar to the effect of conventional heating

causing a temperature rise of 0.3°C–0.4°C. At high rate stimulation of the nerve, the gradual and reversible decrease of amplitude of the test CAPs was retained when the nerve was
exposed to 41.22 and 50.91 GHz. The effect was dependent on the frequency rather than on
the intensity of the irradiation.

The effect of 94 GHz exposure on the assembly/disassembly of neuronal microtubules
in Xenopus spinal cord neurons was studied by Samsonov and Popov (2013). The microtubule array is regulated by a large number of signaling cascades, and may provide information about the biochemical status of neuronal cytoplasm. An exposure at 1.86 W/cm²
increased the rate of microtubule assembly. This effect resulted entirely from the rapid
temperature jump by 8°C induced by the mm wave exposure.

Modulation of calcium oscillations by mm wave irradiation in the mouse embryonic
stem cell-derived neuronal cells was reported by Titushkin et al. (2009). It is evident that
the calcium spiking amplitude, frequency, and spatial distribution are important characteristics of cellular regulatory pathways. Fibroblast cell cultures were exposed to 94 GHz
at 1.86 W/cm² to study the effect of mm wave exposure on actin filament organization
(Titushkin et al., 2009). Millimeter wave irradiation significantly increased the calcium
spiking frequency. The N-type calcium channels, phospholipase C, and actin cytoskeleton appear to be involved in mediating increased calcium spiking. Reorganization of the
actin microfilaments by a 94-GHz field seems to play a crucial role in modulating not only
calcium activity but also cell biomechanics (decrease of cell elasticity). Millimeter wave
exposure for 30 min caused some damage to the actin structure. Many but not all observed
cellular responses to mm wave exposure were similar to thermally induced effects.

Alekseev et al. (1997) presented the results of a study of mm wave effects on the firing
rate of intact pacemaker neurons in the isolated nerve ring of the snail *Lymnaea stagnalis*.
The neurons were exposed to mm waves at a frequency of 75 GHz, and an SAR ranging
from 600 to 4200 W/kg, causing temperature rises of 0.3°C and 2.2°C, respectively. At an
SAR = 4200 W/kg, exposure to mm waves produced biphasic changes in the firing rate,
i.e., a transient decrease in the firing rate within the first 10 s of exposure by 69% below
control, followed by a gradual increase with the time constant of 3.7 min to a new level
exceeding the initial firing rate by 68%. The biphasic changes in the firing rate were reproduced by heating under the condition that the magnitude and the rate of temperature rise
were equal to those produced by the irradiation. It was shown that the transient response
resulted from the hyperpolarization of the neural membrane due to the thermal activation
of the sodium pump. The slow increase in the firing rate was due to the depolarization
of the membrane caused by its elevated permeability to sodium and potassium ions. The
threshold stimulus for a transient response of a neuron found in warming experiments
was a temperature rise rate of 0.0025°C /s. The firing rate changes occurred at temperature
elevations as small as 0.3°C. The phase of transient decrease of the firing rate could be
singled out by varying the exposure pulse duration (Alekseev et al., 2000). Typically, the
decrease in the firing rate occurs when the temperature is decreased. It is not clear what
are the physiological consequences resulting from the transient response of neurons.

Shapiro et al. (2013) showed that 60 GHz mm wave stimulation significantly increased
the action potential firing rate in oocytes coexpressing voltage-gated sodium and potassium channels. The time course of change in the spiking interval upon application of mm
waves paralleled that of the temperature rise. The bulk temperature increases, similar to
those achieved with mm wave exposure, also resulted in a similar acceleration in firing
rate indicating a thermal nature of the mm wave effect. In addition, authors investigated
the response of the sodium-potassium pump to mm wave exposure in oocytes. Upon
application of a 100 s mm wave pulse (64 mW), producing a temperature elevation of about

6°C, the pump current increased by 53% within the first 10s of exposure. The changes in the kinetics and activity level of a sodium-potassium pump were consistent with a thermal mechanism.

Two studies were performed to explore the mm wave effects on electrical activity of organotypic cortical slices (Pikov et al., 2010) and individual neurons of leech ganglia (Romanenko et al., 2014). Pikov et al. (2010) exposed the slices of cortical tissue located in the bottom of the exposure chamber from the top of the bath solution to 60.1 GHz at the highest incident PD of 90 mW/cm². Less than 1 μW/cm² reached the slice level located at 2.2 mm below the solution surface. One-minute exposure caused the reduction of the firing rate, narrowing of the width of the action potential, and decrease of the membrane resistance. These effects were accompanied by mm wave heating of the bath solution by 3°C. The authors compared these changes with the effects of conventional bath heating by 10°C and found that mm wave-induced effects cannot be fully attributed to heating and may involve specific mm wave interaction with tissue. It should be noted that in modeling mm wave heating it is necessary to reproduce not only the magnitude of the temperature rise, but also the temperature rise rate, which plays a significant role in neural responses.

In another study, Romanenko et al. (2014) investigated the effects of 1-min exposures to 60 GHz at the incident power densities of 1, 2, and 4 mW/cm² on the action potential of neurons of the leech ganglia. The firing rate of neurons was slightly suppressed during mm wave exposure while gradual bath heating caused a linear dose-dependent increase in the firing rate. Millimeter wave exposure produced narrowing of the action potentials, which was five times greater at 4 mW/cm² than at equivalent bath heating by 0.6°C. Qualitatively, the changes in the firing rate of leech neurons produced by mm wave exposure were similar to those of snail neurons (Alekseev et al., 1997), i.e., rapid mm wave heating induces a transient decrease of the firing rate followed by a slower increase in the firing rate at longer exposure. The ganglion was exposed from the bottom of a chamber. The exposure beam passed through the polystyrene bottom of a Petri dish 1 mm thick and a paraffin layer 3.2 mm thick before reaching the ganglion. During exposure with the incident PD of 53–212 mW/cm², the bottom of the Petri dish was definitely heated. Due to the high thermal conductivity of paraffin (0.26 W/(m · °C)) the heat could pass from the polystyrene to the ganglion causing heating of the ganglion in addition to the direct effect of mm waves. Therefore, it would be worthwhile to reproduce the study with adequate temperature control.

Most studies showed the changes in the electrical activity and structure of the excitable cells induced by a thermal effect of mm waves. It was shown that the rate of heating plays a significant role in eliciting the electrical response of nerve cells. Some specific effects are apparently not due to a thermal action of mm waves, and require further investigation.

6.1.8 Involvement of Nervous System in Millimeter Wave Effects

Millimeter waves are widely used in Russia, China, and many Eastern European countries for the treatment of more than 30 diseases, including peptic ulcers, pain relief, cardiovascular diseases, and skin disorders (Rojavin and Ziskin, 1998). Positive results were obtained at exposure to very low intensities (usually less than 1 mW/cm²). However, most findings made by scientists in these countries have not been replicated in the West. The systematic comprehensive investigation of hypoalgesic effects of mm waves on humans and animals was carried out in Temple University in the USA.

To evaluate the pain relief effect of mm waves in humans, double-blinded, randomized, crossover, prospective experiments were conducted using cold pressor test as a model of tonic aching pain (Radzievsky et al., 1999). Twelve volunteers participated in the study. They were exposed to 42.25 GHz at the incident PD of 25 mW/cm^2 for 30 min. Millimeter wave exposure produced a significant suppression of pain sensation with an average 37.7% gain in pain tolerance.

The hypoalgesic effect of mm waves on the experimentally induced cold pain in 20 healthy volunteers was studied in a double-blinded crossover investigation by another group of researchers (Partyla et al., 2017). Volunteers were exposed to 42.25 GHz at the intensity of 17.2 mW/cm^2. The hypoalgesic effect of mm waves resulted in a 23%–25% delay in the onset of cold sensation, pain threshold, and beginning of increasing pain compared with baseline condition. However, onsets in the placebo condition did not differ significantly from the exposure condition, only partially confirming the hypoalgesic effect of mm waves. Positive results were obtained in the treatment of chronic pain with mm wave therapy in patients with diffuse connective tissue diseases at the intensities of 2.5 mW/cm^2 (Usichenko and Herget, 2003). It is obvious that appropriate experimental investigations are required using large samples and improved methods of pain stimulation and data acquisition to better evaluate the hypoalgesic effects of mm waves in humans.

The first experiment involving the nervous system in animals revealed that mm wave exposure was able to extend the duration of anesthesia caused by ketamine and chloral hydrate in mice (Rojavin and Ziskin, 1997). In these experiments, mice were exposed to 61.22 GHz at the incident PD of 15 mW/cm^2. Using the cold-water tail-flick test (experimental model of chronic non-neuropathic pain), it was found that the effect was pronounced and comparable to that of 1 mg/kg of morphine (Rojavin et al., 2000). The authors showed that the hypoalgesic effect on mice was proportional to the incident PD. The effect reached the level of about 200% relative to the control, and disappeared after reducing the incident PD to 0.5 mW/cm^2. Radzievsky et al. (2000) compared the hypoalgesic effect of 61.22 GHz mm waves at 15 mW/cm^2 in different sites on the murine body with different innervation densities. They found that the maximal hypoalgesic effect was obtained where the innervation density was the greatest: the nose and paw areas.

The possible involvement of the sciatic nerve in the hypoalgesic effect of mm waves was studied in experiments with the transected nerve (Radzievsky et al., 2001). The murine paw was exposed to 61.22 GHz with the average incident PD of 15 mW/cm^2. Dissection of the nerve resulted in a full loss of the hypoalgesic effect of mm waves. This result directly indicated the involvement of the peripheral nervous system in mm wave-induced hypoalgesia. The pretreatment of mice with naloxone, a nonselective antagonist of opioid receptors, also fully blocked the hypoalgesic effect of mm waves (Rojavin et al., 2000). This result indicated that the antinociceptive effect of mm waves was mediated through endogenous opioids. Moreover, the involvement of δ and κ endogenous opioids in the mm wave-induced hypoalgesia was demonstrated using selective blockers of δ- and κ-opioid receptors and the direct ELISA measurement of endogenous opioids in central nervous system (CNS) tissue (Radzievsky et al., 2008). Thus, a number of endogenous opioids seem to play an important role in the systemic effect of mm waves involving the CNS.

Using an experimental model of chronic non-neuropathic pain, Radzievsky et al. (2008) studied the frequency dependence of the hypoalgesic effect of mm waves. The maximal effect was achieved with exposure of the nasal area of mice with 61.22 GHz mm waves. An equivalent local heating of the same area with a laser did not produce a systemic hypoalgesia (Radzievsky et al., 2004b). Based on these results, the authors concluded that the hypoalgesic effect had a nonthermal nature. However, the initial mechanisms underlying this effect remain unclear. It is suggested that mm waves could stimulate the skin sensory receptors.

Alekseev et al. (2010) studied the mm wave effect on the electrical activity of the sural nerve of mice *in vivo*. The sural nerve innervates the lateral side of the foot along the border between the hairy and glabrous skin. Electrical recordings were made in the nerve region located on the dorsal aspect of the lower leg. Millimeter wave exposure at 42.25 GHz was applied to the receptive field of the sural nerve in the hind paw. Exposure at the peak incident PD of a Gaussian beam ≥45 mW/cm^2 inhibited the spontaneous electrical activity of the nerve. The radiant heat exposure reproduced the inhibitory effect of mm wave exposure indicating the thermal mechanism of the mm wave action. It was shown that the cold sensitive fibers were responsible for the inhibitory effect of mm wave and radiant heat exposures. In addition, the nerve responded to the cessation of mm wave exposure with a transient increase of the firing rate. The threshold peak intensity for this effect was 160 mW/cm^2. The radiant heat exposure did not reproduce this effect. The receptors and mechanisms involved in inducing the transient response to mm wave exposure are not clear. The authors suggested that mast cells were involved in this effect. It should be noted that in this study, the authors selectively tested only one sciatic nerve branch. In order to determine if other skin sensory receptors are affected by mm waves, it is necessary to conduct experiments in which all the branches of the sciatic nerve are involved.

Most studies of the hypoalgesic effect of mm waves were performed at exposure to 61.22 GHz in the near field of antennas at the average incident PD of 13–15 mW/cm^2. Mice were exposed using a horn antenna. The exposure beam had a Gaussian-type distribution and was confined within the antenna aperture with a peak PD of 56 mW/cm^2 (Radzievsky et al., 2004b). The threshold intensity for the inhibitory effect of mm waves (45 mW/cm^2) on cold receptors is within the peak intensities necessary for inducing the hypoalgesic effect. Hence, the cold receptors might be involved directly or indirectly in pain relief produced by mm waves.

Investigations of the reactions of the nervous systems of humans and animals to peripheral mm wave exposure were conducted in double-blind experiments by a number of authors (Lebedeva, 1993, 1997; Lebedeva and Kotrovskaya, 1996; Novikova et al., 2002, 2008a,b; Shanin et al., 2005).

A group of scientists led by Korneva studied the potential of mm waves to stimulate the cutaneous nerve endings of rats using a c-fos immunoreactivity method (Novikova et al., 2002). This method is based on the response of various hypothalamic structures to external stimulation by increased c-fos gene expression, an accepted marker of the activated neurons. Exposure of different parts of the rat body to 42.2 GHz at an output power of 20 mW resulted in activation of hypothalamic neurons. The electrical pain stimulation (EPS) and noxious mechanical stimulation (NMS) increased c-fos gene expression while combined exposure to EPS and mm waves or NMS and mm waves decreased the number of activated neurons (Novikova et al., 2002, 2008a). Millimeter wave irradiation produced a modifying effect consisting of a reduction in the degree of activation of hypothalamic cells evoked by pain stimulations. Moreover, the painful electrical stimulation of the hind limbs of rats caused a reorganization of the central mechanisms that regulate splenic NK cell activity, resulting in a decrease of their cytotoxicity. Millimeter wave exposure protected NK cell activity from the impairment induced by EPS (Shanin et al., 2005). The publications listed above do not provide an adequate assessment of the exposure intensity. However, exposure in the near field of a horn antenna with an output power of 20 mW might be able for the mm waves to thermally activate neurons.

In a study of the mm wave effects on the human nervous system, the sensory reactions of humans were investigated using methods of sensory indications and electroencephalography (Lebedeva, 1993; Lebedeva and Kotrovskaya, 1996). In these experiments, the hands of volunteers were exposed to 37.7, 42.25, and 53.57 GHz at the incident power densities of 5 and 10.5 mW/cm^2. Humans were able to recognize the mm wave stimulation. The predominant modalities of sensations were the pressure, pricking, and thermal reactions. The authors suggested that mm wave action as a stimulus is conveyed through nonspecific excitation pathways. It was speculated that mm-wave perception could involve some types of mechanoreceptors and nociceptors.

Thus, mm waves produce systemic effects on humans and animals. Based on the known biological effects of mm waves, the chain of events initiated by skin exposure to mm waves can be subdivided into four major steps: the initiation phase, the transmission of the signal to the CNS, modulation of the CNS function, and the systemic response (Radzievsky et al., 2008).

6.1.9 Millimeter Wave Effect on Immune System

It has been shown that mm wave irradiation enhances the immune response of organisms (Kabisov, 2000; Pletnev, 2000; Logani et al., 2011). T cells have an impact on practically all aspects of immunity due to their ability to induce specific immune responses. T cells play an important role in the restoration process. Makar et al. (2003, 2006) studied the effects of mm waves on T-cell recovery after suppression by CPA, T-cell activation, proliferation, and effector functions in mice. CPA is an anticancer drug that prevents cell division by cross-linking DNA leading to the reduction of tumor growth (Goodman, 2000; Allison, 2000). Mice were exposed at the nasal area to 42.2 or 61.22 GHz at the peak incident PD of 31.5 mW/cm^2 resulting in temperature elevation of 1.8°C during a 30 min exposure. These studies showed that mm waves can restore production of Interferon gamma and proliferation of T cells suppressed by CPA treatment. No significant changes were observed in the level of IL-10 and proliferation of B cells. These results suggest that mm waves accelerate the recovery process selectively through a T-cell-mediated immune response.

The same group of authors investigated the effect of mm waves on the NK cell activity suppressed by CPA (Makar et al., 2005). NK cells are known to kill a wide variety of tumor cells while sparing normal cells. In these experiments, the authors used the same exposure conditions as described above. Millimeter wave exposure of CPA-treated mice resulted in restoration of CPA-induced suppression of the cytolytic activity of NK cells. It was further demonstrated that mm wave exposure significantly augmented the tumor necrosis factor (TNF-α) production by NK cells suppressed by CPA administration.

Similar results were reported by Novoselova et al. (2002) who studied the effect of mm waves on the immune system of mice with experimental tumors. The whole-body mm wave irradiation (40 GHz, 0.5 μW/cm^2) caused a significant increase in the production of TNF-α, nitric oxide, and NK cell activity at the early stage of tumor development.

Millimeter wave irradiation was able to restore splenic NK cell activity suppressed by painful stimulation of the hind limbs in rats (Shanin et al., 2005). As shown in experiments with neutrophils, the primed rather than intact neutrophils of mice were susceptible to exposure to 41.95 GHz at SAR = 0.45 W/kg (Safronova et al., 2002).

The anti-inflammatory effects of mm waves were studied in mice exposed to 42.2–42.6, 43.0, and 61.22 GHz at intensities of 0.1–0.7 mW/cm^2 (Gapeyev et al., 2008, 2009). Authors used a model of acute zymozan-induced paw edema. A single whole-body exposure of animals to continuous mm waves reduced the exudative edema of inflamed paws by 19%. The anti-inflammatory effects were dependent on both the exposure frequency and modulation frequency.

In the most studies, mm wave effects on immune system were obtained at the thermal intensities of exposure (>10 mW/cm^2). It was suggested that this systemic effect is initiated by stimulation of free nerve endings in the skin (Radzievsky et al., 2008; Alekseev et al., 2010). Then, the signal is conveyed to the CNS where it modulates neural activity resulting in the release of endogenous opioids and development of various biological effects (Logani et al., 2011).

6.1.10 Physiologic Effects of High-Power mm Waves

High intensity mm wave exposure causes overheating of skin and may induce structural protein damage, cell death, stress reactions, acute inflammatory responses, and circulatory dysfunctions.

Human sensory reception (warmth and pain sensations) of high power mm waves was reported in a number of papers. Blick et al. (1997) and Riu et al. (1997) studied the warmth-detection thresholds in human subjects. The pricking pain thresholds in volunteers were investigated by Walters et al. (2000). The cutaneous thresholds for thermal pain was measured during 3 s exposures of each subject's back to 94 GHz at intensities up to 1.8 W/cm^2. The threshold for pricking pain was found to be 43.9°C. The PD required to evoke a threshold sensation of pain was 1.25 W/cm^2 for a 3 s exposure. The results of modeling using a simple thermal model that accounted for heat conduction and penetration depth of mm waves were in good agreement with experimental measurements.

The physiologic effects of whole body exposure of animals to 35 and 94 GHz have been reported (Frei et al., 1995; Ryan et al., 1996, 1997, 2002; Millenbaugh et al., 2006, 2008; Jauchem et al., 2016). The sustained overexposure of rats (~80 min) with intensities of 75 or 90 mW/cm^2 produced significant skin (>46°C) and core heating and subsequent circulatory failure. During irradiation the heart rate increased, mean arterial pressure maintained until skin temperature reached 42°C, at which point mean arterial pressure declined until death. Death occurred at core temperature of 40°C and skin temperature of 48°C. Hypotension was accompanied by vasodilatation in the mesenteric vascular bed. The lethal effect became irreversible when the mean arterial pressure fell to 75 mm Hg even if exposure was ceased. Irradiation induced thermal injury to skin tissue that involved protein damage, oxidative stress, inflammation, immune cell response, and induction of repair processes involving extracellular matrix change. The common mediators involved in several forms of shock such as nitric oxide, platelet-activating factor, and histamine did not play a role in mm wave-induced circulatory collapse. The results indicated that body core heating was the major determinant of induction of circulatory failure. The influence of mm wave heating of the skin and subcutaneous tissues became significant only when a certain threshold rate of heating of these tissues was exceeded. The obtained data suggested that mm waves induced the same thermoregulatory responses as environmental heating.

Xie et al. (2011) evaluated stress reactions in rats exposed to 35 GHz at the average incident power densities ranging from 0.5 to 7.5 W/cm^2. Rats were exposed locally to the back area with an exposure area of 1.8 or 3.6 cm^2. Stress reactions were quantitatively estimated from electroencephalogram (EEG) analysis. The data showed that stress reactions are more intense during the first part of the irradiation than during the later part. The skin temperature elevation produced by mm wave exposure was the main factor responsible for the stress reactions and skin injures.

The direct effect of mm wave exposure on cutaneous melanoma in mice was described in the paper by Szabo et al. (2004). In this case, mm waves were used as the source of hyperthermia. In *in vitro* experiments, keratinocyte and melanoma cell monolayers were exposed from the bottom of a well to 42.25 GHz at an incident PD ranging from 0.78 to 1.48 W/cm^2 producing a maximum temperature rise up to 53°C. Melanoma cells revealed higher susceptibility to hyperthermia than keratinocytes. *In vivo* exposure of cutaneous melanoma at the PD of 1.25 W/cm² for 30 min resulted in a selective tumor destruction without tissue damage of normal skin. Since the penetration depth of mm waves varies with frequency, selective therapeutic heating of tumors at different depths in the body can be performed by choosing an appropriate frequency for the exposure and enforcing air convection near skin surface (Zhadobov et al., 2015).

6.1.11 Mechanisms of mm Wave Action

Many mm wave effects reported in the literature cannot be readily explained solely by the temperature elevation in irradiated objects. Up to now, the mechanisms underlying the nonthermal effects of mm waves are not clear. The resonance theory can be regarded as one of the well-developed hypothesis that is true could be specific for mm waves. As shown by Adair (2003) in his theoretical analysis, the excitation of resonance vibrational modes in molecules is quite feasible due to coupling of the electromagnetic field to their dipoles. However, such mm wave excitable resonances are expected to be strongly damped by energy interchange with other vibrational modes of molecule and of molecules in the surrounding solution. This process cannot allow accumulating enough energy to change the properties of molecules.

Frölich (1968, 1970, 1972, 1978) has suggested another approach to explaining the resonance-type frequency dependence of mm wave effects. His theoretical studies of phase correlations in condensed media show that many dipole moments in a lipid membrane can oscillate coherently. The resonance frequencies of these vibrations depend on the mechanical and structural properties of membranes. They are predicted to lie in the range of 50–150 GHz. It is assumed that vibrations in lipid membranes at resonance frequencies can produce changes in the physical and chemical properties of these membranes resulting in a biological effect. In such a system, the coupling of electromagnetic field greatly increases. However, the increased viscous damping suppresses the resonance effect (Adair, 2003).

For explaining the experimental results, some researchers suggested different nonthermal mechanisms of mm wave action. Beneduci et al. (2013, 2014) studied the effect of mm waves at temperatures close to the phase transition temperature of a membrane using a ²H-NMR spectroscopy. The authors interpreted the decrease of the heavy water quadrupole splitting produced by mm wave exposure by membrane dehydration due to coupling of the mm waves with the fast rotational dynamics of bound water molecules. However, it is not clear how mm waves can interact with bound water or charged phospholipid headgroups, which do not relax in the mm wave range (Klösgen et al., 1996).

Kotnik and Miklavčič (2000) evaluated theoretically the ability of cell membranes to absorb electromagnetic radiation in a wide frequency range. They found that local increase of power dissipation in membranes occurred in the MHz and lower GHz regions. At frequencies above 20 GHz, the power dissipation decreased. The overheating of membranes is excluded due to the effective heat dissipation from thin membranes to the surrounding medium. The authors suggested that high-power dissipation could lead to structural changes in membrane proteins and the lipid matrix. However, the electric field induced in a membrane is too small in comparison with the internal static electric field of the membrane (about 10^5 V/cm) to produce a significant membrane effect.

Deformation of giant phospholipid vesicles reported by Ramundo-Orlando et al. (2009) could be produced by the effect of electrostrictive forces on liposomes arising during mm wave irradiation. Adair (2003) evaluated the magnitude of the electrostrictive forces acting on cells. The electrostrictive pressure is proportional to the permittivity difference between the medium and the cell and to the electric field squared. The calculated electrostrictive pressure at an intensity of 10 mW/cm^2 is about 2×10^{-7} N/m^2, which is much less than the pressure from incident sunlight. Therefore, it is questionable that the electrostrictive pressure at low intensities of mm wave exposure could change the liposome shape.

The multilayer organization of skin might result in a resonance-type absorption of mm waves. As mentioned previously, Feldman et al. (2008) found an enhanced resonance absorption and reflection in the 95–110 GHz range, which was attributed to the coiled sweat ducts in skin acting as helical array antennas to mm waves. However, Alekseev et al. (2008) did not find any sharp resonance-type frequency dependence for either reflection from the human skin measured experimentally, or in the PD and SAR distributions within the skin layers calculated theoretically for frequencies up to 90 GHz. This can be explained by the small difference in permittivity of different human skin layers in this mm wave range.

The thermal effect of mm waves has two distinct features. Millimeter waves cause the temperature elevation in a relatively small volume of exposed matter. Due to the small volume, the rate of heating is high. The fast heating activates the sodium pump of neurons, which induces a fast trans-membrane current and hyperpolarizes the cell membrane inducing a transient decrease in the firing rate (Alekseev et al., 1997). The hyperpolarizing voltage is proportional to the membrane resistance (Carpenter et al., 1968; Carpenter, 1973). In neurons with higher resistance, the greater hyperpolarizing voltage and, hence, a greater transient response is expected. The depolarization of the membrane due to passive ion transport is a relatively slow process resulting in biphasic changes of the firing rate. The results obtained by Alekseev et al. (1997) allow one to draw an important conclusion: to reproduce the thermal effect of mm waves, especially in experiments involving the heating of nerve cells, it is not enough merely to increase the temperature to the maximum level reached, but it is also necessary to warm up an object with a rate of temperature rise equal to that caused by mm wave exposure. If a biological system is regulated by two different mechanisms having different thermal sensitivities and time constants of their thermal reactions, the fast heating that is typical for mm wave exposure may lead to a complex response of the system to exposure.

6.1.12 Indirect Effects of mm Waves

In experiments *in vitro*, different factors can mimic the mm wave effect on biological objects. When a liquid medium is exposed to a narrow mm wave beam, the energy deposition occurs in a very small volume. The rapid temperature rise in this small volume induces a convection current, which occurs in nearly all *in vitro* mm wave experiments, and although undeservedly attracts little attention, is capable of producing biological effects.

A free-type convection appears in a liquid at the temperature gradient of 0.15×10^{-3} °C/m (Landau and Lifshitz, 1986). When physiological solutions are irradiated by 40–70 GHz mm waves, such a temperature gradient is reached within a few seconds after the start of irradiation at an incident PD as small as 10^{-9} W/cm^2 (Khizhnyak and Ziskin, 1996). The background laminar convection can develop in liquid even without mm wave irradiation due to a nonuniform temperature distribution. For example, this convection may result from a lower temperature at the surface of a liquid due to its evaporation. Convection induced by mm waves in a liquid can affect the cellular functioning mimicking the direct mm wave effect on cells. Sharov et al. (1983) discovered the lipid peroxidation in liposomes produced by mm wave exposure at 46.15 GHz and an intensity of 0.5 mW/cm^2. This effect was caused by an increased concentration of oxygen in the liquid due to convectional stirring of different liquid layers. At high intensities (SAR ≥ 4 kW/kg), exposure of a saline solution in a Petri dish can even induce temperature oscillations (Khizhnyak and Ziskin, 1996). Hence, when interpreting the experimental results obtained *in vitro* studies, it is important to take into account the effect of liquid convection. In experiments, stirring liquid during exposure may minimize this effect. In tissues, where the cells and other tissue components are tightly packed, the conditions for convection of fluid are limited.

Frequency-dependent effects of mm waves can be result from the interaction of the irradiated beam of mm waves in the near field of an antenna with an object such as skin or an exposure chamber in *in vitro* experiments. It has been shown that exposure in the reactive zone of horn antennas produces nonuniform heating patterns in irradiated objects. These nonuniform patterns are due to a "geometrical" resonance resulting from a secondary wave-mode interaction between an irradiated object and the corresponding critical cross section of the horn antenna (Khizhnyak and Ziskin, 1994). The location, quantity, number, and size of the local field absorption maxima in irradiated objects are strongly depended on the specific antenna and the frequency of mm wave irradiation. These features of exposure in the near field of an antenna could provide an explanation for a number of frequency-dependent effects of mm wave irradiation.

In experiments *in vitro*, cells are usually exposed in plastic culture plates or dishes filled with a culture medium. When a plastic well filled with liquid is exposed from the bottom of a well, the PD and SAR distribution depend on the irradiation frequency (Alekseev et al., 2017). In this case, a plastic bottom plays the role of a coupler between an antenna and the culture medium. Figure 6.4 demonstrates the dependence of the power reflection coefficient on frequency, as obtained by Alekseev et al. (2017) and extended to THz frequencies. The position and number of maximums and minimums depend on the permittivity of the plastic and thickness of a well bottom. In studying the frequency-dependent biological effects, the measurement of the incident PD is not enough to characterize the exposure intensity. It is necessary to define the PD reaching the cell layers. The frequency-dependent exposure intensities can be calculated using analytical or numerical methods.

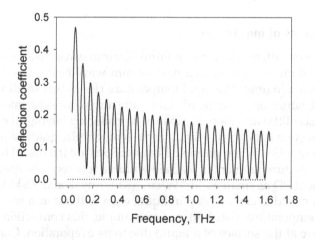

FIGURE 6.4
Frequency dependence of reflection from the polystyrene bottom of a tissue culture well filled with water at 298 K. Permittivity of polystyrene, $\varepsilon^* = 2.56 - j0.003$. Permittivity of water is calculated using the double Debye equation (Equation 6.32) with parameters given by Pickwell et al. (2004a). Dotted line shows the level of zero reflection. The thickness of the polystyrene well bottom is 1.5 mm.

In experiments with mm waves, the temperature measurements can be a challenging problem. The most common devices used for temperature measurements are thermocouples, thermistors, fiber-optic probes, and IR cameras. The IR camera is a useful technique for the measurements of surface temperature. Due to the shallow penetration of mm waves into biological solutions (e.g., 0.34 mm at 58 GHz), the absorbed power is locally concentrated close to the exposed sample surface, inducing a large temperature gradient. This makes it a very difficult task to measure the local temperature in thin cell monolayers, which is an unavoidable step for correct interpretation of experimental biological results. As shown recently, small thermocouples (25 μm in diameter) can be used for accurate temperature measurements (Pakhomov et al., 2000a,b; Zhadobov et al., 2017). On the other hand, fiber-optic probes and thermocouples of greater size (>0.1 mm) are not appropriate for measuring temperature in the thin absorbing layer of a solution because they disturb the temperature distribution in the thin heated area possessing a locally large temperature gradient.

6.1.13 Conclusion

Millimeter waves are entirely absorbed in the epidermis and dermis. Theoretical evaluations of skin heating show that mm wave exposure of skin to 10 mW/cm^2 could increase the skin surface temperature by 1.2°C. Due to effective heat transfer from the superficial regions of skin to deeper tissues, mm wave exposure also results in heating of fat and muscle layers. The fat layer plays the role of an insulator.

The experimental results show that low-intensity (≤10 mW/cm^2) mm wave irradiation does not produce any harmful effect on eyes. However, high-intensity mm wave exposure results in adverse effects on the eye. The ocular damage is induced by the thermal effect of mm waves and depends on the frequency, intensity, and duration of exposure.

Millimeter waves induce a thermal effect on artificial lipid membranes. However, some results obtained in experiments with artificial lipid membranes are inconsistent with a thermal mechanism. The mechanisms underlying these effects are not clear. Furthermore, recent studies do not confirm the nonthermal effects of mm waves on electrical events in cell membranes.

No genotoxic effects were found in cells exposed to mm waves at intensities up to 75 mW/cm^2. Most studies show the absence of the effects of mm waves on gene expression at exposure intensities ≤20 mW/cm^2. Changes in gene expression occur at much higher exposure intensities causing significant temperature elevations in skin.

Millimeter wave irradiation can induce an anticancer effect. However, the data on proliferative effects in different cells is controversial.

Low-intensity mm wave exposure did not reveal changes in functioning of cellular systems. The effects induced by high-power irradiation have most probably been thermal in nature. The data on PS externalization show a new potential of mm wave action on cellular membranes and need further verification in independent studies.

Most studies showed that the changes in electrical activity and structure of excitable cells induced by mm wave irradiation were thermal in origin. The rate of mm wave heating plays a significant role in eliciting the electrical response of nerve cells.

High-power mm wave irradiation of animals produces severe thermal injury to skin tissue, and if the exposed area is sufficiently large, can eventually result in circulatory failure.

Millimeter waves produce systemic effect on humans and animals affecting the immune and nervous systems and involving the endogenous opioids. In most studies, a hypoalgesic effect and an effect on the immune system were obtained at thermal exposure intensities (>10 mW/cm^2). It was suggested that the systemic effect was initiated by stimulation of free nerve endings in the skin. Then the peripheral signal is conveyed to the CNS where it modulates the neural activity resulting in the development of various biological effects.

The possible resonance effect of mm waves has remained a subject of debates. However, independent thorough replications of the claimed resonance effects are required, and more studies are necessary to be conducted to accept the resonance mechanism as a mode of biological action of mm waves.

6.2 Biological Effects of Terahertz Radiation

6.2.1 Introduction

Biological effects of THz radiation have not been studied as extensively as the effects of electromagnetic radiation in microwave and mm wave frequency ranges. This can be explained by the absence of THz sources and detectors available for most researchers for a long time. However, the technology in the THz field has developed rapidly in recent years with its steadily increasing applications in different areas of human activity. Now THz devices are available in many research laboratories. Accordingly, the number of publications on the biological effects of THz radiation has been notably increased during the last 10–15 years (Hintzsche and Stopper, 2012). Nevertheless, it is important that thorough scientific studies of biological effects of THz radiation in the frequency range above 300 GHz be continued.

With increasing use of THz radiation in security scanners, communication, medical applications, and scientific studies, the safety issue becomes very important. The safety limit for the public for the frequency range between 2 and 100 GHz is 1 mW/cm^2 and increases to 10 mW/cm^2 at 300 GHz (IEEE Standard C95.1, 2005). Similar limits are used by ICNIRP and the FDA. These safety standard limits are based on established adverse thermal effects. Safety limits of THz frequencies for the public are 10 mW/cm^2 for whole body exposures and 100 mW/cm^2 for small beams.

The early publications on studies of biological effects at low THz frequencies first appeared in Russian literature over five decades ago. These studies were conducted using specialized backward-wave tube sources. Beginning in 2001, the European countries have been strongly involved in the investigation of biological effects of THz radiation through the large research program "THz-Bridge" (Gallerano, 2004). Among others, the research program is focused on the potential genotoxic effects of THz radiation. To this day, a great number of studies of the effects of THz radiation on molecular and cellular levels, on microorganisms and animals, and mechanisms underlying these effects have been performed. Several comprehensive reviews have been published describing the current state of research on the subject (Fedorov et al., 2003; Siegel, 2004; Wilmink and Grundt, 2011; Hintzsche and Stopper, 2012; Yu et al., 2012; Kirichuk and Ivanov, 2013; Zhao et al., 2014). However, in spite of the great progress in the study of THz biological effects, it is often impossible to draw unequivocal conclusions due to the controversy of the published data.

Besides biological studies, THz radiation is successfully used in time-domain spectroscopy of water and biological molecules (Fischer et al., 2002; Møller et al., 2009). THz time-domain spectroscopy allows measuring the size of the solvation shell around molecules (Arikawa et al., 2008). The THz absorption spectra reflect the low-frequency internal motions or vibrations involving the weakest hydrogen bonds within molecules or between molecules (Globus et al., 2003). The transmitted and reflected THz spectra of materials characterize the vibrational modes and provide information that is not available in other parts of the electromagnetic spectrum.

THz imaging has also been successfully used in medical applications (Woodward et al., 2002; 2003; Humphreys et al., 2004).

In this chapter, the interaction of THz radiation with water and skin, skin heating, and the THz effects on biological objects at different organization as well as the mechanisms underlying these effects are reviewed.

6.2.2 THz Radiation Sources

The most common approach to generate THz frequencies is nonlinear reactive multiplication of lower frequencies from mm wave sources which include the solid-state electronic sources (Gunn diodes, IMPATT devices, tunneling transit time diodes (TUNNETT), and resonant tunneling diodes) and tube sources (BWO, klystrons, carcinotrons). The THz sources using the frequency up-conversion approach are tunable and cover the entire range from 8 GHz to 1000 GHz. These devices provide an output power up to 100 mW at lower frequencies, which drops off between $1/f^2$ and $1/f^3$ with increasing frequency. They operate at room temperature, generate narrow line-width (10^{-6}) CW radiation, and are convenient to use in studies of THz biological effects.

The next most commonly used sources at terahertz frequencies are far-infrared (FIR), electrically-pumped solid state, and quantum cascade lasers. FIR lasers are usually based on grating tuned CO_2 pump lasers injected into a laser cavity with a vacuum envelope container filled with molecular gases (methanol). The high-power CO_2 laser (20–100 W) excites the vibrational levels of gas molecules, which have transition frequencies in the THz spectrum. FIR lasers generate discrete frequencies at output powers up to 100 mW.

Another class of THz sources used in biological experiments is based on electron accelerator devices such as terahertz tubes (BWOs, TWTs, klystrons, and gyrotrons) and free electron lasers (FELs). It is well known that charged particles can radiate electromagnetic (EM) waves only when accelerated. In BWOs, an electron beam is accelerated in the opposite direction to the travelling EM wave. BWOs consist of a strong magnet system (typically 1 T) used to collimate the electronic beam and high-voltage source creating the strong electric field used for accelerating the electronic beam. Typical BWO sources are tunable in the range of 35 GHz to 1.42 THz at output powers up to 100 mW. Orotron-based sources generate radiation in the frequency range of 120–370 GHz with output powers up to 50 mW. They have electronic and mechanical frequency tuning. Other terahertz tubes generate radiation at mW levels.

THz FELs consist of an electron accelerator and a wiggler magnetic array producing undulation of the electron beam. Laboratory FELs can generate tunable THz radiation in the wide range of THz frequencies at output powers up to several tens of W. Due to their large size and complexity, FELs operation requires a qualified staff.

Nowadays, most time-domain devices employ ultrafast lasers. Optical lasers are used for generating pulsed THz radiation by applying the frequency down-conversion technique. Two principal methods are used to generate THz radiation: difference frequency generation and optical rectification.

The principles of THz generation are described in detail elsewhere (Ferguson and Zhang, 2002; Siegel, 2002; Wolbarst and Hendee, 2006; Hosako et al., 2007; Lee and Wanke, 2007; Liu et al., 2007; Tonouchi, 2007; Williams, 2007; Lee 2009; Sirtori, 2009; Wilmink and Grundt, 2011).

The types of THz sources used for exposure of biological objects are usually given in articles on biological effects of THz radiation. It is shown that THz effects may depend on the type of THz source.

6.2.3 Absorption of THz Radiation by Water and Skin

Water is of the greatest importance in the absorption of THz energy. The electrical properties of body tissues in the THz frequencies are mostly determined by the concentration of water, which is ~70% by weight. Also, most biological studies are performed in aqueous media. Therefore, water is of utmost importance in the dosimetric evaluation of absorbed THz energy in objects.

The water molecule forms a tetrahedral structure of hydrogen bonds connected to its neighboring molecules. This facilitates forming the highly dynamic network of interconnected molecules. When a molecule is solvated in water, the water molecules rearrange themselves to accept the molecule. The photon energy of hydrogen bonds is within 0.043–0.22 eV. Thus, as opposed to mm waves, THz radiation can directly excite the vibrational modes of the weakest hydrogen bonds of water and solvated molecules.

If N relaxation processes occur simultaneously with M homogeneously broadened vibrational modes, then the general dielectric function can be expressed according to Møler et al. (2009) as

$$\varepsilon^*(\omega) = \sum_{j=1}^{N} \frac{\Delta\varepsilon_j}{1 - i\omega\tau_j} + \sum_{k=1}^{M} \frac{A_k}{\omega_k^2 - \omega^2 - i\omega\gamma_k} + \varepsilon_\infty \tag{6.31}$$

where $\Delta\varepsilon_j$ is the magnitude of the dispersion and τ_j is the relaxation time of the jth relaxation process, ε_∞ is the optical permittivity, the coefficients A_k are the vibrational amplitudes, $\omega_k/2\pi$ are the resonance frequencies, and γ_k are damping rates of the kth vibrational mode. The complex dielectric function of liquid water at room temperature can be decomposed into four components: a slow relaxation mode at $\tau_1 = 9.4$ ps, a fast relaxation mode at $\tau_2 = 0.25$ ps, an intermolecular stretching vibration mode at ~5 THz, and intermolecular vibration mode at ~15 THz (Kaatze, 1989; Yada et al., 2008). The presentation of N relaxation processes as a sum in which each process is independent of all other processes is not obvious. In some studies, the double Debye theory was used to model the fast and slow relaxation processes of water (Rønne et al., 1997; Buchner et al., 1999; Pickwell et al., 2004a). The best fit to the experimental data was obtained using the double Debye equation:

$$\varepsilon^*(\omega) = \varepsilon_\infty + \frac{\varepsilon_s - \varepsilon_2}{1 + i\omega\tau_1} + \frac{\varepsilon_2 - \varepsilon_\infty}{1 + i\omega\tau_2} \tag{6.32}$$

where ε_s is the static permittivity, ε_∞ is the optical permittivity, ε_2 is an intermediate frequency limit, and τ_1 and τ_2 are the relaxation times of the slow and fast relaxation processes, respectively.

The permittivity of pure water at 298 K calculated using the Equation 6.32 and parameters given by Pickwell et al. (2004a) is presented in Figure 6.1.

Water is a strong absorber at THz frequencies. In a homogeneous medium, the attenuation of the PD of a THz wave is given by

$$\mathrm{PD}(f) = \mathrm{PD}_0(f) \cdot e^{-2a(f)z} \tag{6.33}$$

where f is frequency, $\mathrm{PD}(f)$ is the transmitted intensity, $\mathrm{PD}_0(f)$ is the incident intensity, and z is the sample thickness. The power absorption coefficient $a(f) = 2\alpha(f)$ increases from about 40 up to 580 cm^{-1} following the frequency increase from 0.1 to 3.0 THz (Siegel, 2004). The optical (power) penetration depth decreases from 140 to 40 μm following the frequency increase from 0.1 to 1.6 THz (Jepsen et al., 2007).

Several authors (Fitzgerald et al., 2003; Pickwell et al., 2004b; Sun et al., 2009; Huang et al., 2009; Wilmink et al., 2011b) studied the dielectric properties of skin and other biological tissues at THz frequencies. Because tissues are not 100% water, their absorption coefficients are lower than that of water. For example, the absorption coefficient $a(f)$ for skin, adipose tissue, and striated muscle at 1 THz is around 105, 105, and 130 cm^{-1}, respectively, while for water it is 225 cm^{-1} (Fitzgerald et al., 2003).

Pickwell et al. (2004b) studied the interaction of THz radiation with the forearm and palm skin *in vivo*. The reflection data was simulated using the FDTD model. As the power penetration depth for skin is about 60 μm at 1 THz (Wilmink et al., 2011b), the reflected waveform off the volar forearm is dominated by the reflection from the epidermis whose thickness is about 100 μm. The permittivity data of the epidermis was fitted to the double Debye equation (Equation 6.32). Figure 6.5 demonstrates the real index of refraction of the epidermis calculated using parameters of Equation 6.32 given by Pickwell et al. (2004a,b). The power penetration depth for human skin calculated using the same data given by Pickwell et al. (2004a,b) is shown in Figure 6.6. It should be noted that the calculated values of the index of refraction and penetration depth for human skin and water and those reported in the literature (Jepsen et al., 2007; Nazarov et al., 2008; Wilmink et al., 2011b) are comparable.

Thus, THz radiation is strongly absorbed by water and biological tissues. In the skin, THz radiation with a frequency >0.4 THz is almost entirely absorbed within the epidermis (~0.1 mm) affecting mostly the epidermal cells such as keratinocytes and melanocytes, Langerhans cells as well as free nerve endings. The epidermis does not contain blood

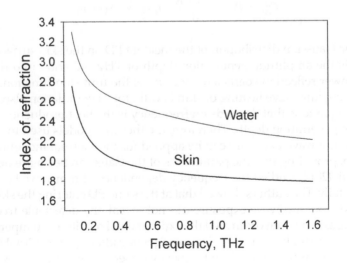

FIGURE 6.5
Real index of refraction for water and skin calculated using double Debye equation (Equation 6.32) with parameters from the papers by Pickwell et al. (2004a,b).

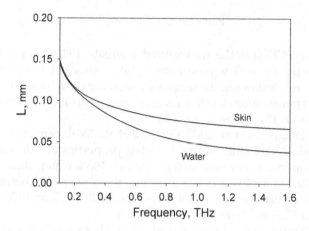

FIGURE 6.6
Frequency dependence of the power penetration depth for water and human skin calculated using the permittivity data from Pickwell et al. (2004a,b).

vessels. Only a small part of THz radiation entering the skin can reach the blood vessels located in the dermis. Therefore, in evaluating the influence of THz radiation on blood components, the *in situ* PD of THz radiation rather than the incident PD should be taken into account to define the threshold intensities of the effects.

6.2.4 THz Radiation Heating of Skin and Water

In experiments with THz radiation, the skin and biological samples are typically exposed to a Gaussian beam. In this case, the heat production due to THz radiation can be defined as follows (Alekseev and Ziskin, 2003):

$$Q(z,r,t) = \frac{2 \cdot (1-R)}{\delta} \cdot I_0 \cdot e^{-\frac{2 \cdot z}{\delta}} \cdot S(r) \cdot u(t) \tag{6.34}$$

where $S(r)$ is the Gaussian distribution of the incident PD on the skin surface, I_0 is the peak PD (W/m²), δ is the amplitude penetration depth of THz radiation into the human skin (m), R is the power reflection coefficient, and $u(t)$ is the unit step function. This equation used for modeling mm wave heating of skin is valid for THz radiation also. The only term in the bio-heat equations that depends on frequency is the heat production, which in turn depends on the penetration depth. Therefore, the thermal models used for calculations of skin heating at mm wave exposure can be applied for the thermal modeling of THz heating of skin also, providing that the parameters of the Gaussian beam are defined.

Alekseev et al. (2012) studied the frequency dependence of mm wave heating of human skin experimentally. The authors showed that at the same PD entering the skin the temperature elevation due to mm wave exposure did not reveal any detectable frequency dependence. Modeling skin heating confirmed the experimental results, i.e., temperature elevation at exposure of skin to high-frequency electromagnetic radiation above 30 GHz is not dependent on the irradiation frequency. The frequency dependence of heating was entirely due to the frequency dependence of reflection of mm waves from the skin. As the absorption of high-frequency irradiation occurs in the thin surface layer of skin, the absorbed energy is concentrated in a small tissue volume. The initial temperature gradient increases rapidly with increasing the frequency due to reducing the penetration depth. This results in a greater heat transfer from the thin heated tissue layer to surrounding tissue. Heat transfer strongly depends on thermal conductivities of tissue layers and blood flow. Therefore, in modeling skin heating at THz frequencies, it is desirable to include in a thermal model all tissue layers in spite of the concentration of absorbed energy in the epidermis.

The heating of skin exposed to THz radiation was modeled in a number of studies (Kanezaki et al., 2008, 2009, 2010; Zilberty et al., 2013, 2014). Kanezaki et al. (2008, 2009, 2010) used a one-dimensional three-layer model (skin, fat, and muscle) to calculate skin heating in the frequency range of 30–300 GHz. The authors found that at the incident PD of 50 mW/cm², the temperature elevations on the surface of skin exposed to 30, 60, 100, and 300 GHz were about 6°C, 7°C, 8°C, and 9.4°C, respectively. The model took into account the reflection of radiation from the skin. The increase of the temperature elevation was probably caused by increasing the exposure intensity due to the reduction of reflection from the skin with increasing frequency. Zilberti et al. (2014) modeled the transient heating of skin exposed to 0.1 and 1.0 THz. In this study, a three-layer model was exploited. It was shown that the skin temperature elevation was significantly higher during the first 1 s of exposure to 1 THz than to 0.1 THz. A parametric analysis showed that the properties of the skin played a major role in the computation of the maximum temperature rise.

Kristensen et al. (2010) theoretically evaluated heating of water exposed to THz radiation. As the biological samples in experiments *in vitro* are filled with culture medium, the assessment of heating of culture medium or water exposed to THz radiation is very important from the point of view of understanding the mechanisms underlying THz effects and dosimetry. The THz source was focused to a spot with a diameter of 0.5 mm. The authors assumed that water was static. The steady-state temperature increase per mW of transmitted power was 1.8°C/mW. Obviously, this is a maximal temperature rise, which is achievable using the static water approach. In reality, heating of water induces convection currents that mix different regions of water possessing different temperatures and tends to smooth down local temperature nonuniformities, thereby reducing the maximal temperature rise. Experimental verification of the model predictions is required before one can rely on the obtained results.

6.2.5 Effects of THz Radiation on Molecules and Membranes

The effects of THz radiation on a molecular level were evaluated by measuring enzyme activities, interaction of enzymes with substrate, spectroscopic changes, and changes in fluorescence spectra of proteins.

The effect of THz radiation on albumin conformation was reported in several papers (Govorun et al., 1991; Cherkasova et al., 2009; Kirichuk and Tsymbal, 2013).

Measuring the circular dichroism (CD) spectra, Govorun et al. (1991) showed the changes in the albumin secondary structure following exposure to pulsed 3.3 THz radiation with pulse energies of 5 mJ. The amount of change was proportional to the number of pulses.

Cherkasova et al. (2009) evaluated the conformational changes of albumin by measuring the characteristic absorption spectra in the UV band and the CD spectra. The irradiation of albumin to 3.6 THz for 60 min with 10 mW (PD was not provided) resulted in statistically significant changes in both spectra resulting from the conformational rearrangements in protein. The observed changes depended on exposure duration and radiation power.

Kirichuk and Tsymbal (2013) measured the absorption and fluorescence spectra of a 2.5% water solution of human albumin. Exposure of samples to 0.129 and 0.150–0.151 THz (nitrogen oxide absorption band) for 30 min resulted in changes of the amplitude rather than the shape of the spectra. The authors attributed these changes to conformational changes of albumin. No PD was reported.

In addition, Govorun et al. (1991) investigated the effects of THz radiation with the parameters given above on the activity of alcohol dehydrogenase, peroxidase, and trypsin. The activity of peroxidase decreased slightly. The other proteins exhibited a nonlinear response.

The interaction of soluble or immobilized calf alkaline phosphatase with the substrate p-nitrophenylphosphate and the interaction between an antibody (mouse monoclonal anti-dinitrophenyl (DNP)) and its antigen DNP were studied in experiments with 0.1 THz irradiation at the PD of 0.008 mW/cm^2 (Homenko et al., 2009). The samples with enzyme and the samples with enzyme and substrate were exposed for 15–90 and 30–120 min, respectively. Irradiation of the enzyme without substrate, or during the enzymatic reaction with substrate, resulted in small but statistically significant reductions in enzyme activity. The immobilized enzyme was not affected. The previously formed substrate-antibody complexes reduced their stability following irradiation. The authors stated that 0.1 THz radiation could induce small but statistically significant alterations in enzyme reactions.

The dependence of the biological effect of THz radiation on the repetition rate of THz pulses was studied by Doria et al. (2004) and Ramundo-Orlando et al. (2007). To investigate the effect of THz radiation on the permeability of artificial membranes, the liposomes were loaded with the enzyme carbonic anhydrase. Its substrate, p-nitrophenyl acetate, was added to the external solution. In the case of a permeability increase or membrane damage, the substrate could penetrate into the liposomes forming the reaction product p-nitrophenolate, which could be detected at the peak of absorbance ($\lambda =$ 400 nm) with the UV spectrometer. In the two sets of exposures, the effect of 0.130 THz was investigated at different pulse repetition rates or pps and power. The FEL generated macropulse duration was about 4 µs. In the first setup, liposomes were exposed for 60 min with the PD of 0.16 mW/cm^2 at pps = 5 Hz or with 0.23 mW/cm^2 at pps = 7 Hz. In the second setup, liposomes were exposed for 2 min at 5.6 mW/cm^2 with pps = 5 Hz, at 7.8 mW/cm^2 with pps = 7 Hz, and at 11.1 mW/cm^2 with pps = 10 Hz. Only exposure at 7.8 mW/cm^2 with pps = 7 Hz for 2 min resulted in a significant increase in enzyme activity. These experiments indicated that the repetition rate of pulsed THz radiation could play an important role in inducing a biological effect. However, the peak power of pulses was not given in the paper.

Ramundo-Orlando et al. (2007) investigated the effect of THz radiation on the same system used in the previous study. Liposomes were exposed to 0.130 THz for 2 min at room temperature (22°C) with different average power densities ranging from 5.2 to 17.1 mW/cm^2 and pps = 5, 7, and 10 Hz. Again, a significant effect was observed only at exposure of the liposomes to 7.7 mW/cm^2 with pps = 7 Hz. CW exposure to 0.130 THz at 6.2 mW/cm^2 did not induce any changes in permeability of liposomes. Thus, the present study confirmed the significance of the repetition rate of THz pulses in eliciting the membrane effect discovered by Doria et al. (2004). The temperature elevations during all exposures did not exceed 0.05°C. For explaining the obtained results, the authors suggested resonance-like mechanisms.

In the studies referred above the molecular systems and liposomes were dissolved or dispersed in a liquid medium. Due to the low penetration depth of THz radiation, the absorption of radiation energy by objects was nonuniform. Therefore, it gives rise to skepticism regarding the direct effect of THz radiation on these systems.

6.2.6 Effects of THz Radiation on the Cellular Level

The effects of THz radiation on cellular systems have been extensively studied using a wide variety of mammalian (keratinocytes, fibroblasts, blood cells, lymphocytes, spleen cells, etc.) and microorganism (yeast, *E. coli*, etc.) cells.

Hadjiloucas et al. (2002) reported results of the study of 0.200–0.350 THz effects on *Saccharomyces cerevisiae* yeast growth. Yeast cells were exposed at room temperature to 5.8 mW/cm^2 for 30, 60, 90, 120, and 150 min. The maximal temperature rise after 2.5 h exposure was 2°C–3°C. The statistically significant enhanced growth rate was observed at 341 GHz. The authors suggested a nonthermal mechanism for explaining their results.

Extensive studies, performed on the effects of THz radiation on human primary keratinocytes were described in two papers (Clothier and Bourne, 2003; Bourne et al., 2008). In the first study, the cells were exposed to pulsed 0.1–2.7 THz radiation with an average power of ~1 mW. The total pulse duration was 20–30 ps. The keratinocyte samples were exposed at room temperature (22°C) for 10, 20, and 30 min at up to 0.45 J/cm^2. Cellular activity and viability was examined using conventional assays. No inhibition or stimulation of cell activity induced by THz radiation was found. The differentiation of cells was also not affected.

In the second paper, the effects of pulsed 0.140–0.150 THz radiation at 0.1–0.25 mW/cm^2 on several human cell lines (human epithelial keratinocytes, corneal, and ND7/23 cells) were reported. The cells were exposed at 22°C for 24 h. The keratinocyte differentiation and viability, morphology, and expression of heat shock proteins and glutathione were tested using conventional assays. No exposed cells exhibited statistically significant changes.

In one paper, the effects of THz radiation on isolated neurons of mollusk *Lymnaea stagnalis* were reported (Ol'shevskaia et al., 2009). Neurons were exposed to 0.7, 2.49, and 3.69 THz at the power densities 0.3–30 mW/cm^2. Irradiation caused significant effects on cellular growth, adhesion (70%–80%), membrane morphology, intracellular structures, and resting membrane potential. Though the temperature elevation during exposure was not measured, it could have been high enough to induce the observed effects.

Munzarova et al. (2013) studied the effects of pulsed 2.205–2.307 THz radiation on the morphology and aggregation of human erythrocytes. The erythrocytes were exposed to 8–10 W/cm^2 for 5–25 s. The power in the 5.6 MHz pulses was about 1 MW. It was found that exposure for 5 s did not cause visible changes in morphology or aggregation of cells. More prolonged exposure (>25 s) resulted in cell lysis. At exposure durations of 10–15 s, the average number of erythrocytes in aggregates was reduced by 10%–15%. The authors measured the intensity of an ultrasound wave in water exposed to THz radiation with the same parameters as used in the biological experiment. The ultrasound wave with a frequency equal to the pulse repetition rate of 5.6 MHz or its first harmonic, 11.2 MHz, was recorded. However, the intensity values of the ultrasound wave were not presented. The authors speculated that the induced ultrasound wave could result in the observed effects.

Demidova et al. (2013) investigated the effect of THz radiation on *E. coli/pKatG-gfp* biosensor cells, which are constructed on the basis of the stress-sensitive promoter of the catalase gene katG. Biosensors are the artificial genetic reporter systems that contain a sensitive element—the promoter of a sensor gene—that is activated in response to external stress. The expression of green fluorescent protein (GFP) is an important indicator of stress in this system. The cell samples (volume 50 μL) were exposed to 1.5, 2.0, and 2.308 THz for 15 min at an average PD of 1.4 W/cm². Peak power in the pulses was ≤1.0 MW. During exposure, the temperature of the cell samples was kept at 35 ± 2°C using the thermal imager and by changing the average emission power. The majority of cells exposed to THz radiation exhibited intense fluorescence signal of the GFP indicating that THz radiation induced the expression of GFP in *E. coli*/pKatG-gfp biosensor cells. No signal was detected in unexposed cells kept at 37°C. The authors did not present the quantitative values of the THz effects. It was suggested that the katG promoter was induced through the oxidative stress pathway.

In a study by Williams et al. (2013), three different cell types were used for THz radiation experiments: human corneal epithelial cells, human retinal pigment epithelial cells, and human embryonic stem cells. The samples were exposed in an incubator at 37°C to broadband coherent synchrotron radiation with a cut off frequency up to ~0.5 THz, for time periods of up to 6 h and multiple 3 h periods. The average PD was in the range of 0.02–0.37 mW/cm². The peak power in the 2 ps pulses was 6 kW. The changes in cell morphology, attachment, proliferation, and differentiation were evaluated. Under all conditions, no statistically significant difference in any of these parameters between irradiated and control cell cultures was observed. Authors suggested that when the cells were grown under ideal conditions, they could compensate for any stimulatory effect of THz radiation.

The effect of CW THz radiation on a rat glial cell line was investigated by Borovkova et al. (2016). The samples were exposed to 0.12–0.18 THz at 3.2 mW/cm² at room temperature for 1, 2, 3, 4, and 5 min. THz irradiation induced a cytotoxic effect, which increased with the increase of exposure duration. The relative number of apoptotic cells increased 1.5 times following 1 min of exposure and this number was doubled after a 3 min exposure. The authors concluded that high-intensity THz irradiation could cause an adverse effect on living organisms.

Thus, the controversial results obtained in the studies of the effects of THz radiation on cellular systems do not allow drawing justifiable conclusions concerning the existence of cytotoxic effects. The experiments in many studies were performed under different conditions with uncertain dosimetry that complicate the evaluation of the obtained results.

6.2.7 Effects of THz Radiation on Cellular Genetic Apparatus

6.2.7.1 Effects on Gene Expression

Early works on the effects of THz radiation on the genetic apparatus of cells are described in detail in the comprehensive review by Wilmink and Grundt (2011). Here, we give only a short description of these publications mainly as reference sources. We will focus our efforts mostly on the description of the late publications on the subject related to the effects on gene expression without direct DNA damage.

Berns and Bewly (1987) and Berns et al. (1990, 1994) investigated the effect of 1.5 THz irradiation on DNA synthesis in different cell lines using a FEL source. Though the energy per 2 μs pulse (2.6 mJ) was relatively high, the temporal average PD was 0.1 mW/cm². The authors found statistically significant increases in inhibition of DNA synthesis. In synchronized cells, the inhibition effect was greater (22%) than in asynchronized cells (17%). The temperature in exposed samples was not measured experimentally. Calculations estimated the temperature rise in samples to be 2.96°C. Nevertheless, the authors concluded that the effect had a nonthermal origin.

A group of authors (Bock et al., 2010; Alexandrov et al., 2011, 2013) performed a systematic study of THz irradiation effects on gene expression in mouse stem cells. In the first study, cells were exposed to broadband THz radiation (centered at 10 THz) at a 1 kHz repetition rate with a peak power in each 35 fs pulse of 30 MW and an average PD of 1 mW/cm^2. Exposure durations were 2, 4, 6, and 9 h. The temperature of cells during exposure was monitored using an IR detector and thermo-sensors glued to the outside of the Petri dish lids. All exposures were performed at an ambient temperature of 26.3°C.

The gene chip survey of gene expression indicated that about 6% of the genes on the array increased more than two times, 5% decreased to the same amount and about 89% did not change. Using reverse transcription polymerase chain reaction (RT-PCR), four selected genes, including the transcription factor peroxisome proliferator-activated receptor gamma (PPARG) were confirmed to be present in the irradiated cells. The authors found out that following a 6-h exposure, lipid droplet-like inclusions appeared in the cellular cytoplasm. They suggested that THz exposure accelerates cell differentiation toward an adipose phenotype by activating PPARG. As the temperature elevation during exposure was low (about 0.3°C) the authors suggested a nonthermal mechanism for explaining the observed effects, namely the direct effect of THz radiation on the DNA conformation.

In the follow-up papers (Alexandrov et al., 2011, 2013), the effect of THz irradiation on the transcriptional activity of heat shock protein (Hsp90, Hsp105, and C-reactive protein) genes was reported. The mouse stem cells were exposed to the same broadband THz radiation (centered at ~10 THz) used in the previous study and to CW THz radiation at 2.52 THz and PD of 1.2 mW/cm^2. The temperature profiles in the Petri dish were calculated and experimentally measured using an IR camera. Temperature elevations at the bottom and at the top of the dish were about 1.5°C and 1.0°C, respectively. Exposure of the cells to the broadband and CW THz radiation for up to 12 h did not activate the heat shock proteins. However, 9 and 12 h exposures to the broadband THz radiation (rather than to CW) activated the expression of Adiponectin, GLUT4, and PPARG.

A group of researchers from the Air Force Research Laboratory conducted comprehensive studies of the effects of THz radiation on the cellular level at high-exposure intensities (Wilmink et al., 2010a,b; Wilmink and Grundt, 2011; Grundt et al., 2011). These studies were performed using optically pumped molecular gas lasers and an adequate dosimetry. Typically, samples were exposed under the controlled temperature conditions at 37°C. The computational dosimetry was performed using a FDTD program. Empirical dosimetry measurements were performed using an IR camera and thermocouples.

In the first two papers, Wilmink et al. (2010a, 2011a) reported the results of investigation of the effects of THz irradiation on human dermal fibroblasts to 2.52 THz at the PD of 84.8 mW/cm^2. The authors evaluated the cellular viability and the transcriptional activation of genes involved in protein and DNA damage pathways. Cellular viability was assessed using the MTT colorimetric assay. The transcriptional activation of heat shock proteins and DNA sensing genes was evaluated using the quantitative polymerase chain reaction (qPCR) technique. For all exposure durations tested (5, 10, 20, 40, and 80 min), more than 90% of cells remained viable. The exposed cells showed a minor increase in the expression of heat shock proteins. None of the DNA repair genes were upregulated. The increases in the expression of heat shock proteins were comparable with those observed in hyperthermic controls.

In the second study, Wilmink et al. (2010b) determined the death thresholds and gene expression profiles in human dermal fibroblast and Jurkat cell lines exposed to 2.52 THz at the PD of 227 mW/cm^2. The MTT data showed that 60% of the Jurkat cells remained viable following 30 min exposure, and only 20% of them survived after the 40 min exposure. Similar results were obtained in the flow cytometry measurements. The data showed that cell death occurred via both apoptotic and necrotic pathways. The microarray data revealed that dermal fibroblasts up-regulated several genes and activated many of the cellular stress response pathways when exposed to THz radiation. The primary genes induced by THz radiation were inflammatory cytokines.

The third study by the same group (Grundt et al., 2011) continued further examination of the cellular effects of THz radiation. Jurkat cells were exposed to 2.52 THz at the PD of 636 mW/cm² for 5, 10, 20, 30, 40, and 50 min. Viability of cells was assessed using the MTT assay. Gene expression was evaluated using an mRNA microarray. The authors found that cell death increased with exposure duration. The median lethal dose was calculated to be ~44 min. THz radiation induced the transcriptional activation of genes associated with cellular proliferation, differentiation, chaperone protein stabilization, and apoptosis. The magnitude of differential expression of genes was comparable with that induced by temperature controls. However, several genes were specifically activated only by THz exposure indicating that this effect was not thermal.

To evaluate spindle disturbances by THz radiation, a human–hamster hybrid cell line was used in experiments *in vitro* (Hintzsche et al., 2011). Monolayer cultures were exposed to 0.106 THz with power densities of 0.043, 0.43 and 4.3 mW/cm² for 0.5 h in an incubator at 36°C. Temperature elevation in cultures exposed to 4.3 mW/cm² was 1.4°C. THz irradiation at 0.43 and 4.3 mW/cm² produced statistically significant spindle disturbances in anaphase and telophase phases of cell division. The authors suggested that the THz radiation induced the effect on the spindle apparatus without directly affecting DNA.

Reported data on the effects of THz radiation on gene expression are controversial. Along with negative results, changes in gene expression were found to occur at low exposure intensities that excluded the thermal effect of irradiation. Alexandrov et al. (2011, 2013) suggested a resonance mechanism of interaction of THz radiation with DNA. The changes in gene expression at high exposure intensities were attributed to a thermal effect of irradiation.

6.2.7.2 *Potential Genotoxic Effects*

Here, we describe the results of studies of the potential genomic and DNA damage induced by THz radiation, mostly in human lymphocytes as well as in human skin cells, in human embryonic stem cells, in human corneal epithelial cells and in bacteria.

Scarfi et al. (2003) investigated the genotoxic effect of THz radiation in human peripheral blood lymphocytes. For exposure of blood samples, a FEL source was used generating a "train" of pulses of about 50 ps duration at a frequency range of 0.120–0.140 THz. The peak power in 4 µs pulses was about 1.5 kW at 0.120 THz. Samples were exposed for 20 min to 1 mW average power. To study micronucleus (MN) frequency and cell proliferation, the cytokinesis block technique was used. The results showed that the THz exposure did not change the cell cycle kinetics or the number of micronuclei, i.e. no direct chromosomal damage to lymphocytes occurred.

Doria et al. (2004) used human lymphocytes for studying genotoxic effects of THz radiation, which was evaluated using the micronucleus (MN) test and comet assay. Lymphocytes were exposed to pulsed 0.13 THz radiation for 20 min. Two experimental conditions were used. In the first set of experiments, an average power was 3.5 mW at a pulse repetition rate of 5 Hz. In the second set of experiments, the pulse repetition rate was 7 Hz at an average power of 5 mW. Both sets of experiments did not reveal chromosome damage (MN assay) or DNA damage (comet assay) in human lymphocytes. When samples were exposed using the second setup in the metal cone a small increase in DNA damage was observed. The authors suggested that the cone played the role of a resonant cavity leading to a significant increase of THz power.

The genotoxic effects of THz radiation on human blood lymphocytes were investigated in another set of experiments using the same exposure system as described in the previous paper (Zeni et al., 2007). The estimated temperature rise during a 20-min exposure of samples at room temperature (23°C) was 0.35°C. Samples were exposed to 0.12 THz at the SAR of 0.4 W/kg and 0.13 THz at the SAR of 0.24, 1.4, and 2 W/kg. Chromosomal damage and cell cycle kinetics were evaluated using the cytokinesis block MN technique. In addition, primary chromosomal damage was tested by applying the alkaline comet assay immediately after exposure. The authors concluded that under the described exposure conditions, DNA damage did not occur and the cell cycle kinetics of lymphocytes did not change.

Korenstein-Ilan et al. (2008) studied the effect of CW 0.1 THz radiation on chromosome number 1, 10, 11, and 17 in human blood lymphocytes using the fluorescence *in situ* hybridization (FISH) method. Exposure was conducted in an incubator at 37°C to 0.031 mW/cm^2 for up to 24 h. The temperature rise in samples during 24 h exposure did not exceed 0.3°C. Chromosomes 11 and 17 were most vulnerable (about 30% increase in aneuploidy after 2 and 24 h of exposure) to THz irradiation while chromosomes 1 and 10 were not affected. The asynchronous mode of replication of all centromeres was increased by 50% after 24-h exposure. The main conclusion of this work made by the authors is that the low-intensity 0.1 THz irradiation induces genomic instability. As noted by Wilmink and Grundt (2011), the total incidence of aneuploidy of all chromosomes in cells following 24-h exposure and sham-exposure reported in paper was 10.6% and 9%, respectively. These indices are within the spontaneous levels reported in literature (Vijayalaxmi and Prihoda, 2008). Thus, the main conclusion of the paper, that low-intensity 0.1 THz irradiation induces genomic instability, is questionable.

Hintzsche et al. (2012) studied the induction of genotoxic effect of THz radiation in two types of human skin cells (HaCaT and human dermal fibroblasts) and in the human–hamster hybrid cell line. The cells were exposed to 0.106 THz with power densities ranging from 0.04 to 2 mW/cm^2 for 2, 8, and 24 h. Genomic damage was evaluated using MN formation. DNA strand breaks and alkali-labile sites were quantified with the comet assay. The exposed cells showed DNA damage levels close to the sham-exposed cells at all exposure durations and power densities. No DNA strand breaks or alkali-labile sites were found.

Genomic damage in human skin cells induced by exposure to 0.380 and 2.520 THz was investigated using the comet assay (Hintzsche et al., 2013). Cells *in vitro* were exposed to power densities ranging from 0.03 to 0.9 mW/cm^2 for 2 and 8 h. DNA damage was not detected at any frequency or exposure duration. In addition, the cell proliferation was quantified and found to be unaffected. According to the authors, they demonstrated for the first time that THz irradiation at higher frequencies (0.380 and 2.520 THz) did not induce genomic damage.

Titova et al. (2013a,b) studied the effects of pulsed THz irradiation on artificial full thickness human skin (EpiDermFT, MatTek) tissues. The top surface of tissue samples was exposed to 0.1–2.0 THz centered at 0.5 THz. THz pulses had a 1.7 ps duration, 1 kHz repetition rate, and peak pulse energy variable from 0.1 to 1 µJ with a PD of 57 mW/cm^2. THz exposure was conducted at room temperature (21°C). The maximal temperature rise was less than 0.7°C. In the first paper, Titova et al. (2013a) used the presence of phosphorylated H2AX as the earliest cellular indicator of double strand breaks in DNA. Exposure to intense THz pulses for 10 min produced a significant induction of H2AX phosphorylation indicating that THz irradiation may cause DNA damage in skin tissue. At the same time, THz irradiation increased the levels of tumor suppressors and proteins responsible for cell-cycle regulation. The authors suggested that DNA damage could be quickly repaired thereby minimizing the genotoxic effect of THz radiation.

In the second paper, Titova et al. (2013b) analyzed gene expression in the artificial skin tissues at the same exposure conditions. Exposure to intense THz pulses produced coordinated changes in gene expression of multiple genes involved in epidermal differentiation. The authors discussed the potential therapeutic applications of high-intensity THz pulses.

Bogomazova et al. (2015) studied the DNA damage and transcriptome responses in human embryonic stem cells (hESC) exposed to narrow-band 2.3 THz irradiation. The hESC samples were exposed through a layer of polystyrene membrane covering the cell chamber. The average PD was 0.14 W/cm^2 at the peak PD of 4 kW/cm^2. The temperature on the surface of the polystyrene membrane was monitored using an IR camera. The temperature on the surface of the polystyrene membrane was kept in the range of 36.5°C–37.5°C by adjusting the shutter aperture. The warming of samples above the room temperature of 24°C was due to the THz exposure. The authors did not find any morphological changes in the exposed cells nor induction of H2AX phosphorylation, which indicated the absence of any genotoxic effect of THz radiation on hESC. The transcription of ~1% of genes was increased insignificantly following exposure.

The expression of heat shock proteins, morphological changes and genotoxic effects were studied following exposure of human corneal epithelial cells to 0.12 THz radiation at a spatially averaged PD of 5 mW/cm^2 (Koyama et al., 2016b). The chamber with cells was maintained under controlled conditions at a temperature of 37°C. The cells were exposed for 24 h. To evaluate genotoxicity, MN frequency was determined. The heat shock protein expression was estimated by Western blotting. Morphological changes were examined using a cell analyzer device. THz exposure produced no statistically significant increase in the MN frequency or morphological changes in cells. Expression of Hsp27, Hsp70, and Hsp90α was unchanged in exposed cells as compared to control. The authors concluded that exposure to 0.12 THz under the experimental conditions produced none or little effect on the genetic apparatus and morphology of cells derived from the human eye.

The data on the induction of genomic damage and telomere length modulation in human primary fetal fibroblasts exposed to 0.1–0.15 THz radiation was reported by De Amicis et al. (2015). The peak output power in 4 μs pulses generated by a FEL was 1.5 kW. The average incident PD was 0.4 mW/cm^2 providing an SAR in the cell medium in the range of 15–20 W/kg. Samples were exposed for 20 min at an ambient temperature of 16°C. The cell culture temperature at the beginning of the irradiation (20°C) was higher than the ambient temperature. During exposure, it asymptotically reached the thermal equilibrium over the 20-min irradiation time. The maximal calculated temperature rise was 0.3°C. DNA damage was evaluated using the Comet assay and phosphorylation of H2AX histone. No DNA damage and telomere length changes in exposed cells were observed. Apoptosis induction or changes in pro-survival signaling proteins were also not found. CREST analysis indicated that THz radiation could induce aneuploidy.

Sergeeva et al. (2016) studied the effect of 2.3 THz irradiation on bacteria Salmonella (S) typhimurium and *E. coli* cells. The samples were exposed to 1.4 W/cm^2 for 5, 10, and 15 min. For the genotoxicity test, the authors measured SOS induction in E. coli PQ37. SOS response is a global response to DNA damage. No significant differences were found between exposed and control cells indicating that THz radiation did not produce a genotoxic effect. Nevertheless, a small increase in total number of *S. typhimurium* after 15 min exposure and an increase in several enzyme activities in E. coli PQ37 were indications that THz radiation affected cell metabolism.

Most studies performed at irradiation intensities of 0.14–5 mW/cm² did not reveal a genotoxic effect of THz radiation in the frequency range of 0.106–2.52 THz. A genotoxic effect at higher intensity (57 mW/cm²) and broadband irradiation was reported by Titova et al. (2013a,b). The data showing a genotoxic effect obtained by Korenstein-Ilan et al. (2008) requires further verification of its validity.

6.2.8 THz Radiation Effects on Skin

Dalzell et al. (2010) evaluated the tissue damage thresholds of THz radiation using computational and experimental approaches. Authors used two exposure setups: short exposure for 2 s to 0.1–1.0 THz with 2–14 W/cm², and long exposure for 60 min to 1.89 THz with 189.9 mW/cm². The short exposure was used in a study of the effect of THz radiation on wet chamois clothes. In this case, the tissue damage threshold (ED50) was determined to be equal to 7.16 W/cm². Computational modeling using an Arrhenius damage model predicted ED50 = 5 W/cm². The long exposure was used in a study of THz effect on freshly excised porcine skin and egg whites. No damage was observed in the porcine skin. Only several egg whites revealed visible signs of coagulation. In this case, the temperature had increased by 10°C–12°C. It is reasonable to suggest that the mechanism underlying the tissue damage was thermal as the temperature in chamois clothes increased up to 60°C by the end of the exposure.

Hwang et al. (2014) studied the inflammatory response in live mice following pulsed THz irradiation using a custom-built laser-scanning confocal microscopy system. The skin of the ear of anesthetized mice was exposed to pulsed THz radiation (2.7 THz, 4 μs pulse width, 61.4 μJ/pulse, 3 Hz repetition rate) for 30 min with an average PD of 260 mW/cm². The beam was focused onto a small spot 300 μm in diameter. The authors could not find any notable temperature change at the surface of the aural skin when the skin was examined with an IR camera. It might be explained by the small size of the irradiation beam. To monitor any potential inflammatory response, resident neutrophils in the area of exposure were repeatedly visualized before and after THz irradiation with a confocal microscope optimized for *in vivo* visualization. No changes in the number of resident neutrophils were observed in nonirradiated control skin areas. However, a massive recruitment of newly infiltrated neutrophils was observed in the exposed skin area 6 h following exposure, indicating the induction of an acute inflammatory response in the skin. The authors suggested that this effect was induced via a nonthermal mechanism.

The histological and molecular changes in the skin of 8-week-old male C57BL/6 mice exposed to an fs-pulsed THz beam were studied by Jo et al. (2014). The skin on the back of mice was exposed to 3-THz radiation with a pulse width of <200 fs and a repetition rate of 1 kHz for 1 h. The THz pulse energy was about 0.26 nJ/pulse. Accumulated energy in the exposed area (1 cm²) for 1 h was ~1.15 J/cm². Skin biopsy samples were taken at 1 and 24 h after exposure. No histological changes were found in either 1 or 24 h post-exposure samples. The authors did not find any inflammatory cells or damaged skin cells such as sunburn cells. The collagen fibers in the dermis were also normal. A microarray analysis revealed that some genes in the exposed skin samples were either biologically activated or suppressed. For instance, the gene transcription of substance P, which is involved in local inflammation, decreased while the transcription of calcitonin gene-related peptide, another neuropeptide that is associated with neurogenic inflammation in eczema, increased significantly. These results are at variance with the histological data. The authors did not provide any explanation for these effects. Any information about the temperature elevation in the exposed skin is also missing.

Kim et al. (2013) investigated wound healing in C57BL/6J and BALB/c nude mice exposed to fs-pulsed THz radiation, as well as the genome-wide expression profile in the exposed mice skin. The frequency spectrum of irradiation ranged up to 2.5 THz. The pulse width was ~310 fs with an energy 0.26 nJ/pulse. The accumulated pulse energy for 1 h was up to 1.15 mJ/cm². Mice were exposed on their dorsal area with a beam 10 mm in diameter and an average PD of 1.15 mW/cm². Within the measurement error of the IR camera (±0.05°C), no temperature rise in the skin during exposure was detected. The authors did not observe any notable changes in the expression of Hsp70 or in the histology of the exposed skin. Microarray analysis of exposed skin samples revealed 149 differentially expressed genes with a mean fold change of signal intensity ≥1.5. Repeated fs-pulsed THz irradiation of a punch wound in the skin significantly delayed the time for wound healing due to up regulation of transforming growth factor beta (TGF-β). The authors suggested that fs-pulsed THz radiation induced a wound-like signal in skin, which inhibited wound healing *in vivo*.

Thus, exposure of skin to high-intensity THz irradiation caused dermal damage and induction of an acute inflammatory response. At lower exposure intensities, there were no histological changes, inflammatory cells, or damaged skin cells detected. However, some genes in exposed skin samples were either biologically activated or suppressed.

6.2.9 THz Radiation Effects on Animals

Due to the limited cross-sectional beam area available in early THz generators, small laboratory animals such as rats and mice were used in the initial studies of THz bioeffects. In these studies, the behavior effects of mice (Bondar et al., 2008) and responses of rats to immobilization stress (Kirichuk et al., 2009; Kirichuk and Tsymbal, 2009) following THz radiation were examined.

Bondar et al. (2008) exposed mice to 3.6 THz with the PD of 23.6 mW/cm² for 15 or 30 min. The behavior of mice was tested for anxiety. THz irradiation increased the anxiety level. The effect was maximum when the mice were in the area of the opening where radiation entered. Mice exposed for 30 min revealed the increased anxiety level on the next day. The observed effect might have resulted from the warmth sensation when the mice were in the area of the opening where the THz radiation intensity was maximum.

A study using albino rats evaluated the effect of 0.150 THz radiation on platelet aggregation and behavioral changes (Kirichuk et al., 2009). Rats were exposed for 15, 30, or 60 min with the PD of 3 mW/cm². Rats were subjected to immobilization stress and then exposed to THz radiation. Immobilization stress enhanced platelet aggregation. Exposure for 60 min produced an increased level of depression and an enhanced level of platelet aggregation even greater than that resulting from the immobilization stress. The mechanism of this effect is not clear.

In another study by Kirichuk and Tsymbal (2009), the effect of THz radiation on the level of lipoperoxidation (LPO) and antioxidant properties of the blood were examined in albino rats subjected to immobilization stress. Animals were exposed to 0.150 THz with the PD of 0.7 mW/cm² for 15 or 30 min. Immobilization stress produced an elevation of stress markers for LPO and antioxidant levels. Irradiation for 30 min reduced the levels of stress markers to control levels. This result contradicted the data reported in (Kirichuk et al., 2009). The authors speculated that the selective absorption of THz radiation by NO molecules was responsible for this effect. However, the mechanism underlying the observed effect, if verified, remains unclear.

The studies of the effects of THz radiation on animals are not numerous. More studies by different groups of researches are required to draw clear conclusions on the reactions of animals to THz radiation.

6.2.10 Mechanisms of Action of THz Radiation

Effects of THz radiation obtained following exposure to high intensities could be reproduced by equivalent temperature elevations indicating a thermal mechanism of THz action. However, in the most of *in vitro* studies the methods used for temperature measurement were not described in detail. Depending on the temperature measuring technique, the result may differ significantly (Zhadobov et al., 2017). For example, with the same THz exposure intensity, the temperature in a cell monolayer may be much higher than that in bulk. Therefore, for the interpretation of the obtained results it is important to define accurately not only the exposure intensities but the temperature elevations also. This could be important for the correct identification of the mechanism of action of THz radiation.

Another problem in identification of mechanisms of THz radiation action is the exploitation of different exposure conditions in different studies. This creates a problem of adequate *in vitro* and *in vivo* dosimetry (Jastrow et al., 2010; Kleine-Ostmann et al., 2014). Moreover, temperature control of cell samples in experiments *in vitro* can be troublesome. The majority of experiments cited in this review were performed at an ambient temperature of 22°C–27°C. It should be noted that the growth of mammalian cells decreases following "cold stress" by lowering the temperature to 25°C–27°C (Wilmink and Grundt, 2011). Moreover, mitochondria can undergo temperature-dependent phase transition at ~23°C (Raison et al., 1971). To avoid these uncertainties, the experiments with cells should be conducted at physiological temperatures.

Effects of THz radiation at low intensities cannot be attributed to a thermal mechanism. They may be caused by a resonance interaction of THz radiation with biomolecules. Using THz time-domain spectroscopy Fisher et al. (2002) investigated absorption spectra of the four nucleobases and corresponding nucleosides forming DNA. They found numerous distinct resonances in the range of 0.5–4.0 THz. The origin of these resonances was interpreted as vibrations of hydrogen bonds between the molecules. Hence, THz radiation may be directly absorbed by DNA at resonance frequencies. Similar results were obtained by Globus et al. (2003).

Based on the data demonstrating DNA involvement in cellular effects of THz radiation, Alexandrov et al. (2010) proposed a hypothesis of the existence of linear and nonlinear resonance interactions of THz radiation with DNA. For describing the local DNA pairing/unpairing (breathing) dynamics, the authors used the Peyrard-Bishop-Dauxois (PBD) model (Peyrard and Bishop, 1989; Dauxois et al., 1993) of double stranded DNA (dsDNA). The THz radiation was implemented in a model without specifying the precise mechanisms of physical coupling to dsDNA. The authors discovered a nonlinear discrete breather mode that resulted from a specific perturbation of the system. This mode can store energy for a long time. The dsDNA molecule had two steady conformational states with different energies and amplitudes. Only in these two states, absorbed energy of an external source compensated for the losses due to friction. One of the states was vibrating at an applied frequency, f(2 THz), and the second was vibrating at $f/2$. A nonlinear mechanism required a spatial perturbation above a certain amplitude threshold. Thus, the model study showed that THz radiation could affect the dsDNA molecule producing large localized openings in the DNA double strand.

Swanson (2011) repeated calculations of the interaction of THz radiation with the dsDNA molecule with parameters including those used by Alexandrov et al. (2010) but varying them in a greater range. Swanson confirmed the previous observation of destabilizing dsDNA breather modes. It was found that parameter variation under reasonable physical conditions could eliminate the breather mode entirely or make it unrealistically strong. The author estimated the amplitude of the electric field necessary to generate breather modes to be 10^9 V/m. This value was much greater than the dielectric breakdown threshold. If these calculations are correct, then the parameters used by Alexandrov et al. (2010) may not be relevant to real situations. To clarify this discrepancy further modeling of THz radiation with DNA is required.

The frequency-dependent effect of THz radiation in experiments *in vitro* could also result from the complex interaction of the incident radiation with the exposure chamber filled with liquid medium. As shown in Figure 6.4, reflection of the incident wave from the bottom of a chamber could drop to zero at some frequencies depositing the maximal radiation energy to a sample while at other frequencies reflection takes on a maximal value (30%–15%) decreasing the deposited radiation energy. This result shows that the comparison of the magnitudes of frequency-dependent changes induced by THz irradiation could be correctly evaluated only with adequate dosimetry.

As demonstrated by Munzarova et al. (2013), high-intensity THz pulses generated an ultrasound wave in a liquid medium with a frequency equal to the repetition rate. Sound waves are generated in liquid or tissues by rapid thermal expansion caused by absorption of THz radiation. Under certain conditions, a sound wave may create a standing wave in the exposed system with a frequency and amplitude determined by the size of the system and its acoustic properties (Lin, 1977a,b). At the coincidence of both frequencies, resonance amplification of the amplitude of the sound wave could occur. It is known that ultrasound exposure at even moderate intensities (0.3 and 0.4 W/cm^2) can produce DNA double-strand breaks (Furusawa et al., 2012). However, the intensity of ultrasound wave generated by THz exposure was not evaluated, and it is not clear whether the intensity of the ultrasound wave was sufficient to produce a biological effect. The generation of an ultrasound wave might explain the bioeffects following some THz exposures.

6.2.11 Conclusion

Reflection and absorption of electromagnetic energy at THz frequencies are well characterized empirically and theoretically. Heating of skin and water by THz irradiation was evaluated only theoretically and need to be confirmed experimentally.

Changes in the molecular systems and liposomes exposed to THz radiation were found in many studies. However, due to the low penetration depth of THz radiation in a liquid medium, the absorption of radiation energy by objects is extremely nonuniform. Therefore, it gives rise to skepticism regarding the direct effect of THz radiation on these systems.

The controversial results obtained in the studies of the effects of THz radiation on cellular systems prevent the drawing of clear-cut conclusions about the existence of the nonthermal THz bioeffects. Moreover, the experiments in many studies were performed under very different conditions and without adequate dosimetry thereby complicating the evaluation of the obtained results.

Reported data on the effects of THz radiation on gene expression are controversial. Along with negative results, gene expression was found to occur at low exposure intensities that excluded the thermal effect of irradiation. To explain a nonthermal effect of THz radiation, Alexandrov et al. (2011, 2013) suggested the resonance mechanism of interaction of THz radiation with DNA. The changes in gene expression at high exposure intensities were attributed to the thermal effect of irradiation.

In spite of the relatively short time of THz studies, the genotoxic effect was investigated in a very comprehensive way. Most studies performed at irradiation intensities of 0.14–5 mW/cm² did not reveal any genotoxic effect of THz radiation in the frequency range of 0.106–2.52 THz. A Genotoxic effect at higher intensity (57 mW/cm²) and broadband irradiation was reported by Titova et al. (2013a,b). The data showing the genotoxic effect obtained by Korenstein-Ilan et al. (2008) requires further verification.

At exposure of skin to high-intensity THz irradiation, dermal damage and induction of an acute inflammatory response were observed. At lower exposure intensities, no histological changes, inflammatory cells, or damaged skin cells were found. However, some genes in exposed skin samples were either biologically activated or suppressed.

The studies of the effects of THz radiation on animals are not numerous. More studies by different groups of researches are required in order to draw clear conclusions on the reactions of animals to THz radiation. Studies regarding the THz radiation interaction with humans are also required.

Three main mechanisms of THz effects were suggested:

1. Thermal mechanism;

2. The nonlinear resonance interaction of THz radiation with DNA;

3. Generation of ultrasound waves in liquid samples by pulsed THz radiation.

The resonance and sound wave hypotheses need to be explored further.

References

Adair, R. K. 2003. Biophysical limits on athermal effects of RF and microwave radiation. *Bioelectromagnetics* 24:39–48.

Alabaster, C. M. 2003. Permittivity of human skin in millimetre wave band. *Electron Lett* 39:1521–1522.

Albini, M., S. Dinarelli, F. Pennella, et al., 2014. Induced movements of giant vesicles by millimeter wave radiation. *Biochim Biophys Acta* 1838(7):1710–1718.

Alekseev, S. I., and M. C. Ziskin. 1995. Millimeter microwave effect on ion transport across lipid bilayer membranes. *Bioelectromagnetics* 16:124–131.

Alekseev, S. I., M. C. Ziskin, N. V. Kochetkova, and M. A. Bolshakov. 1997. Millimeter waves thermally alter the firing rate of the Lymnaea pacemaker neuron. *Bioelectromagnetics* 18:89–98.

Alekseev, S. I., and M. C. Ziskin. 1999. Effects of millimeter waves on ionic currents of *Lymnaea* neurons. *Bioelectromagnetics* 20:24–33.

Alekseev, S. I., M. C. Ziskin, and N. V. Kochetkova. 2000. Effects of millimeter wavelength electromagnetic radiation on neurons: Electrophysiological study. *Crit Rev Biomed Eng* 28(5–6):52–59.

Alekseev, S. I., and M. C. Ziskin. 2001. Distortion of millimeter-wave absorption in biological media due to presence of thermocouples and other objects. *IEEE Trans Biomed Eng* 48(9):1013–1019.

Alekseev, S. I., and M. C. Ziskin. 2003. Local heating of human skin by millimeter waves: A kinetics study. *Bioelectromagnetics* 24:571–581.

Alekseev, S. I., A. A. Radzievsky, I. Szabo, and M. C. Ziskin. 2005. Local heating of human skin by millimeter waves: Effect of blood flow. *Bioelectromagnetics* 26:489–501.

Alekseev, S. I., and M. C. Ziskin. 2007. Human skin permittivity determined by millimeter wave reflection measurements. *Bioelectromagnetics* 28:331–339.

Alekseev, S. I., A. A. Radzievsky, M. K. Logani, and M. C. Ziskin. 2008. Millimeter wave dosimetry of human skin. *Bioelectromagnetics* 29:65–70.

Alekseev, S. I., and M. C. Ziskin. 2009a. Millimeter wave absorption by cutaneous blood vessels: a computational study. *IEEE Trans Biomed Eng* 56(10):2380–2388.

Alekseev, S. I., and M. C. Ziskin. 2009b. Influence of blood flow and millimeter wave exposure on skin temperature in different thermal models. *Bioelectromagnetics* 30:52–58.

Alekseev, S. I., O. V. Gordiienko, A. A. Radzievsky, and M. C. Ziskin. 2010. Millimeter wave effects on electrical responses of the sural nerve in vivo. *Bioelectromagnetics* 31:180–190.

Alekseev, S. I., and M. C. Ziskin. 2011. Enhanced absorption of millimeter wave energy in murine subcutaneous blood vessels. *Bioelectromagnetics* 32(6):423–433.

Alekseev, S. I., M. C. Ziskin, and E. E. Fesenko. 2012. Frequency dependence of heating of human skin exposed to millimeter waves. *Biophysics* 57(1):90–93.

Alekseev, S. I., M. V. Zhadobov, E. E. Fesenko Jr, E. E. Fesenko. 2017. Millimeter wave dosimetry at exposure of cell monolayers. *Biophysics* 62(2):261–264.

Alexandrov, B. S., V. Gelev, A. R. Bishop, A. Usheva, and K. Ø. Rasmussen. 2010. DNA breathing dynamics in the presence of a terahertz field. *Phys Lett A* 374(10):1214–1217.

Alexandrov, B. S., K. Ø. Rasmussen, A. R. Bishop, et al., 2011. Non-thermal effects of terahertz radiation on gene expression in mouse stem cells. *Biomed Opt Express* 2(9):2679–2689.

Alexandrov, B. S., M. L. Phipps, L. B. Alexandrov, et al., 2013. Specificity and heterogeneity of terahertz radiation effect on gene expression in mouse mesenchymal stem cells. *Sci Rep* 3:1184.

Allison, A. C. 2000. Immunosuppressive drugs: the first 50 years and a glance forward. *Immunopharmacol* 47:63–83.

Arikawa, T., M. Nagai, and K. Tanaka. 2008. Characterizing hydration state in solution using terahertz time-domain attenuated total reflection spectroscopy. *Chem Phys Lett* 457:12–17.

Belyaev, I. Ya., Y. D. Alipov, V. A. Polunin, and V. S. Shcheglov. 1993a. Evidence for dependence of resonant frequency of millimeter wave interaction with *Escherichia coli* K12 cells on haploid genome length. *Electromagnetobiology* 12:39–49.

Belyaev, I. Ya., V. S. Shcheglov, Ye. D. Alipov, and S. P. Radko. 1993b. Regularities of separate and combined effects of circularly polarized millimeter waves on *E. coli* cells at different phases of culture growth. *Bioelectrochem Bioenerg* 31:49–63.

Belyaev, I. Ya., Y. D. Alipov, V. S. Shcheglov, V. A. Polunin, and O. A. Aizenberg. 1994. Cooperative response of *Escherichia coli* to the resonance effect of millimeter waves at super low intensity. *Electromagnetobiology* 13:53–66.

Belyaev, I. Ya., V. S. Shcheglov, Y. D. Alipov, and V. A. Polunin. 1996. Resonance effect of millimeter waves in the power range from 10^{-19} to 3×10^{-3} W/cm^2 on *Escherichia coli* cells at different concentrations. *Bioelectromagnetics* 17:312–321.

Beneduci, A., G. Chidichimo, S. Tripepi, and E. Perrotta. 2005a. Transmission electron microscopy study of the effects produced by wide-band low-power millimeter waves on MCF-7 human breast cancer cells in culture. *Anticancer Res* 25(2A):1009–1013.

Beneduci, A., G. Chidichimo, R. De Rose, L. Filippelli, S. V. Straface, and S. Venuta. 2005b. Frequency and irradiation time-dependant antiproliferative effect of low-power millimeter waves on RPMI 7932 human melanoma cell line. *Anticancer Res* 25(2A):1023–1028.

Beneduci, A., G. Chidichimo, S. Tripepi, E. Perrotta, and F. Cufone. 2007. Antiproliferative effect of millimeter radiation on human erythromyeloid leukemia cell line K562 in culture: ultrastructural- and metabolic-induced changes. *Bioelectrochem* 70(2):214–220.

Beneduci, A. 2009. Evaluation of the potential *in vitro* antiproliferative effects of millimeter waves at some therapeutic frequencies on RPMI 7932 human skin malignant melanoma cells. *Cell Biochem Biophys* 55(1):25–32.

Beneduci, A., L. Filippelli, K. Cosentino, M. L. Calabrese, R. Massa, and G. Chidichimo. 2012. Microwave induced shift of the main phase transition in phosphatidylcholine membranes. *Bioelectrochem* 84:18–24.

Beneduci, A., K. Cosentino, and G. Chidichimo. 2013. Millimeter wave radiations affect membrane hydration in phosphatidylcholine vesicles. *Materials* 6:2701–2712.

Beneduci, A., K. Cosentino, S. Romeo, R. Massa, and G. Chidichimo. 2014. Effect of millimeter waves on phosphatidylcholine membrane models: a non-thermal mechanism of interaction. *Soft Matter* 10(30):5559–5567.

Berns, M. W., and W. Bewley. 1987. Inhibition of nucleic acid synthesis in cells exposed to 200 micrometers radiation from the free electron laser. *Photochem Photobiol* 46(2):165–167.

Berns, M. W., W. Bewley, C. H. Sun, and P. Templin. 1990. Free electron laser irradiation at 200 microns affects DNA synthesis in living cells. *Proc Natl Acad Sci USA* 87(7):2810–2812.

Berns, M. W., W. Bewley, C. H. Sun, P. Templin, and A. Karn. 1994. Free electron laser irradiation at 200 μm inhibits DNA synthesis in living cells. *J Laser Appl* 6(7):165–169.

Betsky, O. V. 1993. Millimeter waves in biology and medicine. *Radiotechnica i electronica* 10:1760–1782 (in Russian).

Black, M. M. 1969. A modified radiographic method for measuring skin thickness. *Br J Dermatol* 81:661–666.

Blick, D. W., E. R. Adair, W. D. Hurt, C. J. Sherry, T. J. Walters, and J. H. Merritt. 1997. Thresholds of microwave-evoked warmth sensations in human skin. *Bioelectromagnetics* 18(6):403–409.

Bloom, W and D. W. Fawcett. 1968. *A Textbook of Histology*, 9th edition, pp. 479–509. Philadelphia: Saunders.

Bock, J., Y. Fukuyo, S. Kang, et al., 2010. Mammalian stem cells reprogramming in response to terahertz radiation. *PLoS One* 5(12):e15806.

Bogomazova, A. N., E. M. Vassina, T. N. Goryachkovskaya, et al., 2015. No DNA damage response and negligible genome-wide transcriptional changes in human embryonic stem cells exposed to terahertz radiation. *Sci Rep* 5:7749.

Bondar, N. P., I. L. Kovalenko, D. F. Avgustinovich, A. G. Khamoyan, and N. N. Kudryavtseva. 2008. Behavioral effect of terahertz waves in male mice. *Bull Exp Biol Med* 145(4):401–405.

Borovkova, M., M. Serebriakova, V. Fedorov, et al., 2016. Investigation of terahertz radiation influence on rat glial cells. *Biomed Opt Express* 8(1):273–280.

Bourne, N., R. H. Clothier, M. D'Arienzo, and P. Harrison. 2008. The effects of terahertz radiation on human keratinocyte primary cultures and neural cell cultures. *Altern Lab Anim* 36(6):667–684.

Branchet, M. C., S. Boisnic, C. Frances, and A. M. Robert. 1990. Skin thickness changes in normal aging skin. *Gerontology* 36:28–35.

Buchner, R., J. Barthel, and J. Stauber. 1999. The relaxation of water between 0°C and 35°C. *Chem Phys Lett* 306:57–63.

Carpenter, D. O., and B. O. Alving. 1968. A contribution of an electrogenic Na⁺ pump to membrane potential in *Aplysia* neurons. *J Gen Physiol* 52:1–21.

Carpenter, D. O. 1973. Electrogenic sodium pump and high specific resistance in nerve cell bodies of the squid. *Science* 179:1336–1338.

Caspers, P. J., G. W. Lucassen, and G. J. Puppels. 2003. Combined in vivo confocal Raman spectroscopy and confocal microscopy of human skin. *Biophys J* 85:572–580.

Chahat, N., M. Zhadobov, R. Sauleau, and S. I. Alekseev. 2012. New method for determining dielectric properties of skin and phantoms at millimeter waves based on heating kinetics. *IEEE Trans Microwave Theory Tech* 60(3):827–832.

Chalfin, S., J. A. D'Andrea, P. D. Comeau, M. E. Belt, and D. J. Hatcher. 2002. Millimeter wave absorption in the nonhuman primate eye at 35 GHz and 94 GHz. *Health Phys* 83:83–90.

Chatterjee, I., J. Yoon, R. Wiese, et al., 2013. Millimeter wave bioeffects at 94 GHz on skeletal muscle contraction. *Proc IEEE Topical Conf Biomed Wireless Tech Networks Sensing Systems (BioWireleSS)*, 67–69.

Chen, Q., Q. L. Zeng, D. Q. Lu, and H. Chiang. 2004. Millimeter wave exposure reverses TPA suppression of gap junction intercellular communication in HaCaT human keratinocytes. *Bioelectromagnetics* 25(1):1–4.

Chen, Y., and M. Cui. 2012. Numerical study of deposition of energy of Active Denial Weapon in human skin. *Asia-Pacific Symp Electromagn Compatibil*, 361–364.

Cherkasova, O. P., V. I. Fedorov, E. F. Nemova, and A. S. Pogodin. 2009. Influence of terahertz laser radiation on the spectral characteristics and functional properties of albumin. *Opt Spectrosc* 107(4):566–569.

Chidichimo, G., A. Beneduci, M. Nicoletta, et al., 2002. Selective inhibition of tumoral cells growth by low power millimeter waves. *Anticancer Res* 22(3):1681–1688.

Clothier, R. H., and N. Bourne. 2003. Effects of THz exposure on human primary keratinocyte differentiation and viability. *J Biol Phys* 29(2–3):179–185.

Cohen, I., R. Cahan, G. Shani, E. Cohen, and A. Abramovich. 2010. Effect of 99 GHz continuous millimeter wave electro-magnetic radiation on E. coli viability and metabolic activity. *Int J Radiat Biol* 86(5):390–399.

Crezee, J., and J. J. W. Lagendijk. 1990. Experimental verification of bioheat transfer theories: Measurement of temperature profiles around large artificial vessels in perfused tissue. *Phys Med Biol* 35:905–923.

Crezee, J., J. Mooibroek, J. J. W. Lagendijk, and G. M. J. van Leeuwen. 1994. The theoretical and experimental evaluation of the heat balance in perfused tissue. *Phys Med Biol* 39:813–832.

Dalzell, D. R., J. McQuade, R. Vincelette, et al., 2010. Damage thresholds for terahertz radiation. *Proc SPIE* 7562:1–8.

Dauxois, T., M. Peyrard, and A. R. Bishop. 1993. Dynamics and thermodynamics of a nonlinear model for DNA denaturation. *Phys Rev E Stat Phys Plasmas Fluids Relat Interdiscip Topics* 47(1):684–695.

De Amicis, A., S. D. Sanctis, S. D. Cristofaro, et al., 2015. Biological effects of in vitro THz radiation exposure in human foetal fibroblasts. *Mutat Res Genet Toxicol Environ Mutagen* 793:150–160.

Demidova, E. V., T. N. Goryachkovskaya, T. K. Malup, et al., 2013. Studying the non-thermal effects of terahertz radiation on E. coli/pKatG-GFP biosensor cells. *Bioelectromagnetics* 34(1):15–21.

Di Donato, L., M. Cataldo, P. Stano, R. Massa, and A. Ramundo-Orlando. 2012. Permeability changes of cationic liposomes loaded with carbonic anhydrase induced by millimeter wave radiation. *Radiat Res* 178:437–446.

Doria, A., G. P. Gallerano, E. Giovenale, et al., 2004. THz radiation studies on biological systems at the ENEA FEL facility. *Infrared Phys Tech* 45:339–347.

Ducharme, M. B., and P. Tikuisis. 1991. In vivo thermal conductivity of the human forearm tissue. *J Appl Physiol* 70:2682–2690.

Dykes, P. J., and R. Marks. 1977. Measurement of skin thickness: A comparison of two in vivo techniques with a conventional histometric method. *J Invest Dermatol* 69: 275–278.

El Gammal, S., C. El Gammal, K. Kaspar, et al., 1999. Sonography of the skin at 100 MHz enables in vivo visualization of stratum corneum and viable epidermis in palmar skin and psoriatic plaques. *J Invest Dermatol* 113: 821–829.

Ellison, W. J. 2007. Permittivity of pure water, at standard atmospheric pressure, over the frequency range 0–25 THz and the temperature range 0–100°C. *J Phys Chem Ref Data* 36:1–18.

Emery, A. F., and K. M. Sekins. 1982. Computer modeling of thermotherapy. In J. F. Lehmann (Ed.) *Therapeutic Heat and Cold*, 3rd edition, pp. 133–171. Baltimore/London: Williams and Wilkins.

Fadok, V. A., D. R. Voelker, P. A. Campbell, J. J. Cohen, D. L. Bratton, and P. M. Henson. 1992. Exposure of phosphatidylserine on the surface of apoptotic lymphocytes triggers specific recognition and removal by macrophages. *J Immunol* 148:2207–2216.

FCC. 1996. *Guidelines for Evaluating the Environmental Effects of Radiofrequency Radiation*. Washington, DC: Federal Communications Commission.

Fedorov, V. I., S. S. Popova, and A. N. Pisarchik. 2003. Dynamic effects of submillimeter wave radiation on biological objects of various levels of organization. *Int J Infrared Milli Waves* 24(8):1235–1254.

Feldman, Y., A. Puzenko, P. Ben-Ishai, A. Caduff, and A.J. Agranat. 2008. Human skin as arrays of helical antennas in the millimeter and submillimeter wave range. *Phys Rev Lett* 100(12):128102–128104.

Ferguson, B., and X-C. Zhang. 2002. Materials for terahertz science and technology. *Nat Mater* 1(1):26–33.

Fesenko, E. E., V. I. Geletyuk, V. N. Kazachenko, and N. K. Chemeris. 1995. Preliminary microwave irradiation of water solutions changes their channel-modifying activity. *FEBS Lett* 366:49–52.

Fischer, B. M., M. Walther, and P. U. Jepsen. 2002. Far-infrared vibrational modes of DNA components studied by terahertz time-domain spectroscopy. *Phys Med Biol* 47(21):3807–3814.

Fitzgerald, A. J., E. Berry, N. N. Zinov'ev, et al., 2003. Catalogue of human tissue optical properties at terahertz frequencies. *J Biol Phys* 29(2–3):123–128.

Fornage, B. D., and J. L. Deshayes. 1986. Ultrasound of normal skin. *J Clin Ultrasound* 14: 619–622.

Foster, K. R., H. N. Kritikos, and H. P. Schwan. 1978. Effect of surface cooling and blood flow on the microwave heating of tissue. *IEEE Trans Biomed Eng* 25:313–316.

Foster, K. R., and H. P. Schwan. 1986. Dielectric properties of tissues. In C. Polk and E. Postow (Eds.) *CRC Handbook of Biological Effects of Electromagnetic Fields*, pp. 27–96. Boca Raton, FL: CRC Press.

Foster, K. R., J. A. D'Andrea, S. Chalfin, and D. Hatcher. 2003. Thermal modeling of millimeter wave damage to the primate cornea at 35 GHz and 94 GHz. *Health Phys* 84(6):764–769.

Foster, K. R., H. Zhang, and J. M. Osepchuk. 2010. Thermal response of tissues to millimeter waves: implications for setting exposure guidelines. *Health Phys* 99(6):806–810.

Foster, K. R., M. C. Ziskin, and Q. Balzano. 2016. Thermal response of human skin to microwave energy: A critical review. *Health Phys* 111(6):528–541.

Frei, M. R., K. L. Ryan, R. E. Berger, and J. R. Jauchem. 1995. Sustained 35-GHz radiofrequency irradiation induces circulatory failure. *Shock* 4:289–293.

Fröhlich, H. 1968. Long-range coherence and energy storage in biological systems. *Int J Quant Chem* 2:641–649.

Fröhlich, H. 1970. Long range coherence and the action of enzymes. *Nature* 228:1093.

Fröhlich, H. 1972. Selective long range dispersion forces between large systems. *Phys Lett* 29A:153–154.

Fröhlich, H. 1978. Coherent electric vibrations in biological systems and the cancer problem. *IEEE Trans Microwave Theory Tech MTT* 26:613–617.

Furia, L., D. Hill, and O. P. Gandhi. 1986. Effect of millimeter-wave irradiation on growth of Saccharomyces cerevisiae. *IEEE Trans on Biomed Engineering BME* 33(11):993–999.

Furusawa, Y., Y. Fujiwara, P. Campbell, et al., 2012. DNA double-strand breaks induced by cavitational mechanical effects of ultrasound in cancer cell lines. *PLoS One* 7(1):e29012.

Gabriel, S., R. W. Lau, and C. Gabriel. 1996. The dielectric properties of biological tissues: III. Parametric models for the dielectric spectrum of tissues. *Phys Med Biol* 41:2271–2293.

Gallerano, G. P. 2004. *Tera-Hertz Radiation in Biological Research, Investigations on Diagnostics and Study on Potential Genotoxic Effects*. Frascati: ENEA.

Gandhi, O. P., and A. Riazi. 1986. Absorption of millimeter waves by human beings and its biological implications. *IEEE Trans Microwave Theory Tech* 34:228–235.

Gapeyev, A. B., N. K. Safronova, N. K. Chemeris, and E. E. Fesenko. 1996. Modification of mice peritoneal neutrophil activity at exposure to millimeter waves in near field and far field zones of radiator. *Biophisica* 41(1):205–219 (in Russian).

Gapeyev, A. B., E. N. Mikhailik, and N. K. Chemeris. 2008. Anti-inflammatory effects of low-intensity extremely high-frequency electromagnetic radiation: frequency and power dependence. *Bioelectromagnetics* 29(3):197–206.

Gapeyev, A. B., E. N. Mikhailik, and N. K. Chemeris. 2009. Features of anti-inflammatory effects of modulated extremely high-frequency electromagnetic radiation. *Bioelectromagnetics* 30(6):454–461.

Geletyuk, V. I., V. N. Kazachenko, N. K. Chemeris, and E. E. Fesenko. 1995. Dual effects of microwaves on single Ca^{2+}-activated K^+ channels in cultured kidney cells *Vero*. *FEBS Lett* 359:85–88.

Globus, T. R., D. L. Woolard, T. Khromova, et al., 2003. THz-spectroscopy of biological molecules. *J Biol Phys* 29(2/3):89–100.

Gniadecka, M., and B. Quistorff. 1996. Assessment of dermal water by high-frequency ultrasound: comparative studies with nuclear magnetic resonance. *Br J Dermatol* 135:218–224.

Goodman, M. 2000. Pentostatin (Nipent) and high-dose cyclophosphamide for the treatment of refractory autoimmune disorders. *Semin Oncol* 27:S67–S71.

Gos, P., B. Eicher, J. Kohli, and W-D. Heyer. 1997. Extremely high frequency electromagnetic fields at low power density do not affect the division of exponential phase *Saccharomyces cerevisiae* cells. *Bioelectromagnetics* 18:142–155.

Govorun, V. M., V. E. Tretiakov, N. N. Tulyakov, et al., 1991. Far-infrared radiation effect on the structure and properties of proteins. *Int J Infrared Mili Waves* 12:1469–1474.

Grant, E. H. 1982. The dielectric method of investigating bound water in biological material: An appraisal of the technique. *Bioelectromagnetics* 3:17–24.

Gründler, W., F. Keilmann, and H. Frohlich. 1977. Resonant growth rate response of yeast cells irradiated by weak microwaves. *Physiol Lett* 62A:463–466.

Gründler, W., and F. Keilmann. 1983. Sharp resonance in yeast growth prove nonthermal sensitivity in microwaves. *Phys Rev Lett* 51(13):1214–1216.

Gründler, W., and F. Keilmann. 1989. Resonant microwave effect on locally fixed yeast microcolonies. *Z Naturforsch* 44:863–866.

Gründler, W., F. Kaiser, F. Keilmann, and J. Walleczek. 1992. Mechanisms of electromagnetic interaction with cellular systems. *Naturwissenschaften* 79:551–559.

Grundt, J. E., C. C. Roth, B. D. Rivest, et al., 2011. Gene expression profile of Jurkat cells exposed to high power terahertz radiation. *Proc SPIE* 7897:78970E.

Haas, A. J., Y. Le Page, M. Zhadobov, A. Boriskin, R. Sauleau, and Y. Le Drean. 2016a. Impact of 60-GHz millimeter waves on stress and pain-related protein expression in differentiating neuron-like cells. *Bioelectromagnetics* 37(7):444–454.

Haas, A. J., Y. Le Page, M. Zhadobov, R. Sauleau, and Y. Le Drean. 2016b. Effects of 60-GHz millimeter waves on neurite outgrowth in PC12 cells using high-content screening. *Neurosci Lett* 618:58–65.

Hadjiloucas, S., M. S. Chahal, and J. W. Bowen. 2002. Preliminary results on the non-thermal effects of 200–350 GHz radiation on the growth rate of S. cerevisiae cells in microcolonies. *Phys Med Biol* 47(21):3831–3839.

Hardy, J. D. 1982. Temperature regulation, exposure to heat and cold, and effects of hypothermia. In J. F. Lehmann (Ed.) *Therapeutic Heat and Cold*, 3rd edition, pp. 172–198. Baltimore/London: Williams and Wilkins.

Hintzsche, H., C. Jastrow, T. Kleine-Ostmann, H. Stopper, E. Schmid, and T. Schrader. 2011. Terahertz radiation induces spindle disturbances in human–hamster hybrid cells. *Radiat Res* 75(5):569–574.

Hintzsche, H., and H. Stopper. 2012. Effects of terahertz radiation on biological systems. *Crit Rev Environ Sci Tech* 42(22):2408–2434.

Hintzsche, H., C. Jastrow, T. Kleine-Ostmann, U. Kärst, T. Schrader, and H. Stopper. 2012. Terahertz electromagnetic fields (0.106 THz) do not induce manifest genomic damage in vitro. *PLoS One* 7(9):e46397.

Hintzsche, H., C. Jastrow, B. Heinen, et al., 2013. Terahertz radiation at 0.380 THz and 2.520 THz does not lead to DNA damage in skin cells *in vitro*. *Radiat Res* 179(1):38–45.

Holbrook, K. A., and K. Wolff. 1993. The structure and development of skin. In B. Fitzpatrick, A. Z. Eisen, K. Wolff, I. M. Freedberg, and K. F. Austen (Eds.) *Dermatology in General Medicine*, 4th edition, pp. 97–145. Boston, MA: McGraw-Hill.

Homenko, A., B. Kapilevich, R. Kornstein, and M. A. Firer. 2009. Effect of 100 GHz radiation on alkaline phosphatase activity and antigen–antibody interaction. *Bioelectromagnetics* 30:167–175.

Hosako, I., N. Sekine, M. Patrashin, et al., 2007. At the dawn of a new era in terahertz technology. *Proc IEEE* 95(8):1611–1623.

Huang, S. Y., Y. X. Wang, D. K. Yeung, A. T. Ahuja, Y. T. Zhang, and E. Pickwell-Macpherson. 2009. Tissue characterization using terahertz pulsed imaging in reflection geometry. *Phys Med Biol* 54(1):149–160.

Humphreys, K., J. P. Loughran, M. Gradziel, et al., 2004. Medical applications of terahertz imaging: a review of current technology and potential applications in biomedical engineering. *Conf Proc IEEE Eng Med Biol Soc* 2:1302–1305.

Huzaira, M., F. Rius, M. Rajadhyaksha, R. R. Anderson, and S. Gonzalez. 2001. Topographic variations in normal skin as viewed by in vivo reflectance confocal microscopy. *J Invest Dermatol* 116:846–852.

Hwang, H., J. Yim, J-W. Cho, C. Cheon, Y. Kwon. 2003. 110 GHz broadband measurement of permittivity on human epidermis using 1mm coaxial probe. *IEEE Int MTT-S Micro Symp Dig* 1:399–402.

Hwang, Y., J. Ahn, J. Mun, et al., 2014. *In vivo* analysis of THz wave irradiation induced acute inflammatory response in skin by laser-scanning confocal microscopy. *Opt Express* 22(10):11465–11475.

ICNIRP. 1998. Guidelines for limiting exposure to time-varying electric, magnetic, and electromagnetic fields (up to 300 GHz). *Health Phys* 74(4):494–522.

IEEE Standard C95.1. 2005. IEEE standard for safety levels with respect to human exposure to the radio frequency electromagnetic fields, 3 kHz to 300 GHz.

IEEE C95.3. 2002. IEEE recommended practice for measurements and computations of radio frequency electromagnetic fields with respect to human exposure to such fields, 100 kHz–300 GHz.

Jastrow, C., T. Kleine-Ostmann, and T. Schrader. 2010. Numerical dosimetric calculations for in vitro field expositions in the THz frequency range. *Adv Radio Sci* 8:1–5.

Jauchem, J. R., K. L. Ryan, and T. J. Walters. 2016. Pathophysiological alterations induced by sustained 35-GHz radio-frequency energy heating. *J Basic Clin Physiol Pharmacol* 27(1):79–89.

Jepsen, P. U., U. Moller, and H. Merbold. 2007. Investigation of aqueous alcohol and sugar solutions with reflection terahertz time-domain spectroscopy. *Opt Express* 15(22):14717–14737.

Jo, S. J., S. Y. Yoon, J. Y. Lee, et al., 2014. Biological effects of femtosecond-terahertz pulses on C57BL/6 mouse skin. *Ann Dermatol* 26(1):129–132.

Kaatze, U. 1989. Complex permittivity of water as a function of frequency and temperature. *J Chem Eng Data* 34:371–374.

Kabisov, R. K. 2000. Millimeter radiation in the rehabilitation of oncological patients. *Crit Rev Biomed Eng* 28:29–39.

Kallfass, I., J. Antes, T. Shneider, et al., 2011. All active MMIC-based wireless communication at 220 GHz. *IEEE Trans Terahertz Sci Technol* 1:477–487.

Kanda, M., and D. Orr. 1987. Near-field gain of a horn and open-ended waveguide: Comparison between theory and experiment. *IEEE Trans Antennas Propag* 35(1):33–40.

Kanezaki, A., S. Watanabe, A. Hirata, and H. Shirai. 2008. Theoretical analysis for temperature elevation of human body due to millimeter wave exposure. *Cairo Int Biomed Eng Conf* SB–62.

Kanezaki, A., A. Hirata, S. Watanabe, and H. Shirai. 2009. Effects of dielectric permittivities on skin heating due to millimeter wave exposure. *Biomed Ing Online* 8:20.

Kanezaki, A., A. Hirata, S. Watanabe, and H. Shirai. 2010. Parameter variation effects on temperature elevation in a steady-state, one-dimensional thermal model for millimeter wave exposure of one- and three-layer human tissue. *Phys Med Biol* 55:4647–4659.

Karampatzakis, A., and S. Theodoros. 2010. Numerical model of heat transfer in the human eye with consideration of fluid dynamics of the aqueous humour. *Phys Med Biol* 55(19):5653–5665.

Karampatzakis, A., and S. Theodoros. 2013. Numerical modeling of heat and mass transfer in the human eye under millimeter wave exposure. *Bioelectromagnetics* 34(4):291–299.

Katayev, A. A., A. A. Alexandrov, L. I. Tikhonova, and G. N. Berestovskii. 1993. Frequency-dependent influence of mm-waves on ionic currents of water-plant *Nitellopsis*. The nonthermal effects. *Biofizika* 38:446–462 (in Russian).

Khizhnyak, E. P., and M. C. Ziskin. 1994. Heating patterns in biological tissue phantoms caused by millimeter wave electromagnetic irradiation. *IEEE Trans Biomed Eng* 41:865–873.

Khizhnyak, E. P., and M. C. Ziskin. 1996. Temperature oscillations in liquid media caused by continuous (nonmodulated) millimeter wavelength electromagnetic irradiation. *Bioelectromagnetics* 17:223–229.

Kim, K. T., J. Park, S. J. Jo, et al., 2013. High-power femtosecond-terahertz pulse induces a wound response in mouse skin. *Sci Rep* 3:2296.

Kirichuk, V., N. Efimova, and E. Andronov. 2009. Effect of high power terahertz irradiation on platelet aggregation and behavioral reactions of albino rats. *Bull Exp Biol Med* 148(5):746–749.

Kirichuk, V. F., and A. A. Tsymbal. 2009. Effects of terahertz irradiation at nitric oxide frequencies on intensity of lipoperoxidation and antioxidant properties of the blood under stress conditions. *Bull Exp Biol Med* 148(2):200–203.

Kirichuk, V. F., and A. A. Tsymbal. 2013. Biological effects of THz electromagnetic waves on frequencies of active cell metabolites at a molecular level. *Russian Open Med J* 2:0405.

Kirichuk, V. F., and A. N. Ivanov. 2013. Regulatory effects of terahertz waves. *Russian Open Medical J* 2:0402.

Kleine-Ostmann, T., C. Jastrow, K. Baaske, et al., 2014. Field exposure and dosimetry in the THz frequency range. *IEEE Trans Terahertz Sci Tech* 4(1):12–25.

Kligman, A. M. 1964. The biology of the stratum corneum. In W. Montagana, and W. C. Lobitz (Eds.) *The epidermis*, pp. 387–433. New York: Academic Press.

Klösgen, B., C. Reichle, S. Kohlsmann, and K. D. Kramer. 1996. Dielectric spectroscopy as a sensor of membrane headgroup mobility and hydration. *Biophys J* 71:3251–3260.

Kojima, M., M. Hanazawa, Y. Yamashiro, et al., 2009. Acute ocular injuries caused by 60-GHz millimeter-wave exposure. *Health Phys* 97:212–218.

Kolios, M. C., M. D. Sherar, and J. W. Hunt. 1996. Blood flow cooling and ultrasonic lesion formation. *Med Phys* 23:1287–1298.

Korenstein-Ilan, A., A. Barbul, P. Hasin, A. Eliran, A. Gover, and R. Korenstein. 2008. Terahertz radiation increases genomic instability in human lymphocytes. *Radiat Res* 170(2):224–234.

Kotnik, T., and D. Miklavčič. 2000. Theoretical evaluation of the distributed power dissipation in biological cells exposed to electric fields. *Bioelectromagnetics* 21:385–394.

Koyama, S., E. Narita, Y. Shimizu, et al., 2016a. Effects of long-term exposure to 60 GHz millimeter-wavelength radiation on the genotoxicity and heat shock protein (Hsp) expression of cells derived from human eye. *Int J Environ Res Public Health* 13(8):1–9.

Koyama, S., E. Narita, Y. Shimizu, et al., 2016b. Twenty four-hour exposure to a 0.12 THz electromagnetic field does not affect the genotoxicity, morphological changes, or expression of heat shock protein in HCE-T cells. *Int J Environ Res Public Health* 13(8):E793.

Kristensen, T. T. L., W. Withayachumnankul, P. U. Jepsen, and D. Abbott. 2010. Modeling terahertz heating effects on water. *Opt Express* 18(5):4727–4739.

Kues, H. A., S. A. D'Anna, R. Osiander, W. R. Green, and J. C. Monahan. 1999. Absence of ocular effects after either single or repeated exposure to 10 mW/cm² from a 60 GHz CW source. *Bioelectromagnetics* 20:463–473.

Landau, L. D. and E. M. Lifshitz. 1986. *Theoretical Physics: Fluid Dynamics*, Vol. 6. Moscow: Nauka (in Russian).

Larsen, E. G. 1978. Techniques for producing standard EM fields from 10 kHz to 10 GHz for evaluating radiation monitors. In *Electromagnetic Fields in Biological Systems*, pp. 96–112. Ottawa: Microwave Power Institute.

Lebedeva, N. N. 1993. Sensor and subsensor reactions of a healthy man to peripheral effect of low-intensity millimeter waves. *Millimetrovye Volny v Biologii i Medicine* 2:5–24 (in Russian).

Lebedeva, N. N., and T. I. Kotrovskaya. 1996. Electromagnetic reception and individual specifity of man. *Millimetrovye Volny v Biologii i Medicine* 7:14–20 (in Russian).

Lebedeva, N. N. 1997. Neurophysiological mechanisms of low intensity electromagnetic field effects. *Radiotekhnika* 4:62–66 (in Russian).

Lee, M., and M. C. Wanke. 2007. Applied physics. Searching for a solid-state terahertz technology. *Science* 316(5821):64–65.

Lee, Y-S. 2009. *Principles of Terahertz Science and Technology*. Berlin: Springer.

Le Quement, C., C. N. Nicolaz, D. Habauzit, M. Zhadobov, R. Sauleau, and Y. Le Drean. 2014. Impact of 60-GHz millimeter waves and corresponding heat effect on endoplasmic reticulum stress sensor gene expression. *Bioelectromagnetics* 35(6):444–451.

Li, X., H. Ye, F. Yu, et al., 2012. Millimeter wave treatment promotes chondrocyte proliferation via G1/S cell cycle transition. *Int J Mol Med* 29(5):823–831.

Li, X., C. Liu, W. Liang, et al., 2014. Millimeter wave promotes the synthesis of extracellular matrix and the proliferation of chondrocyte by regulating the voltage-gated K+ channel. *J Bone Miner Metab* 32(4):367–377.

Lin, J. C. 1977a. On microwave-induced hearing sensation. *IEEE Trans Microwave Theory Tech* 25:605–613.

Lin, J. C. 1977b. Further studies on the microwave auditory effect. *IEEE Trans Microwave Theory Tech* 25:936–941.

Liu, H-B., H. Zhong, N. Karpowicz, Y. Chen, X-C. Zhang. 2007. Terahertz spectroscopy and imaging for defense and security applications. *Proc IEEE* 95(8):1514–1527.

Logani, M. K., and M. C. Ziskin. 1996. Continuous millimeter wave radiation has no effect on lipid peroxidation in liposomes. *Radiat Res* 145(2):231–235.

Logani, M. K., and M. C. Ziskin. 1998. Millimeter waves at 25 mW/cm^2 have no effect on hydroxyl radical-dependent lipid peroxidation. *Electro Magnetobiol* 17(1):67–73.

Logani, M. K., I. Szabo, V. R. Makar, A. Bhanushali, S. I. Alekseev, and M. C. Ziskin. 2006. Effect of millimeter wave irradiation on tumor metastasis. *Bioelectromagnetics* 27:258–264.

Logani, M. K., M. K. Bhopale, and M. C. Ziskin. 2011. Millimeter wave and drug induced modulation of the immune system -application in cancer immunotherapy. *J Cell Sci Ther* S5:002.

Makar, V. R., M. K. Logani, I. Szabo, and M. C. Ziskin. 2003. Effect of millimeter waves on cyclophosphamide induced suppression of T cell functions. *Bioelectromagnetics* 24(5):356–365.

Makar, V. R., M. K. Logani, A. Bhanushali, M. Kataoka, and M. C. Ziskin. 2005. Effect of millimeter waves on natural killer cell activation. *Bioelectromagnetics* 26:10–19.

Makar, V. R., M. K. Logani, A. Bhanushali, S. I. Alekseev, and M. C. Ziskin. 2006. Effect of cyclophosphamide and 61.22 GHz millimeter waves onT-Cell, B-Cell, and macrophage functions. *Bioelectromegnetics* 27:458–466.

Martin, S. J., C. P. Reutelingsperger, A. J. McGahon, et al., 1995. Early redistribution of plasma membrane phosphatidylserine is a general feature of apoptosis regardless of the initiating stimulus: Inhibition by overexpression of Bcl-2 and Abl. *J Exp Med* 182:1545–1556.

Mashimo, S., S. Kuwabara, S. Yagihara, and K. Higasi. 1987. Dielectric relaxation time and structure of bound water in biological materials. *J Phys Chem* 91:6337–6338.

Meema, H. E., R. H. Sheppard, and A. Rapoport. 1964. Roentgenographic visualization and measurement of skin thickness and its diagnostic application in acromegaly. *Radiology* 82:411–417.

Mehregan, A. H., K. Hashimoto, D. A. Mehregan, and D. R. Mehregan. 1995. Normal structure of skin. In *Pinkus' Guide to Dermatology*. 6th edition, pp. 5–48. Norwalk, CO: Appleton and Lange.

Millenbaugh, N. J., J. L. Kiel, K. L. Ryan, et al., 2006. Comparison of blood pressure and thermal responses in rats exposed to millimeter wave energy or environmental heat. *Shock* 25:625–632.

Millenbaugh, N. J., C. Roth, R. Sypniewska, et al., 2008. Gene expression changes in the skin of rats induced by prolonged 35 GHz millimeter -wave exposure. *Radiat Res* 169(3):288–300.

Møller, U., D. G. Cooke, K. Tanaka, and P. U. Jepsen. 2009. Terahertz reflection spectroscopy of Debye relaxation in polar liquids [Invited]. *J Opt Soc Am B* 26:A113–A125.

Morimoto, R., A. Hirata, I. Laakso, M. C. Ziskin, and K. R. Foster. 2017. Time constants for temperature elevation in human models exposed to dipole antennas and beams in the frequency range from 1 to 30 GHz. *Phys Med Biol* 62(5):1676–1699.

Munzarova, A. F., A. S. Kozlov, and E. L. Zelentsov. 2013. Effect of terahertz laser irradiation on red blood cells aggregation in healthy blood. *Vestnik NSU: Physics Series* 8(2):117–123 (in Russian).

Naito, S., M. Hoshi, and S. Mashimo. 1997. In vivo dielectric analysis of free water content of biomaterials by time domain reflectometry. *Analyt Biochem* 251:163–172.

Nazarov, M. M., A. P. Shkurinov, E. A. Kuleshov, and V. V. Tuchin. 2008. Terahertz time-domain spectroscopy of biological tissues. *Quant Electron* 38(7):647–654.

Nelson, D. A., M. T. Nelson, T. J. Walters, P. A. Mason. 2000. Skin heating effects of millimeter-wave irradiation-thermal modeling results. *IEEE Trans Microwave Theory Tech* 48(11):2111–2120.

Nelson, D. A., T. J. Walters, K. L. Ryan, et al., 2003. Inter-species extrapolation of skin heating resulting from millimeter wave irradiation: Modeling and experimental results. *Health Phys* 84: 608–615.

Nicolaz, C. N., M. Zhadobov, F. Desmots, et al., 2009a. Absence of direct effect of low-power millimeter-wave radiation at 60.4 GHz on endoplasmic reticulum stress. *Cell Biol Toxicol* 25(5):471–478.

Nicolaz, C. N., M. Zhadobov, F. Desmots, et al., 2009b. Study of narrow band millimeter-wave potential interactions with endoplsmic reticulum stress sensor genes. *Bioelectromagnetics* 30(5):365–373.

Nicolson, S. T., K. H. Yau, S. Pruvost, et al., 2008. A low-voltage SiGe BiCMOS 77-GHz automotive radar chipset. *IEEE Trans Microwave Theory* 56(5):1092–1104.

Novikova, N. S., T. B. Kazakova, V. J. Rogers, and E. A. Korneva. 2002. C-fos gene expression induced in cells in specific hypothalamic structures by noxious mechanical stimulation and its [correction of it's] modification by exposure of the skin to extremely high frequency irradiation. *Neuro Endocrinol Lett* 23(4):315–320.

Novikova, N. S., T. B. Kazakova, V. Rogers, and E. A. Korneva. 2008a. Expression of the c-Fos gene in the rat hypothalamus in electrical pain stimulation and UHF stimulation of the skin. *Neurosci Behav Physiol* 38(4):415–420.

Novikova, N. S., S. V. Perekrest, V. J. Rogers, and E. A. Korneva. 2008b. Morphometric analysis of hypothalamic cells showing c-Fos proteins after movement restriction and EHF-irradiation. *Pathophysiology* 15(1):19–24.

Novoselova, E. G., V. B. Ogaǐ, O. A. Sinotova, O. V. Glushkova, O. V. Sorokina, and E. E. Fesenko. 2002. Effect oh millimeter waves on the immune system in mice with experimental tumors. *Biofizika* 47:933–942 (in Russian).

Odland, G. F. 1971. Histology and fine structure of the epidermis. In E. B. Helwig, and F. K. Mostofi (Eds.) *The Skin*, pp. 28–45. Baltimore: Williams and Wilkins.

Ol'shevskaia, Iu. S., A. S. Kozlov, A. K. Petrov, T. A. Zapara, and A. S. Ratushniak. 2009. Influence of terahertz (submillimeter) laser radiation on neurons in vitro. *Zh Vyssh Nerv Deiat Im I P Pavlova* 59(3):353–359 (in Russian).

Olver, A. D. 1992. *Microwave and Optical Transmission*. New York: John Wiley and Sons.

Pakhomov, A. G., H. K. Prol, S. P. Mathur, Y. Akyel, and C. B. G. Campbell. 1997. Search for frequency-specific effects of millimeter-wave radiation on isolated nerve function. *Bioelectromagnetics* 18:324–34.

Pakhomov, A. G., Y. Akyel, O. N. Pakhomova, B. E. Stuck, and M. R. Murphy. 1998. Current state and implications of research on biological effects of millimeter waves: A review of the literature. *Bioelectromagnetics* 19:393–413.

Pakhomov, A. G., S. P. Mathur, Y. Akyel, J. L. Kiel, and M. R. Murphy. 2000a. High-resolution microwave dosimetry in lossy media. In B. J. Klauenberg, and D. Miklavcic (Eds.) *Radio Frequency Radiation Dosimetry*, pp. 187–197. Dordrecht: Kluwer Academic Publishers.

Pakhomov, A. G., S. P. Mathur, J. Doyle, B. E. Stuck, J. L. Kiel, and M. R. Murphy. 2000b. Comparative effects of extremely high power microwave pulses and a brief CW irradiation on pacemaker function in isolated frog heart slices. *Bioelectromagnetics* 21:245–254.

Papaioannou, A., and T. Samaras. 2011. Numerical model of heat transfer in the rabbit eye exposed to 60-GHz millimeter wave radiation. *IEEE Trans Biomed Eng* 58(9):2582–2588.

Partyla, T., H. Hacker, H. Edinger, B. Leutzow, J. Lange, and T. Usichenko. 2017. Remote effects of electromagnetic millimeter waves on experimentally induced cold pain: A double-blinded crossover investigation in healthy volunteers. *Anesth Analg* 124:980–985.

Pennes, H. H. 1948. Analysis of tissue and arterial blood temperatures in the resting human forearm. *J Appl Physiol* 1:93–122.

Peyrard, M., and A. R. Bishop. 1989. Statistical mechanics of a nonlinear model for DNA denaturation. *Phys Rev Lett* 62(23):2755–2758.

Pickwell, E., B. E. Cole, A. J. Fitzgerald, V. P. Wallace, and M. Pepper. 2004a. Simulation of terahertz pulse propagation in biological systems. *Appl Phys Let* 84(12):2190–2192.

Pickwell, E., B. E. Cole, A. J. Fitzgerald, M. Pepper, and V. P. Wallace. 2004b. In vivo study of human skin using pulsed terahertz radiation. *Phys Med Biol* 49:1595–1607.

Pikov, V., X. Arakaki, V. Harrington, S. E. Fraser, and P. H. Siegel. 2010. Modulation of neuronal activity and plasma membrane properties with low-power millimeter waves in organotypic cortical slices. *J Neural Eng* 7:1–9.

Pletnev, S. D. 2000. The use of millimeter band electromagnetic waves in clinical oncology. *Crit Rev Biomed Eng* 28:573–587.

Radzievsky, A., M. A. Rojavin, A. Cowan, and M. C. Ziskin. 1999. Suppression of pain sensation caused by millimeter waves: A double blind, crossover, prospective human volunteer study. *Anesth Analg* 88:836–840.

Radzievsky, A. A., M. A. Rojavin, A. Cowan, S. I. Alekseev, and M. C. Ziskin. 2000. Hypoalgesic effect of millimeter waves in mice: dependence on the site of exposure. *Life Sci* 66(21):2101–2111.

Radzievsky, A. A., M. A. Rojavin, A. Cowan, S. I. Alekseev, A. A. Radzievsky Jr, and M. C. Ziskin. 2001. Peripheral neuronal system involvement in hypoalgesic effect of electromagnetic millimeter waves. *Life Sci* 68:1143–1151.

Radzievsky, A. A., O. V. Gordiienko, I. Szabo, S. I. Alekseev, and M. C. Ziskin. 2004a. Millimeter wave-induced suppression of B16 F10 melanoma growth in mice: Involvement of endogenous opioids. *Bioelectromagnetics* 25:466–473.

Radzievsky, A., O. Gordiienko, A. Cowan, S. I. Alekseev, and M. C. Ziskin. 2004b. Millimeter wave induced hypoalgesia in mice: Dependence on type of experimental pain. *IEEE Trans Plasma Sci* 32:1634–1643.

Radzievsky, A. A., O. V. Gordiienko, S. I. Alekseev, I. Szabo, A. Cowan, and M. C. Ziskin. 2008. Electromagnetic millimeter wave induced hypoalgesia: frequency dependence and involvement of endogenous opioids. *Bioelectromagnetics* 29:284–295.

Raison, J. K., J. M. Lyons, R. J. Mehlhorn, and A. D. Keith. 1971. Temperature-induced phase changes in mitochondrial membranes detected by spin labeling. *J Biol Chem* 246(12):4036–4040.

Rajadhyaksha, M., S. Gonzalez, J. M. Zavislan, R. R. Anderson, and R. H. Webb. 1999. In vivo confocal scanning laser microscopy of human skin II: Advances in instrumentation and comparison with histology. *Invest Dermatol* 113:293–303.

Ramo, S., J. R. Whinnery, and V. T. Duser. 1993. *Fields and Waves in Communication Electronics*. New York: Wiley and Sons.

Ramundo-Orlando, A., G. P. Gallerano, P. Stano, et al., 2007. Permeability changes induced by 130 GHz pulsed radiation on cationic liposomes loaded with carbonic anhydrase. *Bioelectromagnetics* 28(8):587–598.

Ramundo-Orlando, A., G. Longo, M. Cappelli, et al., 2009. The response of giant phospholipid vesicles to millimeter waves radiation. *Biochim Biophys Acta* 1788(7):1497–1507.

Rhodin, J. A. G. 1967. The ultrastructure of mammalian arteriols and precapillary sphincters. *J Ultrastruct Res* 18:181–223.

Rhodin, J. A. G. 1968. The ultrastructure of mammalian venous capillaries, venules, and small collecting veins. *J Ultrastruct Res* 25:452–500.

Riu, P. J., K. R. Foster, D. W. Blick, and E. R. Adair. 1997. A thermal model for human thresholds of microwave-evoked warmth sensations. *Bioelectromagnetics* 18(8):578–583.

Rojavin, M. A., and M. C. Ziskin. 1997. Electromagnetic millimeter waves increase the duration of anaesthesia caused by ketamine and chloral hydrate in mice. *Int J Radiat Biol* 72:475–480.

Rojavin, M. A., and M. C. Ziskin. 1998. Medical application of millimeter waves. *Q J Med* 91:57–66.

Rojavin, M. A., A. A. Radzievsky, A. Cowan, and M. C. Ziskin. 2000. Pain relief caused by millimeter waves in mice: results of cold water tail flick tests. *Int J Radiat Biol* 76(4):575–579.

Romanenko, S., P. H. Siegel, D. A. Wagenaar, and V. Pikov. 2014. Effects of millimeter wave irradiation and equivalent thermal heating on the activity of individual neurons in the leech ganglion. *J Neurophysiol* 112(10):2423–2431.

Rønne, C., L. Thrane, P. O. Åstrand, A. Wallqvist, K. V. Mikkelsen, and S. R. Keiding. 1997. Investigation of the temperature dependence of dielectric relaxation in liquid water by THz reflection spectroscopy and molecular dynamics simulation. *J Chem Phys* 107(14):5319–5331.

Rosenthal, S. W., L. Birenbaum, I. T. Kaplan, W. Metlay, W. Z. Snyder, and M. M. Zaret. 1976. Effects of 35 and 107 GHz CW microwaves on the rabbit eye. In C. C. Johnson, and M. L. Shore (Eds.) *Biological Effects of Electromagnetic Waves, selected papers of the USNC/URSI annual meeting*, pp. 110–128. Boulder, CO: US Department of Health, Education, and Welfare Publication (FDA) 77–8010.

Ryan, K. L., M. R. Frei, R. E. Berger, and J. R. Jauchem. 1996. Does nitric oxide mediate circulatory failure induced by 35-GHz microwave heating? *Shock* 6:71–76.

Ryan, K. L., M. R. Frei, and J. R. Jauchem. 1997. Circulatory failure induced by 35 GHz microwave heating: Effects of chronic nitric oxide synthesis inhibition. *Shock* 7:70–76.

Ryan, K. L., J. R. Jauchem, M. R. Tehrany, and H. L. Boyle. 2002. Platelet-activating factor does not mediate circulatory failure induced by 35-GHz microwave heating. *Methods Find Exp Clin Pharmacol* 24:279–286.

Safronova, V. G., A. G. Gabdoulkhakova, and B. F. Santalov. 2002. Immunomodulating action of low intensity millimeter waves on primed neutrophils. *Bioelectromagnetics* 23(8):599–606.

Samsonov, A., and S. V. Popov. 2013. The effect of a 94 GHz electromagnetic field on neuronal micro-tubules. *Bioelectromagnetics* 34(2):133–144.

Sandby-Moller, J., T. Poulsen, and H. C. Wulf. 2003. Epidermal thickness at different body sites: relationship to age, gender, pigmentation, blood content, skin type and smoking habits. *Acta Dermatol Venereol* 83:410–413.

Scarfì, M. R., M. Romanò, R. Di Pietro, et al., 2003. Thz exposure of whole blood for the study of biological effects on human lymphocytes. *J Biol Phys* 29:171–177.

Schwan, H. P. 1965. Electrical properties of bound water. *Ann NY Acad Sci* 125:344–354.

Schwan, H. P. 1977. Field interaction with biological matter. *Ann NY Acad Sci* 303:198–213.

Scott, J. A. 1988. A finite element model of heat transport in the human eye. *Phys Med Biol* 33(2):227–241.

Sergeeva, S., E. Demidova, O. Sinitsyna, et al., 2016. 2.3 THz radiation: Absence of genotoxicity/ mutagenicity in Escherichia coli and Salmonella typhimurium. *Mutat Res Genet Toxicol Environ Mutagen* 803–804(6):34–38.

Shafirstein, G., and E. G. Moros. 2011. Modelling millimeter wave propagation and absorption in a high resolution skin model: the effect of sweat glands. *Phys Med Biol* 56(5):1329–1339.

Shanin, S. N., E. G. Rybakina, N. N. Novikova, I. A. Kozinets, V. J. Rogers, and E. A. Korneva. 2005. Natural killer cell cytotoxic activity and c-Fos protein synthesis in rat hypothalamic cells after painful electric stimulation of the hind limbs and EHF irradiation of the skin. *Med Sci Monit* 11(9):BR309–BR315.

Shapiro, M. G., M. F. Priest, P. H. Siegel, and F. Bezanilla. 2013. Thermal mechanisms of millimeter wave stimulation of excitable cells. *Biophys J* 104:2622–2628.

Sharov, V. S., K. D. Kazarinov, V. E. Andreev, A. V. Putvinsky, and O. V. Betsky. 1983. Acceleration of peroxidation of lipids exposed to electromagnetic radiation of millimeter wave range. *Biofizika* 28:146–147 (in Russian).

Sheen, D. M., D. L. McMakin, and T. E. Hall. 2001. Three-dimensional millimeter-wave imaging for concealed weapon detection. *IEEE Trans Microw Theory* 49:1581–1592.

Shneider, M. N., and M. Pekker. 2013. Non-thermal mechanism of weak microwave fields influence on nerve fiber. *J Appl Phys* 114:1–11.

Shneider, M. N., and M. Pekker. 2014. Non-thermal influence of a weak microwave on nerve fiber activity. *J Phys Chem Biophys* 4(5):1–13.

Shuster, S., M. M. Black, and E. McVitie. 1975. The influence of age and sex on skin thickness, skin collagen and density. *Br J Dermatol* 93:639–643.

Siegel, P. H. 2002. Terahertz technology. *IEEE Trans Microwave Theory Tech* 50(3):910–928.

Siegel, P. H. 2004. Terahertz technology in biology and medicine. *IEEE Trans Microwave Theory Tech* 52:2438–2447.

Sirtori, C. 2009. Quantum cascade lasers: Breaking energy bands. *Nature Photonics* 3(1):13–15.

Smith, S. R., and K. R. Foster. 1985. Dielectric properties of low-watercontent tissues. *Phys Med Biol* 30:965–973.

Soubere Mahamoud, Y., M. Aite, C. Martin, et al., 2016. Additive effects of millimeter waves and 2-Deoxyglucose co-exposure on human keratinocytes transcriptome. *PLoS One* 11(8):e0160810.

Stewart, D. A., T. R. Gowrishankar, and J. C. Weaver. 2006. Skin heating and injury by prolonged millimeter-wave exposure: Theory based on a skin model coupled to a whole body model and local biochemical release from cells at supraphysiologic temperatures. *IEEE Trans Plasma Sci* 34(4):1480–1493.

Stolwijk, J. A. J., and J. D. Hardy. 1977. Control of body temperature. In H. K. Douglas (Ed.) *Handbook of Physiology. Section 9. Reactions to Environmental Agents*, pp. 45–69. Bethesda, MD: American Physiological Society.

Sun, Y., B. M. Fischer, and E. Pickwell-MacPherson. 2009. Effects of formalin fixing on the terahertz properties of biological tissues. *J Biomed Opt* 14(6):064017.

Swanson, E. S. 2011. Modeling DNA response to terahertz radiation. *Phys Rev E Stat Nonlin Soft Matter Phys* 83(4 Pt 1):040901.

Sypniewska, R. K., N. J. Millenbaugh, J. L. Kiel, et al., 2010. Protein changes in macrophages induced by plasma from rats exposed to 35 GHz millimeter waves. *Bioelectromagnetics* 31(8):656–663.

Szabo, I., M. A. Rojavin, T. J. Rogers, and M. C. Ziskin. 2001. Reactions of keratinocytes to in vitro millimeter wave exposure. *Bioelectromagnetics* 22(5):358–364.

Szabo, I., M. R. Manning, A. A. Radzievsky, M. A. Wetzel, T. J. Rogers, and M. C. Ziskin. 2003. Low power millimeter wave irradiation exerts no harmful effect on human keratinocytes in vitro. *Bioelectromagnetics* 24(3):165–173.

Szabo, I., S. I. Alekseev, G. Acs, et al., 2004. Destruction of cutaneous melanoma with millimeter wave hyperthermia in mice. *IEEE Trans Plasma Sci* 32:1653–1660.

Szabo, I., J. Kappelmayer, S. I. Alekseev, and M. C. Ziskin. 2006. Millimeter wave induced reversible externalization of phosphatidylserine molecules in cells exposed *in vitro*. *Bioelectromagnetics* 27(3):233–244.

Titova, L. V., A. K. Ayesheshim, A. Golubov, et al., 2013a. Intense THz pulses cause H2AX phosphorylation and activate DNA damage response in human skin tissue. *Biomed Opt Express* 4(4):559–568.

Titova, L. V., A. K. Ayesheshim, A. Golubov, et al., 2013b. Intense THz pulses down-regulate genes associated with skin cancer and psoriasis: a new therapeutic avenue? *Sci Rep* 3:2363.

Titushkin, I. A., V. S. Rao, W. F. Pickard, E. G. Moros, G. Shafirstein, and M. R. Cho. 2009. Altered calcium dynamics mediates P19-derived neuron-like cell responses to millimeter-wave radiation. *Radiat Res* 172(6):725–736.

Tonouchi, M. 2007. Cutting-edge terahertz technology. *Nature Photonics* 1(2):97–105.

Usichenko, T. I., and H. F. Herget. 2003. Treatment of chronic pain with millimeter wave therapy (MWT) in patients with diffuse connective tissue diseases: a pilot case series study. *Eur J Pain* 7(3):289–294.

Vijayalaxmi, M. K. Logani, A. Bhanushali, M. C. Ziskin, and T. J. Prihoda. 2004. Micronuclei in peripheral blood and bone marrow cells of mice exposed to 42 GHz electromagnetic millimeter waves. *Radiat Res* 161(3):341–345.

Vijayalaxmi, and T. Prihoda. 2008. Genetic damage in mammalian somatic cells exposed to radiofrequency radiation: A meta-analysis of data from 63 publications (1990–2005). *Radiat Res* 169:561–574.

Walters, T. J., D. W. Blick, L. R. Johnson, E. R. Adair, and K. R. Foster. 2000. Heating and pain sensation produced in human skin by millimeter waves: Comparison to a simple thermal model. *Health Physics* 78:259–267.

Walters, T. J., K. L. Ryan, D. A. Nelson, D. W. Blick, and P. A. Mason. 2004. Effects of blood flow on skin heating induced by millimeter wave irradiation in humans. *Health Physics* 86:115–120.

Wang, L. V. and H-I. Wu. 2007. *Biomedical Optics: Principals and Imaging*. Hoboken, NJ: Wiley-Interscience.

Welzel, J., C. Reinhardt, E. Lankenau, C. Winter, and H. H. Wolff. 2004. Changes in function and morphology of normal human skin: evaluation using optical coherence tomography. *Br J Dermatol* 150: 220–225.

Williams, B. S. 2007. Terahertz quantum-cascade lasers. *Nature Photonics* 1(9):517–525.

Williams, R., A. Schofield, G. Holder, et al., 2013. The influence of high intensity terahertz radiation on mammalian cell adhesion, proliferation and differentiation. *Phys Med Biol* 58(2):373–391.

Wilmink, G. J., B. D. Rivest, B. L. Ibey, C. L. Roth, J. Bernhard, and W. P. Roach. 2010a. Quantitative investigation of the bioeffects associated with terahertz radiation. *Proc SPIE* 7562:75620L–75620L 10.

Wilmink, G. J., B. L. Ibey, C. L. Roth, et al., 2010b. Determination of death thresholds and identification of terahertz (THz)-specific gene expression signatures. *Proc SPIE* 7562:75620K–75620K-8.

Wilmink, G. J., B. D. Rivest, C. C. Roth, et al., 2011a. In vitro investigation of the biological effects associated with human dermal fibroblasts exposed to 2.52 THz radiation. *Lasers Surg Med* 43(2):152–163.

Wilmink, G. J., B. L. Ibey, T. Tongue, et al., 2011b. Development of a compact terahertz time-domain spectrometer for the measurement of the optical properties of biological tissues. *J Biomed Optics* 16(4):047006.

Wilmink, G. J., and J. E. Grundt. 2011. Invited review article: Current state of research on biological effects of terahertz radiation. *J Infrared Milli Terahz Waves* 32:1074–1122.

Wolbarst, A. B., and W. R. Hendee. 2006. Evolving and experimental technologies in medical imaging. *Radiology* 238(1):16–39.

Woodward, R. M., B. E. Cole, V. P. Wallace, et al., 2002. Terahertz pulse imaging in reflection geometry of human skin cancer and skin tissue. *Phys Med Biol* 47(21):3853–3863.

Woodward, R. M., V. P. Wallace, R. J. Pye, et al., 2003. Terahertz pulse imaging of ex vivo basal cell carcinoma. *J Invest Dermatol* 120(1):72–78.

Wu, T., T. S. Rappaport, and C. M. Collins. 2015. Safe for generations to come: Considerations of safety for millimeter waves in wireless communications. *IEEE Microwave Magazine* 16(2):65–84.

Xie, T., J. Pei, Y. Cui, et al., 2011. EEG changes as heat stress reactions in rats irradiated by high intensity 35 GHz millimeter waves. *Health Phys* 100(6):632–640.

Xu, X., and J. Werner. 1997. A dynamic model of the human/clothing/environment-system. *Appl Hum Sci* 16:61–75.

Yada, S., M. Nagai, and K. Tanaka. 2008. Origin of the fast relaxation component of water and heavy water revealed by terahertz time-domain attenuated total reflection spectroscopy. *Chem Phys Lett* 464:166–170.

Yu, C., S. Fan, Y. Sun, and E. Pickwell-MacPherson. 2012. The potential of terahertz imaging for cancer diagnosis: A review of investigations to date. *Quant Imaging Med Surg* 2:33–45.

Zeni, O., G. P. Gallerano, A. Perrotta, et al., 2007. Cytogenetic observations in human peripheral blood leukocytes following in vitro exposure to THz radiation: A pilot study. *Health Phys* 92(4):349–357.

Zhadobov, M., R. Sauleau, V. Vie, M. Himdi, L. Le Coq, and D. Thouroude. 2006. Interactions between 60-GHz millimeter waves and artificial biological membranes: dependence on radiation parameters. *IEEE Trans Microwave Theory Tech* 54(6):2534–2542.

Zhadobov, M., R. Sauleau, L. Le Coq, et al., 2007. Low-power millimeter wave radiations do not alter stress-sensitive gene expression of chaperone proteins. *Bioelectromagnetics* 28:188–196.

Zhadobov, M., R. Sauleau, Y. Le Dreran, S. I. Alekseev, and M. C. Ziskin. 2008. Numerical and experimental millimeter-wave dosimetry for in vitro experiments. *IEEE Trans Microwave Theory Tech* 56(12):2998–3007.

Zhadobov, M., N. Chahat, R. Sauleau, C. L. Quement, and Y. Le Drean. 2011. Millimeter-wave interactions with the human body: state of knowledge and recent advances. *Int J Microwave Wireless Tech* 3(2):237–247.

Zhadobov, M., S. I. Alekseev, Y. Le Drean, R. Sauleau, and E. E. Fesenko. 2015. Millimeter waves as a source of selective heating of skin. *Bioelectromagnetics* 36:464–475.

Zhadobov, M., S. I. Alekseev, R. Sauleau, Y. Le Page, Y. Le Drean, and E. E. Fesenko. 2017. Microscale temperature and SAR measurements in cell monolayer models exposed to millimeter waves. *Bioelectromagnetics* 38:11–21.

Zhao, L., Y. H. Hao, and R. Y. Peng. 2014. Advances in the biological effects of terahertz wave radiation. *Mil Med Res* 1:26.

Zilberti, L., A. Arduino, O. Bottauscio, and M. Chiampi. 2013. A model to analyze the skin heating produced by millimeter and submillimeter electromagnetic waves. *Proc IEEE Int Conf Electromagnetics Advanced Applications*, 895–898.
Zilberti, L., A. Arduino, O. Bottauscio, M. Chiampi. 2014. Parametric analysis of transient skin heating induced by terahertz radiation. *Bioelectromagnetics* 35(5):314–323.

7

Electroporation

James C. Weaver and Yuri Chizmadzhev*

Massachusetts Institute of Technology

CONTENTS

7.1 Background

In the past decade or so, the electroporation (EP) community has reported a variety of new experimental findings, scientific insights, and promising applications. This includes a new society, ISEBTT (International Society for Electroporation-Based Technologies and Treatments); the purpose, scope, and contact information that is much too long to present here is available online. Overall interest and involvement with EP continues to grow, scientifically and technically. Here, we examine some of the basic concepts and experimental findings that underly present understanding. Accordingly, here, we note some of the advances and new topics that have appeared, or greatly expanded in activity, since the prior edition.

One rather broad example is nonthermal ablation of unresectable cancer tumors, now with four approaches distinguished [1–4]. Each of these citations came early in the recognition and pursuit of a particular approach; since then there have been many publications for those that began many years ago, and of course fewer papers for the recently identified methods. Here, "nonthermal" means only that inescapable Joule heating due to electric field pulsing is not the dominant mechanism of EP. Underlying new ablation methods is increased understanding of cell death. Although many death processes are now viewed

---

* The Electroporation chapter in the 3rd edition was written by both authors. New material and corrections were written by JCW.

as regulated or programmed, "accidental cell death" is a major exception, wherein large physical or chemical perturbations override biological control [5].

Scientific interest in EP has broadened. In addition, some recent experiments involve tremendously extended conditions can be explained, such as 200 kV/cm strength and 6 ns duration [6]. These single pulses that lead to post-pulse responses that exhibit active trans-membrane transport, not simply passive diffusion expected for essentially full plasma membrane (PM) depolarization, an unexpected result. The general view has been that most commonly used pulses create many pores, with their combined conductances sufficient to fully discharge the cell membrane, so that at least for some time the "resting transmembrane voltage" (resting potential) is essentially zero. This recent paper implies otherwise; the intriguing question is "how can this take place?"

Another is revisiting the potential role of lightning in evolution [7,8]. The basic hypothesis is that lightning-induced EP may drive transport of genetic polymers through membranes of protocells [9,10]. This occasional but large transport could significantly augment horizontal gene transport (HGT). A number of early papers have suggested this potentially important role; now, it has been recently reviewed [7,8]. Invited responses to that review resulted in suggestions for additional interpretations and future investigations of the "lightning/electroporation/HGT" hypothesis, including one that uses an analog of the Drake equation to estimate the order of magnitude of lightning-induced HGT, and that suggests that lightning probably contributed before biotic HGT evolved [11].

Still another new topic is a set of reports that describe the phenomena of CANCAN (cancelation of cancelation) [12,13] with the relatively unexplored bipolar cancelation (BPC); a key phenomenon that is observed for EP by very large but also short (submicrosecond) electric field pulses. In BPC, a unipolar pulse is followed by a pulse of opposite polarity, with this pair of pulses termed a bipolar pulse. The spacing between the two components of a bipolar pulse ranges from the shortest technically possible, limited by the effective slew rate from the first peak magnitude to the second opposite polarity peak magnitude. An intriguing feature is that BPC is difficult to reconcile with existing models of EP. We have described a new mechanism hypothesis based on entry of occluding molecules into pores, and this provides a possible explanation for the decreased tracer molecule entry into cells during the second part of a bipolar pulse [14].

Cells and tissues contain multiple, spatially distributed barriers that compartmentalize charged and large molecules. These barriers are largely constructed out of lipids, usually phospholipids. For this reason, only very small molecules with effective high lipid solubility penetrate cells and their organelles (single or double phospholipid bilayers [15]), which have a large variety of channels and transporters that facilitate transport of particular ions and molecules. Other significant barriers consist of one or more layers of cells connected by tight junctions around bladders and ducts (retention of specialized fluids), and the tough, flexible stratum corneum of mammalian skin (prevention of water loss, entry of toxic molecules and infectious agents). Electroporation results in an essentially universal physical reduction of such barriers by creating membrane-spanning aqueous pathways. Aqueous pathways (large dielectric constant $\epsilon_w \approx 80$) across lipid-containing (small dielectric constant $\epsilon_1 \approx 2$) barriers greatly favor transport of even small, monovalent ions [16,17].

Applied electric field pulses with dominant frequency content below ~300 MHz cause concentration of voltage across membranes of isolated cells, [18–20] and groups of cells spaced close together in a tissue [21]. If the time-dependent transmembrane voltage, $U_m(t)$, becomes sufficiently large, then stochastic rearrangements of membrane phospholipid molecules hypothesized to occur at a high rate, such that water-containing defects ("pores") measurably alter the membrane's transport properties. This is electroporation.

The simplest statement is that electroporation "creates new aqueous pathways" through lipid-based barriers. Almost all electroporation studies to date have focused on bilayer membranes (BLMs), both artificial planar bilayer membranes and cell membranes. In bilayer membranes, electroporation occurs under biochemically mild conditions, usually with a small temperature rise. For most easily observable phenomena such as cell transfection and molecular uptake, electroporation-related phenomena are believed to depend nonlinearly on the transmembrane voltage, $U_m(t)$. An exposure time-dependent onset within the range $\sim 0.2 < U_m < \sim 1$ V is usually found for single short (1 µs to 10 ms pulses).

Both dramatic electrical behavior ("reversible electrical breakdown" = REB for cells) and significant molecular transport occur. Most interest to date has focused on the electropermeabilization that coincides with REB conditions, which involves a large increase in membrane permeability for many all ions and molecules (particularly for longer pulses). Other consequences of electroporation are electrofusion of cells to other cells or tissue, and electro-insertion of membrane proteins into cell membranes.

The ability of a lipid-containing sheet to exclude ions and charged molecules is fundamental, and is a result of the change in "Born energy" associated with moving a charge from a medium with a large permittivity (e.g., water) to a region with a low permittivity (e.g., the interior of a phospholipid BLM). Here, the Born energy is the electrostatic energy of an ionic charge embedded in a medium with permittivity ϵ, written here in terms of the electric field, E, and $\epsilon = K\epsilon_0$ (K is the dielectric constant and $\epsilon_0 = 8.85 \times 10^{-12}$ Fm^{-1}) [22].

$$W_{\text{Born}} = \int_{\text{all space but ion}} \frac{1}{2}\epsilon E^2 \, dV \tag{7.1}$$

The essential barrier function of cell membranes can be represented by a thin sheet of lipid. This allows the magnitude of the Born energy barrier, ΔW_{Born}, to be computed by the following process: a charged sphere (representing the ion or molecule) is initially located in water far from the lipid sheet ($W_{\text{Born,i}}$) and then moved to the center of the sheet ($W_{\text{Born,f}}$), which requires the expenditure of energy. The corresponding barrier height, $\Delta W_{\text{Born}} = W_{\text{Born,f}} - W_{\text{Born,i}}$, is large even for small monovalent ions (e.g., Na$^+$ and Cl$^-$), is still larger for multivalent charged molecules, and also depends on the membrane thickness, sphere radius, and the amount and distribution of charge within the sphere.

For a single, isolated charge such as a small ion (e.g., Na$^+$), the largest contribution to ΔW_{Born} arises from the region close to the ion. The small diameter of an ion (solute) of type "s" is typically ($2r_s \approx 0.4$ nm is significantly smaller than a typical membrane thickness of $d_{m,1} \approx 4$ nm) for the lipid hydrocarbon chains (The corresponding full thickness is $d_m \approx 5$ nm, which includes the phospholipid's headgroups). As noted above, ΔW_{Born} can be estimated by calculating the change in energy to move the ion from bulk water is significantly less than a typical membrane thickness ($d_{m,1}$); smaller values for some artificial planar bilayer membranes, larger for cell membranes). This allows ΔW_{Born} to be estimated by neglecting the membrane thickness, and instead considering bulk lipid. This is justified, because the greatest contribution to the electric field is in the volume near the ion. This estimate yields

$$\Delta W_{\text{Born}} \approx \frac{e^2}{8\pi\epsilon_0 r_s}\left[\frac{1}{K_m} - \frac{1}{K_w}\right] \approx 100 \, kT \tag{7.2}$$

where the relevant temperature is $T = 37°C = 310$ K. Numerical solutions to the electrostatic problem for a thin low dielectric constant sheet immersed in water yields relatively small corrections. A barrier of this size is surmounted at a negligible rate by thermal fluctuations (spontaneous ion movement). Moreover, a transmembrane voltage, $U_{m,direct}$, which is much larger than physiological values would be needed to provide this energy. Uncharged molecules that can partition into the membrane, and then cross the membrane by diffusion; these species are not significantly affected by ΔW_{Born}. Instead, their transport is governed by a passive permeability due to the combined effect of dissolution and diffusion.

Spontaneous barrier crossing is therefore negligible. An early calculation considered not only the case of "intact sheet" but also the case of a fixed cylindrical pore [16,17]. Both aqueous configurations lowered ΔW_{Born}, but the greater reduction was achieved by the pore. The basic pore structure, penetration of the lipid membrane by an aqueous pathway, is of course the essence of channels based on proteins. It is also the basis of the "transient aqueous pore" theory of electroporation, but with the significant difference that the fluctuating and expandable electroporation aqueous pathways can be created rapidly (time scale of ns), but are metastable, with pore lifetimes reported to range from "ms" to many "s."

To our knowledge, the first experimental observations of electroporation-related phenomena were the irreversible [23] and reversible [24] "breakdown" of the excitable membrane of the node of Ranvier. Almost a decade later, nonthermal killing of microorganisms by electric field pulses was reported, [25–27] followed a few years later by the observation of a large, field-induced molecular permeability increase in natural vesicles [28]. Increasing numbers of experimental reports involving electrical behavior of field-pulsed cell membranes came in the next few years [29–31]. Artificial planar bilayer membranes [32,33] exhibited dramatic electromechanical behavior: the first pore-based theory advanced to explain the fate of pulsed planar membranes, [34–40] and then in a series of further experimental [41–43] and additional theoretical studies [44–46]. Other reports confirmed and extended observation of cell membrane transport due to increase in field-induced permeability [47–50]. This included introduction of "inactive" DNA into red blood cells, [51] followed by the critically important demonstration of transformation of cells by electrically mediated DNA uptake [52].

An important feature of artificial and cell membranes is that they concentrate electric field pulses with slow rise times (relative to the membrane charging time) because of the large membrane resistance relative to that of the extracellular and intracellular media [18–20,53,54]. This form of field amplification can be regarded as voltage concentration due to a spatially distributed voltage divider effect within a single or multicellular system. In this case of current injection (current clamp) conditions, field amplification can also arise from current density concentration, arising from multiple cells in close proximity or nearby insulating objects. In the case of cell and organelle membranes providing the predominant barriers, fast pulses with rise times smaller than ~3 ns (significant frequency content above ~300 MHz) spatially distributed dielectric voltage division emerges, electric fields tend toward approximate uniformity, and voltage concentration at membranes is much smaller [21].

However, most electroporation studies and applications have utilized pulses with rise times that exceed a typical cell charging time. In the case of artificial planar bilayer membranes, the membrane completely blocks the current pathway, so that the entire voltage across the experimental apparatus electrodes appears (after a characteristic charging time, $\tau_{CHG} \approx 10^{-6}$ s) across the membrane. In the case of cells, the situation is more complicated, but an approximate guide is obtained for the case of a spherical cell for which $U_{m,max} \approx 1.5 E_{app} r_{cell}$, which shows that the change in transmembrane voltage is given approximately by the product of the electric field and the cell size.

Conventional pulse conditions involve large electric field magnitudes and relatively long rise times (relatively low frequencies). Field pulses applied in aqueous extracellular media typically have magnitudes of $1 kV\ cm^{-1}$ (mammalian cells) to $10 kV\ cm^{-1}$ (bacteria). As discussed below, most cells have characteristic linear dimensions of $L_{cell} \approx 1$–10 µm, although skeletal muscle and nerve cells are typically much larger. Such pulses result in $U_m(t)$ reaching 0.2–1.5 V in times of order 1 µs to 10 ms. The widely used "exponential pulse" is often specified only by its decay ($E = E_0 \exp - t/\tau_{pulse}$) with the rise time probably longer than τ_{CHG} but usually not reported. Square (rectangular; actually trapezoidal in the approximation that rise and fall times are linear) pulses ($E = E_0$ or 0) are less frequently employed, but usually have pulse widths (durations) of 1–100 µs, and sometimes longer. Overall, other waveforms (multiple pulses, bipolar pulses, and gated RF pulses) have still received relatively little attention.

7.2 Pore Models of Planar Lipid Bilayer Electromechanical Behavior

Artificial planar BLMs are widely used to investigate basic aspects of the bilayer portion of cell membranes [32,33]. Laboratory conditions provide an electric field amplification by the factor $A_{BLM} = L_{elec}/d_m$, where L_{elec} is the electrode separation and d_m is the membrane thickness. Within a charging transient characterized by a time constant $\tau_m = R_e C_m$ (resistance of the electrolyte on both sides and the membrane capacitance), the electric field within a passive (fixed) membrane reaches $E_m = U_m/d_m$. For example, if one-half volt is applied to the electrodes, U_m reaches 0.5 V within about a τ_m of several microseconds. An advantage of such membranes for mechanism studies is that several measurements can be made on the same preparation. These attributes allow short pulse studies to be carried out in which the pulse duration is the same order of magnitude as τ_m or even faster. During the charging transient, the full electrode voltage does not appear across the membrane, and the resistance of the charging pathway should be included. For pulses with rise times shorter than about 3 ns, the dielectric properties of the bathing electrolytes should be included by assigning a capacitance with the dielectric constant of the electrolyte [21] in parallel with R_e.

Creation of artificial planar membranes originally involved use of relatively large amounts of organic solvent [32,33]. Significant improvement was subsequently achieved by using two (different, if desired) previously formed monolayers on aqueous solutions [55]. Unlike their cellular counterparts, these membranes are essentially macroscopic, typically spanning a circular aperture ($D_{ap} \approx 1$ mm; corresponding membrane area is in an electrically insulating septum). The convenient access to the chambers on both sides of the septum allows electrical measurements to be readily made, and the macroscopic chamber size results in a small electrolyte electrical resistance (sum of resistances on both sides, $R_e \approx 100$ V) between the membrane and macroscopic electrodes located about 1 cm away on each side. BLMs have a capacitance per area of about $C_{area} \approx 1$ µF/cm, and therefore a typical BLM has a capacitance of order $C_{BLM} \approx 3 \times 10^{-8}$ F. As a result $\tau_m \approx 3$ µs.

The bulk charge relaxation time of an aqueous electrolyte is $\tau_e = \varepsilon_e/\sigma_e = K_e \varepsilon_0 \rho_e$. For physiological saline, this basic relaxation time is small compared to the characteristic times of conventional electroporation pulses. Using a resistivity $\rho_{sal} = 0.83$ Ω m and a dielectric constant $K_{sal} = 72$, the relaxation time is $\tau_e \approx 0.5$ ns. This is much less than the charging times of typical BLM (and of cell membranes). For this reason, BLM experiments often have excellent time resolution for electrical measurements.

The measurement of a BLM transmembrane current, $I(t)$, following a step change in the applied electrode voltage, V_0, allows the induced membrane conductance to be followed. In such experiments, it is found that during its lifetime a membrane can pass through up to four distinguishable stages. The first stage is a simple charging of the membrane, governed by τ_m given above. The second stage is characterized by a constant voltage and associated (small) current. The third stage has a fluctuating current, but sometimes in this stage, the membrane reverts to a quiet, steady current state. If a large voltage is applied to the membrane for a short time, then the intact membrane often makes a transition into a peculiar long-lived (tens of minutes) excited state that is characterized by a large conductance and pronounced current fluctuations, even at low U_m. This peculiar state was termed a "stress state" [56]. A fourth stage is often reached in which $I(t)$ exhibits a drastic irreversible increase to saturation. Visual inspection shows that upon saturation the membrane has ruptured; the membrane material no longer spans the aperture and instead has collected on the aperture rim.

If a new BLM is created and an experiment repeated, then the next $I(t)$ is qualitatively reproduced, but the membrane lifetime, τ_m, the time from step voltage application to onset of a drastic current rise, is usually different. Both the character of the fluctuations and their duration are different. In short, the lifetime exhibits stochastic behavior. This characteristic feature of the membrane response can be explained by the hypothesis of transient aqueous pores.

The dependence of the mean membrane lifetime, $\bar{\tau}_m$, on various factors was studied to clarify the mechanism of membrane rupture [34,41–43]. The effect of varying U_m was most revealing. Over the range 300–600 mV the dependence of $\log_{10} \bar{\tau}_m$, on U_m is usually almost linear, e.g., an increase in U_m by 100 mV causes a tenfold decrease in $\bar{\tau}_m$. At larger U_m, the decrease in $\bar{\tau}_m$ becomes less pronounced. If, for example, U_m is increased from 200 mV to 1.4 V the mean lifetime changes by more than six orders of magnitude, decreasing to about 10 μs. This highly nonlinear dependence on U_m is not expected for electrostrictive mechanisms and provides key support for the transient aqueous pore hypothesis. Rupture (irreversible breakdown) was also studied by the charge injection technique [41]. In this method, a short (e.g., 400 ns) square pulse of moderate amplitude is applied to the membrane, with the result that $U_m(t)$ rises quickly to about 0.4 V. After 300–400 μs, U_m drops to zero over about 50 μs because of rupture. Many features of rupture following charge injection can be described quantitatively by a transient aqueous pore model [34,57,58].

One of the most dramatic aspects of electroporation is "reversible electrical breakdown" (REB), which is actually a high conductance state that acts to protect the membrane through a rapid discharge [57]. Planar membranes made of oxidized cholesterol have been studied using the charge injection method. If such membranes are charged to about 1 V in about 400 ns, the membrane resistance reversibly decreases by nearly nine orders of magnitude [41]. In typical experiments, U_m reached 0.9–1.2 V. Significantly, the value $U_m \approx 1.2$ V cannot be exceeded by further increasing the pulse amplitude. This includes experiments on cell membranes [59–61]. After a rapid discharge, the membrane survives, remains mechanically stable, and can be recharged. This was the first observation of REB in planar BLMs. Later, REB was also studied using a voltage-clamp method.

Significantly, REB of cell membranes is similar to the behavior of oxidized cholesterol membranes [41,42] or UO_2^{2+} planar BLMs [62]. An important experimental observation is that such planar membranes can exhibit either rupture or REB, depending only on the charging procedure. A moderate pulse of injected charge leads to destruction, with $U_m(t)$ decreasing in a two-stage, sigmoidal curve: following an initial post pulse decay, $U_m(t)$ begins to level off, but then decays further as the membrane ruptures.

In contrast, for large pulses, $U_m(t)$ reaches significantly higher values and then suddenly drops rapidly. Still bigger pulses led to even more rapid membrane discharge. These very different outcomes can be quantitatively described by a transient aqueous pore model [57,58].

7.3 Cell Membrane Electromechanical Phenomena

A cell membrane is much more complex than an artificial planar BLM. But even if the detailed biochemical composition is neglected, there are still important physical differences. These include the membrane's nonplanar shape, the closed membrane topology, the nonzero trans-membrane voltage due to pump activity, the presence of membrane proteins, and membrane cytoskeleton interactions [63]. Although real cells range from spherical to elongated cylinders to irregular three-dimensional shapes, a local membrane area can often be regarded as a small subsystem with a planar geometry. Consider the most commonly treated cell shape (spherical) for the small electric field case. As is well known, for small fields a spherical cell develops a change in transmembrane voltage, ΔU_m, which varies in position over the membrane and also with time:

$$\Delta U_m = \frac{1.5 E_e r_{cell}}{1 + r_{cell} G_m (\rho_{e,ext})} \left[1 - \exp(-t/\tau_{m,cell}) \right] \cos\theta \qquad (7.3)$$

where r_{cell} is the spherical cell radius, $\rho_{e,int}$ and $\rho_{e,ext}$ are the resistivities of the intracellular and extracellular electrolytes, respectively, G_m is the (constant; no electroporation) cell membrane conductance, θ is the angle between the applied electric field, $\vec{E}_{app} = \vec{E}_0 e^{jwt}$, and the site on the cell membrane at which U is measured. In this classic case, the response field, $\vec{E}_{res}$, differs significantly from $\vec{E}_{app}$, in that $\vec{E}_{res}$ goes around the cell. In contrast $\vec{E}_{app}$ is uniform, as it is the field that would exist if the cell were removed and only aqueous electrolyte was present. Finally, the time constant associated with charging the fixed cell membrane is

$$\tau_{m,cell} = \frac{r_{cell} G_m (\rho_{e,int} + 0.5 \rho_{e,ext})}{1 + r_{cell} G_m (\rho_{e,int} + 0.5 \rho_{e,ext})} \qquad (7.4)$$

Typical mammalian cells with $r_{cell} \approx 10$ μm have $\tau_m \approx 1$ μs. For $t \gg \tau_m$ and G_m essentially zero, Equation 7.3 reduces to the widely used simple form

$$\Delta U_m = 1.5 E_e r_{cell} \cos\theta \qquad (7.5)$$

However, Equations 7.3–7.5 are not valid for electroporation, because these equations do not hold if the membrane conductivity varies with position. Specifically, with electroporation, G_m varies dramatically with time at the sites of large U_m, but hardly at all at other sites. This has been convincingly established experimentally by submicrosecond fluorescence measurements with membrane dyes that respond to the transmembrane voltage [59–61]. Moreover, for suspended cells with significantly different extracellular and intracellular medium conductivity, membrane deformation is expected [64–66], and has been observed experimentally [67]. With this in mind, theoretical models that use Equations 7.3 and 7.4 under conditions with significant electroporation should be viewed with suspicion.

Two irreversible cell membrane electroporation processes have been identified at the cellular level. First, mechanically bounded small regions of the cell membrane, e.g., regions bounded by cytoskeletal elements and attached to the cytoskeleton by membrane proteins [63], may behave like a small planar membrane and may therefore exhibit prompt rupture even though the plasma membrane typically has a low surface tension [68,69] compared to an artificial planar BLM [34,70]. Surface tension tends to expand a pore once it has formed;

therefore, rupture is much less likely in cell plasma membranes unless the cell is osmotically swollen and thus has an elevated tension. In this case, the behavior of a BLM is relevant. A topologically closed membrane, e.g., a vesicle, is not expected to rupture globally. Unlike a BLM, there is no boundary at which membrane phospholipids can accumulate by expansion of one or a few large pores. The cell membrane surface tension, Γ_{cell}, is also important, and is expected to be small for some cell or vesicle membranes. But for some vesicles and intracellular organelles Γ is large [71].

In the case of BLM, the tension is due to the meniscus at the aperture and is a constant during pore expansion. For cells and vesicles, however, the membrane tension is associated with osmotic pressure difference, $\Delta\Pi$, through Laplace's law. Following electroporation, $\Delta\Pi$ (if it exists) goes to zero, and the tension, Γ, also tends to zero. In this case, pore evolution is more complicated and involves the laws of colloid osmotic lysis. In the second case, reversible electroporation may be accompanied by significant molecular transport between the extracellular and intracellular volumes, with the resulting chemical imbalance leading to cell stress and eventual lysis. This is an example of the importance of considering biochemical change due to field exposures (see *BBA*, Chapter 5).

Minimum size pores are believed to be small, of order $r_{p,min} \approx 0.8$ nm [72–74] or in erythrocytes about a factor of 2 smaller. However, significantly larger (several nanometer radii) pores are believed to evolve for longer, e.g., 100 μs electroporating pulses that are used to deliver ~1 kDa drug molecules such as bleomycin into cells. In this case, cell membranes discharge during reversible electrical breakdown (REB) through the pores, and the cellular or vesicular membrane returns to its initial state, except for consequences of net ionic or molecular transport through the transient aqueous pore population. The inability to promptly rupture via critical pores to directly lyse a cell is expected to apply to unswollen cells.

Cell membranes are believed to exhibit REB, i.e., a tremendous increase in electrical conduction which can be inferred from transmembrane voltage measurements [59–61], and which is believed due to ionic conduction through transient aqueous pores. Electric field pulses that cause U_m to rapidly rise into the range 0.5–1.5 V cause onset of REB with essentially no dependence on membrane composition. For this reason, the onset of electroporation involving REB is believed to be universal, and it has been observed for a wide variety of cell types. The behavior of the transmembrane voltage, $U_m(t)$, during membrane charging and the subsequent appearance and evolution of a pore population, is intimately connected with the number and size of pores. The success of a transient aqueous pore model in providing a quantitative description of $U_m(t)$ under these conditions gives confidence that electroporation is a valid concept. Significantly, a large increase in molecular transport across cell membranes is generally observed for essentially the same pulse conditions (cell exposures) that cause REB.

7.4 Nonpore Theories of Electromechanical Phenomena

One early approach to explaining membrane destabilization for an elevated U_m involved "punch through" [75], whereas another was based on electromechanical collapse due to compression of the membrane [76]. Electrocompression models have several important attributes. First, it is deterministic, predicting a critical transmembrane voltage, $U_{m,c}$, above which rupture occurs. However, for realistic values of membrane compressibility for solvent-free membranes this model predicts $U_{m,c} \approx 5\,V$, which is about an order of magnitude too large. Further, the absence of a marked change in membrane capacitance, C_m, before rupture argues strongly against large-scale electrocompression, as an increase in C_m is an inevitable consequence of a decrease in membrane thickness, d_m. Moreover, the observed stochastic nature of rupture is in direct conflict with the concept of a deterministic critical voltage. Neither the stochastic nature nor the strong lifetime dependence on U_m is expected for an electromechanical rupture mechanism. Finally, the fate of the membrane in this model depends only on U_m, but experiments also show a dependence on pulse duration.

Electrohydrodynamic models based on viscoelastic behavior have also been advanced [77], but are intimately related to electrocompression theories. The only difference is that the electrocompression model attributes the increase in system energy to elastic compression energy of the membrane, whereas in the electrohydrodynamic model, it corresponds to the work required to form new membrane surface. In both types of deterministic models, the development of instability ("irreversible electric breakdown" or "rupture") represents a nonlocal process that occurs simultaneously over a large area of the membrane. In contrast, pore models involve highly localized events that involve only a small fraction of the total membrane area for conventional electroporation used for molecular uptake. At another extreme, however, pulses that cause intracellular effects by organelle electroporation are hypothesized to involve supra-electroporation that involves a very large pore density; see Section 7.11.

7.5 Pore Theories of Electromechanical Phenomena

We first provide a qualitative description of how a membrane is believed to respond to an applied pulse. This is illustrated by the example of $U_m(t)$ given in Figure 7.1. The spontaneous rate of pore formation due to thermal fluctuations is very small. The pore creation rate depends on a Boltzmann factor with an energy contribution that decreases as u_m^2 (Equation 7.6). Even at a resting potential of $U_{m,rest} \approx -60\,mV$ (nerve membrane) to $-200\,mV$ (inner mitochondrial membrane), a minimum size pore will only occasionally appear in a membrane [74]. Application of an external electric field pulse begins by charging local membrane areas. Initially, displacement currents flow as the membrane charges through the extracellular and intracellular electrolyte. In the case of a spherical cell membrane, the polar regions (Equation 7.3; θ small) first reach voltages at which pore creation becomes significant. When U_m exceeds $\sim 0.5\,V$, pore creation becomes significant. As more pores rapidly appear and U_m rises further, the newly acquired local membrane conductance begins to discharge the membrane through the evolving pore population. When U_m reaches $\sim 1\,V$, there has been a huge increase in the local pore density and U_m begins to decrease even though the applied field may itself still be increasing. This is reversible electrical breakdown (REB), the high conductance state associated with significant electropermeabilization of the local membrane area. If the pulse continues after REB, the transmembrane voltage may continue at about the same value (a plateau in U_m), or may increase again before reaching a plateau. At the end of the pulse, many local areas in the polar region are so conductive that U_m quickly drops to ~ 0. According to what is known, a population of metastable pores remains, with individual pores assumed to vanish stochastically due to local thermal fluctuations.

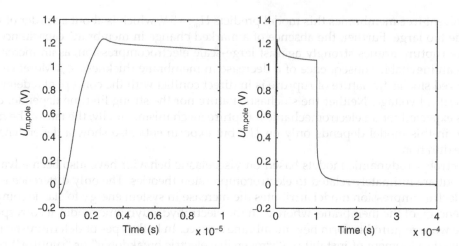

FIGURE 7.1
Illustration of the time-dependent transmembrane voltage, $U_m(t)$, for electroporation. This example shows the behavior at the pole of a two-dimensional cell model for conditions that cause electroporation and reversible electrical breakdown (REB) at $U_m \approx 1.2\,V$. A qualitative description of what is believed to occur is given in the text. This example uses a conventional electroporation electric field pulse of magnitude 1100 V/cm and a trapezoidal waveform with 1 μs rise and fall times and a 98 μs flat peak. Left panel: 10 μs timescale showing the initial passive charging of the membrane, followed by the spike at which pore conduction onset is so rapid that it arrests the voltage rise and causes a decrease even though the pulse is still on. Right panel: 400 μs timescale showing REB followed by a transmembrane voltage plateau during the pulse and then a decay when the pulse ends. This model has a distributed resting potential source and membrane resistance that together generate a resting transmembrane voltage of $U_{m,rest} = -90\,mV$ [80]. This description uses the asymptotic membrane electroporation model assigned to a circular cell with organelle models (Gowrishankar et al., unpublished results).

Molecular transport is believed to occur during the pulse when the pore population changes rapidly, first expanding in pore size and number, and then shrinking mainly in pore size as U_m eventually decreases, with pore number decreasing more slowly. Transient aqueous pore models for artificial planar BLMs [57,58] and cell membranes are consistent with this view [78–81].

Initial quantitative theories and models used analytical methods to estimate the creation and destruction rates of pores, based on nucleation theory in which pores are regarded as membrane defects [34]. Molecular dynamics (MD) simulations were possible only recently, and these support some of the basic transient aqueous pore concepts [82,87]. For example, a toroidal-like geometry is spontaneously achieved (Figure 7.2).

However, computer limitations presently restrict the model volume to be small, imposing a significant limitation on the concentration of soluble ions and molecules that are candidates for transport through a membrane by passing through a transient pore. Entry of water and aqueous electrolytes (large dielectric constant) into a fluid BLM (small dielectric constant) is increasingly favored as the electric field within the lipid region of the bilayer becomes larger. This is the basis of the transient aqueous pore theoretical model, originally introduced in a series of seven back-to-back papers [34–40]. With similar pore creation, mechanisms independently proposed several years later [44,45]. Nucleation theory is based on the absolute rate equation and involves an estimate of the free energy change, $(\Delta W)_p(r_p, U_m)$, associated with formation of a large dielectric constant aqueous pore within the small dielectric constant lipid portion of the membrane. The initial, simplest form neglected the "spreading resistance" (access resistance) and "Born energy change for ion insertion" (partitioning), which were included in some later versions, and gave (see Figure 7.3)

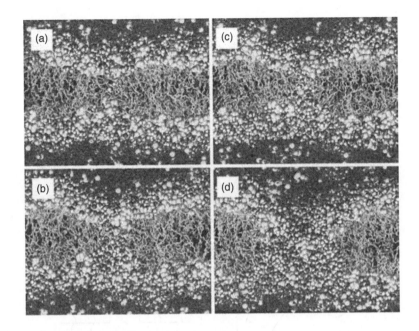

FIGURE 7.2
Snapshots of pore creation according to a molecular dynamics simulation. An important, partial test of electroporation was obtained by imposing a constant electric field, $E = 0.5$ V/nm (5×10^6 V/cm) throughout a small volume that contains aqueous electrolyte and a small area of phospholipid bilayer membrane (Tieleman, D.P. *BMC Biochem.*, 5, 10, 2004). The phospholipid headgroups are white, the hydrocarbon chains are gray, and water is dark gray. The chloride and sodium ions are somewhat difficult to make out in this gray-scale reproduction, so the reader is referred to the original paper for a color depiction. The snapshots are at times (a) 5.33, (b) 5.45, (c) 5.50, and (d) 5.70 ns from starting the simulation. As described in the original paper (Tieleman, D.P. *BMC Biochem.*, 5,10, 2004) initially, water molecules stochastically enter into the bilayer interior, leading to "formation of single-file like water defects penetrating into the bilayer." These and other MD results [82–87] show that pores can form on a nanosecond time scale, and are hydrophilic, with phospholipids present on the interior of the fluctuating pore. These hourglass or toroidal-like pores are reminiscent of the simple drawings used to motivate early models of electroporation. Present MD models are "noisy" in the sense that for a typical computational volumes and times only a few transported ions are involved. However, this approach has great promise, depending on improved computational power.

$$(\Delta W)_p (r_p, U_m) = 2\pi\gamma r_p - \pi\Gamma r_p^2 - 0.5 C_{1 \rightarrow w} U_m^2 \pi r_p^2 \tag{7.6}$$

where γ is the line tension associated with a pore edge, Γ is the surface tension of a pore-free planar membrane, and $C_{1 \rightarrow w} = \varepsilon_0 [\varepsilon - \varepsilon_1]/d_m$ is the difference in specific capacitance due to replacement of lipid by water. At zero transmembrane voltage $(\Delta W)_p(r_p, U_m)$ is a parabola with a maximum of ~100 kT, consistent with infrequent spontaneous BLM rupture.

The initial suggestion that pore formation could occur and lead to membrane rupture did not involve electrical behavior. The basic idea was that a "cookie cutter" model for a pore formation energy at zero membrane potential, $(\Delta W)_p(r_p)$ could be used, based on a gain in "edge energy," $2\pi r_p \gamma$, as a pore is created, and a simultaneous reduction in surface energy, $\pi r_p^2 \Gamma$, due to the loss of a circular patch of membrane [88]. The interpretation is simple: a pore-free membrane is envisioned, then a circular region is cut out of the membrane, and the difference in energy between these two states calculated and identified as $(\Delta W)_p(r_p)$. The change in pore energy due to an elevated transmembrane voltage is contained in the third term of the right-hand side of Equation 7.6. The membrane is regarded as a capacitor,

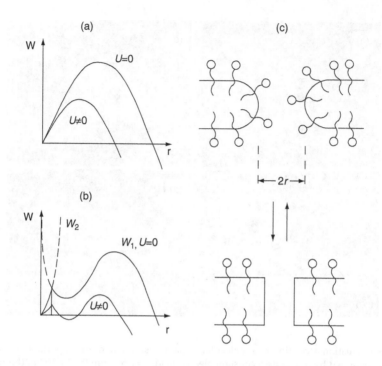

FIGURE 7.3

Drawing of imagined pore structures and associated pore creation energy. Early transient aqueous pore theory was based on two related concepts, hydrophilic pores and hydrophobic pores, with some models considering both and others only hydrophilic pores. (a) Hydrophilic pore creation energy, W, plotted as a function of pore radius, r, for zero transmembrane voltage ($U=0$) at which W is maximal, and a representative elevated voltages, at which W is decreased (favoring hydrophilic pore formation). (b) More complicated energy landscape for the hypothesis that small hydrophobic pores (curve W_2 at $U=0$) form first, followed by thermal activation to hydrophilic pores (curve W_1 at $U=0$). For elevated U, the overall energy decreases, with two peaks, which favors increased hydrophobic pore formation and also transitions to hydrophilic pores. Dependent on time and U, hydrophilic pores can surmount the right-most barrier and expand to rupture the membrane (expected for artificial planar bilayer membranes, much less plausible for cell membranes with small surface tension). (c) Envisioned transitions between hydrophobic pores (bottom) and hydrophilic pores (top). In this simple view, hydrophobic pores are imagined to be cylindrical, with an interior surface characterized by a hydrocarbon–water interface (large surface energy), and hydrophilic pores are "inverted," with phospholipid head groups lining the pore interior. Recent molecular dynamics simulations show that hydrophilic pores are expected, and the precursor membrane conformations involve water entry, achieving a water chain (analogous to a hydrophobic pore) that penetrates the membrane before a phospholipid-lined pore forms.

with the U_m-dependent term representing the change in electrical energy resulting from replacing membrane material with dielectric constant ε_1 by water with dielectric constant ε_w in a cylindrical pore of radius r_p. In other words, creation of a hydrophilic pore (hereafter simply "pore") is described as a change in specific capacitance, $C_{1 \to w}$ in the region occupied by the pore. However, for small hydrophilic pores, even if bulk electrolyte exists within the pores, the permittivity would be $\varepsilon \approx 70\varepsilon_0$, only about ten percent smaller than for pure water. Moreover, the pore interior resistance would still be large, $R_{p,int} \approx \rho_e d_m / \pi r_p^2$ compared to the spreading resistance (see below), so the voltage across the pore would be very close to U_m. Although each of the "ingredients" of the pore model is plausible, if they are combined to represent a complete experimental situation, the overall model is too complex to solve in closed form. Other membrane deformations, conformational changes, and hypothesized pore structures are shown in Figure 7.4 [89].

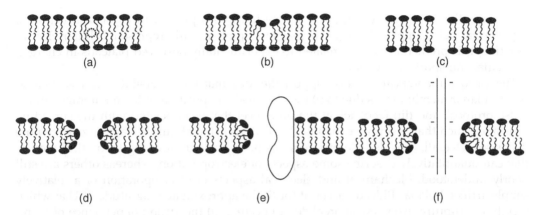

FIGURE 7.4

Hypothesized pore structures. Illustrations of hypothetical structures of both transient and metastable membrane conformations that may be involved in electroporation. Hypothetical bilayer membrane structures related to electroporation: (a) membrane free volume fluctuation; (b) aqueous protrusion into the membrane ("dimple"); (c) hydrophobic pore proposed by Chizmadzhev and coworkers [34]; (d) hydrophilic pore proposed by Litster and by Taupin and coworkers, usually regarded as the "primary pores" through which ion and molecules pass during electroporation; (e) composite pore with one or more proteins at the pore's inner edge; (f) composite pore with "foot-in-the-door" charged macromolecule inserted into a hydrophilic pore. Although the actual transitions are not known, the transient aqueous pore model assumes that transitions from A → B → C or D occur with increasing frequency as U_m increases. Type E may form by entry of a tethered macromolecule when U_m is large, and then persist after U_m has decayed by pore conduction. These hypothetical structures have not been directly observed, but are consistent with a variety of experimental observations and with theoretical models. (Reproduced from Weaver, *J. Cell. Biochem.* 51, 426–35, 1993. With permission.)

Such models are, however, now routinely solved numerically on computers to generate qualitative and quantitative predictions, and these results can be compared with experimental observations. Solutions for artificial planar BLMs have been developed, and these produce reasonable, but not completely correct, quantitative descriptions of measurable quantities such as the transmembrane voltage, $U_m(t)$ the pore size distribution, and also the membrane conductance, G_m, which increases tremendously during REB. The transport of small ions and small molecules can also be predicted approximately (see Section 7.6). In general agreement with experimental observation [41], a model solved for different pulse magnitudes also predicts the four distinguishable outcomes that are found experimentally for an oxidized cholesterol planar membrane subjected to a 400 ns second square charging pulse: (i) simple, passive charging of the membrane capacitance for small pulses; (ii) charging to about 0.5 V, followed by a sigmoidal decay of U_m as the membrane ruptures for a moderate pulse; (iii) incomplete reversible electrical breakdown in which the membrane achieves a high conductance state, but not enough to discharge the membrane fully to zero, for a larger pulse; and (iv) reversible electrical breakdown due to a still larger but transient high conductance that discharges the membrane completely [57]. This behavior reflects the interplay between the rapidly changing electrical conductance and the mechanical expansion and contraction of the individual pores in a heterogeneous, dynamic pore population.

An extension of the single artificial planar BLM to two identical membranes in series can be used as a very simple model of a "cubic cell" [90]. By using a very low value of Γ, the inability of a spherical membrane to rupture can be approximated, and this allows the behavior of cell membranes to longer pulses to be explored. Such an approach is ongoing and generates predictions of $U_m(t)$ and the transport of small charged molecules of type "s", $\vec{n}_s$ that are reasonable. Investigation of a planar membrane has also generated a surprise; the prediction of an approximate intrapulse plateau in U_m as a function of exponential pulse amplitude [58]. Whereas too simple to fully represent cellular electroporation, this prediction may be related to experimentally observed plateaus in charged molecular transport (see Section 7.6).

The various theoretical models support the idea that the reversibility of electroporation in planar membranes is due to (i) the chemical composition of the membrane, (ii) the pulse protocol, and (iii) feedback at the pore level that is associated with the spreading resistance, such that as a pore expands, the local transmembrane voltage across the pore decreases. Overall, considerable progress has been made in devising theoretical models that can quantitatively describe some aspects of electroporation, whereas others are still poorly understood. Mechanical and electrical aspects of electroporation of a relatively simple artificial planar BLM do account for (i) the approximate magnitude of U at which membrane rupture (irreversible breakdown) occurs, (ii) the strong dependence of membrane lifetime on U_m, and (iii) the stochastic nature of rupture. Moreover, a reasonable but not exact quantitative description of U_m is given by a transient aqueous pore theory, and the maximum fractional aqueous area of the membrane during reversible electroporation [58] agrees with limited experimental observations [59,60]. There has been some progress in predicting molecular transport, but much remains to be done, and the mechanisms of membrane recovery, cellular stress, and the determinants of cell survival or death are essentially not understood. Moreover, single pulse electroporation has been emphasized by theories and models to date, and relatively little is known about the importance of pulse shape, repetition, and spacing of multiple pulses. The challenge is to understand what changes persist and therefore represent the state of the membrane when second, and then additional pulses are applied.

7.6 Molecular and Ionic Transport

Greatly enhanced molecular and ionic transport is the basis of most all applications of electroporation. DNA introduction into cells for transfection was first reported about 25 years ago [52] and "transfection" has almost become synonymous with "electroporation" in some areas of biological research [91–94]. Delivery of drugs, proteins, and fluorescent indicators into cells and tissues is a basic manipulation that is also widely used in research, and is being adopted for clinical treatment of local cancer tumors [95–97]. Accordingly, by now numerous potential applications in biology, biotechnology, and medicine have been suggested, and many other applications are explored. The basic idea is qualitatively simple: application of one or more electrical pulses leads to elevated U_m, which if sufficiently high and long leads to membrane pore formation and subsequent expansion to transport water-soluble molecules under the influence of local driving forces (Figure 7.5). Quantitatively, however, surprisingly little is established theoretically using cell and tissue models. In the case of potential biomedical applications involving *in vivo* electroporation, more research will be needed to understand both efficacy and side effects.

Early studies of transport reported molecular release from biological vesicles due to a field-induced permeability increase [28]. Red blood cells were subsequently used to demonstrate DNA delivery into a cell that was associated with dielectric breakdown of the cell membrane [51]. This experiment did not, however, involve the critical demonstration of cell transfection. This achievement was reported several years later [52,98]. Molecular uptake

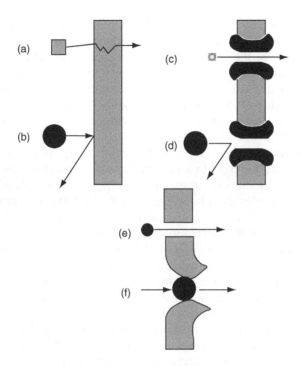

FIGURE 7.5

Schematized drawing of molecular transport pathways. These pathways are envisioned to exist in the intact or permeabilized lipid bilayer portion of a cell membrane or of an artificial bilayer membrane. The membrane may contain preexisting channels or induced pores. This cartoon can, with some restriction, be considered valid for multilayer structures, e.g., in the skin's stratum corneum. (a) Hydrophobic molecule, which is shown as a gray square can cross the lipid bilayer via partitioning and diffusion. (b) Hydrophilic molecule (large black dot), which is repelled from the lipid phase, cannot overcome a hydrophobic barrier. (c) Small ions (gray dot) can cross a membrane through narrow preexisting defects or proteinous channels. (d) Large polar molecules (large black dot) cannot pass through ion channels evolved to regulate small ion transport. (e) Electropores are large enough to provide effective transport of ions and polar particles of moderate size, with the size dependent on evolution of pores during a particular electrical pulse. (f) Bigger charged molecule (large black dot), e.g., plasmid DNA, can be forced by the local electric field to enlarge an electropore and then move across the membrane.

into cells has now been widely reported, with experiments typically using a large number of cells. These measurements determine the average molecular transport per cell by measuring a total cell population effect. Examples of delivered molecules in such experiments include antibodies [99–101], enzymes [47], and small molecules [1,102–105]. A few experiments obtained calibrated measurements that yielded that approximate number of molecules delivered into individual cells [1,102–105], with quantitative results needed for the development of theories and models for transport. Some of these experiments show that there is significant cell–cell variation in molecular transport.

Taken together these studies show that significant molecular transport occurs under approximately the same conditions that cause REB. This is an important finding, but does not address the question of how much molecular transport occurred for various pulsing conditions, nor was the question of cell–cell variation considered. One particularly interesting study showed that uptake of a first fluorescence-labeled molecule (fluorescence-labeled dextran; 19 kDa) was a reliable indicator for the uptake of a second, larger fluorescent molecule (phycoerythrin, 240 kDa) [106]. This report is consistent with the idea that electroporative molecular transport is a physical process (movement through aqueous pathways), which is relatively nonspecific if the pathway is not too close to the molecule's size. As mentioned earlier, studies with artifical planar BLMs show that electroporation depends on the history of the transmembrane voltage, $U_m(t)$. This implies that physical factors which govern field-induced change in U_m over a cell membrane should be important, i.e., the shape, size and orientation of cells with respect to the cells with respect to the local electric field. In addition to isolated cell models, a didactic multicellular model of a hypothetical local tissue region shows that individual cells can experience significantly different changes in U_m over each cell membrane [21].

Biological systems are also well known to be variable, e.g., displaying cell-to-cell variation in many properties ("biological variability"). At a nanometer scale, electroporation is believed to arise from fluctuations of water molecules and phospholipid molecules and also nearby ions or molecules that are transported through the membrane in the presence of an average elevated U_m. This view intrinsically arises in molecular dynamics (MD) simulations of artificial membrane electroporation [82–87] and is consistent with stochastic models based on analytic estimates [34,44,45,107]. For both analytic and MD analysis, the overall process of forming pores is fundamentally stochastic. Existing continuum models that exhibit REB have significant internal feedback between pore population ionic conduction and $U_m(t)$. This intrinsic regulation of the local transmembrane voltage is missing from the present MD analysis of electroporation.

Pore formation is expected to become more deterministic for pulses significantly shorter than 1 ns or for pores created in spatially restricted regions of a cell membrane, e.g., small phospholipid regions within the mitochondrial inner membrane [108]. However, conditions favoring deterministic pore creation have been uncommon to date. With this in mind, electroporation-related phenomena are expected to exhibit significant cell–cell variability. This in turn supports the idea that quantitative molecular transport determinations at both the population level and the individual cell level are important to understanding the magnitude and mechanisms of molecular transport.

Of the many possible molecular transport measurement methods, optical methods have the best combination of sensitivity, specificity, and speed. Both image analysis (quantitative microscopy) and flow cytometry make quantitative measurements at the individual cell level. This allows measurement of the number of molecules present by light absorbance (least sensitive) and by fluorescence or luminescence (most sensitive). With corrections for background and nonspecific binding to external cell surfaces, measurements can determine the number of molecules of type "s" taken up (or released), n_s, from individual cells. Image analysis and flow cytometry are generally complimentary. Flow cytometry makes spatially unresolved individual cell measurements at rates of 10^2–10^4 cell/s, and therefore routinely analyzes large cell populations. Image analysis excels at measurements with spatial resolution (of order 1 μm) but with increasingly improved temporal resolution that is best (fastest) for gated (strobed) image acquisition and generally less (slower) for rastered image acquisition. Both flow cytometric and image-based molecular uptake measurements are at their best when using molecular probes such as propidium iodide (PI) that exhibits major changes in fluorescence upon binding. Such test molecules are attractive because wash steps are avoided and measurement speed is governed by molecular (ionic) transport and binding kinetics combined with optical signal-to-noise ratio considerations. If confocal or two-photon microscopy were used with sufficiently large cells that a portion of the intracellular region can be volumetrically resolved, then molecular transport into an intracellular volume could be quantitatively monitored during the uptake process.

Image analysis also provides information about localization of molecular transport [109–112]. This has allowed observation of the degree of cellular uptake asymmetry.

In the case of suspended spherical cells the instantaneous transmembrane voltage, $U_m(t)$, at the two poles (consider $\theta = 0$, π in Equations 7.3 and 7.5 for pre-electroporated cells). These equations suggest that U_m will be increased at one pole and diminished at the other. A mammalian cell's resting potential (transmembrane voltage) is $U_{m,rest} \approx 60\text{–}90\,\text{mV}$ (cell interior negative with respect to exterior). Qualitatively, it could be expected that $U_{m,rest}$ adds at one pole and subtracts at the other. Quantitatively, this has been addressed by describing U_m during electroporation and finding that the fractional change is small except within the equatorial region [78]. Electroporation asymmetry can also be hypothesized as arising from a metabolically driven ionic current that passes through membrane leaks (the passive cell membrane resistance) to establish $U_{m,rest}$ and to also estimate changes due to electroporation shunting current through electropores [80]. Consideration of U_m alone is not expected to provide a full explanation. Whereas some experiments measure U_m [60,61], other experiments reporting asymmetry involve molecular transport observations [109–112], and in these cases, net transport should be understood.

An example of quantitative, individual cell level molecular transport determinations involved yeast cells in a medium containing $80\,\mu\text{M}$ PI (668 Da; charge of $z = +2$). Without electroporation there is negligible uptake. This is expected because of the large Born energy barrier (Equation 7.1) for small charged molecules, and doubly charged PI is a well-established "membrane exclusion dye" that is routinely used to test for cell membrane integrity [113]. However, a single square electric field pulse within the electrolyte ($E_e = 5 \times 10^3$ V/cm for a pulse with duration $t_{pulse} = 50\,\mu\text{s}$) results in a significant average uptake, viz. $\bar{n}_{PI} \approx 10^8$ molecules per cell. Flow cytometric fluorescence measurement is aided by PI binding to doubly stranded nucleic acids within the cell, which significantly increases PI fluorescence [103]. But for typical experimental conditions, PI fluorescence is weaker than calcein. Accordingly, in a subsequent example, red blood cell ghosts were suspended in an aqueous electrolyte with the green fluorescent polar tracer molecule, calcein (623 Da; net charge of $z = -4$) at a concentration of $1\,\text{mM}$. Calcein-exposed cells emit only very slight green fluorescence if unpulsed. This control case fluorescence is attributed to weak surface binding and autofluorescence. However, if a single "exponential pulse" $E_e(t) = E_{e,0}\exp{-t/\tau_{pulse}}$ with $\tau_{pulse} \approx 3$ ms and $E_{e,0} > 3 \times 10^3$ V/cm^{-1}, then a plateau in molecular uptake $\bar{n}_{Cal} \approx 7 \times 10^4$ molecules per ghost is observed. For the same conditions, but with fluorescence-labeled macromolecules $10\,\mu\text{M}$ lactalbumin (14.5 kDa; $z \approx -15$) and $10\,\mu\text{M}$ bovine serum albumin (BSA; 68 kDa; $z \approx -25$), an uptake plateau is also found, $\approx 7 \times 10^4$ molecules per ghost [114]. Surprisingly, for these single exponential pulse experiments, the plateau uptake per ghost is well below the estimated equilibrium value obtained by multiplying the supplied extracellular concentration and the ghost volume, $\bar{n}_{s,equi} = c_{ext} V_{ghost}$. Extension of these experiments to multiple pulses for BSA uptake shows that the plateau value for $\bar{n}_{BSA}$ increases with pulse number, but remains well below $\bar{n}_{BSA,\,equi}$. Finally, observation of an uptake plateau well below equilibrium holds for yeast experiments in which the effective partition coefficient between the extracellular medium and cell interior for calcein was estimated experimentally, [115] and for other experiments in which calcein uptake and clonal growth were both measured at the individual cell level [105].

The variation in individual cell uptake can also be determined and is significant. Yeast uptake of PI by a 50 μs square pulse and erythrocyte ghost uptake of calcein, fluorescence-labeled lactalbumin, and fluorescence-labeled BSA due to single ~1 ms exponential pulses show broad population distributions in the amount of uptake per cell without distinct subpopulations. In contrast, molecular uptake of calcein by a (*Saccharomyces cerevisiae*) subjected to a single ~1 ms exponential pulse exhibits several subpopulations that change markedly as the pulse amplitude is increased from an approximate threshold

$E_{e,0} \approx 1 \times 10^3$ V/cm and above threshold to $\sim 7 \times 10^3$ V/cm [115]. In spite of this significant heterogeneity, the average uptake per cell, $\bar{n}_{Cal}$ exhibits plateaus, with separate plateaus found for both a "major uptake subpopulation" and a "minor uptake subpopulation." Surprisingly, for these single exponential pulse experiments with yeast (elongated, budding), the plateau uptake per cell is well below (more than the order of magnitude smaller) than $\bar{n}_{equi}$, even after the intracellular or extracellular partition coefficient is included. In summary, several single pulse experiments have found uptake plateaus corresponding to nonequilibrium amounts. These results suggest that the plateau may be a consequence of molecular transport driven by local electric fields, e.g., electrophoresis. An approximate plateau in U_m is predicted by a transient aqueous pore model for an exponential pulse that causes electroporation [58]. If molecular transport is dominated by electrophoresis (or electro-osmosis) through rapidly changing pores during a pulse, then nonequilibrium net transport may therefore result. If instead molecular transport is dominated by diffusion during and after a pulse [116], then net transport can approach equilibrium values or can be less, depending on the number of pores and their lifetime. The total intracellular and extracellular volumes of the system, which is usually quite different for *in vitro* and *in vivo* conditions, (Equation 7.7) is also important [117].

Presently, quantitative molecular transport measurements at the individual cell level have been made on (i) red blood cell ghosts, for which the uptake per ghost was determined for calcein, lactalbumin, and BSA due to a single exponential pulse with a ~1 ms time constant and (ii) intact yeast (*S. cerevisiae*) *cells*, for which the uptake per cell was determined for PI because of a single 50 μs square pulse, and calcein, lactalbumin, and BSA because of an exponential pulse with a 1 ms time constant. It is therefore not yet established whether nonequilibrium uptake is a general feature, particularly for small charged molecules. Similarly, it is not yet known whether multiple pulses, pulses of other shapes, or certain features of the transported molecules are particularly important. In short, the mechanism of molecular transport is not yet understood in detail. For small molecules, the creation of a pore population probably occurs independently of molecular transport, but for larger molecules, particularly highly charged macromolecules such as DNA, electrically created pores may be significantly enlarged by interaction with approaching molecules driven by the local field (Figure 7.4).

In addition to electrophoresis through pores involving local, inhomogeneous electric fields, and time-dependent diffusion through pores, pulsed cells may be stimulated by presently unknown mechanisms to take up molecules by endocytosis [118]. External additional driving forces such as a pressure difference due to simultaneous or subsequent centrifugation may act to both enlarge primary (electric field-created) pores and to drive flow through the enlarged pores. Quantitative uptake measurements were also reported for mammalian cell experiments with submicrosecond (10–100 ns) megavolt-per meter scale (150 kV/cm) pulses in which extracellular media with smaller conductivity were used [67]. For these conditions with low extracellular conductivity media, significant cell deformation occurs. Cell deformation increases the challenge of understanding molecular transport through pores. Overall, the strongest evidence to date supports involvement of electrical drift (electrophoresis) for moving small charged molecules through pores, with diffusion contributing to both neutral and charged molecules. The interpretation of experiments that introduce highly charged DNA is consistent with local electrophoresis.

Moreover, a transient aqueous pore theoretical model involving only electrophoretic transport through a dynamic pore population created by a single exponential pulse, predicts some of the plateau behavior found for red blood cell ghosts and yeast cells. A tentative interpretation is that electroporation involves a rapid interaction between the membrane conductance due to pores, and the transmembrane voltage, $U_m(t)$. A slight increase in U_m results in rapid creation of many pores, which by a voltage divider effect tends to reduce U_m. This tendency to a nearly constant U_m seems to prevail during much, but not all, of the pulse duration, and this is qualitatively consistent with a local transmembrane electrophoretic transport that is independent of the pulse magnitude once a significant number of pores exist. Given the central importance of molecular transport to applications, considerably more development of basic insight into molecular transport mechanism is needed. Both the average and the variation in molecular uptake or release per cell is of basic importance to cellular electroporation, yet has even now received relatively little attention.

7.7 Electrotransfection

The delivery of DNA into cells *in vitro* is the predominant application of electroporation [91–94,119,120] and is extremely important. Molecular transport of DNA into cells by electric field pulsing was first reported in 1976 [51], but only as a demonstration of principle, since it did not alter cell function. Indeed, the first electrically induced gene transfer *in vitro* with subsequent expression was demonstrated in 1982 [52], and this stimulated a large number of papers demonstrating the applicability of electrotransfection to mammalian, plant, bacterial, and yeast protoplasts and cells. Electrotransfection has significant advantages: it is physical and therefore universal, effective, and often is the only method that gives positive results. For this reason, electrotransfection is actively pursued for human gene therapy based on two general approaches: (i) cells treated *in vitro* followed by reimplantation into the body [94,121–123] and (ii) cells transfected either in isolated tissues (e.g., plant tissue) or mammalian tissue *in vivo* [94,120,124–127]. For maximum utility, the efficiency of introduction of active DNA and cell survival must be simultaneously optimized, but understanding mechanisms involved in electroporation and downstream events remains inadequate.

Many investigators have reported a correlation between electroporation and electrotransfection. This could be interpreted as support for the role of electropores as the actual pathways for DNA transport. However, primary pores caused solely by an increased U_m by a short pulse are too small ($r_{p,min} \approx 10$ nm [73]) to accommodate DNA. Passive entry and diffusion through a moderately large pore ($r_p \approx 10$ nm) may allow DNA entry [128]. The frequency-of-occurrence of large pores ($r_p > 10$ nm) [58,129,130] and the possibility that entering DNA drives enlargement of a pore should also be considered. In any case, DNA uptake is usually not due to passive diffusion. Instead, the following driving forces were considered: (i) flow of water occurring due to the colloid-osmotic cell swelling following electropermeabilization [131], (ii) electro-osmotic flow through a pore with a charged interior surface [132], (iii) electrophoretic transfer of DNA through pores [133,134], and (iv) electrophoretically driven adsorption of DNA onto the membrane, followed by endocytosis which engulfs the DNA [118,135]. Other relatively recent experiments support the mechanism of electrophoresis by local electric fields focused (by the spreading resistance) through pores, such that DNA is carried into and through a pore that is actively enlarged by the electrically driven DNA [133,134].

The introduction of DNA by electroporation also increases the uptake of dextrans > 20 kDa supplied after pulsing. This occurs even if the dextran is added a few minutes after pulsing, implying a pore lifetime of 10–100 s. Moreover, the larger the DNA fragment, the greater the increase in permeability to the dextrans. The interpretation is that the use of a two-pulse technique (a large first pulse to create pores, a second long but much smaller to cause electrophoresis) provides separation of the primary electroporation process and subsequent field-driven transport through long lifetime pores. A DNA molecule may also prevent a DNA-occupied pore from closing, a foot-in-the-door mechanism that may lead to prolonged pore lifetimes. A fluctuating pore temporarily occupied by a macromolecule can allow small molecules to continue to be transported [89]. The introduction of highly charged heparin into the skin's stratum corneum by pulses believed to cause electroporation results in cotransport of small molecules that are consistent with this possibility [136].

An associated theory predicts that DNA in the electroporating electric field exerts high pressure on the membrane, which can then induce structural rearrangements of the membrane [137]. In this view, electrophoresis is the transport mechanism for DNA uptake, as it brings DNA to the cell surface and then drags DNA through the membrane, initially entering preexisting pores, which are then enlarged and deformed in course of translocation. This is an example of a process that leads to secondary pores, which are significantly different from the primary pores that arise solely by the interaction of the electric field with the membrane.

Molecular electroinsertion is distinct from transport of ions or molecules through a membrane. Experiments have shown that certain macromolecules can be inserted stably into cell membranes by pulses associated with electroporation [138–142]. A qualitative picture is that transient openings in the cell membrane provide an opportunity for such macromolecules to partially enter a pore and then become trapped as the pore shrinks. Perhaps one end of a membrane-spanning molecule is loosely bound to part of the membrane, such that the molecule can rotate into a pore, only to become trapped as the pore shrinks and eventually vanishes. Electroinsertion is such a fascinating event that it deserves conceptual emphasis, even though relatively few studies have been made since its discovery.

Electrofusion provides somatic hybridization of cells [121,122,143–149]. This has led to demonstrations of cell–tissue fusion [150,151], hybridomas for antibody production [92,152], individual cell and vesicle manipulation [153,154], tumor vaccine production [155,156], and other applications [91,93,157]. But the mechanism of cell electrofusion is still not fully understood. The understanding we do have comes from different types of studies. Experiments using model systems consisting of two planar lipid bilayers have provided significant insight [70]. After pressure application, the bilayers reach a state of close contact. Close proximity is usually necessary for cell electrofusion. The distance between bilayers is determined by the equilibrium of all acting forces: molecular, electrostatic, hydrostatic pressure, and hydrational. After a lag time, one or more bridges (stalks) form spontaneously between two adjacent monolayers. These bridges then expand, leading to a so-called trilaminar structure, which contains a single bilayer in contact with two bilayers along a perimeter. A trilaminar structure is rather stable, but after a voltage pulse is applied, electroporation occurs, followed by an irreversible rupture of the contact bilayer with its transition to so-called membrane tube. This stage of the process results in fusion because now there are joined lipid phase and water compartments. It is important to note that two different structural rearrangements take place: (i) stalk (or bridge) formation between adjacent monolayers and (ii) pore formation in contact bilayer with measurable time lag. Note that the first stage is essentially spontaneous, and that the electric field is involved only during the second stage of the fusion process.

Additional insight follows from noting that the probability of stalk formation depends on its energy, which in turn is determined by the favorable molecular geometry of phospholipid molecules. From the viewpoint of continuous media mechanics, this implies a dependence on the spontaneous curvature of monolayers. This theory was compared with the results of experiments in which lag times were measured for membranes with different spontaneous curvatures. Good agreement was obtained, supporting the view that the stalk mechanism is involved in lipid bilayers fusion.

Cell fusion is much more complicated. Attempts to find evidence for trilaminar structures in electrically pulsed cell suspensions have not been successful. For this reason, another fusion mechanism and the interaction of coaxial electropores at adjacent membranes have been considered [158]. In this case, it was shown that attractive forces due to the Maxwell tension between two parallel bilayers with coaxial pores are large enough to almost bend the membranes and to bring the pores together until a fusion of pore edges is achieved. These two mechanisms differ in their sequence of events: (i) monolayer fusion and followed by electroporation (the first case; see above) and (ii) electroporation followed by fusion of pore edges (the second case). Significantly, it has been experimentally demonstrated [159,160] that fusion can also proceed using a protocol in which pulsing precedes cell contact. This supports the mechanism of fusion through electropores. Additional understanding of electrofusion should therefore depend on further developments in the understanding of electroporation.

Extension of cell–cell electrofusion *in vitro* to cell–tissue *in vivo* has been briefly described [150,151] and offers the prospect of many applications in research and medicine. In this case, critical issues involve making contact between the introduced cells or vesicles to the target tissue and then causing a high probability of fusion while retaining the viability of both the introduced cells and the target tissue.

7.8 Membrane Recovery

Membrane recovery after pulsing is fundamentally important to understanding whether an electroporation protocol is reversible at the membrane level and at the cellular level. Terminology includes "resealing" and "pore lifetime." According to the transient aqueous pore hypothesis, recovery is expected to involve shrinkage and disappearance of pores, with some models further assuming that pores shrink to a minimum size before stochastically vanishing. However, quantitative data that constrain membrane recovery mechanisms remain relatively scarce and are often indirect. For example, molecular uptake observations are often used, which depend on more than pore shrinkage and destruction.

The scientific literature contains reports with widely varied membrane recovery times, from nanoseconds to minutes at room temperature to 37°C and even longer at low temperatures. Here, we cite several examples, beginning with several papers with data relevant to membrane barrier recovery. These include molecular and ionic uptake on human erythrocytes ($\tau_p \approx 1$–10 h and strongly dependent on temperature, with much longer resealing at 3°C than at 37°C), on isolated rat skeletal muscle cells ($\tau_p \approx 500$ s) [161], PI uptake by electropermeabilized myeloma cells ($\tau_p \approx 100$ s) [162], dye uptake ($\tau_p \approx 120$ s) [163], Ca^{2+} influx into vesicles ($\tau_p \approx 165$ ms) [111], and into adherent cultured cells (τ_p timescale of milliseconds to seconds) [164]. As these examples illustrate, there is a wide range of membrane recovery timescales for molecular uptake, but with artifical membranes often faster than cellular membranes. Electrical measurements can also be used and have the advantage that the transported species (small ions at a high concentration: Na^+, K^+, and Cl^-) are preexisting throughout cells, so they do not require delivery by mixing and diffusion to reach cell membranes. Examples are electrical measurements on isolated frog-muscle cell membranes [165] ($\tau_p \approx 500$ s), on cell suspensions and cell pellets, and on artificial planar BLM. Molecular dynamics simulations of electroporation are relatively recent and suggest pore lifetimes of a only few nanoseconds [86], which is difficult to reconcile with experimental values based on ionic and molecular transport.

Both reversible and irreversible electroporation lead rapidly (typically 1–100 µs) to a high conductance state, which discharges the membrane after pulsing or provides a small membrane resistance that participates in a voltage divider effect to reduce the transmembrane voltage, even during the pulse [58]. By definition, irreversible behavior has no physical membrane recovery, and recovery by biological repair of significant membrane openings due to large magnitude or longlasting pulses has not yet been investigated. In considering what is known about membrane recovery, it was noted above that both electrical and molecular assessments of membrane barrier function can be made.

Early experiments used electrical measurements and planar membranes to show that after a decrease in the voltage, there is a very rapid (<5 µs) decrease in the membrane conductance [62,166]. Initially, this result was interpreted as reflecting rapid resealing of pores [166]. It was later shown, however, that a rapid decrease in conductance is associated with the nonlinear behavior of a pore's current–voltage curve [56,167,168]. The number and the mean radius of the pores were unchanged on a timescale of microseconds, but in the timescale of 1–10 ms, the decrease in conductance is governed by a change in the size of the pores. For artificial planar BLMs, pores disappear from the membrane on a timescale of milliseconds. For cell membranes, the timescale for the disappearance of pores is much longer, ranging from seconds to hours [56].

Electrical assessment of recovery has the advantage of speed and convenience, but testing for restoration of membrane barrier function by probing with molecules of different sizes and charges may fundamentally be more revealing as to the extent and kinetics of recovery. Indeed, several studies have reported the results of delayed addition experiments, with probe molecules supplied to pulsed cells at different times after pulsing. As expected, the qualitative observation from experiments using total population measurements is that significantly less uptake occurs if molecules are added to the extracellular medium after the pulse. Typically, the added molecules are small [169], but sometimes macromolecules, including DNA, were used [134]. An important finding is that if analytical techniques with individual cell level capability (microscopy, flow cytometry, image analysis) are used, then subpopulations with uptake of delayed addition molecules are observed [115,152,170,171]. Factors affecting membrane recovery kinetics have not yet been thoroughly investigated. However, some experiments show that reduced temperatures lead to much longer membrane recovery times [172]. This is not surprising, as the diffusive pore shrinking that is expected as the membrane discharges are expected to have this qualitative temperature dependence. Moreover, most physical and chemical processes of multi-molecular systems are characterized by one or more rates that have Boltzmann factors, with their strong, nonlinear reduction in rate at lower temperature.

Pulses that lead to pore formation and evolution are expected to involve a dynamic pore population with time-dependent pore size distributions [57,58]. For this reason, the change with time of the membrane's ability to exclude molecules of different sizes and charge should provide additional insight into the membrane recovery process. Indeed, experiments have shown that if molecules are first presented to cells at increasing time delays after pulsing, then a decreasing fraction of cells have a persistent ability to take up molecules [170]. This suggests that a subpopulation of cells has metastable pores with a distribution of pore lifetimes. Enhanced recovery by adding certain surfactants has been demonstrated [173,174]. The discovery of enhancement both challenges our understanding of what membrane recovery is and offers promise as a therapy for electrical injury that involves nonthermal membrane damage by otherwise irreversible electroporation.

7.9 Cell Stress and Survival

Most *in vitro* applications of electroporation benefit from some understanding of cell survival, but for *in vivo* applications, it is becoming essential. *In vitro* electroporation often focuses on delivery of molecules into the cytosol, but for some research studies [175–177] related to nonthermal electrical injury [174,178,179] and harvesting of cellular products [180] release of molecules is sought.

A general observation over many experiments is that as the field magnitude is increased for a given pulse shape, phenomena such as molecular uptake become significant at a "fuzzy threshold" (dependent on pulse shape, including pulse duration), and then increase. However, at about the same "fuzzy threshold," cell viability begins to decrease, with almost all cells getting killed as the electric field is increased. Although the mechanism of cell killing by electroporation is not fully established, a plausible hypothesis is that cell survival or death is mainly due to the degree of molecular exchange between cells and their environment and the resulting cell stress due to chemical imbalances [170,181,182]. This is consistent with the observation that cell killing can occur without significant heating [25–27,174,183] and that a tremendous increase in membrane permeability and associated molecular transport occurs.

A transient pore population and also possibly a small number of metastable pores are expected, and all may contribute to stress-inducing transport. Thus, reversible membrane electroporation (complete resealing or pore disappearance) may still lead to net transport (uptake or release). This means that relatively nonspecific molecular exchange may occur between the intracellular and extracellular volumes and can lead to stress-inducing chemical imbalances. Depending on the ratio of intracellular and extracellular volumes, the composition of the extracellular medium and the cell type, a cell may not recover from the associated biochemical imbalance (stress) and will therefore die. Both reversible and irreversible electroporations result in transient openings (perforations) of the membrane, which are often large enough that the pores are not selective. In this case, molecular transport is expected to be nonspecific. It is plausible that a portion of the cell membrane behaves much like a small planar membrane and undergoes rupture (irreversible electroporation). Just as in the case of reversible electroporation, significant molecular transport between the intracellular and extracellular volumes may lead to a significant chemical imbalance. If this imbalance is too large, recovery may not occur, resulting in cell death. It has been hypothesized [182] that the volumetric ratio

$$F_{vol} = \frac{V_{extracellular}}{V_{intracellular}} \tag{7.7}$$

should correlate with cell survival or death. In this equation, $V_{extracellular}$ is the volume of liquid medium outside the cell and $V_{intracellular}$ is the volume of liquid in the cell interior. The idea is that, for a given cell type and extracellular medium composition, $F_{vol} \gg 1$ (typical of *in vitro* conditions such as cell suspensions and anchorage-dependent cell culture) should tend to favor cell death. The other extreme is typical of *in vivo* tissue conditions ($F_{vol} \approx 0.15$, a higher interstitial fluid fraction) and this should favor cell survival. The dilution of released molecules is governed by F_{vol} and partitioning between the extracellular and intracellular environments [115]. For example, if the partition coefficient is one, the maximum *in vivo* initial dilution factor in solid tissue should be $1/0.15 \approx 7$, whereas the expected dilution is several orders of magnitude larger for typical *in vitro* conditions. This suggests that for the same degree of electroporation, significantly less damage may occur in tissue than in body fluids or under most *in vitro* conditions. With time, however, released molecules can diffuse within the interstitial space, be cleared by blood perfusion, and then distributed by the systemic circulation. The ultimate fate of released molecules is governed by excretion, metabolism, and storage, which is traditionally described by pharmacokinetics.

Cell viability of culturable cells can be stringently tested by clonal growth assays, whereas diffentiated cells are often assessed by assaying particular functions, such as membrane exclusion dyes. However, caution should be exercised in assessing cell viability after electroporation protocols. After all, there is little *a priori* justification for using membrane-exclusion dyes (e.g., trypan blue [960 D, $z = -4$], PI [668 D, $z = +2$]), because electroporation causes the membrane permeability to significantly increase by unknown amounts for unknown times. Membrane-exclusion dyes are generally larger than some small ions and molecules (e.g., Ca^{2+}). Uptake or release of such ions and molecules may occur even if membrane recovery has progressed to the point that membrane-exclusion dyes are excluded by the membrane. Without validation, it cannot be assured that the cell membrane has recovered sufficiently that fatal chemical imbalances are avoided. Instead, relevant functional tests should be considered. If electroporation is to be optimally used, a significantly better understanding of the mechanism of cell death will be needed.

7.10 Tissue Electroporation and *In Vivo* Delivery

A purposeful electroporation of tissue *in vivo* and *in vitro* has been motivated by therapeutic interventions such as tumor treatment by delivery of anticancer drugs [97,184], gene therapy by delivery of DNA, and other genetic material [94,126,127,185], and delivery of various sized molecules into and across the skin [184,186–188]. Undesirable consequences of tissue electroporation have also been identified. A major insight is that tissue electroporation is the source of a nonthermal contribution to electrical injury [174,178,179,183]. Tissue electroporation has also been identified as a side effect to defibrillation interventions [72,189–191]. Finally, tissue electroporation may be relevant to neuromuscular incapacitation (stunning) pulses [192].

Describing the response of many closely spaced cells to an applied pulse is central to understanding electroporation of solid tissue. A fundamental attribute of cells is that applied electric fields result in response fields that are largest in lipid-based membranes, which have an effective high resistivity even in the presence of many ion channels. This is the basis of the amplification associated with Equation 7.3. Although well established at the cellular level [19,20,54], the corresponding concentration of electric fields in tissues has received less attention [21]. Here we emphasize that this voltage-concentrating effect means that electroporation of other lipid-based barriers should occur preferentially. For preferential electroporation, two features should be sought: (i) tissue barriers comprised mainly of lipids and (ii) mechanical deformability (compliance) of membranes comprise of the particular lipids so that the electrostatically favored entry of water into a deform-able phospholipid-based membrane results in the creation of aqueous pathways.

In many solid tissues, there are significant spaces between most cells, such that for small electric fields the electrical currents at low frequencies flow mainly between the cells. In this case, tissue electroporation consists of electroporation of individual cells whose behavior is expected in many respects to be similar to the electroporation of isolated cells, but with two major differences: (i) the local extracellular electric field depends in a complicated way on many other neighboring cells [21,193] and (ii) the ratio of the extracellular to intracellular volumes (Equation 7.7) is usually small, just the opposite of most *in vitro* electroporation conditions. This means that if chemical exchange between the intracellular and extracellular volumes is the main cause of cell stress and therefore cell death, tissue electroporation may be intrinsically less damaging than most *in vitro* electroporation conditions.

Tumor tissue is an important example of tissue for which many cells have intercellular aqueous pathways. Even without electroporation, there is a significant physiological resistance to entry of anticancer drugs because of limited blood perfusion, elevated interstitial pressure, and relatively large distances to blood vessels [194]. Not only does electroporation greatly reduce the main barrier (that of a cell membrane itself), tissue electroporation should also reduce these physiological resistances. For typical cancer chemotherapy conditions, blood perfusion delivers the anticancer drug to sites within a tumor and the drug then diffuses across the avascular regions. Local tissue electroporation should create aqueous pathways that assist drug movement and that may also relieve pressure, but the fourth power dependence of volumetric flow on pathway size implies that significant water flow may be more difficult than diffusion and drift of small drugs. But if the primary pores created electrically subsequently expand, then flow may be successful in reducing the pressure, and perfusion should increase. Diffusional barriers should also be reduced because of the new aqueous pathways. Striking results have, in fact, been reported in experimental tumor systems, mainly using the drug bleomycin, which is a potent drug that ordinarily does not cross the membrane readily [119,195–197]. Importantly, clinical use has been vigorously pursued [95,97,198–200]. Initial results were often obtained by treating surface tumors (nodules) [95]. More generalized use requires electrode access to provide localized electric field pulses to the targeted tumors [201–203]. As a partial guide, the use of electrical impedance measurements or even electrical impedance imaging can be considered [204,205].

Interestingly, there is a significant economic barrier to a general approach to local tumor treatment and ECT-specialized drugs (e.g., molecules with significant charge) that do not passively cross the cell membrane. Almost all approved anticancer drugs (the striking exception is bleomycin) readily cross the cell membrane, actively or passively. Accordingly, such molecules do not enjoy a tremendous increase in delivery by electroporation. Thus, even though it should be fundamentally attractive to use tissue electroporation with cell membrane-impermeant drugs, e.g., an established drug with several charge groups added that are quickly cleaved by intracellular enzymes to greatly reduce side effects, the modified drug will be regarded as new; the expensive and lengthy approval process for new drugs is a significant disincentive.

Tissues that are comprised of one or more monolayers of cells in which the cells are connected by tight junctions are somewhat favored to experience voltage concentration across their membranes. Such tissues form the linings of organs and other specialized structures, such as the lining of sweat gland ducts [206]. An example of such behavior is found in a didactic, multicellular model [21,193]. Qualitatively, the main barrier of each cell monolayer consists of two cell membranes in series and can therefore be regarded approximately as two planar BLMs in series. In fact, some tissues such as frog skin and toad bladder are plausible approximations to an ideal single cell monolayer tissue, in which a single cell monolayer is the main barrier. For this reason, such tissues provide a convenient experimental system that allows a convenient investigation of electrical behavior of tissue electroporation [207]. In contrast, recent experiments have focused on molecular transport into or through epithelia [208–211]. More complicated and realistic models of regions of a tissue with a layer of cells connected by tight junctions are now becoming available [21,193].

Transdermal drug delivery has long been of interest, with both chemical and physical "enhancers" being pursued [188]. Skin electroporation is one of the approaches based on physical intervention [184,186,187]. Mammalian skin is a complicated tissue. It has both the specialized barrier structure, the stratum corneum (SC), and appendages, sweat ducts and hair follicles, which perforate the SC [212–214]. The SC is the skin's main barrier. It is a dead tissue whose barrier properties are often described by using a "brick wall model" [215]. The "bricks" are corneocytes, which contain cross-linked keratin and increase in volume by up to a factor of 5 if the SC is hydrated, the usual condition for transdermal drug delivery. The "mortar" is the intervening lipid, which surrounds the corneocytes, and exists as mostly parallel bilayers made of special (nonphospholipid) lipids, with about 5–6 bilayers between each of the approximately 20 rows of corneocytes. The SC is mechanically flexible but tough, essentially impenetrable to most infectious microorganisms and very impermeable to water-soluble molecules, particularly charged molecules, as the lipids are present as about 100 bilayers in series. The corneocytes are residual entities, left over from cells that migrated outwards to form the SC, with the multilamellar lipid bilayer providing most of the barrier function of the skin. Clearly, this very effective barrier has evolved to provide protection, but it also presents a major barrier to potential medical interventions, viz. transdermal drug delivery [188] and extraction of chemical analytes, e.g., glucose within the subcutaneous interstitial fluid, for minimally invasive sensing [216–218].

The skin's appendages (sweat gland ducts and hair follicles) are usually lined with an extension of the SC, or, deeper within the skin, by a double layer of living cells connected by tight junctions [206]. Both the appendageal barriers and the SC barrier are candidates for electroporation, but at very different transbarrier voltages, U_{barrier}. The double cell lining of sweat ducts should experience electroporation at about $U_{\text{barrier}} \approx 2$–$4\,\text{V}$, but the approximately 100 multilamellar bilayers of the SC need $U_{\text{barrier}} \approx 50$–$100\,\text{V}$ for pulses with duration of $100\,\mu\text{s}$ to $1\,\text{ms}$, i.e., about 0.5–1 V per lipid bilayer [219–222].

Electroporation of skin and other tissues can be studied *in vitro* using a well-established apparatus, a permeation chamber [223], which is a version of the Ussing chamber originally used for molecular flux and electrical studies of epithelial tissues [224]. Two- and four-electrode systems can be used for electrical stimulation and measurement, and in addition, molecular transport measurements can be made by supplying molecules in the donor chamber and removing aliquots at intervals from the acceptor chamber for chemical assay. Experiments of this type with human skin show that if exponential pulses with $U_{\text{SC},0} \approx 50$–$300\,\text{V}$ and time constant $\tau_{\text{pulse}} \approx 1$ ms are applied every 5 s for 1 h, then there is an enhancement by up to a factor of 10^4 in the flux of charged molecules of up to about 1 kDa [186,225]. Companion electrical impedance measurements show a rapid (≤ 25 ms) decrease in skin resistance [226], and both molecular flux and electrical measurements show that either reversible or irreversible behavior occurs, depending on the transdermal pulse amplitude, $U_{\text{SC},0}$. Several *in vivo* experiments show that transdermal delivery can be achieved with minimal damage [186,227–229]. This is consistent with the theoretical estimates of associated heating within the nearby viable epidermis [230].

Extension of this type of *in vitro* method to almost continuous measurement of transdermal molecular flux uses a sampling stream and quantitative, computer-controlled spectrofluorimetry to measure two fluorescent molecule concentrations at alternating intervals, so that with deconvolution, two molecular fluxes and passive electrical properties can be determined for each skin preparation [231]. A faster responding, single flux version of the same method allows the demonstration of both the large magnitude and the rapid onset and cessation of the flux of calcein (623 D, $z = -4$) and supports the view that skin electroporation can deliver small pharmaceuticals with rapid delivery onset [232]. Such methods provide a flexible approach to characterize new aqueous pathways created by skin electroporation.

Gene therapy based on physical introduction of genetic material into cells *in vivo* is of great and growing interest and includes tissue electroporation [94,126,127,185,233]. Electroporation-based gene therapy is related to electrochemotherapy of tumors by introduction of bleomycin or other anticancer drugs, but with the significant difference that gene therapy requires delivery of large molecules (e.g., DNA), whereas traditional anticancer drugs are small. This is consistent with the use of smaller, longer electroporating pulses in gene therapy [129,130,234]. If the desired therapy does not require that all cells in a tissue be modified, local tissue electroporation can be used to treat some cells. The modified cells can, for example, secrete a therapeutic molecule. An early, partial demonstration was based on subcutaneous injection of DNA followed by surface electrodes for *in vivo* electroporation, leading to transformation of some cells [124]. Major advances have since occurred [94,126,127,185]. As with all new technologies, undesired side effects must be considered and understood along with possible uses.

Thus, the possibility of tissue damage must also be considered. Fortunately, major advances in understanding the role of electroporation in tissue damage has been achieved, through a series of studies motivated by the hypothesis that electroporation can account for a nonthermal permeabilization of cell membranes [174,178,179]. Although electrical injury to tissue has in the past been interpreted as a thermal denaturation phenomenon, more recent studies make a convincing case that electroporation can be a significant factor, particularly for the larger cells such as skeletal muscle cells and nerve cells [183]. Moreover, the demonstration that certain surfactants can significantly accelerate membrane barrier function recovery has offers a basis for therapy after electrical shock injury [173,174,235]. Not only have surfactants such as Poloxamer–188 been pursued as a damage-minimizing therapeutic for electrical injury, this polymer is active against damage due to ionizing radiation that also causes cell membrane permeabilization [236] (see Chapter 10 in *BMA*). Damaging consequences of tissue electroporation are also relevant to the strong electrical pulses which are widely used to stimulate fibrillating hearts [72,189–191], and this is an active research area. In this case, alteration of electrical behavior has often been emphasized.

Tissue electroporation thus has compelling potential advantages for medical interventions. A general attribute is that it achieves chemical results, transport of molecules into desired sites, without leaving another chemical residue such as the transdermal drug delivery enhancer dimethyl sulfoxide. Perhaps even more important, however, is the fact that electroporation is caused electrically, and the tissue experiencing electroporation can be rapidly assessed electrically, e.g., by impedance measurements. This means that much better control of molecular transport for drug delivery and analyte extraction may be possible. In spite of tremendous progress, it is nevertheless true that a better fundamental understanding of electroporation mechanism is needed. The characteristics of such pathways need to be better established quantitatively, in terms of both molecular transport and electrical properties. Also, the potential side effects of possible tissue damage must be confronted, and the trade-off between desired and undesired consequences understood. This is a classic challenge.

Several potential applications of tissue electroporation have now been identified and are vigorously pursued [94,97,126,127,184]. Understanding tissue electroporation thus has several motivations. Unintended exposure to electric fields such as those due to lightning and contact or close approach to electrical power sources or distribution wiring can cause nonthermal tissue damage [174,178,179]. Stunning (neuromuscular incapacitation) devices may also cause tissue electroporation or membrane channel denaturation. Although some acute side effect possibilities have been considered [192,237–240], the spatially distributed fields within the body should be investigated to obtain a thorough understanding of both efficacy and potential side effects.

7.11 Electroporation of Organelles

Most models of cells focus on the outer, plasma membrane. At low frequencies and small applied-field amplitudes, the response field is excluded from the cell interior and the site of organelles with their own single or double membranes. However, very-short field pulses have high-frequency content and can lead to displacement currents and associated transient intracellular electric fields [80,81,241]. A recent analysis shows that absolute rate theory can plausibly account for pore creation on a nanosecond timescale at a transmembrane voltage of $U_m \approx 1.2\,V$. This supports the use of spatially distributed cell models that are based on the asymptotic model of membrane electroporation [80,81]. Such models show that extensive poration occurs for submicrosecond, megavolt-per-meter pulses. Further, the area pore density is exceptionally large. In the plasma membrane, this leads to intracellular ionic conduction currents and associated large fields within the cell [61,80,81]. According to initial cell models involving the supraelectroporation hypothesis [80,81], an extremely large pore density (pores per area) is predicted for the cell's outer plasma membrane and also internal organelle membranes. This means that pores are extremely close together, and this in turn suggests that deterministic membrane deformation should be expected [108] to create a large membrane conductance that limits the magnitude of U_m to ~1 V [61].

The supraelectroporation hypothesis predicts that for very large intracellular fields, the membranes of organelles should also electroporate [81]. Indeed, a striking experimental observation shows that intracellular granules take up calcein from the cytosol [242], with organelle membrane electroporation as the likely cause. Following this report of *in situ* organelle electroporation, there have been a growing number of studies supporting the view that extremely large field pulses cause intracellular effects.

Many of these investigations find evidence for apoptosis, not the prompt necrosis that is consistent with a large increase in plasma membrane permeability by conventional electroporation [243–253]. These experiments involve electric field pulses of durations between 7 and 300 ns and with intensities from 360 to 10 kV/cm. Such pulses cause intracellular effects such as cytochrome *c* release, caspase activation, phosphatidylserine (PS) translocation, disruption of nuclear DNA, vesicle membrane electroporation, and molecular uptake into subcellular granules [242,244–252,254]. It is important to note that apoptosis and necrosis are distinguished as the two major types of cell death [255–259]. Prompt necrosis is known to be an outcome of excessive conventional electroporation when the pulses are sufficiently long, intense, or repeated enough times [108,174,179,260–262]. Apoptosis (programmed cell death) is usually stimulated by biochemical perturbation of molecular signaling pathways [258,263–267] and not by the application of electrical fields. Indeed, apoptosis has only occasionally been reported to follow conventional electroporation [268,269]. Although significant phosphatidylserine (PS) translocation occurs in the plasma membrane (PM) of red blood cells for conventional electroporation pulses (kV/cm^{-1}) [270–272], some of these recent studies with extremelylarge (~100 kV/cm^{-1}) field pulses show extensive PS translocation [252,273]. Nevertheless, some experiments report insignificant uptake of membrane integrity dyes such as PI and that plasma membrane electroporation is minimal or has not occurred [243,245,246,248,250–252,273,274]. This suggests that the PM permeabilization for at least some molecules is only minimally increased by these pulses. Even though the applied fields are extremely strong, their effects are nonthermal due to the limited pulse duration (from 7 to 300 ns). Often, the pulse intensity is adjusted to limit the Joule heating per pulse to $\sigma_e E_{app}^2 \Delta t \sim 1.7$ J/mL, where σ_e is the electrolyte conductivity, E_{app} is the applied field intensity, and Δt is the pulse duration. In this case, the corresponding adiabatic (assumption of zero heat conduction; a worst case) temperature rise is only ~0.4°C per pulse.

The use of these ultrashort (submicrosecond), extreme (10–300 kV/cm) pulses is relatively new, but has generated intense interest. The mechanism underlying the observed intracellular effects has not yet been established. One hypothesis is that ultrashort, extreme pulses cause irreversible effects at the membrane level, either membrane rupture or electrically based membrane protein denaturation [85,275–279]. Supraelectroporation is another hypothesis. It predicts that there is a massive creation of transient pores, which expand negligibly because of the short pulse duration, and this leads to full reversibility at the membrane level [80,81]. This is qualitatively consistent with avoiding prompt necrosis, because most ions and molecules should be retained by membranes with minimum size (~0.8 nm) pores. The observed irreversible effects at the cellular level then arise from ionic and molecular transport through pores, which includes phospholipid translocation and other downstream events. As noted above, a contribution to irreversibility may also arise from electro-denaturation (long-lived membrane channel conformational changes induced by the supraphysiologic transmembrane voltage; ~0.3 V) [280–282], a magnitude that is achieved by both conventional and supraelectroporation. However, the duration of $U_m \approx 1$ V decreases by several orders of magnitude in going from conventional to supraelectroporation, and the kinetics of the membrane protein conformational changes are not yet known. In any case, the basic idea is that for the largest of these fields, a very large number of pores are created in all of a cell's membranes, such that the field penetrates into the cell interior and also the organelle membranes, with the intracellular electric field nearly equal to the applied electric field, even after displacement currents have decayed [80]. That is, poration is so extensive that ionic current flows through the cell's membrane, in marked contrast to low-field responses in which current flows predominantly around the cell [80,81]. This opens the conceptual possibility of distinct effects due to electroporation of various types of organelles. For example, if pore lifetimes are long (as often inferred from conventional electroporation experiments), then it may be possible to gate open the mitochondrial permeability transition pore (MPTP) [108], which appears to require depolarizing the inner mitochondrial membrane (IMM) for many seconds [283]. However, other mechanism hypotheses are proposed. At the time of this writing, the cause of intracellular effects by extreme field pulses has not yet been established, but is likely to involve electroporation.

Acknowledgments

This study is supported partially by NIH grant RO1-GM63857 and an AFOSR/DOD MURI grant on "Subcellular Responses to Narrowband and Wideband Radio Frequency Radiation," administered through Old Dominion University.

References

1. B. Poddevin, S. Orlowski, J. Belehradek Jr., and L.M. Mir. Very high cytotoxicity of bleomycin introduced into the cytosol of cells in culture. *Biochem. Pharmacol.*, 42(Suppl.):567–575, 1991.
2. R.V. Davalos, L.M. Mir, and B. Rubinsky. Tissue ablation and irreversible electroporation. *Ann. Biomed. Eng.*, 33:223–231, 2005.
3. R. Nuccitelli, U. Pliquett, X. Chen, W. Ford, R.J. Swanson, S.J. Beebe, J.F. Kolb, and K.H. Schoenbach. Nanosecond pulsed electric fields cause melanomas to self-destruct. *Biochem. Biophys. Res. Comm.*, 343:351–360, 2006.
4. S.K. Frandsen, H. Gissel, P. Hojman, T. Tramm, J. Eriksen, and J. Gehl. Direct therapeutic applications of calcium electroporation to effectively induce tumor necrosis. *Cancer Res.*, 72:1336–1341, 2012.
5. L. Galluzzi, J.M. Bravo-San Pedro, and G. Kroemer. (108 authors total) Essential versus accessory aspects of cell death: Recommendations of the NCCD 2015. *Cell Death Diff.*, 22:58–73, 2015.
6. E. Sözer, Z.A. Levine, and P.T. Vernier. Quantitative limits on small molecule transport via the electroper- meome measuring and modeling single nanosecond perturbations. *Sci. Rep.*, 7:57–1–57–13, 2017.
7. T. Kotnik. Lightning-triggered electroporation and electrofusion as possible contributors to natural horizontal gene transfer. *Phys. Life Rev.*, 10:351–370, 2013.
8. T. Kotnik. Prokaryotic diversity, electrified DNA, lightning waveforms, abiotic gene transfer, and the Drake equation: Assessing the hypothesis of lightning-driven evolution. *Phys. Life Rev.*, 10:384– 388, 2013.
9. D.W. Deamer and J.P. Dworkin. Chemistry and physics of primitive membranes. *Top. Curr. Chem.*, 259:1–27, 2005.
10. J.C. Blain and J.W. Szostak. Progress toward synthetic cells. *Ann. Rev. Biochem.*, 83:615–640, 2014.
11. J.C. Weaver. Estimating the contribution of lightning to microbial evolution: Guidance from the Drake equation *Comment on Lightning-triggered electroporation and electrofusion as possible contributors to natural horizontal gene transfer by Tadej Kotnik. Phys. Life Rev.*, 10:373–376, 2013.
12. B.L. Ibey, J.C. Ullery, O.N. Pakhomova, C.C. Roth, I. Semenov, H.T. Beier, M. Tarango, S. Xiao, K.H. Schoenbach, and A.G. Pakhomov. Bipolar nanosecond electric pulses are less efficient at electrop- ermeabilization and killing cells than monopolar pulses. *Biochem. Biophys. Res. Commun.*, 443:568–573, 2013.
13. A.G. Pakhomov, I. Semenov, S. Xiao, O.N. Pakhomova, B. Gregory, K.H. Schoenbach, J.C. Ullery, H.T. Beier, S.R. Rajulapati, and B.L. Ibey. Cancellation of cellular responses to nanoelectroporation by reversing the stimulus polarity. *Cell. Mol. Life Sci.*, 22:4431–4441, 2014.
14. T.R. Gowrishanker, J.V. Stern, K.C. Smith, and J.C. Weaver. Nanopore occlusion by external moleclues: A biophysical mechanism for bipolar cancellation in cell membrances. *Biochem. Biophys. Res. Commun.* pii: S0006-291X(18)31519-5, 2018. doi:10.1016/j.bbrc.2018.07.024. [Epub ahead of print].
15. J. Darnell, H. Locish, and D. Baltimore. *Molecular Cell Biology*. Scientific American Books, New York, 1986.
16. V.A. Parsegian. Energy of an ion crossing a low dielectric membrane: Solutions to four relevant electrostatic problems. *Nature*, 221:844–846, 1969.
17. V.A. Parsegian. Ion-membrane interactions as structural forces. *Ann. NY Acad. Sci.*, 264:161–174, 1975.

18. K.R. Foster and H.P. Schwan. Dielectric properties of tissues. In C. Polk and E. Postow, Eds., *Handbook of Biological Effects of Electromagnetic Fields*, 2nd ed., CRC Press, Boca Raton, 1996, pp. 25–102.

19. J. Gimsa and D. Wachner. A polarization model overcoming the geometric restrictions of the Laplace solution for spheroidal cells: Obtaining new equations for field-induced forces and transmembrane potential. *Biophys. J.*, 77:1316–1326, 1999.

20. T. Kotnik and D. Miklavcic. Second-order model of membrane electric field induced by alternating external electric fields. *IEEE Trans. Biomed. Eng.*, 47:1074–1081, 2000.

21. T.R. Gowrishankar and J.C. Weaver. An approach to electrical modeling of single and multiple cells. *Proc. Natl. Acad. Sci. USA*, 100:3203–3208, 2003.

22. M. Zahn. *Electromagnetic Field Theory: A Problems Solving Approach*. Wiley & Sons, New York, 1979.

23. R. Stampfli and M. Willi. Membrane potential of a Ranvier node measured after electrical destruction of its membrane. *Experientia*, 8:297–298, 1957.

24. R. Stampfli. Reversible electrical breakdown of the excitable membrane of a Ranvier node. *Ann. Acad. Brasil. Ciens.*, 30:57–63, 1958.

25. A.J.H. Sale and A. Hamilton. Effects of high electric fields on microoranisms: I. killing of bacteria and yeasts. *Biochem. Biophys. Acta*, 148:781–788, 1967.

26. W.A. Hamilton and A.J.H. Sale. Effects of high electric fields on microorganisms: II. Killing of bacteria and yeasts. *Biochim. Biophys. Acta*, 148:7789–8000, 1967.

27. A.J.H. Sale and W.A. Hamilton. Effects of high electric fields on microorganisms: III. Lysis of erythrocytes and protoplasts. *Biochim. Biophys. Acta*, 163:37–43, 1968.

28. E. Neumann and K. Rosenheck. Permeability changes induced by electric impulses in vesicular membranes. *J. Membr. Biol.*, 10:279–290, 1972.

29. U. Zimmermann, J. Schultz, and G. Pilwat. Transcellular ion flow in *Escherichia coli* and electrical sizing of bacterias. *Biophys. J.*, 13:1005–1013, 1973.

30. U. Zimmermann, G. Pilwat, and F. Riemann. Dielectric breakdown of cell membranes. *Biophys. J.*, 14:881–899, 1974.

31. H.G.L. Coster and U. Zimmermann. Dielectric breakdown in the membranes of *Valonia utricularis:* The role of energy dissipation. *Biochim. Biophys. Acta*, 382:410–418, 1975.

32. H.T. Tien. *Bilayer Lipid Membranes (BLM): Theory and Practice*. Marcel Dekker, New York, 1974.

33. H.T. Tien and A. Ottova. The bilayer lipid membrane (BLM) under electric fields. *IEEE Trans. Dielect. Elect. Ins.*, 10:717–727, 2003.

34. I.G. Abidor, V.B. Arakelyan, L.V. Chernomordik, Yu.A. Chizmadzhev, V.F. Pastushenko, and M.R. Tarasevich. Electric breakdown of bilayer membranes: I. The main experimental facts and their qualitative discussion. *Bioelectrochem. Bioenerg.*, 6:37–52, 1979.

35. V.F. Pastushenko, Yu.A. Chizmadzhev, and V.B. Arakelyan. Electric breakdown of bilayer membranes: II. Calculation of the membrane lifetime in the steady-state diffusion approximation. *Bioelectrochem. Bioenerg.*, 6:53–62, 1979.

36. Y.A. Chizmadzhev, V.B. Arakelyan, and V.F. Pastushenko. Electric breakdown of bilayer membranes: III. Analysis of possible mechanisms of defect origin. *Bioelectrochem. Bioenerg.*, 6:63–70, 1979.

37. V.F. Pastushenko, Y.A. Chizmadzhev, and V.B. Arakelyan. Electric breakdown of bilayer membranes: IV. Consideration of the kinetic stage in the case of the single-defect membrane. *Bioelectrochem. Bioenerg.*, 6:71–79, 1979.

38. V.B. Arakelyan, Y.A. Chizmadzhev, and V.F. Pastushenko. Electric breakdown of bilayer membranes: V. consideration of the kinetic stage in the case of the membrane containing an arbitrary number of defects. *Bioelectrochem. Bioenerg.*, 6:81–87, 1979.

39. V.F. Pastushenko, V.B. Arakelyan, and Y.A. Chizmadzhev. Electric breakdown of bilayer membranes: VI. A stochastic theory taking into account the processes of defect formation and death: Membrane lifetime distribution function. *Bioelectrochem. Bioenerg.*, 6:89–95, 1979.

40. V.F. Pastushenko, V.B. Arakelyan, and Yu.A. Chizmadzhev. Electric breakdown of bilayer membranes: VII. A stochastic theory taking into account the processes of defect formation and death: Statistical properties. *Bioelectrochem. Bioenerg.*, 6:97–104, 1979.

41. R. Benz, F. Beckers, and U. Zimmermann. Reversible electrical breakdown of lipid bilayer membranes: A charge-pulse relaxation study. *J. Membr. Biol.*, 48:181–204, 1979.
42. R. Benz and U. Zimmermann. Relaxation studies on cell membranes and lipid bilayers in the high electric field range. *Bioelectrochem. Bioenerg.*, 7:723–739, 1980.
43. R. Benz and F. Conti. Reversible electrical breakdown of squid giant axon membrane. *Biochim. Biophys. Acta*, 645:115–123, 1981.
44. J.C. Weaver and R.A. Mintzer. Decreased bilayer stability due to transmembrane potentials. *Phys. Lett.*, 86A:57–59, 1981.
45. I.P. Sugar. The effects of external fields on the structure of lipid bilayers. *J. Physiol. Paris*, 77:1035–1042, 1981.
46. V.F. Pastushenko and Y.A. Chizmadzhev. Stabilization of conducting pores in BLM by electric current. *Gen. Physiol. Biophys.*, 1:43–52, 1982.
47. U. Zimmermann, F. Riemann, and G. Pilwat. Enzyme loading of electrically homogeneous human red blood cell ghosts prepared by dielectric breakdown. *Biochim. Biophys. Acta*, 436:460–474, 1976.
48. K. Kinosita Jr. and T.Y. Tsong. Survival of sucrose-loaded erythrocytes in circulation. *Nature*, 272:258–260, 1978.
49. J. Teissie and T.Y. Tsong. Electric field induced transient pores in phospholipid bilayer vesicles. *Biochemistry*, 20:1548–1554, 1981.
50. U. Zimmermann, P. Scheurich, G. Pilwat, and R. Benz. Cells with manipulated functions: New perspectives for cell biology, medicine and technology. *Angew. Chem. Int. Ed. Engl.*, 20:325–344, 1981.
51. D. Auer, G. Brandner, and W. Bodemer. Dielectric breakdown of the red blood cell membrane and uptake of SV 40 DNA and mammalian cell RNA. *Naturwissenschaften*, 63:391, 1976.
52. E. Neumann, M. Schaefer-Ridder, Y. Wang, and P.H. Hofschneider. Gene transfer into mouse lyoma cells by electroporation in high electric fields. *EMBO J.*, 1:841–845, 1982.
53. H. Fricke. The electric permittivity of a dilute suspension of membrane-covered ellipsoids. *J. Appl. Phys.*, 24:644–646, 1953.
54. H. Pauly and H.P. Schwan. Über die Impedanz einer Suspension von kugelförmigen Teilchen mit einer Schale. *Z. Naturforsch.*, 14B:125–131, 1959.
55. M. Montal and P. Mueller. Formation of bimolecular membranes from lipid monolayers and a study of their electrical properties. *Proc. Natl. Acad. Sci. USA*, 60:3561–3566, 1972.
56. L.V. Chernomordik and Y.A. Chizmadzhev. Electrical breakdown of BLM: Phenomenology and mechanism. In E. Neumann, A. Sowers, and C. Jordan, Eds., *Electroporation and Electrofusion in Cell Biology*. Plenum Press, New York, 1989, pp. 83–96.
57. A. Barnett and J.C. Weaver. Electroporation: A unified, quantitative theory of reversible electrical breakdown and rupture. *Bioelectrochem. Bioenerg.*, 25:163–182, 1991.
58. S.A. Freeman, M.A. Wang, and J.C. Weaver. Theory of electroporation for a planar bilayer membrane: Predictions of the fractional aqueous area, change in capacitance and pore-pore separation. *Biophys. J.*, 67:42–56, 1994.
59. K. Kinosita Jr., I. Ashikawa, N. Saita, H. Yoshimura, H. Itoh, K. Nagayma, and A. Ikegami. Electroporation of cell membrane visualized under a pulsed-laser fluorescence microscope. *Biophys. J.*, 53:1015–1019, 1988.
60. M. Hibino, M. Shigemori, H. Itoh, K. Nagyama, and K. Kinosita. Membrane conductance of an electroporated cell analyzed by submicrosecond imaging of transmembrane potential. *Biophys. J.*, 59:209–220, 1991.
61. W. Frey, J.A. White, R.O. Price, P.F. Blackmore, R.P. Joshi, R. Nuccitelli, S.J. Beebe, K.H. Schoenbach, and J.F. Kolb. Plasma membrane voltage changes during nanosecond pulsed electric field exposures. *Biophys J.*, 90:3608–3615, 2006.
62. L.V. Chernomordik, S.I. Sukharev, I.G. Abidor, and Y.A. Chizmadzhev. The study of the BLM reversible electrical breakdown mechanism in the presence of UO_2^{2+}. *Bioelectrochem. Bioenerg.*, 9:149–155, 1982.
63. M. Edidin. Lipids on the frontier: A century of cell-membrane bilayers. *Nat. Rev. Mol. Cell Biol.*, 4:414–418, 2003.

64. M. Winterhalter and W. Helfrich. Deformation of spherical vesicles by electric fields. *J. Colloid. Interface. Sci.*, 122:583–586, 1988.

65. E. Neumann and S. Kakorin. Electrooptics of membrane electroporation and vesicle shape deformation. *Curr. Opin. Colloid Interface Sci.*, 1:790–799, 1996.

66. R.P. Joshi, Q. Hu, K.H. Schoenbach, and H.P. Hjalmarson. Theoretical prediction of electrome-chanical deformation of cells subjected to high voltages for membrane electroporation. *Phys. Rev. E*, 65:021913-1–021913-10, 2002.

67. K.J. Müller, V.I. Sukhorukov, and U. Zimmermann. Reversible electropermeabilization of mammalian cells by high-intensity, ultra-short pulses of submicrosecond duration. *J. Membr. Biol.*, 184:161–170, 2001.

68. J. Dai and M.P. Sheetz. Regulation of endocytosis, exocytosis, and shape by membrane tension. *Cold Spring Harb. Symp. Quant. Biol.*, 60:567–571, 1995.

69. N. Gov, A.G. Zilman, and S. Safran. Cytoskeleton confinement and tension of red blood cell membranes. *Phys. Rev. Lett.*, 90:228101-1–118101-4, 2003.

70. L.V. Chernomordik, G.B. Milikyan, and Y.A. Chizmadzhev. Biomembrane fusion: A new con-cept derived from model studies wing two interacting planar lipid bilayers. *Biochim. Biophys. Acta*, 906:309–352, 1987.

71. Y.A. Chizmadzhev, D.A. Kumenko, P.I. Kuzmin, L.V. Chernomordik, J. Zimmerberg, and F.S. Cohen. Lipid flow through fusion pores connecting membranes of different tensions. *Biophys. J.*, 76:2951–2965, 1999.

72. K.A. DeBruin and W. Krassowska. Electroporation and shock-induced transmembrane poten-tial in a cardiac fiber during defibrillation strength shocks. *Ann. Biomed. Eng.*, 26:584–596, 1998.

73. J.C. Neu and W. Krassowska. Asymptotic model of electroporation. *Phys. Rev. E*, 59:3471–3482, 1999.

74. K.C. Melikov, V.A. Frolov, A. Shcherbakov, A.V. Samsonov, Y.A. Chizmadzhev, and L.V. Chernomordik. Voltage-induced nonconductive pre-pores and metastable pores in unmodi-fied planar bilayer. *Biophys. J.*, 80:1829–1836, 2001.

75. H.G.L. Coster. A quantitative analysis of the voltage-current relationships of fixed charge membranes and the associated property of "punch-through". *Biophys. J.*, 5:669–686, 1965.

76. J.M. Crowley. Electrical breakdown of bimolecular lipid membranes as an electromechanical instability. *Biophys. J.*, 13:711–724, 1973.

77. D.S. Dimitrov and R.K. Jain. Membrane stability. *Biochim. Biophys. Acta*, 779:437–468, 1984.

78. K.A. DeBruin and W. Krassowska. Modeling electroporation in a single cell: I. Effects of field strength and rest potential. *Biophys. J.*, 77:1213–1224, 1999.

79. K.A. DeBruin and W. Krassowska. Modeling electroporation in a single cell: II. Effects of ionic concentration. *Biophys. J.*, 77:1225–1233, 1999.

80. D.A. Stewart, T.R. Gowrishankar, and J.C. Weaver. Transport lattice approach to describing cell electroporation: Use of a local asymptotic model. *IEEE Trans. Plasma Sci.*, 32:1696–1708, 2004.

81. K.C. Smith, T.R. Gowrishankar, A.T. Esser, D.A. Stewart, and J.C. Weaver. Spatially distributed, dynamic transmembrane voltages of organelle and cell membranes due to 10 ns pulses: Predictions of meshed and unmeshed transport network models. *IEEE Trans. Plasma Sci.*, 34:1394–1404, 2006.

82. D.P. Tieleman, H. Leontiadou, A.E. Mark, and S.-J. Marrink. Simulation of pore formation in lipid bilayers by mechanical stress and electric fields. *J. Am. Chem. Soc.*, 125:6382–6383, 2003.

83. D.P. Tieleman. The molecular basis of electroporation. *BMC Biochem.*, 5:10, 2004.

84. H. Leotiadou, A.E. Mark, and S.J. Marrink. Molecular dynamics simulations of hydrophilic pores in lipid bilayers. *Biophys. J.*, 86:2156–2164, 2004.

85. Q. Hu, S. Viswandham, R.P. Joshi, K.H. Schoenbach, S.J. Beebe, and P.F. Blackmore. Simulations of transient membrane behavior in cells subject to a high-intensity ultrashort electric pulse. *Phys. Rev. E*, 71:03194-1–03194-9, 2005.

86. M. Tarek. Membrane electroporation: A molecular dynamics simulation. *Biophys. J.*, 88:4045–4053, 2005.

87. Q. Hu, R.P. Joshi, and K.H. Schoenbach. Simulations of nanopore formation and phos-phatidylserine externalization in lipid membranes subjected to high-intensity, ultrashort elec-tric pulse. *Phys. Rev. E*, 72:031902-1–031902-10, 2005.

88. J.D. Litster. Stability of lipid bilayers and red blood cell membranes. *Phys. Lett.*, 53A:193–194, 1975.

89. J.C. Weaver. Electroporation: A general phenomenon for manipulating cells and tissue. *J. Cell. Biochem.*, 51:426–435, 1993.

90. T.E. Vaughan and J.C. Weaver. A theoretical model for cell electroporation: A quantitative description of electrical behavior. In F. Bersani, Ed., *Electricity and Magnetism in Biology and Medicine*. Plenum, New York, 1999, pp. 433–435.

91. J.A. Nickoloff. Ed. *Methods in Molecular Biology, Electroporation Protocols for Microorganisms*, vol. 47. Humana Press, Totowa, 1995.

92. J.A. Nickoloff, Ed. *Animal Cell Electroporation & Electrofusion Protocols*, Methods in Molecular Biology, vol. 48. Humana Press, Totowa, 1995.

93. J.A. Nickoloff, Ed. *Plant Cell Electroporation & Electrofusion Protocols*, Methods in Molecular Biology, vol. 55. Humana Press, Totowa, 1995.

94. M.J. Jaroszeski, R. Gilbert, and R. Heller, Eds., *Electrically Mediated Delivery of Molecules to Cells: Electrochemotherapy, Electrogenetherapy and Transdermal Delivery by Electroporation*. Humana Press, Totowa, 2000.

95. M. Belehradek, C. Domenge, B. Luboinski, S. Orlowski, J. Belehradek Jr., and L.M. Mir. Electrochemotherapy, a new antitumor treatment. First clinical phase I-II trial. *Cancer*, 72:3694–3700, 1993.

96. R. Heller, M. Jaroszeski, L.F. Glass, J.L. Messina, D.P. Rapport, R.C. DeConti, N.A. Fenske, R.A. Gilbert, L.M. Mir, and D.S. Reintgen. Phase I/II trial for the treatment of cutaneous and subcutaneous tumors using electrochemotherapy. *Cancer*, 77:964–971, 1996.

97. A. Gothelf, L.M. Mir, and J. Gehl. Electrochemotherapy: Results of cancer treatment using enhanced delivery of bleomycin by electroporation. *Cancer Treat. Rev.*, 29:371–387, 2003.

98. T.K. Wong and E. Neumann. Electric field mediated gene transfer. *Biochem. Biophys. Res. Commun.*, 107:584–587, 1982.

99. I. Uno, K. Fukami, H. Kato, T. Takenawa, and T. Ishikawa. Essential role for phosphatidylinositol 4,5-bisphosphate in yeast cell proliferation. *Nature*, 333:188–190, 1988.

100. D.L. Berglund and J.R. Starkey. Isolation of viable tumor cells following introduction of labelled antibody to an intracellular oncogene product using electroporation. *J. Immunol. Methods*, 125:79–87, 1989.

101. M. Rui, Y. Chen, Y. Zhang, and D. Ma. Transfer of anti-TFAR19 monoclonal antibody into HeLa cells by *in situ* electroporation can inhibit apoptosis. *Life Sci.*, 71:1771–1778, 2002.

102. L.M. Mir, H. Banoun, and C. Paoletti. Introduction of definite amounts of nonpermeant molecules into living cells after electropermeabilization: Direct access to the cytosol. *Exp. Cell Res.*, 175:15–25, 1988.

103. D.C. Bartoletti, G.I. Harrison, and J.C. Weaver. The number of molecules taken up by electroporated cells: Quantitative determination. *FEBS Lett.*, 256:4–10, 1989.

104. M.R. Prausnitz, B.S. Lau, C.D. Milano, S. Conner, R. Langer, and J.C. Weaver. A quantitative study of electroporation showing a plateau in net molecular transport. *Biophys. J.*, 65:414–422, 1993.

105. E.A. Gift and J.C. Weaver. Simultaneous quantitative determination of electroporative molecular uptake and subsequent cell survival using gel microdrops and flow cytometry. *Cytometry*, 39:243–249, 2000.

106. L. Graziadei, P. Burfeind, and D. Bar-Sagi. Introduction of unlabeled proteins into living cells by electroporation and isolation of viable protein-loaded cells using dextran-fluorescein isothiocyanate as a marker for protein uptake. *Anal. Biochem.*, 194:198–203, 1991.

107. K.T. Powell and J.C. Weaver. Transient aqueous pores in bilayer membranes: A statistical theory. *Bioelectrochem. Bioelectroenerg.*, 15:211–227, 1986.

108. J.C. Weaver. Electroporation of biological membranes from multicellular to nano scales. *IEEE Trans. Dielect. Elect. Ins.*, 10:754–768, 2003.

109. W. Mehrle, U. Zimmermann, and R. Hampp. Evidence for asymmetrical uptake of fluorescent dyes through electro-permeabilized membranes of *Avena* meosphyll protoplasts. *FEBS Lett.*, 185:89–94, 1985.

110. E. Tekle, R.D. Astumian, and P.B. Chock. Electroporation using bipolar oscillating electric field: An improved method for DNA transfection of NIH3T3 cells. *PNAS*, 88:4230–4234, 1991.

111. E. Tekle, R.D. Astumian, W.A. Fraiuf, and P.B. Chock. Asymmetric pore distribution and loss of membrane lipid in electroporated DOPC vesicles. *Biophys. J.*, 81:960–968, 2001.

112. M. Golzio, J. Teissie, and M.P. Rols. Direct visualization at the single-cell level of electrically mediated gene delivery. *Proc. Natl. Acad. Sci. USA*, 99:1292–1297, 2002.

113. H.M. Shapiro. *Practical Flow Cytometry*, 3rd ed. Wiley-Liss, New York, 1995.

114. M.R. Prausnitz, C.D. Milano, J.A. Gimm, R. Langer, and J.C. Weaver. Quantitative study of molecular transport due to electroporation: Uptake of bovine serum albumin by human red blood cell ghosts. *Biophys. J.*, 66:1522–1530, 1994.

115. E.A. Gift and J.C. Weaver. Observation of extremely heterogeneous electroporative molecular uptake by *Saccharomyces* cerevisiae which changes with electric field pulse amplitude. *Biochim. Biophys. Acta*, 1234:52–62, 1995.

116. M. Puc, J. Kotnik, L.M. Mir, and D. Miklavcic. Quantitative model of small molecules uptake after *in vitro* cell electropermeabilization. *Bioelectrochemistry*, 60:1–10, 2003.

117. J.C. Weaver. Electroporation of cells and tissues. *IEEE Trans. Plasma Sci.*, 28:24–33, 2000.

118. S. Satkauskas, M.F. Bureau, A. Mahfoudi, and L.M. Mir. Slow accumulation of plasmid in muscle cells: Supporting evidence for a mechanism of DNA uptake by receptor-mediated endocytosis. *Mol. Ther.*, 4:317–323, 2001.

119. L.M. Mir. Therapeutic perspectives of in vivo cell electropermeabilization. *Bioelectrochemistry*, 53:1–10, 2001.

120. F. Andre and L.M. Mir. DNA electrotransfer: Its principles and an updated review of its therapeutic applications. *Gene Ther.*, 11(Suppl. 1):S33–S42, 2004.

121. E. Neumann, A.E. Sowers, and C.A. Jordan, Ed., *Electroporation and Electrofusion in Cell Biology*. Plenum Press, New York, 1989.

122. D.C. Chang, B.M. Chassy, J.A. Saunders, and A.E. Sowers, Ed., *Guide to Electroporation and Electrofusion*. Academic Press, New York, 1992.

123. L.H. Li, P. Ross, and S.W. Hui. Improving electrotransfection efficiency by post-pulse centrifugation. *Gene Ther.*, 6:364–372, 1999.

124. A.V. Titomirov, S. Sukharev, and E. Kistoanova. *In Vivo* electroporation and stable transformation of skin cells of newborn mice by plasmid DNA. *Biochim. Biophys. Acta*, 1088:131–134, 1991.

125. R.L. Harrison, B.J. Byrne, and L. Tung. Electroporation-mediated gene transfer in cardiac tissue. *FEBS Lett.*, 435:1–5, 1998.

126. T. Goto, T. Nishi, T. Tamura, S.B. Dev, H. Takeshima, M. Kochi, K. Yoshizato, J. Kuratsu, T. Sakata, G.A. Hofmann, and Y. Ushio. Highly efficient electro-gene therapy of solid tumor by using an expression plasmid for the herpes simplex virus thymidine kinase gene. *Proc. Natl. Acad. Sci. USA*, 97:354–359, 2000.

127. D.J. Wells. Gene therapy progress and prospects: Electroporation and other physical methods. *Gene Ther.*, 11:1361–1369, 2004.

128. P.-G. de Gennes. Passive entry of a DNA molecule into a small pore. *Proc. Natl. Acad. Sci. USA*, 96:7262–7264, 1999.

129. J.C. Neu, K.C. Smith, and W. Krassowska. Electrical energy required to form large conducting pores. *Bioelectrochemistry*, 60:107–114, 2003.

130. K.C. Smith, J.C. Neu, and W. Krassowska. Model of creation and evolution of stable electropores for DNA delivery. *Biophys. J.*, 86:2813–2826, 2004.

131. H. Stopper, H. Jones, and U. Zimmermann. Large scale transfection of mouse L-cells by electropermeabilization. *Biochim. Biophys. Acta*, 900:38–44, 1987.

132. D.S. Dimitrov and A.E. Sowers. Membrane electroporation-fast molecular exchange by electroosmosis. *Biochim. Biophys. Acta*, 1022:381–392, 1990.

133. V.A. Klenchin, S.I. Sukharev, S.M. Serov, L.V. Chernomordik, and Y.A. Chizmadzhev. Electrically induced DNA uptake by cells is a fast process involving DNA electrophoresis. *Biophys. J.*, 60:804–811, 1991.

134. S.I. Sukharev, V.A. Klenchin, S.M. Serov, L.V. Chernomordik, and Y.A. Chizmadzhev. Electroporation and electrophoretic DNA transfer into cells. The effect of DNA interaction with electropores. *Biophys. J.*, 63:1320–1327, 1992.

135. L.V. Chernomordik, A.V. Sokolov, and V.G. Budker. Electrostimulated uptake of DNA by liposomes. *Biochim. Biophys. Acta*, 1024:179–183, 1990.

136. J.C. Weaver, R. Vanbever, T.E. Vaughan, and M.R. Prausnitz. Heparin alters transdermal transport associated with electroporation. *Biochem. Biophys. Res. Commun.*, 234:637–640, 1997.

137. V.P. Pastushenko and Y.A. Chizmadzhev. Energetic estimations of the deformation of translocated DNA and cell membrane in the course of electrotransformation. *Biol. Mem.*, 6:287–300, 1992.

138. Y. Mouneimne, P-F. Tosi, Y. Gazitt, and C. Nicolau. Electro-insertion of xeno-glycophorin into the red blood cell membrane. *Biochem. Biophys. Res. Commun.*, 159:34–40, 1989.

139. M. Zeira, P-F. Tosi, Y. Mouneimne, J. Lazarte, L. Sneed, D.J. Volsky, and C. Nicolau. Full-length CD4 electro-inserted in the erythrocyte membrane as a long-lived inhibitor of infection by human immunodeficiency virus. *Proc. Natl. Acad. Sci. USA*, 88:4409–4413, 1991.

140. C. Nicolau, Y. Mouneimne, and P-F. Tosi. Electroinsertion of proteins in the plasma membrane of red blood cells. *Anal. Biochem.*, 214:1–10, 1993.

141. K.E. Ouagari, J. Teissie, and H. Benoist. Glycophorin a protects K562 cells from natural killer cell attack. *J. Biol. Chem.*, 270:26970–26975, 1995.

142. S. Raffy, C. Lazdunski, and J. Teissie. Electroinsertion and activation of the C-terminal domain of colicin A, a voltage gated bacterial toxin, into mammalian cell membranes. *Mol. Membr. Biol.*, 21:237–246, 2004.

143. P. Scheurich, U. Zimmermann, M. Mischel, and I. Lamprecht. Membrane fusion and deformation of red blood cells by electric fields. *Z. Naturforsch.*, 35:1801–1805, 1980.

144. J. Teissie, V.P. Knutson, T.Y. Tsong, and M.D. Lane. Electric pulse-induced fusion of 3t3 cells in monolayer culture. *Science*, 216:537–538, 1982.

145. U. Zimmermann. Electric field-mediated fusion and related electrical phenomena. *Biochim. Biophys. Acta*, 694:227–277, 1982.

146. U. Zimmermann and G. Küppers. Cell fusion by electromagnetic waves and its possible relevance for evolution. *Naturwissenschaften*, 70:568–569, 1983.

147. A.E. Sowers. Movement of a fluorescent lipid label from a labeled erythrocyte membrane to an unlabeled erythrocyte membrane following electric-field-induced fusion. *Biophys. J.*, 47:519–525, 1985.

148. D.A. Stenger and S.W. Hui. Kinetics of ultrastructure changes during electrically-induced fusion of human erythrocytes. *J. Membr. Biol.*, 93:43–53, 1986.

149. I.P. Sugar, W. Forster, and E. Neumann. Model of cell electrofusion. Membrane electroporation, pore coalescence and percolation. *Biophys. Chem.*, 26:321–335, 1987.

150. J.R. Grasso, R. Heller, J.C. Cooley, and E.M. Haller. Electrofusion of individual animal cells directly to interaction corneal epithelial tissue. *Biochim. Biophys. Acta*, 980:9–14, 1989.

151. R. Heller and R.J. Grasso. Transfer of human membrane surface components by incorporating human cells into interaction animal tissue by cell-tissue electrofusion *in vivo*. *Biochim. Biophys. Acta*, 1024:185–188, 1990.

152. I. Tsoneva, T. Tomov, I. Panova, and D. Strahilov. Effective production by electrofusion of hybridomas secreting monoclonal antibodies against hc-antigen of *Salmonella*. *Bioelectrochem. Bioenerg.*, 24:41–49, 1990.

153. D.T. Chiu, C.F. Wilson, F. Ryttsen, A. Stromberg, C. Farre, A. Karlsson, S. Nordholm, A. Gaggar, B.P. Modi, A. Moscho, R.A. Garza-Lopez, O. Orwar, and R.N. Zare. Chemical transformations in individual ultrasmall biomimetic containers. *Science*, 283:1892–1895, 1999.

154. A. Stromberg, F. Ryttsen, D.T. Chiu, M. Davidson, P.S. Eriksson, C.F. Wilson, O. Orwar, and R.N. Zare. Manipulating the genetic identity and biochemical surface properties of individual cells with electric-field-induced fusion. *Proc. Natl. Acad. Sci. USA*, 97:7–11, 2000.

155. K.T. Trevor, C. Cover, Y.W. Ruiz, E.T. Akporiaye, E.M. Mersh, D. Landais, R.R. Taylor, A.D. King, and R.E. Walters. Generation of dendritic cell-tumor cell hybrids by electrofusion for clinical vaccine application. *Cancer Immunol. Immunother.*, 53:705–714, 2004.

156. W.T. Lee, K. Shimizu, H. Kuriyama, H. Tanaka, J. Kjaergaard, and S. Shu. Tumor-dendritic cell fusion as a basis for cancer immunotherapy. *Otolaryngol. Head Neck Surg.*, 132:755–764, 2005.

157. S.W. Hui, N. Stoicheva, and Y.-L. Zhao. High-efficiency loading, transfection, and fusion of cells by electroporation in two-phase polymer systems. *Biophys. J.*, 71:1123–1130, 1996.

158. P.L. Kuzmin, V.P. Pastushenko, I.G. Abidor, S.I. Sukharev, A.V. Barbul, and Y.A. Chizmadz-hev. Electrofusion of cells: Theoretical analysis. *Biol. Membr.*, 5:600–612, 1988.

159. A.E. Sowers. A long lived fusogenic state is induced in erythrocytes ghosts by electric pulses. *J. Cell. Biol.*, 102:1358–1362, 1986.

160. J. Teissie and M.-P. Rols. Fusion of mammalian cells in culture is obtained by creating the contact between cells after their electropermeabilization. *Biochem. Biophys. Res. Commun.*, 140:258–264, 1986.

161. M. Bier, S.M. Hammer, D.J. Canaday, and R.C. Lee. Kinetics of sealing for transient electropores in isolated mammalian skeletal muscle cells. *Bioelectromagnetics*, 20:194–201, 1999.

162. C.S. Djuzenova, U. Zimmermann, H. Frank, V.L. Sukhorukov, E. Richter, and G. Fuhr. Effect of medium conductivity and composition on the uptake of propidium iodide into electropermeabilized myeloma cells. *Biochim. Biophys. Acta*, 1284:143–152, 1996.

163. E. Neumann, K. Toensing, S. Kakorin, P. Budde, and J. Frey. Mechanism of electroporative dye uptake by mouse B cells. *Biophys. J.*, 74:98–108, 1998.

164. M.N. Teruel and T. Meyer. Electroporation-induced formation of individual calcium entry sites in the cell body and processes of adherent cells. *Biophys. J.*, 73:1785–1796, 1997.

165. M. Bier, W. Chen, T.R. Gowrishankar, R.D. Astumian, and R.C. Lee. Resealing dynamics of a cell membrane after electroporation. *Phys. Rev. E*, 66:062905-1–062905-4, 2002.

166. R. Benz and U. Zimmermann. The resealing process of lipid bilayers after reversible electrical breakdown. *Biochim. Biophys. Acta*, 640:169–178, 1981.

167. L.V. Chernomordik, S.I. Sukharev, I.G. Abidor, and Yu.A. Chizmadzhev. Breakdown of lipid bilayer membranes in an electric field. *Biochim. Biophys. Acta*, 73:203–213, 1983.

168. Yu.A. Chizmadzhev and I. Abidor. Bilayer lipid membranes in strong electric fields. *Bioelectrochem. Bioenerg.*, 7:83–100, 1980.

169. G. Pilwat, U. Zimmermann, and F. Riemann. Dielectric breakdown measurements of human and bovine erythrocyte membranes using benzyl alcohol as a probe molecule. *Biochim. Biophys. Acta*, 406:424–432, 1975.

170. J.C. Weaver, G.I. Harrison, J.G. Bliss, J.R. Mourant, and K.T. Powell. Electroporation: High frequency of occurrence of the transient high permeability state in red blood cells and intact yeast. *FEBS Lett.*, 229:30–34, 1988.

171. S. Kwee, H.V. Nielsen, and J.E. Celis. Electropermeabilization of human cultured cells grown in monolayers: Incorporation of monoclonal antibodies. *Bioelectrochem. Bioenerg.*, 23:65–80, 1990.

172. K.P. Mishra and A.B. Singh. Temperature effects on resealing of electrically hemolysed rabbit erythrocytes. *Indian J. Exp. Biol.*, 24:737–741, 1986.

173. R.C. Lee, L.P. River, F.-S. Pan, L. Ji, and R.L. Wollmann. Surfactant induced sealing of electropermeabilized skeletal muscle membranes *in vivo*. *Proc. Natl. Acad. Sci. USA*, 89:4524–4528, 1992.

174. R.C. Lee, D. Zhang, and J. Hannig. Biophysical injury mechanisms in electrical shock trauma. *Ann. Rev. Biomed. Eng.*, 2:477–509, 2000.

175. M.R. Prausnitz, J.D. Corbett, J.A. Grimm, D.E. Golan, R. Langer, and J.C. Weaver. Millisecond measurement of transport during and after an electroporation pulse. *Biophys. J.*, 68:1864–1870, 1995.

176. U. Pliquett, M.R. Prausnitz, Y. Chizmadzhev, and J.C. Weaver. Measurement of rapid release kinetics for drug delivery. *Pharm. Res.*, 12:546–553, 1995.

177. P.E. Marszalek, B. Farrell, P. Verdugo, and J.M. Fernandez. Kinetics of release of serotonin from isolated secretory granules. I. Amperometric detection of serotonin from electroporated granules. *Biophys. J.*, 73:1160–1168, 1997.

178. D.C. Gaylor, K. Prakah-Asante, and R.C. Lee. Significance of cell size and tissue structure in electrical trauma. *J. Theor. Biol.*, 133:223–237, 1988.

179. D.L. Bhatt, D.C. Gaylor, and R.C. Lee. Rhabdomyolysis due to pulsed electric fields. *Plast. Reconstr. Surg.*, 86:1–11, 1990.

180. V. Ganeva, B. Galutzov, N. Eynard, and J. Teissie. Electroinduced extraction of ß-galactosidase from *Kluyveromyces lactis*. *Appl. Microbiol. Biotechnol.*, 56:411–413, 2001.
181. M.R. Michel, M. Elgizoli, H. Koblet, and Ch. Kempf. Diffusion loading conditions determine recovery of protein synthesis in electroporated p3x63 ag8 cells. *Experientia*, 44:199–203, 1988.
182. J.C. Weaver. Molecular basis for cell membrane electroporation. *Ann. NY Acad. Sci.*, 720:141–152, 1994.
183. R.C. Lee and R.D. Astumian. The physiochemical basis for thermal and nonthermal "burn" injury. *Burns*, 22:509–519, 1996.
184. A.R. Denet, R. Vanbever, and V. Preat. Skin electroporation for transdermal and topical delivery. *Adv. Drug Deliv. Rev.*, 56:659–674, 2004.
185. R. Heller, M. Jaroszeski, A. Atkin, D. Moradpour, R. Gilbert, J. Wands, and C. Nicolau. *In vivo* gene electroinjection and expression in rat liver. *FEBS Lett.*, 389:225–228, 1996.
186. M.R. Prausnitz, V.G. Bose, R. Langer, and J.C. Weaver. Electroporation of mammalian skin: A mechanism to enhance transdermal drug delivery. *Proc. Natl. Acad. Sci.*, 90:10504–10508, 1993.
187. J.C. Weaver and R. Langer. Electrochemical creation of large aqueous pathways: An approach to transdermal drug delivery. *Prog. Dermatol.*, 33:1–10, 1999.
188. M.R. Prausnitz, S. Mitragotri, and R. Langer. Current status and future potential of transdermal drug delivery. *Nat. Rev. Drug Discov.*, 3:115–121, 2004.
189. O. Tovar and L. Tung. Electroporation and recovery of cardiac cell membrane with rectangular voltage pulses. *Am. J. Physiol.*, 263:H1128–H1136, 1992.
190. D.K. Cheng, L. Tung, and E.A. Sobie. Nonuniform responses of transmembrane potential during electric field stimulation of single cardiac cells. *Am. J. Physiol.*, 277:H351–H362, 1999.
191. E.R. Cheek and V.G. Fast. Nonlinear changes of transmembrane potential during electrical shocks: Role of membrane electroporation. *Circ. Res.*, 94:208–214, 2004.
192. R.M. Fish and L.A. Geddes. Effects of stun guns and tasers. *Lancet*, 358:687–688, 2001.
193. T.R. Gowrishankar, C. Stewart, and J.C. Weaver. Electroporation of a multicellular system: Asymptotoic model analysis. In *Proceedings of the 26th Annual International Conference of the IEEE EMBS*, San Francisco, 2004.
194. R.K. Jain. Physiological resistance to the treatment of solid tumors. In B.A. Teicher, Ed., *Drug Resistance in Oncology*. Marcel Dekker, New York, 1993, pp. 87–105.
195. M. Okino and H. Mohri. Effects of a high-voltage electrical impulse and an anticancer drug on *in vivo* growing tumors. *Jpn. J. Cancer Res.*, 78:1319–1321, 1987.
196. L. Mir, S. Orlowski Jr., J. Belehradek, and C. Paoletti. *In Vivo* potentiation of the bleomycin cytotoxicity by local electric pulses. *Eur. J. Cancer*, 27:68–72, 1991.
197. L.M. Mir, S. Orlowski, J. Belehradek, J. Teissie, M.P. Rols, G. Sersa, D. Miklavcic, R. Gilbert, and R. Heller. Biomedical applications of electric pulses with special emphasis on antitumor electrochemotherapy. *Bioelectrochem. Bioenerg.*, 38:203–207, 1995.
198. C. Domenge, S. Orlowski, B. Luboinski, T. De Baere, G. Schwaab, J. Belehradek, and L.M. Mir. Antitumor electrochemotherapy: New advances in the clinical protocol. *Cancer*, 77:956–963, 1996.
199. I. Entin, A. Plotnikov, R. Korenstein, and Y. Keisari. Tumor growth retardation, cure, and induction of antitumor immunity in B16 melanoma-bearing mice by low electric field-enhanced chemotherapy. *Clin. Cancer Res.*, 9:3190–3197, 2003.
200. M. Hyacinthe, M.J. Jaroszeski, V.V. Dang, D. Coppola, R.C. Karl, R.A. Gilbert, and R. Heller. Electrically enhanced drug delivery for the treatment of soft tissue sarcoma. *Cancer*, 85:409–417, 1999.
201. R.A. Gilbert, M.J. Jaroszeski, and R. Heller. Novel electrode designs of electrochemotherapy. *Biochim. Biophys. Acta*, 1334:9–14, 1997.
202. D. Sel, S. Mazeres, J. Teissie, and D. Miklavcic. Finite-element modling of needle electrodes in tissue from the perspective of frequent model computations. *IEEE Trans. Biomed. Eng.*, 50:1221–1232, 2003.
203. S.B. Dev, D. Dhar, and W. Krassowska. Electric field of a six-needle array electrode used in drug and DNA delivery *in vivo*: Analytical verus numerical solutions. *IEEE Trans. Biomed. Eng.*, 50:1296–1300, 2003.

204. R.V. Davalos, B. Rubinsky, and D.M. Otten. A feasibility study for electrical impedance tomography as a means to monitor tissue electroporation for molecular medicine. *IEEE Trans. Biomed. Eng.* 49:400–403, 2002.
205. R.V. Davalos, B. Rubinsky, L.M. Mir, and D.M. Otten. Electrical impedance tomography for imaging tissue electroporation. *IEEE Trans. Biomed. Eng.*, 51:761–767, 2004.
206. M.J. Berridge and J.L. Oschman. Transporting Epithelia. Academic Press, New York, 1972.
207. K.T. Powell, A.W. Morgenthaler, and J.C. Weaver. Tissue electroporation: Observation of reversible electrical breakdown in viable frog skin. *Biophys. J.*, 56:1163–1171, 1989.
208. E.B. Ghartey-Tagoe, J.S. Morgan, K. Ahmed, A.S. Neish, and M.R. Prausnitz. Electroporation-mediated delivery of molecules to model intestinal epithelia. *Int. J. Pharm.*, 270:127–138, 2004.
209. J.L. Kirby, L. Yang, J.C. Labus, R.J. Lye, N. Hsia, R. Day, G.A. Cornwall, and B.T. Hinton. Characterization of epidymal epithelial cell-specific gene promotors by *in vivo* electroporation. *Biol. Reprod.*, 71:613–619, 2004.
210. H.E. Abud, P. Lock, and J.K. Heath. Efficient gene transfer into the epithelial cell layer of embryonic mouse intestine using low-voltage electroporation. *Gastroenterology*, 126:1779–1787, 2004.
211. E.B. Ghartey-Tagoe, J.S. Morgan, A.S. Neish, and M.R. Prausnitz. Increasing permeability of intestinal epithelial monolayers mediated by electroporation. *J. Control. Release*, 103:177–190, 2005.
212. L.A. Goldsmith, Ed. *Physiology, Biochemistry, and Molecular Biology of the Skin*, 2nd ed. Oxford University Press, New York, 1991.
213. H. Schaefer and T.E. Redelmeier. *Skin Barrier: Principles of Percutaneous Absorption*. Karger, Basel, 1996.
214. K.C. Madison. Barrier function of the skin "la raison d'etre" of the epidermis. *J. Invest. Dermatol.*, 121:231–241, 2003.
215. A.S. Michaels, S.K. Chandrasekaran, and J.E. Shaw. Drug permeation through human skin: Theory and *in vitro* experimental measurements. *AIChEJ*, 21:985–996, 1975.
216. J.A. Tamada, N.J.V. Bomannon, and R.O. Potts. Measurement of glucose in diabetic subjects using noninvasive transdermal extraction. *Nat. Med.*, 1:1198–1202, 1995.
217. R.T. Kurnik, B. Berner, J. Tamada, and R.O. Potts. Design and simulation of a reverse iontophoretic glucose sensor. *J. Electrochem. Soc.*, 145:4119–4125, 1998.
218. R.O. Potts, J.A. Tamada, and M.J. Tierney. Glucose monitoring by reverse iontophoresis. *Diabetes Metab. Res. Rev.*, 18:S49–S53, 2002.
219. Yu.A. Chizmadzhev, V. Zarnytsin, J.C. Weaver, and R.O. Potts. Mechanism of electroinduced ionic species transport through a multilamellar lipid system. *Biophys. J.*, 68:749–765, 1995.
220. Y. Chizmadzhev, A.V. Indenbom, P.I. Kuzmin, S.V. Galinchenko, J.C. Weaver, and R. Potts. Electrical properties of skin at moderate voltages: Contribution of appendageal macropores. *Biophys. J.*, 74:843–856, 1998.
221. Y. Chizmadzhev, P.I. Kuzmin, J.C. Weaver, and R. Potts. Skin appendageal macropores as possible pathway for electrical current. *J. Invest. Dermatol. Symp. Proc.*, 3:148–152, 1998.
222. J.C. Weaver, T.E. Vaughan, and Y. Chizmadzhev. Theory of electrical creation of aqueous pathways across skin transport barriers. *Adv. Drug Deliv. Rev.*, 35:21–39, 1999.
223. D.R. Friend. *In vitro* permeation techniques. *J. Control. Release*, 18:235–248, 1992.
224. H.H. Ussing. *The Alakli Metal Ions in Biology*. Springer-Verlag, Berlin, 1960.
225. D. Bommannan, L. Leung, J. Tamada, J. Sharifi, W. Abraham, and R. Potts. Transdermal delivery of lutenizing hormone releasing hormone: Comparison between electroporation and iontophoresis *in vitro*. *Proceedings of the International Symposium Controlled Release on Bioactive Materials*, vol. 20, pp. 97–98, 1993
226. U. Pliquett, R. Langer, and J.C. Weaver. Changes in the passive electrical properties of human stratum corneum due to electroporation. *Biochim. Biophys. Acta*, 1239:111–121, 1995.
227. R. Vanbever, D. Fouchard, A. Jadoul, N. De Morre, V. Preat, and J.-P. Marty. *In vivo* noninvasive evaluation of hairless rat skin after high-voltage pulse exposure. *Skin Pharmacol. Appl. Skin Physiol.*, 11:23–34, 1998.
228. R. Vanbever, G. Langers, S. Montmayeur, and V. Preat. Transdermal delivery of fentanyl: Rapid onset of analgesia using skin electroporation. *J. Control. Release*, 50:225–235, 1998.

229. A. Sharma, M. Kara, F.R. Smith, and T.R. Krishnan. Transdermal drug delivery using electroporation: II. Factors influencing skin reversibility in electroporative delivery of terazosin hydrochloride in hairless rats. *J. Pharm. Sci.*, 89:536–544, 2000.

230. G. Martin, U. Pliquett, and J.C. Weaver. Theoretical analysis of localized heating in human skin subjected to high voltage pulses. *Bioelectrochemistry*, 57:55–64, 2002.

231. U. Pliquett and J.C. Weaver. Electroporation of human skin: Simultaneous measurement of changes in the transport of two fluorescent molecules and in the passive electrical properties. *Bioelectrochem. Bioenerg.*, 39:1–12, 1996.

232. M.R. Prausnitz, U. Pliquett, R. Langer, and J.C. Weaver. Rapid temporal control of transdermal drug delivery by electroporation. *Pharm. Res.*, 11:1834–1837, 1994.

233. L.M. Mir, M.F. Bureau, J. Gehl, R. Rangara, D. Rouy, J.-M. Caillaud, P. Delaere, D. Brannellec, B. Schwarts, and D. Scherman. High-efficiency gene transfer into skeletal muscle mediated by electric pulses. *Proc. Natl. Acad. Sci. USA*, 96:4262–4267, 1999.

234. J.C. Neu and W. Krassowska. Modeling postshock evolution of large electropores. *Phys. Rev. E*, 67:021915-1–021915-12, 2003.

235. R.C. Lee, E.G. Cravalho, and J.F. Burke, Eds., *Electrical Trauma: The Physiology, Manifestations and Clinical Management*. Cambridge University Press, Cambridge, 1992.

236. G. Greenebaum, K. Blossfield, J. Hannig, C.S. Carrilo, M.A. Beckett, R.R. Weichselbaum, and R.C. Lee. Poloxamer 188 prevents acute necrosis of adult skeletal muscle cells following high-dose irradiation. *Burns*, 30:539–547, 2004.

237. M.N. Robinson, C.G. Brooks, and G.D. Renshaw. Electric shock devices and their effects on the human body. *Med. Sci. Law*, 30:285–300, 1990.

238. S. Anders, M. Junge, F. Schulz, and K. Puschel. Cutaneous current marks due to a stun gun injury. *J. Forensic Sci.*, 48:1–3, 2003.

239. W.C. McDaniel, R.A. Strabucker, M. Nerheim, and J.E. Brewer. Cardiac safety of neuromuscular incapacitating defensive devices. *Pacing Clin. Electrophysiol.*, 28(Suppl. 1):S284–S287, 2005.

240. P.J. Kim and W.H. Franklin. Ventricular fibrillation after stun-gun discharge. *N. Engl. J. Med.*, 353:958–959, 2005.

241. K.R. Foster. Thermal and nonthermal mechanisms of interaction of radio-frequency energy with biological systems. *IEEE Trans. Plasma Sci.*, 28:15–23, 2000.

242. K.H. Schoenbach, S.J. Beebe, and E.S. Buescher. Intracellular effect of ultrashort pulses. *Bioelectromagnetics*, 22:440–448, 2001.

243. S.J. Beebe, P.M. Fox, L.J. Rec, K. Somers, R.H. Stark, and K.H. Schoenbach. Nanosecond pulsed electric field (nsPEF) effects on cells and tissues: Apoptosis induction and tumor growth inhibition. *IEEE Trans. Plasma Sci.*, 30:286–292, 2002.

244. S.J. Beebe, P.M. Fox, L.J. Rec, L.K. Willis, and K.H. Schoenbach. Nanosecond high intensity pulsed electric fields induce apoptosis in human cells. *FASEB J.*, 17:1493–1495, 2003.

245. P.T. Vernier, Y. Sun, L. Marcu, S. Salemi, C.M. Craft, and M.A. Gundersen. Calcium bursts induced by nanosecond electric pulses. *Biochem. Biophys. Res. Commun.*, 310:286–295, 2003.

246. J. Deng, K.H. Schoenbach, E.S. Buescher, P.S. Hair, P.M. Fox, and S.J. Bebe. The effects of intense submicrosecond electrical pulses on cells. *Biophys. J.*, 84:2709–2714, 2003.

247. P.S. Hair, K.H. Schoenbach, and E.S. Buescher. Sub-microsecond, intense pulsed electric field applications to cells show specificity of effects. *Bioelectrochemistry*, 61:65–72, 2003.

248. S.J. Beebe, J. White, P.F. Blackmore, Y. Deng, K. Sommers, and K.H. Schoenbach. Diverse effects of nanosecond pulsed electric fields on cells and tissues. *DNA Cell Biol.* 22:785–796, 2003.

249. M. Stacey, J. Stickley, P. Fox, V. Statler, K. Schoenbach, S.J. Beebe, and S. Buescher. Differential effects in cells exposed to ultra-short, high intensity electric fields: Cell survival, DNA damage, and cell cycle analysis. *Mutat. Res.*, 542:65–75, 2003.

250. J.A. White, P.F. Blackmore, K.H. Schoenbach, and S.J. Beebe. Stimulation of capacitive calcium entry in HL-60 cells by nanosecond pulsed electric fields (nsPEF). *J. Biol. Chem.*, 279:22964–22972, 2004.

251. N. Chen, K.H. Schoenbach, J.F. Kolb, R.J. Swanson, A.L. Garner, J. Yang, R.P. Joshi, and S.J. Beebe. Leukemic cell intracellular responses to nanosecond electric fields. *Biochem. Biophys. Res. Commun.*, 317:421–427, 2004.

252. P.T. Vernier, Y. Sun, L. Marcu, C.M. Craft, and M.A. Gundersen. Nanoelectropulse-induced phosphatidylserine translocation. *Biophys. J.* 86:4040–4048, 2004.
253. K.H. Schoenbach, R.P. Joshi, J.R. Kolb, N. Chen, M. Stacey, P.F. Blackmore, E.S. Buescher, and S.J. Beebe. Ultrashort electrical pulses open a new gateway into biological cells. *Proc. IEEE*, 92:1122–1137, 2004.
254. E. Tekle, H. Oubrahim, S.M. Dzekunov, J.F. Kolb, and K.H. Schoenbach. Selective field effects on intracellular vacuoles and vesicle membranes with nanosecond electric pulses. *Biophys. J.*, 89:274–284, 2005.
255. G. Chen and D.V. Goeddel. TNF-R1 signaling: A beautiful pathway. *Science*, 296:1634–1635, 2002.
256. H. Wajant. The Fas signaling pathway: More than a paradigm. *Science*, 296:1635–1636, 2002.
257. J.-S. Kim, L. He, and J.J. Lemasters. Mitochondrial permeability transition: A common pathway to necrosis and apoptosis. *Biochem. Biophys. Res. Commun.*, 304:463–470, 2003.
258. N.N. Danial and S.J. Korsmeyer. Cell death: Critical control points. *Cell*, 116:205–219, 2004.
259. E.E. Varfolomeev and A. Ashkenazi. Tumor necrosis factor: An apoptosis JuNKie? *Cell*, 116:491–497, 2004.
260. R.C. Lee and M.S. Kolodney. Electrical injury mechanisms: Electrical breakdown of cell membranes. *Plast. Reconstr. Surg.*, 80:672–679, 1987.
261. B. Bagriel and J. Teissie. Control by electrical parameters of short- and long-term cell death resulting from electropermeabilization of Chinese hamster ovary cells. *Biochim. Biophys. Acta*, 1266:171–178, 1995.
262. C.R. Keese, J. Wegner, S.R. Walker, and I. Giaver. Electrical wound-healing assay for cells *in vitro*. *Proc. Natl. Acad. Sci. USA*, 101:1554–1559, 2004.
263. D.R. Green and J.C. Read. Mitochondria and apoptosis. *Science*, 281:1309–1312, 1998.
264. M.O. Hengartner. The biochemistry of apoptosis. *Nature*, 407:770–776, 2000.
265. G.I. Evan and K.H. Vousden. Proliferation, cell cycle and apoptosis in cancer. *Nature*, 411:342–348, 2001.
266. S. Orrenius, B. Zhivotosky, and P. Nicotera. Regulation of cell death: The calcium-apoptosis link. *Nat. Rev. Mol. Cell Biol.*, 4:552–565, 2003.
267. L. Scorrano and S.J. Korsmeyer. Mechanisms of cytochrome c release by proapoptotic BCL-2 family members. *Biochem. Biophys. Res. Commun.*, 304:437–444, 2003.
268. F. Hofmann, L.H. Scheller, W. Strupp, U. Zimmermann, and C. Jassoy. Electric field pulses can induce apoptosis. *J. Membr. Biol.*, 169:103–109, 1999.
269. J. Piñero, M. Lopez-Baena, T. Ortiz, and F. Cortes. Apoptotic and necrotic cell death are both induced by electroporation in HL60 human promyeloid leukaemia cells. *Apoptosis*, 2:330–336, 1997.
270. V. Dressler, K. Schwister, C.W.M. Hast, and B. Deuticke. Dielectric breakdown of the erythrocyte membrane enhances transbilayer mobility of phospholipids. *Biochim. Biophys. Acta*, 732:304–307, 1983.
271. L.Y. Song, J.M. Baldwin, R. O'Reilly, and J.A. Lucy. Relationship between the surface exposure of acidic phospholipids and cell fusion in erythrocytes subjected to electrical breakdown. *Biochim. Biophys. Acta*, 1104:1–8, 1992.
272. C.W.M. Haest, D. Kamp, and B. Deuticke. Transbilayer reorientation of phospholipid probes in the human erythrocyte membrane. Lessons from studies on electroporated and resealed cells. *Biochim. Biophys. Acta*, 1325:17–33, 1997.
273. P.T. Vernier, L.I. Aimin, L. Marcu, C.M. Craft, and M.A. Gundersen. Ultrashort pulsed electric fields induce membrane phospholipid translocation and capase activation: Differential sensitivities of Jurkat T lymphoblasts and rat glioma C6 cells. *IEEE Trans. Dielect. Elect. Ins.*, 10:795–809, 2003.
274. P.T. Vernier, Y. Sun, L. Marcu, C.M. Craft, and M.A. Gundersen. Nanosecond pulsed electric fields perturb membrane phospholipids in T lyphoblasts. *FEBS Lett.*, 572:103–108, 2004.
275. R.P. Joshi and K.H. Schoenbach. Electroporation dynamics in biological cells subjected to ultrafast electrical pulses: A numerical simulation study. *Phys. Rev. E*, 62:1025–1033, 2000.

276. R.P. Joshi, Q. Hu, R. Aly, K.H. Schoenbach, and H.P. Hjalmarson. Self-consistent simulations of electroporation dynamics in biological cells subjected to ultrashort pulses. *Phys. Rev. E*, 64:011913-1–011913-10, 2001.
277. R.P. Joshi, Q. Hu, K.H. Schoenbach, and H.P. Hjalmarson. Improved energy model for membrane electroporation in biological cells subjected to electrical pulses. *Phys. Rev. E*, 62:041920-1–041920-8, 2002.
278. R.P. Joshi and K.H. Schoenbach. Mechanism for membrane electroporation irreversibility under high-intensity, ultrashort pulse conditions. *Phys. Rev. E*, 66:052901-1–052901-4, 2002.
279. R.P. Joshi, Q. Hu, K.H. Schoenbach, and S.J. Beebe. Energy-landscape-model analysis for irreversibility and its pulse-width dependence in cells subjected to a high-intensity ultrashort electric pulse. *Phys. Rev. E*, 69:051901-1–051901-10, 2004.
280. W. Chen and R.C. Lee. Altered ion channel conductance and ionic selectivity induced by large imposed membrane potential pulses. *Biophys. J.*, 67:603–612, 1994.
281. W. Chen, Y. Han, Y. Chen, and D. Astumiam. Electric field-induced functional reductions in the K+ channels mainly resulted from supramembrane potential-medicated electroconformational changes. *Biophys. J.*, 75:196–206, 1998.
282. W. Chen. Supra-physiological membrane potential induced conformational changes in K+ channel conducting system of skeletal muscle fibers. *Bioelectrochemistry*, 62:47–56, 2004.
283. C. Loupatatzis, G. Seitz, P. Schonfeld, F. Lang, and D. Siemen. Single-channel currents of the permeability transition pore from the inner mitochondrial membrane of rat liver and of a human hepatoma cell line. *Cell Physiol. Biochem.*, 12:269–278, 2002.

8

Musculoskeletal Effects and Applications of Electromagnetic Fields

Joseph A. Spadaro

New York Upstate Medical Center

CONTENTS

8.1 Introduction

The intent of this chapter is to summarize the last 10 years' work on the responses of musculo-skeletal tissues and cells to exogenous electromagnetic fields (EMFs) and their clinical applications to bone and cartilage. In addition, it is intended to be a resource for anyone wishing to quickly access the most recent research and clinical reports along with expert commentary.

There have been five decades of modern laboratory research in this area and four decades of clinical application. Readers of the third edition of this handbook have the benefit of an extensive chapter by Arthur Pilla on the subject (Pilla, 2006). His bibliography contained 397 citations through 2006 and was particularly detailed on the question of biophysical mechanisms and models. Since then, at least 253 papers have been published as revealed by National Library of Medicine (Medline) searches.

In order to provide the reader a sense of how the science has progressed, 16 recent high-quality reviews were chosen as guides for this chapter. They focus on musculoskeletal cells and tissues and cover *in vitro*, animal, and clinical studies utilizing a fairly wide range of EMF characteristics, but mostly magnetic fields of low frequency and intensity. The reader is directed to these reviews and their bibliographies for a more detailed study of their particular area or system and the specific published reports on which they are based. Table 8.1 contains a listing of the reviews that form the backbone of this chapter. A brief summary of the findings is given below for each review. While some overlap and repetition is unavoidable, each review contributes a somewhat different perspective. The goal is to enable the reader to estimate the "health" of the current research and clinical

TABLE 8.1

Published Reviews of Electromagnetic Field (EMF) Effects on Skeletal Tissues Described in this Chapter

Main Target Area	Authors, Year PMID (see Ref.)	Subject Emphasis	Years Covered	Comments
Cell studies and mechanisms	Maziarz et al. (2016) PMID 27086866	Stem cells (MSCs)	2007–2015	Extensive tabulation of EMF parameters and +/− responses
	Ross et al. (2015) PMID 26042793	Stem cells (hBMSCs) differentiation	1975–2015	Table of pulsed EMF parameters 2008–2015
	Fini et al. (2013) PMID 23339690	Articular chondrocytes and cartilage explants	1991–2012	Tabulated 17 studies in cartilage models; EMF suppresses inflammation; tissue engineering
	Pall (2013) PMID 23802593	VGCCs in a wide array of tissue cells	1990–2011	VGCCs triggered by EMFs Ca/calmodulin, NO, kinase G pathways

(Continued)

TABLE 8.1 (*Continued*)

Published Reviews of Electromagnetic Field (EMF) Effects on Skeletal Tissues Described in this Chapter

Main Target Area	Authors, Year, PMID (see Ref.)	Subject Emphasis	Years Covered	Comments
Fracture healing— Methodology and clinical trials	Cadossi et al. (2017) Markov, ISBN-1482248514	EMF Mechanisms and clinical examples: bone and cartilage	1791–2014	Good background and mechanisms, diagrams; table of TGFb/BMP responses for EMFs
	Cook et al. (2015) PMID 25440417	Overview clinical EMF technol. & applications	1957–2014	Wide ranging applications of EMF (incl. LIPUS); non-union data weak
	Behrens et al. (2013) Medscape 778366_1	Overview: technol. & data on fracture healing	1744–2012	Tabulates evidence for fracture healing; Defines "Levels of evidence"
	Griffin et al. (2011) PMID 21491410	Systematic review: RCTs of EMFs for delayed union	1980–2011	Only 4 RCTs qualified; EMF response not significant
	Mollon et al. (2008) PMID 18978400	Meta-analysis of delayed union RCTs of EMFs	1980–2008	Only 4 RCTs qualified; EMF response not significant
Osteoporosis— Basic and clinical	Zhu et al. (2017) PMID 28665487	5 EMF clinical studies;	1990–2013	Tables very useful. Clinical RCTs inconsistent
		12 animal, 21 cell studies	2002–2017	Animal studies heterogeneous
	Wang, R. et al. (2016) PMID 27356174	Molecular mechanisms, 3 pathways, MSC differentiation	1990–2015	EMF can restore osteo-adipogenic balance; Study heterogeneity limits progress
Oseotoarthritis & cartilage— Basic and clinical	Ganesan et al. (2009) PMID 20329696	Overview EMF and cells; animal models; clinical trials	1974–2009	EMF Mechanisms, anti-inflammatory effects; clinical trials (function, pain) inconclusive
	Ryang We et al. (2013) PMID 22504115	Systematic clinical review. 14 RCTs, 482 patients, knee osteoarthritis	1990–2011	Good tabulation of trials and EMFs. High qual. RCTs, PEMF effective for pain, function @ 8 week
	Li, S. et al. (2013) PMID 24338431	Systematic clinical review. 9 RCTs, 636 pts., most knee osteoarthritis	1994–2013	EMF: 15% decrease in pain; not different from placebo in function or quality of life
Wound healing	Aziz & Cullum (2015) PMID 26134172	Systematic review of RCTs of EMFs for leg ulcers	1990–2014	Only 3 RCTs qualified; EMF response not significant; (inconclusive benefit)
	Saliev et al. (2014) PMID 25319486	Cell & animal studies related to dermal wounds+EMF	1990–2013	18 directly related studies most in last decade. Other novel applications of EMF

Abbreviations: EMF, electromagnetic field; PEMF, pulsed EMF; MSC, mesenchymal stem cells; hBMSC, human bone marrow stem cells; VGCC, voltage-gated calcium channel; LIPUS, low-intensity pulsed ultrasound; RCT, randomized controlled trials; PMID, PUBMED ID# for easy retrieval.

applications and to discern where and how this application of EMFs to biology can be advanced.

8.2 A Brief Historical Perspective

The use of EMFs to improve bone and cartilage repair was an outgrowth of the original research on the electrical properties of bone and injured tissues and the subsequent attempts to stimulate repair and regeneration using weak electrical currents (Yasuda and Sata, 1955; Bassett et al., 1964; Becker and Spadaro, 1972). This may help explain what may appear to some as a strange initial application of bioelectromagnetics to bone, in contrast, for example, to cancer research, neurophysiology, or immunology. On the other hand, it was several innovative orthopedic surgeons who led the way: Robert O. Becker MD, C. Andrew L. Bassett MD, Carl T. Brighton MD, PhD, E. Yasuda MD, Zachary Friedenberg MD, and their many colleagues. The present author also had the good fortune to be associated with the development of electromagnetic interventions for the application to skeletal regeneration and repair from the early years as a graduate student under Becker, C. H. Bachman PhD, and David G. Murray MD and in collaboration with Andrew Marino PhD and others. He also had the opportunity to collaborate with Arthur Pilla for whose assistance and enthusiasm he will ever be grateful. Pilla was instrumental in the theory and development of low-frequency pulsing EMF as a noninvasive stimulus until his untimely death in 2015.

The natural clinical targets for the surgeons and researchers were at first the failures of bone fracture healing, delayed union and nonunion, that are estimated to occur approximately 5% of the time on average, depending strongly on circumstances and location. More recently, the targets of EMF have grown to include the manipulation of stem cell proliferation and differentiation aimed at the repair of articular cartilage in osteoarthritis and the healing of difficult or chronic soft tissue wounds.

The most fundamental biophysical mechanisms thought to be involved in coupling of time-varying EMFs to molecular systems and cells is better discussed by experts and may be found in earlier chapters of this handbook and Pilla's review in the previous edition (Pilla, 2006). This would include issues such as signal to thermal noise ratio, high-frequency effects vs. low-frequency effects, submolecular fields, and cyclotron resonance. Instead, the present chapter will only outline the cellular and molecular pathways thought by the review authors to be activated by the applied fields. For the most part, these fields are low-frequency pulses or sinusoidal waves of low magnitude (nonthermal), although some new studies are using low-frequency pulse-modulated MHz "carrier" waves of low amplitude. The reason for the predominance of low-frequency modulation is likely partly historic, partly for convenience, but mostly because they are similar to endogenous fields and currents seen during development, wound repair or neuromuscular activities. In the most recent decade, inductive (magnetic) coupling has been the most frequently used methodology, presumably because it provides a convenient, noninvasive way to introduce electric currents (and magnetic fields) *in vitro* and *in vivo*. As time went on, a large number of low-frequency, magnetic, and electric experiments appeared to offer evidence of positive EMF responses, even though this evidence, as will be seen, is somewhat inconsistent and incomplete.

Largely because of the wide variety of electromagnetic field frequencies, pulse rates, intensities, waveforms, and application times used in the many research reports represented by the reviews, this chapter will use "electromagnetic field" (EMF) or if plural (EMFs) to represent them, with distinctions made as needed. EMF is used here to include static and time-varying magnetic and electric stimuli. (The pulsed magnetic field subtype is often denoted 'PEMF' in the literature.) RCT is used to denote "randomized controlled trial" (plural, RCTs). Most acronyms are defined when introduced. Familiar molecular abbreviations are often used without definition.

8.3 Bibliographic Perspective

Most of the reviews described on here were identified using PubMed searches of the NLM Medline database in June 2017. An initial search from 1975 to the present yielded 634 citations, retrieved under bone, cartilage, or wound healing coupled within the major topic, "electromagnetic fields." These were then filtered for "reviews." Others were found by hand review of bibliographies. Of a total of 28 reviews, 16 were selected for inclusion as more recent and best quality in each category. Each had 50–100 literature citations. To examine the trend in total publication and research activity in EMFs and musculoskeletal cells, tissues, and clinical trials, the number of citations per year from 1975 to 2017 from the above search was used as a sample (Figure 8.1). This showed a relative increase in activity during the 1980s and another increase after 2000. The first increase coincided with the development and use of pulsed EMF technology.

An earlier bibliographic analysis of the first three decades also showed a publication increase in the 1980s, although the collection was less restrictive and performed mostly by "hand" (Spadaro, 1993). The citations from the last decade (2007–2017) show a general continuation of the number of annual publications/year.

8.4 Cell and Molecular Mechanisms of EMFs

8.4.1 EMF Responses and Mechanisms in Stem Cells (Maziarz et al., 2016)

The review by Maziarz et al. (2016) covers the experimental literature from the most recent decade on the effects of EMFs on the proliferation and differentiation of an assortment of adult stem cells. Most of the papers reviewed (17/22) used bone marrow-derived, mesenchymal stem cells (BM-MSCs) and 13/22 used low-frequency, pulsed magnetic fields, while the rest employed low-frequency sinusoidal or static/sine combination EMFs. After an explanation of the fundamental roles of stems cells, the authors justify the likely role of

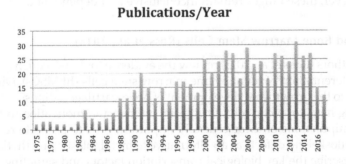

Publications/Year

FIGURE 8.1
Using a PUBMED search as an estimate of papers published between 1975 and 2017 on the subjects of electromagnetic fields and bone or cartilage or wound healing, 634 papers were retrieved. From 2007 to 2017 alone, it was estimated that 253 were published (about 23/year). This compares to an average of 22/year for the previous decade. (The number for 2017 was estimated since the test was performed at midyear. Also, MEDLINE subject classifications typically lag for the last year.)

exogenous EMFs based on earlier findings of endogenous EMFs in embryogenesis, adult homeostasis, cell migration and wound healing.

On 3 pages, the authors tabulate 22 studies of exogenous, low-frequency, low-intensity EMFs, separated by whether sinusoidal or pulsed EMFs are used. They point out that human stem cells appear to exhibit a strong increase in proliferation (20%–60%) after EMF exposure, with longer S-phase and shorter G1 phase in the cell cycle, independent of whether sinusoidal or pulsed EMFs are used. Much of the evidence also shows differentiation effects at different stages of the life cycle, and with different culture conditions and media. Overall, however, the MSC responses to EMF appear to be inconsistent from study to study. Null or negative findings (e.g., reduced proliferation or differentiation) have been reported in some cases and conditions (their figure 2). The expression of various markers is also inconsistent between observers.

In an attempt to find clues to the relationship of cellular response type to EMF frequency and field intensity, the authors provide a useful graphical map, showing sinusoidal and pulsed waveform results separately. In addition, they map the distribution of waveforms in the recent studies by reference number for easy retrieval. They conclude that the inconsistencies do not allow a clear explanation of how EMF parameters affect stem cell differentiation. Nevertheless, several interesting observations were made: MSC derivatives, bone and cartilage, are not the only cells that seem to be sensitive to low-frequency EMFs. Evidence for neurogenic and cardiogenic cell proliferation and/or differentiation has been reported. Also, interesting changes in stem cell morphology after EMF exposure have been seen, such as cell compaction, increased size, polygonal shape change, and expression of heat shock proteins hsp27 and hsp70.

The authors emphasize that to date, the mechanisms of EMF responses remain unclear, although those mentioned by other reviewers appear likely: changes in plasma membrane polarization and deformation in molecules controlling ion channel conduction. They also mention intracellular and extracellular reactive oxygen species formation as possible agents. The latter are liable to be inhibitive second messengers at high concentrations or induce beneficial signaling pathways at lower concentrations. Microthermal processes may also play a role.

In summary, Maziarz et al., suggest that cell proliferation appears more likely to result at 50 Hz/5 mT for sinusoidal EMFs and for 15–75 Hz/1.8–3 mT with pulsed EMFs. They suggest that cell differentiation is likely at slightly higher frequencies and similar intensities. In reality, however, these ranges remain inconclusive and dependent on many variables.

8.4.2 EMFs and Bone Marrow Stem Cells (Ross et al., 2015)

Ross and co-authors (Ross et al., 2015) review the evidence for low-frequency EMF enhancement of the differentiation of human bone marrow stem cells (hBMSCs). Differentiation of hBMSCs is key to the growth and development of bone, cartilage, adipose cells, and stromal cells supporting hematopoietic cells. Of special interest and motivation to the authors are the *in vitro* manipulations of these crucially important cells to promote regeneration and repair of musculoskeletal defects as an alternative to metal/plastic prosthetic implants. The authors first describe the key biological transcription factors and signaling molecules that are now known to allow differentiation of the multi-potent hBMSCs into bone, cartilage, or adipose tissues. Transcription factors CBFA-Runx2 and Osterix (Sp7) drive bone formation, while Sox9 and Wnt/b-catenin pathways drive chondrogenesis. During natural development and regeneration, electric fields from endogenous ionic currents appear to impact tissue growth and shape as emphasized in the early work of Becker (1961). Currently, Ross et al., suggest these currents are the basis of the responses of cells and tissues to exogenous EMFs by altering membrane permeability and voltage-gated calcium channels in patterned ways that have yet to be discovered. They act as triggers for downstream pathways that couple to key transcription factors. Numerous experiments have observed increases in expression of osteogenic markers (proteins or mRNAs) after EMF exposure of hBMSCs or other osteoblast precursor cells *in vitro*. The markers include alkaline phosphatase, RUNX/CBFA1, TGF-b1, osteopontin, osteonectin, collagen I, collagen III, bone morphogenetic proteins (BMP-2,4), and bone extracellular mineral deposition. According to Ross et al., some have reported that decreases in the frequency of intracellular Ca^{2+} oscillations play a key role in EMF induced hBMSC osteogenic differentiation. It is noteworthy that persistent tissue level Ca^{2+} flux changes have been observed in mouse calvarial bone *in vivo* after 15 Hz pulsed, 2 mT EMF was applied (Spadaro and Bergstrom, 2002).

As for EMF stimulus specificity, the review by Ross et al., presents an interesting table of frequencies and intensities of pulsed EMFs from 11 studies showing effects on hBMSCs *in vitro*. The frequency range is 5–150 Hz, with seven studies using 15 Hz. All but one study showed characteristics and markers for osteogenic differentiation. On the other hand, low-frequency pulsed EMFs can cause chondrocytic differentiation and proliferation under favorable culture conditions or when the stem cells are already committed to this phenotype. Finally, the authors comment that most investigators rarely say why they selected electrical parameters for their experiments.

8.4.3 Voltage-Gated Calcium Channels (Pall, 2013)

Another review of cell mechanisms by Pall (2013) gives very convincing arguments that voltage-gated calcium channels (VGCCs) on the cell plasma membrane are the most likely primary targets for exogenous EMFs effects on stem cells, osteoblasts, chondrocytes, neutrophils, neural cells, etc. The author (a biochemist) reviews 23 studies to support this hypothesis. The evidence from these studies revolves around showing that specific VGCC blockers (or inhibition of their downstream pathways) inhibit EMF effects. Also, lots of other studies are cited that implicate changes in intracellular calcium concentrations after EMF exposure, some very rapid (seconds, minutes) and some slower (days, weeks). An increase of intracellular Ca^{2+} stimulates calcium/calmodulin-dependent nitric oxide (NO) synthases and elevates levels of NO. The subsequent elements of the pathway, according to Pall, involve increases in cGMP and protein kinase G activity. On the other hand, the author also found evidence of "pathophysiological" responses to EMFs via the same VGCC channels and the synthesized NO combining with superoxide, forming peroxynitrite and free-radical oxidants. This could result in DNA single strand breaks or other cellular damage and inflammation.

In addition, Pall cited a recent report by Pilla (2012) who found a substantial Ca/calmodulin-dependent increase in nitric oxide in less than 5 s after the onset of a 2-Hz pulsed EMF (27 MHz RF, 2.5 μT). The NO response was seen in MN9D neuronal-type cells and human fibroblasts when previously challenged by serum depletion and heat shock, and was nullified by calmodulin antagonist WF-7. Pall suggests that the rapidity of the NO response in this experiment is strong evidence of a VGCC pathway mechanism for the EMF. The strength of Pall's review is its focus on the VGCC mechanism as a common element, despite a wide variety of EMF waveform and frequencies (static, RF, pulses, ELF, electric field, magnetic field, etc.) and equally wide range of secondary cellular/tissue responses. While the apparent lack of EMF waveform specificity may bring renewed skepticism in nonthermal applications of EMF, on balance the volume of accumulated laboratory observations favoring the sensitivity of VGCC's seems to be a positive way forward.

(Note: this may be compared to Pilla's emphasis on the Ca/calmodulin activation as the essential common initial step in EMF activation.)

8.4.4 EMFs in Tissue Engineering and Cartilage (Fini et al., 2013)

Fini et al. (2013) have provided a substantial review of the current situation with regard to the roles and mechanisms that exogenous EMFs can play in tissue engineering of hyaline cartilage repair in arthritic joints. In the process, she and her colleagues document 11 studies that investigated the constituents of the inflammatory microenvironment near a cartilage lesion or after surgical intervention (dominated by inflammatory cytokines IL-1b and TNF-a). More importantly, the authors summarize the results of no less than 17 laboratory studies of human and animal chondrocytes or cartilage explants cultured *in vitro* and treated with EMFs (15 pulsing waveforms, 1 sinusoidal, and 1 static magnetic field).

The two main EMF effects seen in this array of studies are (a) anabolic effects on the chondrocytes, including cell proliferation, matrix production, collagen II synthesis, proteoglycan (PG) synthesis, and (b) a suppression of inflammatory cytokine activity and their catabolic effects. Significantly, the anti-inflammatory effects seem to occur in part by upregulation of cell membrane adenosine receptors (A2a-ARs) by biophysical mechanisms still to be explained. The ARs are linked to G-protein components at the membrane and stimulate an increase in cAMP molecules that inhibit production of TNF-a and IL-1b inflammatory cytokines. Also, in chondrocytes and synovial cells, A2a-AR has been shown to inhibit the transcription factor, nuclear factor-kappa beta (NF-kB), notorious for mediating inflammatory pathways. In addition, the EMF anabolic stimulation of the chondrocytes matrix is thought to help strengthen the cells against the destructive effect of excess inflammation.

In recent years, there has been a concerted effort to engineer biological replacements for damaged human joint cartilage using human cells and various scaffolds as a solution to osteoarthritis. Because of the noninvasive nature and positive findings described above, EMFs would likely play a role in the *in vitro* formation of the constructs and then in the postsurgical phase to strengthen and protect the transplants.

8.5 EMF Methodology for Bone and Cartilage Healing

8.5.1 Overview of EMFs in Bone and Cartilage Repair (Cadossi et al., 2015)

Cadossi et al. (2015) have assembled an excellent review that includes a description of the cellular mechanisms currently thought to be operative in each type of EMF stimulation of bone and cartilage (inductive pulsed EMF, capacitively coupled EMF and also pulsed ultrasound). The mechanisms, covered elsewhere in this chapter, emphasize the calcium signaling pathways originating in the plasma membrane and/or the endoplasmic reticulum (ER) and their effects on precursor cell differentiation, proliferation, and matrix production. According to the authors, many previous experimental studies show that inductive EMFs appear to trigger primarily Ca^{2+} release from the ER, while capacitive coupling stimulates calcium channels in the plasma membrane. A table is provided, listing 16 key cell and tissue studies and their observed responses. A number of studies of bone and cartilage cells exposed to various EMFs are referenced from the last decade to strengthen the earlier evidence.

The authors then provide an overview of the important studies and trials showing clinical benefits of EMFs in bone healing in nonunions, articular cartilage lesions, presurgical and postsurgical osteoarthritis and on osteonecrosis of the hip. Most of these are not randomized and inadequately placebo controlled. The authors, however, add several recent clinical trials not apparently referenced by other reviewers, particularly in the area of osteoarthritis treatment, and one double blind study of EMF therapy for osteoporotic vertebral fracture, all with positive findings.

8.5.2 Bone Stimulator Technology (Cook et al., 2015)

Cook et al. (2015) in their recent comprehensive clinical review, "Healing in the New Millennium: Bone stimulators," provide an outline of the chief EMF methodologies developed for bone healing, how they have been used, an evaluation of the success rates and an extensive bibliography. Also included is an evaluation of pulsed ultrasound bone growth stimulation, a method beyond the scope of this chapter. The central EMF methods are direct currents (DC) (the forerunner) where electrodes are inserted into the fracture site and microampere currents applied; capacitive coupling (CC) for which bare or insulated electrodes are placed on the skin and kHz currents are applied; and inductive coupling (IC) in which pulsed, low-frequency magnetic fields induce currents in the tissues using portable, battery operated coil transducers. Although the latter type, often called "PEMF," is currently the most popular, all three are FDA approved for marketing for the treatment of nonunions and delayed unions. Cook et al., give the rationale for the additional uses of EMFs for the prevention of nonunion after injury or surgery in high-risk procedures such as ankle fusions (arthrodesis), repair of osteochondral lesions, the treatment of arthritis/inflammatory disease, osteoporosis, and chronic leg ulcers. (Some of these will be discussed below.) As is also discussed elsewhere in this chapter, EMFs mechanism of action on clinical fracture healing is still largely a matter of speculation and research. It has been that way for over 30 years.

8.6 Evaluation of Clinical Trials of EMFs for Bone Healing

8.6.1 Fracture Treatment—Evidence Levels (Behrens et al., 2013)

To evaluate the efficacy of EMFs for fracture healing, one can turn to other recent reviews, especially systematic reviews and meta-analyses. Behrens et al. (2013) incorporate information in their review on the "levels of evidence" measure of clinical trials in their evaluations. To evaluate the quality of evidence from clinical trials and develop recommendations, surgeons and researchers typically use the scale shown in Table 8.2.

According to Behrens et al., direct current (DC) methodology has no Level I evidence available for treatment of nonunions and the majority of studies are case series (Level IV) even though successful union rates of 70%–80% have been reported. Inductive coupling (IC, or pulsed EMF) treatment for delayed unions and fracture nonunions has a plethora of trials reported (Behrens references 7 previous studies), but no Level I evidence is available and most evidence is Level IV. Capacitive coupling (CC) treatment has several Level II studies

TABLE 8.2

Levels of Evidence in Clinical Trials

Levels of Evidence	Derived from....
Level I	RCTs with a significant difference between arms, or if without significant difference, with narrow confidence intervals. (Also included are systematic reviews or meta-analyses of Level I trials.)
Level II	Prospective cohort studies, RCTs of poor quality. (Also included are systematic reviews of Level II trials or nonhomogeneous Level I trials.)
Level III	Case-control studies, retrospective cohort trials (and systematic reviews of Level II trials).
Level IV	Case series without control groups or with only historical controls.
Level V	Consists in expert opinion.

Source: Behrens et al. (2013).
Note: Level I is the highest level, carrying the highest recommendation for use.
Abbreviation: RCT, randomized clinical trial.

for delayed unions or nonunions and reported healing rates were in the 60%–78% range. A related fourth method of EMF therapy involving both static and low-frequency magnetic fields is applied simultaneously. In theory, this EMF method couples to calcium or other ions and is referred to as "combined magnetic fields" (CMF) or "ion resonance." Despite a number of laboratory studies and commercialization supporting this idea, Behrens et al., indicate that no human studies to date demonstrate the efficacy of CMF in nonunions and delayed unions. One double-blinded trial of CMF on patients undergoing a posterior spinal fusion, however, showed a faster healing after 9 months compared to controls.

8.6.2 EMF Fracture Treatment—Systematic Review (Griffin et al., 2011)

A meta-analysis by Griffin et al., and cited by Behrens et al., was able to include only four double-blinded RCTs (three pulsed EMF and one CC) for nonunion or delayed union despite thousands of patients treated with EMFs worldwide since its debut around 1978. Searching the medical literature databases (MEDLINE, EMBASE, Cochrane, etc.) revealed that RCTs of high quality and control are very rare. Only 125 patients (subjects) were included in the combined data. The primary outcome was satisfactory radiographic healing of the fracture (3 cortices bridged) by a fixed time (24 weeks from entry). The results of the analysis showed that there was a small nonsignificant positive effect size (relative risk 1.6) and large heterogeneity. Although three of four trials showed slightly positive effects the results nevertheless are considered "inconclusive" for fracture healing.

8.6.3 EMF Fracture Treatment—Meta-Analysis (Mollon et al., 2008)

A similar meta-analysis by Mollon et al., three years earlier, gave essentially the same result. In this case, of 2,546 trial citations found, 32 were reviewed in full, and 11 met the inclusion criteria. After removal of trials with inadequate blinding, group imbalances, etc., only four RCTs remained in the analysis—the same four that appeared again in the Griffin study. The level of evidence claimed in this analysis was Level II. The relative risk effect size was 1.76, and the results are considered "inconclusive" At the present writing, there does not appear to be any additional RCT, systematic reviews, or meta-analyses that would change this evaluation for nonunion or delayed union treated with EMFs.

8.7 EMFs for Osteoporosis Treatment

8.7.1 EMF for Postmenopausal Osteoporosis (Zhu et al., 2017)

This review by Siyi Zhu et al., from the West China Hospital, P.R. China appears to be an important contribution to the literature on the potential application of EMFs to the treatment or prevention of osteoporosis. In several places in this chapter, substantial evidence is presented for the anabolic effects of EMFs on bone, the increase of osteoblastic proliferation and differentiation, and its effects in reducing inflammatory cytokines. This would seem to imply that an EMF applied locally and noninvasively would be able to prevent or reverse bone weakening and density loss and prevent fracture. Yet this possibility seems to have been largely ignored by researchers and clinicians. During the last 10 years, however, there has been a rapid expansion of interest and experimental work on this and it has largely come from China.

The authors first describe 5 small clinical trials, 4 of which were placebo controlled involving a total of 224 subjects with osteoporosis or disuse osteopenia treated with pulsed EMF. Only one of the studies showed a significant increase in bone mineral density (BMD). Another showed an increase in physical exercise function. Obviously, this is too small a data set from which to draw conclusions. In addition, each used a different pulsed EMF stimulus and regimen. The only randomized, double blind, sham placebo controlled trial showed no significant difference between pulsed EMF (15 Hz pulse burst, 2 mT) and sham after 8–24 weeks follow-up (Spadaro et al., 2011).

Turning to basic science the authors tabulate 12 studies using animal models of osteoporosis, again with a variety of pulsed EMF waveforms, frequencies and most using an ovariectomized rat model. All studies showed a positive increase in BMD or histological μCT parameters of bone strength. What is especially interesting is the relatively narrow range of treatment waveforms; all but one study were in the 8–15 Hz frequency range and 1–4 mT magnetic field amplitude. Data included, μCT measurement parameters, DXA, bone formation and resorption markers, and mRNA expression for key genes.

Finally, the authors tabulate and summarize a list of 22 laboratory studies (last 10 years) on bone and bone cells (or analogs) in cultures treated with low-frequency pulsed EMF with evidence on the proliferation, differentiation, formation, resorption, and mineralization of bone *in vitro*. The analyses include gene expression and or proteins produced by the cells in response to the stimulus, indicating changes in their stage of development.

From this body of *in vitro* work and the animal studies above, the authors draw the following conclusions:

1. The pulsing EMF that seems to be the most efficient in stimulating bone formation and reducing resorption and thus likely to improve bone density is in a pulse rate window of 7.5–50 Hz, an intensity window (peak) of 0.1–3.8 mT, and treatment times of 0.7–8 h/day for up to 12 weeks. Several groups (including their own) found 8 Hz pulse rate, 3.8 mT peak magnetic field intensity and 0.7 h/day for 12 weeks to be most efficient.

2. The likely mechanisms by which a pulsed EMF could be expected to enhance osteogenesis are by the Wnt signaling pathway, since elements of this were upregulated in the cell experiments.

3. The OPG/RANK/RANKL signaling pathway is also known to be important and the evidence supports this. Specifically, an increase in the OPG/RANKL protein ratio, produced by osteoblasts and osteocytes, would favor bone formation over resorption. Pulsed EMFs have been shown to elevate OPG.

4. As mentioned by others, pulsed EMFs are able to increase the activation of the adenosine receptors on various cells, reducing the effects of inflammatory cytokines that can lead to bone resorption by osteoclasts.

5. The combined use of pulsed EMFs with other agents may give an increased efficacy and needs to be investigated.

6. The safety of using EMFs for osteoporosis treatment and prevention needs to be verified.

8.7.2 Systematic Review of Osteoporosis and EMF (Wang et al., 2016)

While not as detailed as the Zhu review, Wang et al., present a good synopsis of the scientific rationale and using EMFs for counteracting osteopenia and osteoporosis. They cite a number of recent and classical papers showing how low-frequency EMFs increase the proliferation of MSCs and bias their differentiation toward the osteoblast phenotype and away from the adipocyte phenotype. In addition, they cite recent studies on how this appears to depend on cell state, cell type, and EMF characteristics (frequency, waveform, intensity, and time). EMFs also affect the balance between the activation of osteoclastic resorption and bone formation via the expression of RANKL or osteoprotegerin (OPG), respectively. In this regard, pulsed EMF studies in the 8–15 Hz, 2–3.5 mT range have been found to decrease RANKL and increase OPG, favoring osteoblastic bone formation over resorption and preserving bone mass in ovariectomized rat models. Similar waveforms have been found to positively influence bone architecture and reduce disuse bone loss in animal osteoporosis models produced by hind limb unloading.

Clinical controlled trial data on osteoporosis is fairly scarce as indicated above, but related studies of EMF treatment effectiveness for chronic pain ("bone pain" or low back pain), at least in the short term, have been more forthcoming.

As for cellular mechanisms for EMFS ameliorating osteoporosis, the authors diagram first the familiar modulation of Ca/calmodulin binding discussed by Pilla and others (Pilla, 2015), and its resulting modulation of nitric oxide (NO) via the NO synthases. These lead ultimately in bone cells or precursors, to the production of bone anabolic proteins and growth factors. They also diagram an alternative pathway involving RAS/RAF/MAP-K eventually leading to a similar result.

8.8 EMFs for Cartilage Repair and Arthritis: Overview

8.8.1 Arthritis & EMF—Overview (Ganesan et al., 2009)

A summary of the review by Ganesan et al., is included because it deals with the subject of EMF application to the treatment of osteoarthritis and the experimental basis for it. It is also a comprehensive review of the background and the various forms of EMF stimuli, the cellular mechanisms, and the evidence for clinical efficacy. It is a good starting point for those investigating the use of EMF for the prevention and treatment of arthritis and cartilage repair and regeneration.

After some historical background, the authors begin with a brief discussion of the properties of the noninvasive "low-frequency" pulsed EMF stimuli ("signals") that have typically been used, looking at ranges of "frequencies, intensities, durations, and waveforms." Noninvasive coupling methods (capacitive or inductive), but not modulated RF fields, were included. In discussing *in vitro* evidence they include a table of observed "beneficial" effects of EMF observed on cells involved in the etiology of osteoarthritis (chondrocytes, osteoblasts, osteoclasts, fibroblasts, lymphocytes, and neutrophils). The evidence is persuasive and includes bone formation, chondrocyte regeneration, matrix synthesis, reduction of osteoclast maturation, and reduction of inflammation. The authors review the proposed evidence for EMF signal transduction mechanisms, with the various cells. In the case of bone cells, the prominent examples are (1) the mobilization and redistribution of surface receptors and protein kinase C activity, resulting in increased Ca^{2+} influx and mobilization and downstream changes in signaling cascades, and (2) in the case of inflammatory cells, there is evidence that the same membrane Ca^{2+} mechanism may be at work, as well as changes to the membrane cytoskeleton and alterations in protein kinase activity. The result is an anti-inflammatory effect, such as a reduction in lysosomal enzyme activity and cartilage matrix damage. Recent papers cited also give evidence of a modulation of MSC differentiation by the EMF as well as increases in stem cell proliferation. Both effects are important in the regenerative repair of joint cartilage and bone, as noted previously.

In examining the evidence of EMF treatment or prevention in "clinical trials," the authors cite a few studies where the EMF reduced pain, and increased mobility in arthritic patients. On the other hand, some clinical trials could not demonstrate a symptomatic benefit and a 2006 systematic review showed EMFs to be of "little value." These authors conclude that the research is presently only about half way toward understanding the mechanisms by which EMF can restore injured joint tissue and only part way toward selection of optimal stimulation regimes.

8.8.2 Osteoarthritis—Clinical Systematic Review (Ryang We et al., 2013)

This is a recent systematic review of 14 screened, randomized, placebo-controlled studies (RCTs) of EMFs with a total of 930 patients with knee osteoarthritis (OA). It was the most recent review found using quality selection filtering and meta-analysis techniques. Given the current situation alluded to by Ganesan et al., and others, in which conflicting findings on pulsed EMF efficacy in osteoarthritis are common, systematic and objective reviews are welcome.

The RCTs used widely accepted scoring methods for pain (visual analog scale (VAS)) and function (Western Ontario & McMaster osteoarthritis index (WOMAC)), at time periods out to 16 weeks. Most of the trials used six weeks of daily treatments with pulsed EMF, half of the subjects receiving active EMF units. The placebo controls were generally well designed but varied in method. Subjects, therapist, and assessor were blinded in many of the trials. The EMFs details are described in a table and varied widely in pulse frequency, flux density, etc. Three trials used pulse-modulated carrier waves (27 MHz) and the rest were low-frequency pulses (1–50 Hz). While measures of subject heterogeneity were considered adequate for the analysis, this did not apparently include the EMFs, which varied in waveform, intensity, and daily exposure time.

The results as a whole (both pain and function) showed that EMF was not more effective than placebo. When knee function was examined, EMF was more effective only at the

8 week time period. When trials with sufficient blinding, low attrition rates, and higher methodological quality were considered, EMF was more effective in reducing pain than placebo treatment at four and eight weeks after the start of treatment. No significant differences were seen in adverse events. The authors point out some technical weaknesses in several of the trials; including their poor standardization of the EMF stimulus protocols (timing and type), and a poor description of the placebo used.

8.8.3 Osteoarthritis—Clinical Cochrane Review (Li et al., 2013)

Another contemporary systematic review by Li et al. (2013) of clinical trials of EMF treatment for osteoarthritis should be mentioned. While previous reviews appeared to confirm the Ryang et al. (2013) review's findings that there is a marginal, but unproven benefit in either reducing pain or improving joint function with EMF field application, the review by Li et al., seems a bit more positive. Nine RCT studies with 636 participants in total showed a moderate benefit in pain relief (15%) but with no significant effect on physical function. (This review had some overlap in study inclusion with the Ryang paper.) Due to weaknesses in design reporting and some possible biases, according to the authors, the results do not appear to significantly shift the assessment of clinical benefit away from the "possible, moderate" category. This suggests the need for more definitive studies perhaps by determining optimal EMF waveforms and regimens for osteoarthritis treatment before reliable improvements in outcome can be expected.

In other recent developments in osteoarthritis treatment with EMFs, Nelson et al. (2013) have also shown a very positive clinical result in a pilot RCT of early knee arthritis treated with a 1 Hz, 7 ms pulse-modulated 6.8 MHz carrier wave applied for 30 min/day for up to 42 days. A 50% reduction in VAS pain score was seen in EMF treated vs. sham. In another similar study reported by Bagnato et al. (2016), 60 patients with documented knee osteoarthritis were treated with a 1 kHz, 100 μs pulsed, 27 MHz carrier wave EMF with a 9.8 mW peak power amplitude, applied over the knee for 12 h/day. After 1 month, those treatment with active devices resulted in a 25% reduction in pain scores (VAS) vs. a 3.7% reduction in those with placebo control devices ($p < 0.001$). Knee function scores (WOMAC) likewise improved ~18% with the EMF ($p < 0.02$). A similar pulsed radio frequency (PRF) waveform used by Pilla (2015) to trigger NO production in fibroblasts via a calmodulin/NO/cGMP pathway was a 2 Hz, 2 ms pulse modulated 27 MHz carrier wave that seems to be more able to reduce inflammation and pain. If confirmed and refined by additional studies, this type of pulse-modulated microwave EMF (or PRF) may lead to future improvements in the non-pharmacologic treatment of osteoarthritis.

8.8.4 EMFs in Tissue Engineering and Cartilage (Fini et al., 2013)

This previously discussed review by Fini et al. (2013) is also very appropriate to revisit here in that it deals with tissue engineering to repair and regenerate cartilage damaged by osteoarthritis. In the application of EMFs to the *in vitro* and surgical phases of the use of engineered constructs, the anti-inflammatory effects triggered by EMFs are an advantage as discussed above. On the other hand, during the direct treatment of patients with early phase osteoarthritis, the authors emphasize that the observed anti-inflammatory activity of EMFs become very important. This is because reducing inflammation should relieve pain and reduce further damage and prolong the useful life of the natural joint tissues. The authors cite a few clinical trial reports in which application he applications of EMFs had both short- and long-term benefits in terms of pain and function.

8.9 EMFs for Aiding Wound Healing

8.9.1 Venous Ulcer Treatment (Aziz and Cullum, 2015)

Much of what has already been said of EMF and stem cells, MSCs, fibroblasts, myofibrocytes, and tendon cells applies also to soft tissue wound healing. The cells are of the same origin and several of the authors previously cited include some information on them. Deficient wound healing is a major medical problem, exemplified by ischemic and pressure ulcers, diabetic neuropathy, stasis wounds after spinal cord injury (paralysis), and burn wounds. In the search for additional interventions, low-frequency EMF stimulation has been proposed over the years. The clinical evidence, however, is scant as indicated by the Cochrane systematic review by Aziz and Cullum (2015). A wide database search yielded only "three" RCTs of EMFs for treating venous leg ulcers in a total of 94 patients. Because of heterogeneity, possible bias, and other limitations, these trials were not of methodologically suitable quality and the data could not be pooled. Aziz and Cullum concluded that there is *insufficient quality evidence* at present to show a clinical beneficial effect in speeding healing of leg ulcers or reducing pain.

8.9.2 Wound Healing and Tissue Engineering (Saliev et al., 2014)

Saliev et al. (2014) provide a review predominantly of laboratory studies related to soft tissue healing as well as to other cellular/tissue responses to EMFs in neurodegenerative diseases and tissue engineering applications. The experimental literature is considerably more robust than for the clinical trials. The authors cite 18 studies directly involving EMF effects on wound healing aspects, most from the most recent decade. The reader interested in following the wound healing applications would be well served to examine these citations. The authors conclude that, given the great clinical potential and therapeutic capacity for noninvasive EMF in wound care and in tissue regeneration, one can expect a future complimentary development of both. They also call for more clinical investigations, carried out with caution because of possible mutagenic adverse effects.

8.10 Discussion

8.10.1 Overview of the Decade

Pilla's (2006) handbook chapter closed with the following main points and projections:

- An abundance of experimental evidence and clinical experience demonstrates that exogenous EMFs of fairly low intensity and frequency can have profound effects on healing processes in musculoskeletal tissues. The application of EMFs to the treatment of arthritis, cartilage repair, and wound healing is growing.
- The clinical findings on EMFs have been validated by well-designed, well-controlled clinical trials.
- There is an increase in understanding the mechanism(s) of action of EMF to the point that specific waveform designs can be made *a priori* for particular conditions.
- The potential applications of EMFs therapeutics go well beyond the musculoskeletal area.

A decade later, the current reviews and literature generally continue to support most of these conclusions. Experimental evidence has increased, the evidence of low-intensity, low-frequency effects has continued to be produced, and in many cases results appear more robust. Cell effects with EMFs, especially with stem cells (MSCs) can now more easily be measured using molecular techniques. Also seen is a recent burst of positive osteoporosis findings for EMFs in animal models. Spurred by the interest in regenerative methods of treating osteoarthritis using cultured stem cell transplants, EMFs seem to provide a boost to proliferation, while at the same time reducing inflammation when applied *in vivo*. On mechanisms, it is fair to say that in the last decade, there has been some clarification and confirmation of the Ca^{2+} transport first messenger as the leading contender, and more authors have investigated pathways involving ROS formation. It is also fair to add that progress in this area is somewhat dependent on the progress in understanding of the biology of the cells themselves, without the exogenous EMFs. Witness in this regard the discoveries of the role of osteocytes in controlling bone remodeling and the roles of sclerostin and Wnt signaling. Finally, going beyond bone and cartilage repair, additional evidence has emerged that EMFs may enhance the differentiation of MSCs into neural cells. There is increased evidence that the anti-inflammatory responses of EMFs seem to have role in arthritis treatment, and other conditions that can reduce the use of systemic drugs.

Upon reflection, however, there are several qualifications and comments that need to be made concerning progress in the most recent decade, which follow below.

8.10.2 The Heterogeneity Problem

First, the heterogeneity of experiments, models, experimental conditions, and EMF characteristics leads to confusion and lack of confidence. Most of the reviewers have pointed out that that many contradictory findings occur, even among what appear to be well-done studies. Among cell studies, the experimental conditions (media, sources, life cycle stages, extraction procedures, etc.) likely account for this. Additionally, from this author's observations, it is rare for experiments to be verified by replication. Non-reproducibility in science has become a major problem (Baker, 2016). This is serious enough in conventional circles, but in a controversial field like bioelectromagnetics, it can be fatal. Some researchers, in addition, do not have valid repetitions within one study, relying on multiple wells from the same culture instead of repeat cultures. Many authors do not justify their choices of experimental conditions in order to be able to relate their results to those of others. This is especially true with regard to EMF waveforms, intensities, and application timing.

8.10.3 Clinical Trial Findings

It appears that Pilla's characterization of the clinical picture of EMFs as validated and well designed (Pilla, 2006) is not well supported by the reviews, specifically the systematic and meta-analyses currently available for nonunion or delayed union fracture treatment. Very few adequately performed trials have been reported (none are Level I evidence) and this has not changed in the last decade. The few trials available were inconclusive, with the possible exception of capacitively coupled EMF trials (Level II evidence). In recent reviews of EMF treatment of osteoarthritis, some evidence for pain relief was evident and there were only suggestive findings for improvement in function. Although levels of evidence were not specifically rated, no Level I studies seem to have been found. It is possible, then, that the EMFs currently used clinically for bone and cartilage are only marginally effective at best.

What might explain the discrepancy with Pilla's assessment? Clearly, many thousands of patients have been treated following the FDA approval of the marketing of EMF bone growth stimulators in the United States about 35 years ago. While some technological improvements in transducer design have streamlined its use, it is apparent that properly conducted trials for EMF fracture healing appear to have ceased and only some informal or nonpublic data may be available. This suggests that the continued development and testing of new waveforms and EMF regimes for bone and fracture healing has been hampered by the requirements and costs of FDA approval and commercialization in the United States. The less strict regulatory environment in Europe and Asia may allow for continued progress (Cadossi et al., 2015) but with less verification of clinical efficacy. Osteoarthritis treatment and prevention using EMF appears to have great potential, and hopefully it may avoid a similar fate. The same may be said of EMF treatment of wound healing and cutaneous ulcers. Commercial bias is also a strong factor in EMF translational research and must be recognized and counteracted by all.

8.10.4 EMF Waveforms and Mechanisms

During the last decade, there has been a continued heterogeneity in EMF characteristics in the published cell and animal experiments and to some extent in clinical uses. The focus is now generally on low frequency, time-varying magnetic stimuli, generally assumed to interact primarily via induced electric fields (and currents) within tissues and cells. (Direct interaction of cells with a weak magnetic field *per se* is less likely, but cannot be ruled out.) Most authors provide little rational for their choices of EMF waveforms. Some investigators may not appreciate the higher frequency components present due to rapid signal rise and fall times. The pulse repetition rate and amplitude alone may not be sufficient descriptors.

As for EMF interaction mechanisms, the molecular targets have been refined somewhat although intracellular calcium remains key. Pilla, Brighton, and others have left us several excellent hypotheses (Pilla, 2006, 2015). The shifting of ions, molecules, or receptors by the induced electric fields is thought to modulate binding kinetics along key cellular pathways. The plasma membrane voltage-gated calcium channel (VGCC) and intracellular Ca/calmodulin binding are prime suspects. The activation of nitric oxide and reactive oxygen species (ROS) are more recent findings, considered rapid second messengers. The ability of EMFs to modulate inflammation pathways is also a remarkable development. Changes appear to be able to occur rapidly (0.1 s to several min.) although older evidence exists that EMF exposure effects on Ca fluxes can persist for a day or two *in vivo* (Spadaro and Bergstrom, 2002). Certainly, other targets are possible. Current evidence seems to suggest that EMF is a rather "blunt instrument" at present and most of the reviewers felt that more investigation of the basic mechanisms is sorely needed.

Pilla's approach to EMF waveform design (Pilla, 2015) was through interaction modeling and has been very successful. On the other hand, empirical approaches are also valid and need to be expanded, but without some rationale for choice, systematic variation of EMF parameters, or control of other variables, progress will be limited. A "mini-Manhattan project" for waveform testing using a standard tissue model may be fruitful.

8.10.5 Beyond Bone

This review did not examine applications of EMFs outside the musculoskeletal tissues. Nevertheless, as discoveries of the multi-potency of stem cells such as MSCs continue, it is likely that EMF responsiveness will also be found in the differentiation, proliferation, and activity of their specific progeny. Even more likely may be the combination of a pharmacological agent and an EMF, where the EMF may act to potentiate the effect of a drug at a local site. An example may be in the treatment of osteoporosis where an antiresorptive agent is given at low dose while an EMF is applied over the hip region to achieve an increase in bone density and strength, with less risk from the drug's side effects. The same strategy could apply to local pain relief. The apparent very low-risk profile of EMFs used clinically makes new applications feasible. Pilla (2015) states,

> The predictions of the proposed model open a host of significant possibilities for configuration of non-thermal EMF signals for clinical and wellness applications that can reach far beyond fracture repair and wound healing. Active studies are underway to assess the utility of the known anti-inflammatory activity of PRF [pulsed radio frequency fields] for the treatment of traumatic brain injury, neurodegenerative diseases, cognitive disorders, degenerative joint disease, neural regeneration, and cardiac and cerebral ischemia.

8.11 Conclusions

The preceding decade has seen continued interest in basic research in low-frequency, low-intensity EMF for bone and cartilage repair, but very few clinical trials. Investigations of its possible application to osteoporosis and osteoarthritis have increased with positive findings. Some new evidence emerged supporting proposed mechanisms, mostly based on EMF modulation of intracellular calcium ion binding, channel fluxes, and NO release. Most observers call for more studies on mechanisms as well as an organized approach to reducing study heterogeneity and increasing replication. High-level evidence of clinical effectiveness is surprisingly sparse, but adverse events seem to have been rare. The prospect of reducing pharmacological treatments to upregulate regenerative processes is anticipated to be a driver for a renewal of worldwide interest in EMF applications in biology and medicine.

Acknowledgments

Many thanks to Donald Bridy and Robert Rudolph for their assistance in preparing the manuscript and to Mary Spadaro for her constant support.

References

Aziz Z, Cullum N. 2015. Electromagnetic therapy for treating venous leg ulcers. *Cochrane Database Syst Rev* (7): CD002933.

Bagnato GL, Miceli G, Marino N, Sciortino D, Bagnato GF. 2016. Pulsed electromagnetic fields in knee osteoarthritis: a double blind, placebo-controlled, randomized clinical trial. *Rheumatology* (Oxford) 55(4): 755–62.

Baker M. 2016. 1,500 scientists lift the lid on reproducibility. *Nature* 533(7604): 452–4.

Bassett CA, Pawluk RJ, Becker RO. 1964. Effects of electric currents on bone in vivo. *Nature* 204: 652–4.

Becker RO. 1961. The bioelectric factors in amphibian-limb regeneration. *J Bone Joint Surg Am* 43-A: 643–56.

Becker RO, Spadaro JA. 1972. Electrical stimulation of partial limb regeneration in mammals. *Bull N Y Acad Med* 48(4): 627–41.

Behrens SB, Deren ME, KO M. 2013. A review of bone growth stimulation for fracture treatment. *Curr Orthop Pract* 24(1): 84–91.

Cadossi R, Cadossi M, Setti S. 2015. Physical regulation in cartilage and bone repair. In: Markov M (ed.) *Electromagnetic Fields in Biology and Medicine.* Boca Raton, FL: CRC Press, pp. 253–72.

Cook JJ, Summers NJ, Cook EA. 2015. Healing in the new millennium: bone stimulators: an overview of where we've been and where we may be heading. *Clin Podiatr Med Surg* 32(1): 45–59.

Fini M, Pagani S, Giavaresi G, De Mattei M, Ongaro A, Varani K, Vincenzi F, Massari L, Cadossi M. 2013. Functional tissue engineering in articular cartilage repair: is there a role for electromagnetic biophysical stimulation? *Tissue Eng Part B Rev* 19(4): 353–67.

Ganesan K, Gengadharan AC, Balachandran C, Manohar BM, Puvanakrishnan R. 2009. Low frequency pulsed electromagnetic field—a viable alternative therapy for arthritis. *Indian J Exp Biol* 47(12): 939–48.

Griffin XL, Costa ML, Parsons N, Smith N. 2011. Electromagnetic field stimulation for treating delayed union or non-union of long bone fractures in adults. *Cochrane Database Syst Rev* (4): CD008471.

Li S, Yu B, Zhou D, He C, Zhuo Q, Hulme JM. 2013. Electromagnetic fields for treating osteoarthritis. *Cochrane Database Syst Rev* (12): CD003523.

Maziarz A, Kocan B, Mariuz B, Budzik S, Cholewa M, Ochiya T. 2016. How electromagnetic fields can influence adult stem cells: positive and negative impacts. *Stem Cell Res Ther* 7:54 12 pp.

Mollon B, da Silva V, Busse JW, Einhorn TA, Bhandari M. 2008. Electrical stimulation for long-bone fracture-healing: a meta-analysis of randomized controlled trials. *J Bone Joint Surg Am* 90(11): 2322–30.

Nelson FR, Zvirbulis R, Pilla AA. 2013. Non-invasive electromagnetic field therapy produces rapid and substantial pain reduction in early knee osteoarthritis: a randomized double-blind pilot study. *Rheumatol Int* 33(8): 2169–73.

Pall ML. 2013. Electromagnetic fields act via activation of voltage-gated calcium channels to produce beneficial or adverse effects. *J Cell Mol Med* 17(8): 958–65.

Pilla AA. 2006. Chapter 11: Mechanisms and therapeutic applications of time-varying and static magnetic fields. In: Barnes FS, Greenebaum B (eds.) *Handbook of Biological Effects of Electromagnetic Fields,* 3rd Edition. Boca Raton, FL: CRC Press.

Pilla AA. 2012. Electromagnetic fields instantaneously modulate nitric oxide signaling in challenged biological systems. *Biochem Biophys Res Commun* 426(3): 330–3.

Pilla AA. 2015. Pulsed electromagnetic fields; from signaling to healing. In: Markov M (ed.) *Electromagnetic Fields in Biology and Medicine.* Boca Raton, FL: CRC Press, pp. 29–48.

Ross CL, Siriwardane M, Almeida-Porada G, Porada CD, Brink P, Christ GJ, Harrison BS. 2015. The effect of low-frequency electromagnetic field on human bone marrow stem/progenitor cell differentiation. *Stem Cell Res* 15(1): 96–108.

Ryang We S, Koog YH, Jeong KI, Wi H. 2013. Effects of pulsed electromagnetic field on knee osteoarthritis: a systematic review. *Rheumatology* (Oxford) 52(5): 815–24.

Saliev T, Mustapova Z, Kulsharova G, Bulanin D, Mikhalovsky S. 2014. Therapeutic potential of electromagnetic fields for tissue engineering and wound healing. *Cell Proliferation* 47(6): 485–93.

Spadaro JA. 1993. 30 Years of bioelectrical repair and growth: A bibliographic analysis. In: Blank M (ed.) *Electricity and Magnetism in Biology and Medicine; Proceedings of the First World Congress.* San Francisco, CA: San Francisco Press, pp. 289–90.

Spadaro JA, Bergstrom WH. 2002. In vivo and in vitro effects of a pulsed electromagnetic field on net calcium flux in rat calvarial bone. *Calcif Tissue Int* 70(6): 496–502.

Spadaro JA, Short WH, Sheehe PR, Hickman RM, Feiglin DH. 2011. Electromagnetic effects on fore-arm disuse osteopenia: a randomized, double-blind, sham-controlled study. *Bioelectromagnetics* 32(4): 273–82.

Wang R, Wu H, Yang Y, Song M. 2016. Effects of electromagnetic fields on osteoporosis: a systematic literature review. *Electromagn Biol Med* 35(4): 384–90.

Yasuda I, Noguchi K, Sata T. 1955. Dynamic callus and electric callus. *J Bone Joint Surg Am* 37: 1292–1293.

Zhu S, He H, Zhang C, Wang H, Gao C, Yu X, He C. 2017. Effects of pulsed electromagnetic fields on postmenopausal osteoporosis. *Bioelectromagnetics* 38(6): 406–24.

9

Thermal Therapy Applications of Electromagnetic Energy

P.R. Stauffer
Thomas Jeffereson University

D.B. Rodrigues
University of Maryland School of Medicine

D. Haemmerich
Medical University of South Carolina

C.-K. Chou
C-K. Chou Consulting

CONTENTS

9.1 Introduction

Since the 1940s, diathermy has been used in rehabilitation medicine to relieve pain from sprains and strains. To accomplish therapy, radiofrequency (RF), microwave (MW), and ultrasound (US) energy have been used for deep tissue heating to increase blood flow and collagen tissue extensibility as well as to decrease joint stiffness and muscle spasm [1]. Since the mid-1970s, moderate temperature hyperthermia (40–45°C for 30–60 min) has been applied in combination with ionizing radiation and/or chemotherapy to treat cancer [2–7]. Due to widely varying requirements for controllably heating tissue in the head, thorax, pelvis, and extremities, equipment for heating tumors located near the surface or deep in the body continues to evolve to this day [8–10]. External heating systems generally rely on deposition of electromagnetic (EM) energy via electric fields radiated or capacitively coupled into the body, magnetic fields inductively coupled into the body, or ultrasound acoustic pressure fields conducted into the body. In the 1980s, there was extensive development of miniature implantable heat sources based on resistively or capacitively coupled RF currents, circular or linear polarization MW antennas, optical fiber mounted laser-illuminated diffuser crystals, or various hot source techniques all designed to produce moderate temperature rise in tumor when implanted in a closely spaced array of sources [11]. Over the next decade, these same implanted heat sources were adapted to apply higher powers to achieve complete tissue necrosis, or thermal ablation, at tissue temperatures between 50°C and 100°C for clinical applications like treating cardiac arrhythmias [12–14], and soon thereafter also for malignant tumors [15–17]. Diathermy, hyperthermia, and ablation all use the same EM energy deposition fundamentals to achieve different tissue temperature profiles that address unique clinical conditions and diseases. Other medical applications using the propagating characteristics of EM fields, such as radiofrequency telemetry to couple sound signals to implanted hearing devices [18,19], electroporation [20], microwave radiometry for temperature monitoring [21–24], active microwave imaging [25,26], and low frequency RF for wound healing, nerve regeneration, or nonthermal wave propagation applications are not discussed further in this review.

   In this chapter, EM heating mechanisms are first explained, followed by a discussion of the relationship between EM power deposition and tissue temperature rise. While engineering developments and supporting laboratory and animal studies are beyond the scope of this review, representative technologies that are available for heating human tissue with EM fields are discussed both for moderate temperature hyperthermia treatments and for higher temperature thermal ablation applications. Finally, clinical trial results published over the past 20 years are summarized for the most common treatment sites.

9.1.1 Electromagnetic Heating Mechanisms

Most of us have experienced shocks from touching leaky 50/60 Hz household appliances. The human body, although not as good a conductor as most metals, is not a good insulator either; thus, current flows in tissue in response to an applied electric field. At frequencies below about 10 kHz, electric fields induce currents in the body that noticeably stimulate excitable tissues (i.e., nerves, muscle, and heart tissues) and are perceived as nerve stimulation or pain. As frequency increases, the perception threshold of electro-stimulatory effects increases and thermal perception threshold decreases. At higher frequencies above 100 kHz, thermal perception becomes dominant, so one may experience an RF burn rather than electric stimulation or shock. To understand how RF energy causes tissue heating, it is necessary to understand how EM energy interacts with tissue. When an EM field impinges on the human body, some energy is reflected at the body surface and some penetrates into the body. The amount of reflection and penetration depends on frequency, dielectric permittivity of tissue, and coupling (or impedance match) of applicator to tissue surface.

In general, biological tissues can be classified into two major categories. High water content tissues such as muscle, skin, and internal organs have higher dielectric constants and electrical conductivities than tissues with low water content, such as fat and bone. Lung and bone marrow tissues contain intermediate amounts of water, and have dielectric constants and conductivities that fall between the other two groups. In the RF range, tissues with high water content and high conductivity conduct electrical current well, because of the ions and polar water molecules. Tissues with low water content, such as fat and bone, have mostly bound charges that do not easily support conduction currents. Furthermore, the dielectric properties of tissue are a function of frequency. The dielectric constant decreases, while the conductivity increases with increasing frequency. Gabriel et al. have published extensive dielectric property data for 43 tissues [27,28] along with a parametric model for interpolating dielectric constant and conductivity of tissues across a broad frequency range [29]. See also Chapter 4 in *BBA*.

The action of EM fields on tissues produces two types of effects: (i) the oscillation of free charged particles (i.e., ions), and (ii) the rotation of polar molecules at the frequency of the applied field [30]. Attenuation of free charge motion occurs due to electrical resistance of tissue. At radio frequencies below ~10–30 MHz, an alternating electric field induces a net movement of ions. Resistive (ohmic) losses associated with the induced current causes "joule heating." This is the mechanism of capacitively coupled heating between RF plate electrodes typically at 8–30 MHz [31,32], and also for RF ablation heating using 500 kHz–27 MHz RF current electrodes [17,33–36]. At frequencies above about 100 MHz, the radiative mode of electromagnetic propagation and dielectric losses in tissue predominate over conduction current losses. Under these conditions, heating results primarily from friction caused by mechanical interactions between adjacent polar water molecules that oscillate in an attempt to maintain alignment with the time varying electric field. This is the primary heating mechanism of microwave applicators used in hyperthermia treatment of cancer as well as microwave ovens used to cook food. Resistive and friction losses are the basis of EM energy absorption, which produces heat in tissue [5,7,9,37].

9.1.2 Temperature Rise Due to EM Heating

The rate of temperature rise (heating rate—HR) in tissue from an applied EM field is related to the rate of energy absorption (specific absorption rate—SAR) by Equation (9.1). SAR is dependent on the electric field in tissue and tissue conductivity as shown by Equation (9.2). The final tissue temperature is defined by a balance of heat sources and heat sinks and is most often calculated using the Pennes [38] Bioheat Equation (Equation 9.3) as a function of deposited energy, metabolic heating rate (Q_m), heat losses from thermal conduction $k\nabla^2 T$, and blood flow induced thermal convection $c_b \omega_b (T - T_a)$.

$$HR = \frac{SAR}{69.77c} (°C/min) \tag{9.1}$$

$$SAR = \frac{\sigma}{\rho} E^2 (W/kg) \tag{9.2}$$

$$\rho c \frac{\partial T}{\partial t} = k\nabla^2 T - c_b \omega_b (T - T_a) + Q_m + \rho SAR \tag{9.3}$$

where
   HR is heating rate in tissue (°C/min)
   SAR is specific absorption rate (W/kg)
   c is the specific heat capacity of tissue (J/kg/K)
   E is the root-mean-square value of the induced electric field strength in tissue (V/m)
   ρ is the density of tissue (kg/m³)
   σ is the dielectric conductivity of tissue (S/m)
   T is the tissue temperature (°C)
   k is the thermal conductivity of tissue (W/m/K)
   Q_m is the metabolic heat generation rate (W/kg)
   c_b is the blood specific heat capacity (J/kg/K)
   ω_b is the blood perfusion rate (kg/m³/s)
   T_a is the temperature of incoming arterial blood (°C).

In a typical clinical hyperthermia treatment of soft tissue tumor using about 100 watts output power of an external microwave applicator, the temperature, T, will increase as shown in Figure 9.1. Initially, there is a linear increase in T lasting about 3 min. In normal tissue, after this initial period of linearly increasing temperatures proportional to applied power, there is a period of nonlinear temperature rise usually lasting another 7–10 min, where HR falls off due to increasing heat dissipation related to the temperature gradient (conduction) and blood perfusion (convection). In tissues with severely compromised perfusion, like the necrotic core of a tumor, temperature will monotonically approach a steady state value dictated by the magnitude of SAR and thermal properties of surrounding tissue, as shown on the upper curve in Figure 9.1, with thermal equilibrium established when $\rho SAR = -k\nabla^2 T$ (heat diffusion). For most living tissues, a marked increase in blood perfusion normally occurs as the temperature reaches 42°C–44°C due to the vasodilatation response of blood vessels to carry extra heat away from the region, as shown in Figure 9.1. This characteristic is relied upon during hyperthermia treatments to increase blood flow and tissue oxygenation to the tumor cells and to provide extra protection for normal tissues within the treated area.

During hyperthermia treatment, the blood flow in many tumors is vigorous at the periphery and sluggish in the center [39,40]. Since tumor growth often damages the vasculature

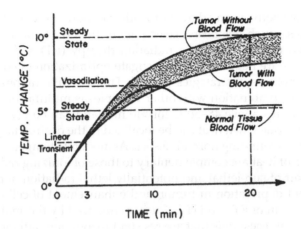

FIGURE 9.1
Temperature change in tumor and normal tissues following application of RF energy (reprinted with permission) [6].

producing hardened nonelastic blood vessels, there is no vasodilatation during heat treatment in portions of the tumor. Thus, the final temperature of the tumor core is higher than that of the surrounding tissues after steady state conditions are reached. The shaded area in Figure 9.1 indicates the range of temperature rise in tumors. The lower temperatures are generally near the higher perfusion periphery of the tumor whereas the upper curve represents temperature of tissues near the central core with lower blood perfusion.

The rate of energy absorption, SAR, must be sufficiently high so that a therapeutic temperature level can be maintained over a significant treatment duration, typically 60 min. If too little power is applied, the temperature elevation will not be high enough or the duration long enough for clinical benefit. If too much power is applied, safe normal tissue temperatures may be exceeded for too long, resulting in complications such as tissue blisters or burns. For hyperthermia treatment, pain sensors in the skin are generally a reliable means for alerting the patient of an unsafe temperature. If the applied power level is set so that only mild discomfort is experienced by the patient, vasodilatation and blood perfusion cooling should be sufficient to limit tissue temperatures to a range of 40–45°C that is both tolerable and therapeutically effective. For thermal ablation treatments, higher SAR is required to raise tissue temperatures at least 15–20°C above normal, usually for a shorter duration (10–25 min for tumor ablation, and <1 min for cardiac ablation) in order to produce tissue necrosis directly. The short duration of heating minimizes the onset of higher cooling from increased tissue perfusion, making temperature rise correlate more directly with SAR. Use of high-temperature thermal ablation, sometimes considered "thermal surgery," is generally restricted to smaller volumes of tissue lacking temperature related pain receptors, where treatment can be localized to the diseased tissue and avoid heating extended volumes of critical normal tissues.

9.2 Hyperthermia Therapy for Cancer

Hyperthermia (HT) is a cancer treatment whereby tissue temperature is elevated to moderate temperatures in the range of 40–45°C for 30–60 min either locally, regionally, or throughout the whole body as an adjuvant to either radiotherapy or chemotherapy. Over the last four decades, much has been learned about the effects of heat on cells and the interactions between heat and ionizing radiation therapy (RT) and chemotherapy (CT) [2–4,41]. Recent efforts are beginning to investigate optimization of combinations of heat with various immunotherapy strategies [42–45]. The scientific rationale for heating tissue either alone or in combination with other therapies is multifactorial. Heat is directly cytotoxic at temperatures above 48–50°C for >10 min and can be used alone for thermal ablation of diseased tissue when heat can be localized to the desired target while avoiding excessive heating of surrounding normal tissues. At moderate temperatures between 40°C and 45°C, the effects of heat are complementary to those of ionizing radiation with regard to inhibition of repair of sub-lethal and potentially lethal radiation damage, reduction of hypoxia and nutrient deprivation in tumor, and enhancement of cell-cycle sensitivity to radiation. The synergism of RT and HT is further enhanced by thermal killing of hypoxic and S phase (DNA syntheses) cells that are resistant to ionizing radiation alone.

The biological rationale for using HT in combination with chemotherapy is equally compelling [2,46–49]. First, modestly increased temperature (e.g., >39°C) induces a variety of physiologic responses in tissue, including increased blood perfusion, oxygenation, and cellular metabolism. Additionally, a moderate temperature rise increases permeability of the vascular wall and cellular membranes, which enhance transfer of drug from the vasculature to the tumor environment and into the tumor cells [50]. Increasing the amount of blood flowing through a tumor combined with enhanced drug uptake by thermally excited cells enhances the amount of DNA damage, inhibits repair of potentially lethal DNA damage, and can reverse drug resistance, thereby increasing the potency of many drugs. Recent investigations in gene therapy have also reported effective use of HT for targeted, localized induction of gene therapy using the heat shock promoter [51–54].

Although both *in vitro* and *in vivo* animal studies provide strong biological rationale for the clinical application of HT, implementation in treating human tumors remains challenging. The therapeutic temperature range of hyperthermia therapy is extremely narrow, only a 5°C range between 40°C and 45°C. Direct cell killing is minimal at the lower temperatures whereas at temperatures above 45°C for typical 60 min treatments, normal cells are killed indiscriminately along with tumor cells. Indiscriminate killing of normal tissue surrounding a tumor volume is unacceptable in many tissue sites. Minimizing trauma to surrounding normal tissue is especially important for superficial tumors located in or just under the skin, since skin must not be damaged in order to maintain an effective shield against infection. Successful hyperthermia therapy is thus dependent on heating tumors within a narrow therapeutic window. Numerous factors affect the clinical results of hyperthermia treatments. The foremost problem in HT is the generation and precise control of heat within irregularly shaped tumors buried in heterogeneous tissue regions of complex anatomy. Early clinical use of HT was hampered by a lack of adequate equipment to controllably deliver uniform heating of deep-seated and large superficial lesions, and by a lack of thermometry to provide reliable feedback to control the heat distribution within the narrow therapeutic range. Considerable progress in recent years has added more effective treatment planning [55,56] and improved equipment capabilities [9,10] that include more extensive real time monitoring and control of hyperthermia treatments.

The goal of treatment planning and real-time temperature monitoring is to produce a uniform thermal dose distribution that is within the therapeutic range throughout the tumor. Thermal dose accumulates as a function of temperature and time [57]. Thermal dosimetry measures most often reported in the literature include (i) temperature parameters—T_{max}, T_{min}, T_{ave}, T_{90}, and T_{10}; (ii) time parameters—cumulative time above 40°C, 41°C, 42°C, and

43°C; and (iii) thermal dose parameters—cumulative equivalent minutes at 43°C (CEM43) and cumulative equivalent minutes at 43°C for the T_{90} temperature (CEM43T_{90}) [58]. In this nomenclature, T_{90} represents 10th percentile temperature of a distribution, or the tissue temperature exceeded by 90% of all temperature measurements. While uncertainties remain in calculating thermal dose at ablative temperatures exceeding about 60°C, the most accurate and commonly used method of quantifying thermal damage to tissue in the hyperthermic range is the thermal isoeffect dose relationship which shows that cell killing doubles for every 1°C rise in temperature above 43°C; killing is reduced by about one quarter for every 1°C below 43°C [59]. This leads to the following expression for calculating thermal dose:

$$CEM43 = \sum_{i=1}^{n} t_i \cdot R^{43-T_i} \qquad (9.4)$$

where CEM43 is the cumulative number of equivalent minutes at 43°C, t_i is the i-th time interval in min, R is a factor that accommodates different rates of cell death above and below the 43°C breakpoint in the Arrhenius plot (i.e., $R = 1/4$ for $T < 43$°C and $R = 1/2$ for $T > 43$°C), and T is the average tissue temperature in °C over the treatment interval t_i at that measurement point. To quantify heterogeneous thermal dose distributions within a tumor volume, the calculation of tumor dose combines the concepts of thermal dose accumulated at each point with 10th percentile tumor temperature (T_{90}). This allows calculation of a volumetric tumor thermal dose by calculating CEM43 thermal dose over $t_i = 1$ minute intervals based on the average T_{90} temperatures over each of those intervals, and summing together all one minute thermal doses to obtain the total treatment thermal dose in CEM43T_{90} [57,58].

During hyperthermia treatments, tumor temperature and the accumulated thermal dose distribution are dependent on EM energy deposition pattern and heat redistribution from conduction and convection (see Equation 9.3). Energy deposition is a complex function of frequency, intensity, polarization of the applied fields, applicator size and geometry, as well as size, depth, geometry, and dielectric properties of the tumor [5,9,60–62]. The material, thickness, and dimensions of a cooling waterbolus, a pliable container of water placed between the source and the skin, also influence the applicator power deposition pattern as well as skin cooling, which adjusts the depth of maximum temperature [63–68]. In spite of numerous technical difficulties, there are now over 38 published clinical trials of hyperthermia in human cancer patients as summarized in this chapter's clinical results section [47]. The vast majority is randomized trials that demonstrate a positive statistically significant increase in complete response or survival endpoints with the addition of HT to RT or CT. Dewhirst et al. [2] pointed out that as technology improves, the benefits from this form of therapy are also improving.

9.2.1 Methods of Heating Tissue with EM Energy

Available methods for heating tumors may be classified as either whole body hyperthermia, deep regional hyperthermia, deep local hyperthermia, superficial hyperthermia, or interstitial/intracavitary hyperthermia. Whole body hyperthermia is generally achieved via thermal conduction heating of skin from hot air, hot water, or infrared radiation. Regional heating is generally produced with heated blood or fluid perfusion of partial body regions, or with 70–150 MHz phased array RF fields for regionally localized heating deep in the pelvis, torso, or limbs [69–74]. Due to the large wavelength of RF frequencies that penetrate well in the human body, focused local heating of deep tissue targets is generally not possible with EM fields. Alternatively, deep local heating of small tissue volumes is possible with highly focused ultrasound arrays that spread power deposition over large areas of skin to achieve an intense focal region at depth (e.g., $2 \times 2 \times 7$ mm^3 volume) that can be scanned mechanically or electronically to achieve larger zones of heating [75,76]. Moreover, numerous technologies are available for intense heating around miniature RF electrodes, microwave antennas, laser irradiated crystal diffusers, tubular ultrasound radiators, or hot sources that are implanted interstitially through needles or catheters, or via natural body cavities into tumors at depth [11,77–79]. Figure 9.2 shows four examples of interstitial and intracavitary ablation devices used for deep local heating applications. For heating superficial tumors located within 3–4 cm of the skin surface, typical methods include microwave antennas [63,64,80–87], unfocused ultrasound transducer arrays [88,89], RF capacitively coupled surface electrodes [31,32,90,91], and recently introduced thermographic camera controlled large area infrared radiators [92].

The electromagnetic energy used to produce HT is usually distinguished by frequency as either RF or microwave. Strictly speaking, the RF spectrum is between 3 kHz and 300 GHz, but for hyperthermia applications RF generally refers to frequencies below 300 MHz. Commonly used RF frequencies are 8, 13.56, and 27.12 MHz, which have been widely used in diathermy and capacitively coupled RF current HT [31,93–96]. RF current heating has also been applied at frequencies from 500 kHz to 27 MHz using interstitial electrodes to

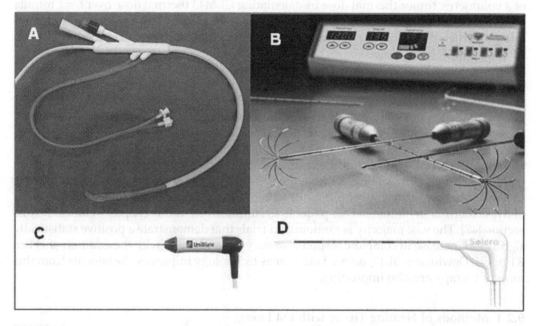

FIGURE 9.2
Example interstitial and intracavitary EM thermal ablation sources. (A) Multi-port catheter-mounted helical coil microwave antenna for transurethral heating of prostate disease (courtesy of Urologix LLC, Minneapolis, Minnesota). (B) LeVeen needle RF electrodes that deploy into an umbrella shape after insertion for producing large (2–5 cm diameter) thermal lesions (courtesy of Boston Scientific Corp., Natick, Massachusetts). (C) Uniblate electrode for CT guided RF ablation of scalable 1–3 cm length by 1–2.5 cm diameter regions in tissues such as non-resectable liver tumors or bone metastasis (courtesy of AngioDynamics, Latham, New York). (D) Solero 2.45 GHz microwave antenna with water cooling of tip for ablative treatment of soft tissue tumors (courtesy of AngioDynamics, Latham, New York.)

localize heating at depth [34,97–100]. Even lower RF frequencies from 50 kHz to 13 MHz have been used for inductive coupling of magnetic fields into the body for direct tissue heating [101–103] or for coupling energy into implanted ferromagnetic seed materials [104–108]. Frequencies between 300 MHz and 300 GHz are considered microwave. The most commonly used microwave frequencies for HT are 433, 915, and 2450 MHz, which are designated ISM (industrial, scientific, and medical) frequencies in the United States and Europe (433 MHz in Europe only). Frequencies higher than 2450 MHz have little practical value for HT due to their limited penetration in lossy tissue. At frequencies below 433 MHz, field penetration is deeper but the applicator must be larger and thus focusing becomes difficult due to the long wavelength compared to human body and tumor dimensions.

For localized heating of superficial (<4 cm deep) tumors, 433 MHz is generally considered to provide the best compromise of applicator size and field penetration and is most used in Europe and Asia. Figure 9.3 (left) shows a commercial hyperthermia system with interchangeable gently contoured 433 MHz applicators for treating superficial tumors. Producing ~15% less penetration [109], 915 MHz applicators are most common in the United States due to Federal Communications Commission (FCC) regulations. A typical superficial microwave hyperthermia patient treatment setup is shown in Figure 9.3 (right) for a 915 MHz waveguide applicator coupled to chestwall disease with 1 cm thick conformal waterbolus. Although air-cooling of skin can be used, a deionized waterbolus with dielectric constant ($\varepsilon_r = 80$) closer to tissue ($\varepsilon_r = 50$) is usually placed between the applicator and skin surface to couple microwaves effectively into tissue while maintaining skin temperatures below 45°C to minimize pain. For treating deep disease > 4 cm depth, more penetrating lower frequencies must be used to deliver RF energy to the tumor. At 5–30 MHz, RF conduction currents can be capacitively coupled into the body placed between two external plate electrodes. While currents naturally split and flow in multiple paths through the body with higher current flowing in paths of lower resistance, some steering of the heating pattern at depth is possible using differential size electrodes, whereby

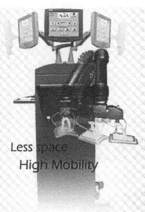
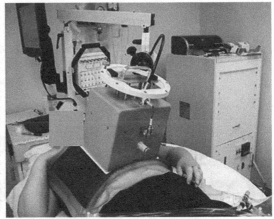

FIGURE 9.3
Superficial microwave hyperthermia. HT system with one of several different size 433 MHz antennas suspended from a variable position support arm (left). Temperature monitoring and control interface shown on treatment screen. (Courtesy of Alba Hyperthermia System, Rome, Italy.) 915 MHz waveguide applicator over custom conformal waterbolus treating recurrent chestwall disease with BSD500 microwave hyperthermia system (right).

current density is reduced under the larger electrode. Because the highest current density always occurs at the electrode-skin interface, cooling boluses must be used to protect the skin. Since fat heats significantly more than underlying lower resistance tissues due to low specific heat and dielectric properties, RF capacitive heating is generally applicable only for thin patients with tumors in specific locations that allow natural concentration of current into the tissue target region.

For controllable localized heating of large tumors deep in the body, RF multi-antenna phased array methods are generally used [69–71,74]. The system shown in Figure 9.4 is a recent commercial implementation of the four 70 MHz waveguide phased array system pioneered at AMC Medical Center (Amsterdam, The Netherlands). During treatment, large waterboluses inflate around the patient to couple radiated fields into tissue and the phases and amplitudes of the waveguides are adjusted by the operator to steer a large heat focus to the desired target at depth. Thermal feedback is generally provided by temperature sensors placed in natural body cavities such as bladder, rectum, and vagina to monitor deep tissue temperatures close to the tumor target. The system shown in Figure 9.5 consists of an annular array of 100 MHz dipole antennas in three concentric rings of eight antennas intended to treat 8–12 cm diameter tumors inside the torso or legs. By varying relative amplitudes and phases of the antennas, the large region of heat focus can be steered around within the body to center on specific targets such as bladder, cervix, or rectum. Noninvasive temperature monitoring of this hyperthermia/magnetic resonance hybrid system has been validated in a heterogeneous phantom [72,110,111]. Details of RF heating technology for local, regional, and whole body hyperthermia have been published previously [8–10,61–63,112].

It is impossible for a single piece of equipment to fulfill the clinical requirements for effective hyperthermia treatment of all patients. HT practitioners should have the option to choose most appropriate equipment from a wide range of technology that can optimize heat delivery based on specific location and tissue properties of the tumor and environment, and general physical condition of the patient. Uniform and safe heating of entire tumors located in complex heterogeneous patient anatomy is challenging and should be

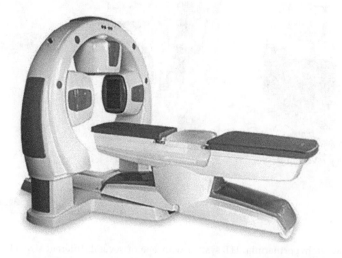

FIGURE 9.4
Alba 4D deep regional hyperthermia system with four 70 MHz waveguide applicators placed concentrically around the body and coupled to tissue with inflatable waterboluses. (Courtesy of Alba Hyperthermia Systems, Rome, Italy.)

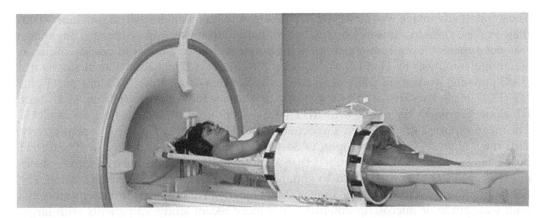

FIGURE 9.5
BSD-2000/3D/MR deep regional hyperthermia system. Combining deep regional heating and MRI 3D treatment monitoring provides the capability to monitor changes in tissue temperature and perfusion, and even necrosis that develops between multiple heat treatments. (Courtesy of Pyrexar Medical, Salt Lake City, Utah.)

applied only by individuals well trained in the theory and practical application of hyperthermia treatment. Minimum qualifications for treatment personnel have been defined [113]. Due to the complexity of coupling RF energy to human tumors, careful heating pattern studies should be performed on all exposure geometries prior to treatment to assure the best treatment setup for the patient. Quality assurance guidelines have been published recently [114–118] that update the extensive literature describing still appropriate quality assurance considerations for clinical hyperthermia [74,119–129]. While the distribution of blood perfusion in and around the tumor is highly variable with time, position, and temperature, treatment planning of EM power deposition and thermal redistribution of energy from conduction and perfusion is now possible with increasingly accurate EM and thermal simulation software that now incorporate realistic 3D patient models [56,130]. Regardless of planning, accurate thermometry is critical in all phases of clinical hyperthermia.

9.2.2 Clinical Trials of Hyperthermia for Cancer Therapy

Datta et al. [47,131,132] recently reviewed the results of 33 published randomized and non-randomized clinical trials (RCTs) looking at the benefit of hyperthermia when added to either chemotherapy or radiotherapy. The following is condensed from those comprehensive reviews. The nomenclature used in the clinical studies is as follows: radiotherapy (RT), hyperthermia (HT), chemotherapy (CT), radiation plus hyperthermia (RHT), chemotherapy plus hyperthermia (CHT), radiation plus chemotherapy (RCT), and radiation with chemotherapy plus heat (RCHT).

9.2.2.1 Breast Cancer

Breast cancer is the most widely investigated cancer site for adjuvant HT. In the 1990s, five randomized Phase III trials of inoperable primary or recurrent breast cancer were combined for a total of 306 patients randomized to either RT alone or RHT [133]. With differing methods, the five trials demonstrated a significant overall improvement in complete response (CR) rate for patients receiving RHT (59%) compared with RT alone (41%).

The greatest advantage was observed in patients with recurrent lesions in previously irradiated areas, since maximum tolerable re-irradiation dose was low. A survival advantage was not apparent, even though complete responders enjoyed improved quality of life. A recent meta-analysis by Datta et al. included 8 two-arm (627 patients) and 24 single-arm (1,483 patients) studies of locally recurrent breast cancers using either RT alone or RT plus HT [132]. In the two-arm studies, a CR of 60.2% was achieved with RHT vs. 38.1% with RT alone. Similarly, the single-arm RHT studies produced an overall CR rate of 63.4%. The mean reported grades 3 and 4 toxicities with RHT were 14.4% and 5.2%, respectively. This meta-analysis had a time span of 34 years and inherent variability in RT and HT doses. However, the study concluded that without adding to morbidity, moderate doses of HT with RT could be expected to enhance CR by 22% compared with RT alone. The EM techniques used in this meta-analysis were mostly external microwave hyperthermia with waveguide or microstrip antennas. In a more recent study, 73 patients with large-sized breast cancer recurrences were treated with thermographic camera controlled water filtered infrared-A irradiators with hypofractionated re-irradiation [134]. A CR of 61% was achieved with only grade 1 toxicities, which was a very positive result for this heavily pretreated late-stage disease.

9.2.2.2 Cervical Cancer

Datta et al. [135] performed a network meta-analysis (NMA) of four different treatment regimens for cervical cancer: RT, RHT, RCT, and RCHT. This NMA covered 23 clinical trials including 1,160 patients. Those treated with RHT had superior outcomes when compared with RT with an overall odds ratio (OR) of 2.67 for CR, where OR is the probability of CR occurring divided by the probability of CR not occurring. Acute and late toxicities were comparable for both arms. In a randomized trial with 30 patients per arm investigating trimodality therapy for cervix [136], a CR of 83.3% was obtained for RCHT compared with 46.7% in the RT only arm. The NMA showed a significant advantage of RCHT over RT (OR: 4.52) and over RCT (OR: 2.91) for achieving CR. A second endpoint—patients alive at the end of the study period—was analyzed in 12 comparative studies comprising a total of 807 patients, of whom 596 patients were alive at the end of the study period. Again, RCHT provided a significant advantage over RCT (OR: 2.65) or RT alone (OR: 5.57). As an example of long-term improvement from HT, at the 12-year follow-up, local control remained better in the RHT group (56%) vs. RT alone (37%). And the survival advantage persisted over 12 years: 37% (RHT) vs. 20% (RT) [137]. A wide range of EM heating devices were used for these studies including regional heating with either capacitive or radiative RF systems, or intracavitary heating with custom-built coaxial TEM applicators.

9.2.2.3 Head and Neck Cancer

Another systematic review and meta-analysis was conducted to evaluate controlled clinical trials in head and neck cancer [131]. Only two-arm studies were considered, yielding 451 patients from six studies of which five were randomized. The overall CR with RT alone was 39.6% (range 31.3–46.9%), and it increased to 62.5% (range 33.9–83.3%) in the RHT arm. The OR was 2.92 favoring the combined treatment with RHT over RT alone. The EM techniques used in these studies included RF capacitive and microwave waveguide hyperthermia systems.

Three randomized trials studied the effects of trimodality RCHT vs. conventional RCT for treating nasopharyngeal carcinoma [138–140]. All studies showed significantly improved outcomes with added EM hyperthermia. Local control rates increased from 12.2% (RCT) to 19.2% (RCHT); 5-year survival increased from 7.9% to 18.4% with HT; 5-year progression-free survival (PFS) increased 9.6% [138]; 5-year disease-free survival (DFS) increased 30.8% [139]; and average DFS increased from 37.5 to 78 months [140]. In two studies that evaluated CR, the addition of HT increased CR from 81.1% to 98.6% in one study [138] and from 62.8% to 81.6% in the other [139]. Quality of life (QoL) was assessed by Zhao et al. and patients that received hyperthermia showed significantly improved QoL scores [140].

9.2.2.4 Rectal Cancer

A 2009 Cochrane review studied six randomized trials with 520 patients [141]. Four studies (424 patients) reported significantly improved 2-year overall survival (OS) in the RHT group though differences disappeared after 3 years. No significant differences in acute toxicity were observed. Rectal heating was accomplished with either intracavitary microwave or coaxial TEM sources or external RF array applicators. In a retrospective study of 106 patients [142], pathological complete response (pCR) was seen in 6.7% of patients in the RCT group and 16.4% in the RCHT group. Patients who received at least four hyperthermia treatments achieved a significantly higher pCR rate of 22.5%. Furthermore, adding HT appeared to reduce distant metastasis, increase disease-free survival, and improve overall survival in a subgroup that received lower radiation doses.

9.2.2.5 Melanoma and Other Superficial Malignancies

In a Radiation Therapy Oncology Group (RTOG) study published in 1991 [143], 307 patients were treated with either RHT or RT alone. Approximately, half had head and neck tumors, one-third had breast carcinoma or chest wall recurrence, and the remaining patients had a variety of superficial malignancies. There was no limit on tumor size specified in the protocol. In this widely variable disease population, complete response rates were not significantly different between those treated with RHT (32%) or RT alone (30%). However, a subgroup analysis revealed significant improvement in complete response and duration of local control in patients with tumors smaller than 3 cm in maximal extent, and in those with breast or chest wall recurrences. For lesions larger than 3 cm, there was no difference in outcome which related to the fact that larger tumors exceeded the effective treatment capabilities of microwave applicators available in the 1980s for that trial. Heating techniques and thermal dosimetry documentation varied widely between institutions and a lack of quality assurance led subsequently to the development of RTOG-sponsored guidelines for performing quality hyperthermia treatments [119,120,123,144].

In a subsequent multicenter randomized trial, 128 metastatic or recurrent malignant melanoma lesions in 68 patients were randomized to receive RT or RHT [145]. Although there were generally higher temperatures, quality assurance was still a concern in this trial with only 14% of treatments achieving the protocol objective of 43°C for 60 min. Even so, the trial demonstrated a significant benefit for the addition of HT, with a 2-year local control (LC) of 46% (RHT) vs. 28% (RT). A similar increase was observed in CR: 62% (RHT) vs. 35% (RT). Addition of heat did not significantly increase acute or late radiation reactions. Jones et al. [146] performed a randomized trial with a rigorous thermal dose prescription (minimum of 10 CEM43T_{90}) that pooled 109 patients with widely variable superficial tumors including breast carcinoma, melanoma, head and neck cancers, and others. Addition of HT to RT led to a significant increase in CR: 66.1% for RHT vs. 42.3% for RT alone. As in other studies, pre-irradiated patients received the highest benefit: 68.2% (RHT) vs. 23.5% (RT). Although some early work [147] used capacitive plate RF hyperthermia, most clinical treatments of superficial tissue disease involved the use of 915 or 433 MHz microwave antennas.

9.2.2.6 Bladder Cancer

The use of HT in the treatment of bladder cancer has a dedicated special issue in the International Journal of Hyperthermia [148]. In 1994, Masunaga et al. randomized 49 bladder cancer patients to RT or RHT [149]. Tumor response was evaluated in terms of down-staging and it achieved 48% with RT and 57% with RHT. However, the patients in the RHT group that achieved higher tumor temperatures ($T_{mean} > 41.5°C$) achieved 83% tumor down-staging, demonstrating the importance of adequate temperature. Van der Zee reported a subgroup of 101 patients achieving a CR of 51.0% with conventional RT and 73.1% with added heat. The corresponding 3-year local control increased from 33% to 42%, and 3-year survival increased from 22% to 28% [150]. In a more recent trial, high-risk T1 and T2 bladder cancers were treated with transurethral resection followed by RCHT (n = 45). After a median follow-up of 34 months, the OS was 89% [151], demonstrating safety and efficacy of this quadrimodal therapy regimen.

With most trials accomplishing bladder hyperthermia with externally applied regional RF capacitive or radiative devices, Colombo et al. conducted a multicenter, randomized trial comparing CT alone to CT plus 915 MHz intravesical microwave applicator heating of non-muscle invasive bladder cancer (n = 83) [152]. At 2-year follow-up, the recurrence rate after CT alone was several-fold higher than that of CHT: 57.5% vs. 17.1%. After a long follow-up (median: 90 months), recurrences were noted in 40% of CHT patients and 80% of patients treated with CT alone [153]. The 10-year DFS was estimated at 52.8% for CHT vs. 14.6% for CT alone [154].

9.2.2.7 Esophageal Cancer

Three randomized studies demonstrated an advantage for the addition of HT to CT or RCT in the treatment of esophageal cancer [155–157]. In one study of 53 patients, HT was delivered using an intracavitary RF electrode and histopathologic response was significantly improved in the trimodality arm: 66.7% vs. 38.5%. In a follow-up study [156], an additional 40 patients were treated with CT alone or combined with HT yielding a histopathologic response of 18.8% vs. 41.2% for the combined treatment. A third randomized trial used an intracavitary microwave applicator for heating and produced a 3-year survival rate of 42.4% in the RHT group vs. 24.2% for RT alone [157]. Kuwano et al. conducted the largest clinical trial to date (n = 243) studying the effects of hyperthermia, chemotherapy and irradiation on esophageal cancer [158]. Both pCR (8.4% vs. 19.1%) and 5-year OS (13.7% vs. 22.3%) were significantly higher in the RCHT group. More recent single-arm studies of adjuvant heat have further validated extended survival in esophageal cancer patients with 5-year OS of 50.0% (n = 24) [159] and 3-year OS of 42.5% (n = 50) [160]. Toxicities were reported to be tolerable and limited to grade 2 or 3 in all studies.

9.2.2.8 Lung Cancer

Only a few studies have investigated the role of RHT in the treatment of non-small cell lung cancer (NSCLC). Karasawa et al. [161] compared 19 patients treated with RHT with a historical control group of 30 patients treated with RT alone. The RT group had 0% CR, whereas the RHT group achieved 26.3% CR. This was accompanied by a significant increase in OS: 6.7% (RT) vs. 37.0% (RHT). A small case-control study of 26 lung cancer patients with bone invasion demonstrated a large improvement for RHT over RT alone in terms of both 2-year LC (76.1% vs. 16.9%) and OS (44.4% vs. 15.4%) [162]. Despite these promising results, a more recent multi-institutional prospective randomized trial of locally advanced NSCLCs showed no significant difference of OS, local response, or treatment-related toxicity [163], although a significantly higher 1-year PFS was seen 29.0% (RT) vs. 67.5% (RHT). All these studies employed RF capacitive heating systems with somewhat uncertain ability to localize heating effectively in lung.

The addition of heat to chemotherapy appears to present better results for the treatment of NSCLC than the previously inconclusive dual-therapy RHT. Shen et al. randomized 80 patients to CHT or CT alone [164]. Although there was no significant difference in response rates, the clinical benefit response (a clinical index used with incurable tumors to assess improvement in quality of life) was significantly higher in the CHT group: 82.5% vs. 47.5%. Wang et al. [165] performed a similar clinical study in 119 patients with advanced NSCLC, but adding a third treatment arm with radiation. A remarkable curative rate was achieved with trimodality treatment: 90.7% (RCHT) vs. 72.8% (RCT) and 62.2% (RT). Although toxicity increased in the RCHT group, toxicity was reported to be tolerable or readily alleviated with short-term symptomatic treatment. Overall, patients treated in the trimodality arm achieved significant improvement in alleviation of tumor oppression syndrome and higher quality of life.

9.2.2.9 Prostate Cancer

The feasibility of adding HT to RT/CT in the treatment of prostate cancer has been evaluated only in phase I/II clinical trials. Tilly et al. [166] reported 6-year OS of 95% for primary carcinoma and 60% for recurrences using RHT in a 22-patient trial. Similarly, a 5-year OS of 87% was observed with limited toxicity (≤grade 2) in a phase II study of 144 patients with high-risk or locally advanced disease treated with RHT and antihormonal therapy [167]. All studies used external RF array applicators operating between 70 and 120 MHz.

9.2.2.10 Sarcomas

Issels et al. reported a large phase III multicenter European Organization of Research and Treatment of Cancer (EORTC) trial in localized high-risk-soft-tissue sarcoma. A total of 341 patients were randomized to receive a three-drug-regimen alone or with regional HT [168]. Treatment response was significantly improved in the CHT group with 28.8% responders compared to 12.7% for the aggressive CT regimen alone. The results indicate that regional HT from RF array applicator combined with the three-drug-regimen can be given safely with moderate and acceptable toxicity, accompanied by significantly improved clinical response. Evidence of combining HT with radiation in the treatment of sarcomas is scarce, with a few small trials showing minor benefit to the addition of heat [169,170].

9.2.2.11 Glioblastoma Multiforme

Seventy-nine patients with glioblastoma multiforme were randomized following external beam RT and chemotherapy to receive brachytherapy alone or combined with interstitial HT via placement of helical-coil MW antennas [171]. Both time-to-tumor progression and survival were significantly improved for patients in the adjuvant heat arm. Median survival increased from 18 to 20 months and 2-year survival more than doubled (from

15% to 31%) with the addition of heat to best available treatment, a statistically significant benefit for added heat with acceptable toxicity. Similarly, Stea et al. [172] reported a statistically significant survival benefit in 62 patients with high grade gliomas treated with either brachytherapy plus interstitial ferromagnetic seed hyperthermia or brachytherapy alone, reaching a median survival of 23 months and 2-year survival of 47% with combined treatment vs. 18% for brachytherapy alone. Maier-Hauff et al. [106] performed a clinical trial in 59 recurrent glioblastoma patients, which showed a median survival of 13.4 months from time of recurrence, which when added to the initial response produced overall survival of 23.2 months after primary tumor diagnosis.

9.2.2.12 Pancreatic Cancer

A recent systematic review compared 14 phase I/II clinical studies (n = 395) on locally advanced and/or metastatic pancreatic cancer patients that used adjuvant HT [173]. Patients were treated with regional capacitive/radiative RF HT (n = 189), intracavitary MW HT (n = 39) or whole-body hyperthermia using an infrared radiant heat device (n = 20), combined with chemotherapy, radiotherapy or both. Six studies included a control group and showed a longer OS in the hyperthermia groups than in the control groups (11.7 vs. 5.6 months). Overall response rate, reported in three studies with a control group, was also better for the hyperthermia groups (43.9% vs. 35.3%).

9.2.2.13 Summary of Clinical Trials

Results of the above published EM-based hyperthermia clinical trials are intriguing. Apart from two early RTOG trials using first generation heating systems with inadequate quality assurance, the overwhelming clinical evidence demonstrates substantial benefit from the addition of HT to RT and/or CT. These clinical trials span several decades. As a result, there is an inherent lack of uniformity across trials concerning HT delivery and treatment schedules, as well as RT treatment protocols, dose, and technique. The trials strongly advocated for improved quality of heat treatment, which led to a string of quality assurance guidelines covering technical requirements of heating devices and clinical requirements. Despite these difficulties, the generally positive character of these trials suggests that the future of HT is extremely promising and that technological advances should continue to produce even more positive results.

9.3 Thermal Ablation Therapy

Hyperthermia is typically employed as adjuvant therapy combined either with radiation or chemotherapy since moderate temperature hyperthermia as a sole treatment is not sufficient to produce durable complete responses [174]. This early conclusion has been confirmed with laboratory [58,175] and clinical data [176–179] that continue to demonstrate our inability to attain sufficiently high thermal doses throughout large tumors to produce sustained tumor response.

Thermal ablation refers to the localized destruction of a tissue region by heat-induced coagulation necrosis and uses temperatures well above the hyperthermic temperature range, typically from 50°C to 100°C. Above 50°C, cells undergo coagulation necrosis in less than 4–6 min; at temperatures greater than 60°C, necrosis occurs within seconds [180]. At these higher temperatures thermal cell kill is effective independent of cell type, meaning that thermal ablation can create a zone of complete cell kill as long as adequate temperatures are obtained. Central parts of larger tumors are often poorly perfused with blood, leading to hypoxic (i.e., low oxygen) conditions. It is known that hypoxic tumor regions are often resistant to radiation and/or chemotherapy, whereas thermal ablation works particularly well in tissue regions with reduced blood flow due to the lack of perfusion mediated cooling.

The goal of thermal ablation is to directly kill (ablate) tumor volumes in carefully targeted regions that do not include critical normal tissues like skin, nerves, or major blood vessels. Unlike hyperthermia, which relies on modest physiology-modifying thermal doses applied to large regions including normal tissue around a tumor, ablative treatments are restricted to just the tumor target with minimal normal tissue margin, and no critical normal tissues. Thus, the clinical targets for thermal ablation and hyperthermia therapy are quite different. While hyperthermia is generally directed toward large tumors that are distributed within or wrapped around critical normal tissues that cannot be destroyed, thermal ablation applications usually involve treatment of smaller tissue volumes located in organs or regions that lack strong temperature-based pain response and can withstand the loss of some surrounding normal tissue to ensure complete necrosis of tumor cells. Most often used in the hands of interventional radiologists with noninvasive computed tomography, ultrasound, or magnetic resonance imaging guidance, clinical applications include tumor ablation, cardiac and spinal ablations to block tissue/nerve conduction, intravascular ablations for plaque removal or varicose vein therapy, and larger tissue ablations in the prostate, brain, and liver [12,181–185]. Thermal ablation is usually carried out under conscious sedation or light general anesthesia, with limited hospital stay (0–2 days), and usually very few side effects.

EM fields employed for thermal ablation therapy are based primarily on two methods: Radiofrequency Ablation (RFA), which employs EM waves in the lower-frequency range of 450–500 kHz; and Microwave Ablation (MWA), which employs EM in the range of 0.915–2.45 GHz. While RFA is based on resistive heating due to ionic currents, MWA takes advantage of dielectric losses from the rotation of water dipoles present in soft tissues. Both methods require the insertion of a small diameter applicator—either an RF electrode for RFA or microwave antenna for MWA—into or adjacent to the tissue region to be heated. Examples of RFA and MWA applicators are shown in Figure 9.2. Applicator placement is performed manually by the treating physician and is typically guided by real-time medical imaging, such as ultrasound or computed tomography imaging. RFA found its first clinical application for the treatment of cardiac arrhythmia (i.e., irregular heartbeat) in the 1980s by very localized destruction of tissue regions in the heart responsible for the arrhythmias [12]. In the 1990s, RF ablation was increasingly used for cancer therapy by destroying malignant tumor cells with heat [186,187]. Today, thermal ablation is used to treat a wide variety of diseases, such as varicose veins and uterine bleeding [188,189].

9.3.1 Biophysics of Radiofrequency Ablation

In contrast to hyperthermia, which elevates tumor temperature to less than 45°C, radiofrequency ablation applies RF electric fields (450–500 kHz) to produce ionic currents in tissue and cause resistive heating to at least 50°C. Direct heating is limited to tissue in close proximity to the RF electrode, while more distant tissue is indirectly heated through thermal conduction (Figure 9.6). Temperatures greater than 100°C are generally avoided to

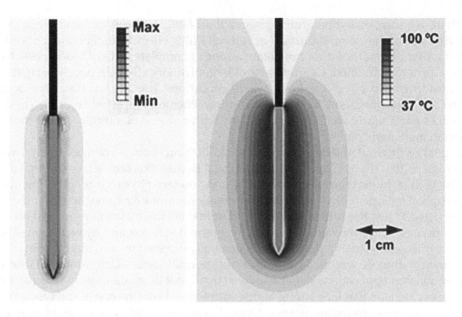

FIGURE 9.6
Simulated electric field in close vicinity to an RF electrode (left) and corresponding temperature distribution which extends further out into soft tissue (right). The electrode has an internal cooling mechanism, where water is circulated during ablation to cool the tissue next to the applicator to prevent tissue charring.

prevent tissue boiling, vaporization, and carbonization. These phenomena cause a large increase in tissue impedance around the electrode that restricts RF current and limits further extent of heating. Therefore, the goal of RFA is to achieve and maintain a temperature in the range of 50–100°C throughout the target volume. This therapeutic window is much larger than the 40–45°C window for hyperthermia, thus requiring less uniform distribution of power deposition than for hyperthermia applications. Still, the power applied to the RF electrode must be controlled to maintain tissue temperatures in this desired range. Often, a temperature sensor (thermistor or thermocouple) is integrated into the electrode to allow monitoring of electrode temperature, and applied power is adjusted based on surface temperature of the electrode. Other approaches include application of a prescribed constant power level for a given time period, or the use of tissue impedance as measured between the RF electrode and the dispersive electrode (ground pad) for feedback control signal. Typical power levels for RFA devices are in the range of 100–250 W. Figure 9.6 depicts the electric field strength and corresponding temperature distribution surrounding an internally-cooled RF electrode inserted in soft tissue like muscle or tumor.

The heat produced by RF energy depends on the electrode geometry, applied voltage, and electrical conductivity of surrounding tissue. Conductivity varies depending on tissue type, with bone, fat and aerated lung having considerably lower conductivity than soft tissues, which can limit heating during RF ablation from an implanted electrode (Table 9.1). In addition, conductivity varies with temperature (~2%/°C), and changes if tissue is removed from the body [190].

9.3.2 Biophysics of Microwave Ablation

Microwaves fall between ~300 MHz and 300 GHz in the electromagnetic spectrum, and the Federal Communications Commission (FCC) permits unrestricted use of a few frequencies

TABLE 9.1

Electrical Conductivity of Tissue at Typical RFA Frequency of 500 kHz

Tissue Type	Electrical Conductivity σ (S/m)	Reference
Normal liver (rat, *in vivo*)	0.36	[191]
Liver tumor (rat, *in-vivo*)	0.45	[191]
Myocardium (porcine, *in vivo*)	0.54	[192]
Lung inflated (porcine, *ex vivo*, 37°C)	0.1	[193]
Fat (porcine, *ex vivo*, 22°C)	0.02	[194]
Bone (porcine, *ex vivo*, 20°C)	0.03	[193]
Blood (rabbit, *ex vivo*, 20°C)	0.7	[195]
Vaporized tissue	$\sim 10^{-15}$	Assumed same as air

for industrial, scientific and medical purposes. The most commonly used frequencies for MWA devices are 915 MHz and 2.45 GHz. MWA antennas used for ablation are often based on predicate devices that have been used for interstitial MW hyperthermia, and are often similar in construction (Figure 9.7). Common antenna designs include slot antennas, monopoles, dipoles, triaxial designs, choked antennas, and helical coil antennas [11,196]

At frequencies employed for MWA, displacement currents dominate rather than the conduction currents that dominate at lower RFA frequencies. These displacement currents result from rotation of polar tissue molecules, primarily water. Thus, the dielectric tissue properties at microwave frequencies are to a large extent dictated by water content [204,205]. Table 9.2 lists the dielectric properties of various tissues at 1 and 10 GHz. A more extensive listing of dielectric properties for a broad range of *in vivo* and *in vitro* tissues over a frequency range of 10 Hz to 20 GHz is given by Gabriel et al. [27,28] including a parametric model [29] for interpolating values. In addition to dependency on frequency and water content, dielectric properties change as a function of temperature [190], which can reduce heating efficiency at higher temperatures. Use of MWA for tumor ablation has received increasing attention in recent years due to several advantages over RFA: (1) faster heating rate; (2) larger zone of direct tissue heating, with deeper penetration of EM field and thus less reliance on thermal conduction—as a result, ablation times are often shorter; (3) higher temperatures are possible due to independence on tissue charring and steam formation; and (4) does not require a dispersive electrode (ground pad). There is also some evidence that MWA performs better close to vasculature compared to RFA [206], and performs better in lung since not limited by high impedance of aerated tissue [207].

9.3.3 Tumor Ablation Devices

The goal of tumor ablation is to expose the tumor to cytotoxic temperatures (i.e., above ~50°C). Unless otherwise indicated, this must include at least a 0.5–1.5 cm ablative margin of seemingly normal tissue for large tissue targets in liver and lung, though a smaller margin may be adequate in some tumor sites (e.g., kidney) [183]. Initial RFA devices based on single needle electrodes were limited to ablation zone diameters of about 1.6 cm. Since tumors are often considerably larger, in the range of ~3–5 cm, subsequent RFA devices used various strategies to enlarge the ablation zone. Some devices employed multiple deployable tines or needle clusters (Figure 9.8). Other devices used cooling of the RF needle to limit adjacent tissue temperature and thus increase the ablation zone [208,209]. Pulsing of radio frequency energy to allow time for thermal dissipation of peak temperatures near the electrode has also proven useful to reduce overheating of adjacent tissue and thereby

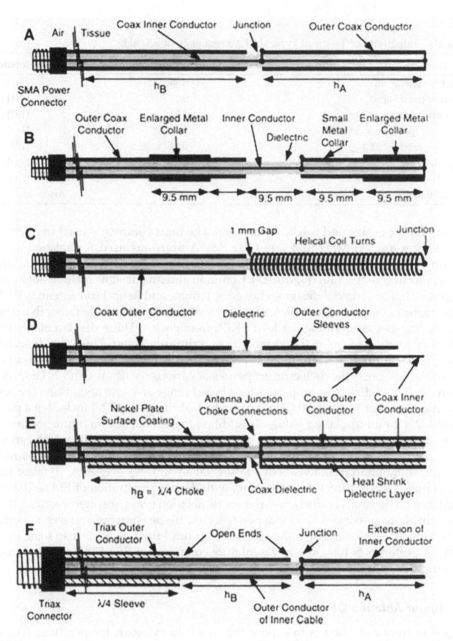

FIGURE 9.7
Schematic drawings of coaxial cable mounted interstitial microwave antennas intended for insertion into lossy tissue inside insulating catheters. (A) Dipole antenna showing extension of the coax inner conductor (h_A) and implanted length of outer conductor (h_b), separated at the "junction" [197]. (B) Dipole with enlarged diameter collars for increased capacitive coupling through the catheter wall, which helps extend the heating pattern axially away from the junction [198]. (C) Helical coil antenna with fine wire coil ~1 turn per mm axial length. The coil attaches to the inner conductor at the tip and has a 1-mm separation gap to the outer conductor [199,200]. (D) Multinode antenna [201] with short sections of outer conductor removed to expose inner conductor "nodes" for extending the heating pattern axially. (E) Dipole antenna with quarter-wavelength chokes made from metallic coating on the outer dielectric surface over both the h_A and h_b antenna sections [202]. (F) Sleeve dipole antenna with quarter-wavelength sleeve and transformed open end [203]. (Figure reprinted with permission of Springer Verlag from [11].)

TABLE 9.2

Dielectric Properties of Tissue at Microwave Frequencies [27,28]

Tissue	1 GHz		10 GHz	
	ε_r	σ	ε_r	σ
Adipose (fat)	5.45	0.05	4.6	0.59
Bone (cortical)	12.4	0.16	8.12	2.14
Breast	5.41	0.05	3.88	0.74
Kidney	57.9	1.45	40.3	11.6
Liver	46.4	0.90	32.5	9.39
Lung (inflated)	21.8	0.47	16.2	4.21
Muscle	54.8	0.98	42.8	10.6

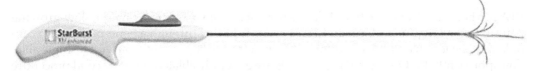

FIGURE 9.8
The StarBurst XLi-RFA device that incorporates metal tine electrodes that deploy out into surrounding tissue after percutaneous insertion to the target combined with controlled infusion of cooled saline that promotes complete ablation of tumors up to 7 cm in diameter. The RF electrode device features real-time, multi-point temperature feedback system from the seven active arms. (Courtesy of RITA Medical Systems, Mountain View, California.)

increase effective heating volume. For example, a combined approach that involves use of a multi-probe cluster of internally cooled electrodes with pulsing has demonstrated larger lesion size than those achieved by any method alone [208]. Current RFA devices can generate ablation zones in the range of 3–5 cm, with heating durations of 12–25 min. The newer MWA devices can generate similar size ablation zones with single MW antennas in typically shorter duration of ~10 min [196]. For tumors that cannot be ablated with a single electrode, either multiple sequential ablations are performed or multiple electrodes/antennas are inserted and activated simultaneously, depending on device and indication.

9.3.4 Oncological Applications of Thermal Ablation

9.3.4.1 Liver Cancer

Surgical resection is the only curative treatment for liver cancer but only 10–20% of patients with liver tumors can be treated by surgery [210]. For this reason, minimally invasive RFA and MWA have become widely used cancer therapies for the liver [211,212]. Since tumor RFA was introduced more than 20 years ago [213], there has been extensive work on liver tumor RFA [214,215], and only more recently with MWA [216]. Studies of over 3000 RFA-treated patients have shown the efficacy of percutaneous RFA for small (<3 cm) primary liver tumors. Complete local response averages 70–75% in tumors between 3 and 5 cm, but drops to <25% in larger tumors. With successful ablation, 5-year survival rates of 51–76% have been reported [211]. This pattern of excellent local control for small primary liver tumors with significant long-term nonlocal recurrence is also true in RFA of hepatic metastases. Livraghi et al. concluded that RF ablation is a relatively low-risk procedure for focal liver tumor treatment based on results with 3,554 lesions [217]. However, to date there are no randomized prospective controlled studies comparing liver RFA to standard surgical resection in any population.

9.3.4.2 Kidney Cancer

Standard radical or partial nephrectomy may be excessively invasive for small kidney tumors, and RFA can offer an alternative minimally invasive treatment [211,218]. Similar to applications in liver, RFA is most effective in treating kidney tumors less than 3 cm in diameter [218]. With increasing size, there is an increased risk of local recurrence. The number of patients treated is relatively small. However, early short-term results suggest a 70–90% success rate in small kidney tumors [211].

9.3.4.3 Bone Cancer

RFA has been used for more than 15 years to treat osteoid osteoma, a benign, slow-growing painful lesion [219]. To perform an RFA, a probe is placed through a bone-penetration cannula into the lesion and activated for 4–6 min at 90°C [220]. Success rates for a single ablation approach 100%. Occasional recurrences are generally ablated with a second procedure [221]. Lanza et al. [222] performed a systematic review of the literature in 2014 and found 95% success clinically in 1772 patients. Overall, treatment of osteomas by RFA is considered highly effective, safe and allows early return to function with minimal morbidity. In addition, there is strong evidence suggesting the utility of RFA for treatment of painful metastatic bone tumors [223].

9.3.4.4 Lung Cancer

For patients with inoperable lung cancer, percutaneous RFA using computed tomography guidance represents a minimally invasive treatment option with potential patient benefit, in particular when combined with radiotherapy [224,225]. In the lung, MWA has advantages over RFA, since power deposition from MWA is not limited by the lower conductivity of aerated lung tissue [207,226].

9.3.4.5 Breast Cancer

RFA for breast cancer has been studied in patients starting around 1999 [227]. A recently published retrospective study in 386 patients treated at 10 institutions suggests that RFA in breast cancer is a safe and promising minimally invasive therapy for small tumors <1 cm in diameter. Ipsilateral breast tumor recurrence 5 years after RFA was 3% for tumors <1 cm, but increased to 94% for tumors 1–2 cm [228].

9.3.4.6 Other Tumors

While RFA has only been applied in limited fashion in prostate tumors [182], both MWA and RFA have been employed more widely for adrenal tumors [229,230].

9.3.5 Non-Oncologic Clinical Applications of EM Heating

Outside the world of cancer therapy, there are numerous clinical applications for EM heating with RF and MW sources, using either moderate temperature hyperthermia or high-temperature thermal ablation techniques. The following sections offer a brief overview of several approaches that are representative of the wide range of non-oncologic uses of heat.

9.3.5.1 Cardiac Arrhythmia Treatment

Thermal ablation is widely used as therapy for cardiac arrhythmia (i.e., irregular heart beat) that is resistant to drug-based treatment. For certain cardiac arrhythmias, RFA has become the treatment of choice with success rates close to 100%, such as for several types of tachycardia (i.e., heart beating too fast, >150 beats per minute); it is also widely used for some types of atrial fibrillation (i.e., disorganized, quivering contraction of the atria). Most often, RFA rather than MWA is employed, and when applied in the heart is termed "cardiac radiofrequency catheter ablation." Cardiac RFA is typically carried out by specialized cardiologists (electrophysiologists) trained in the treatment of cardiac arrhythmia. The procedure uses a specially equipped laboratory that includes the ability to perform imaging during the procedure, usually fluoroscopy (i.e., x-ray imaging supplemented by a contrast agent to visualize vascular structures and the heart chambers). The RFA catheter (Figure 9.9) is introduced into the patient's vasculature through a vein or artery, and steered into the heart to the target site where it delivers RF energy to ablate diseased heart tissue surrounding the electrode tip (Figure 9.10). Additional catheters that record the electrical activity of the heart assist in locating the source of the arrhythmia and positioning the electrode accordingly. Ablation zone sizes are usually small (<1 cm diameter), with short ablation times of less than 1 min.

9.3.5.2 Pain

By ablating nerves, RFA can provide rapid pain relief (in hours to days) for patients with pain resistant to conventional forms of palliation. One of the more common applications is for RFA denervation of spinal nerves in the cervical and lumbar region to address lower back pain [185]. There is also long-term experience with other indications such as trigeminal neuralgia [231].

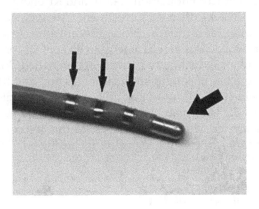

FIGURE 9.9
Cardiac RFA catheter (2.3 mm diameter), with ablation electrode (large arrow) and additional electrodes for recording electrical heart activity (small arrows.)

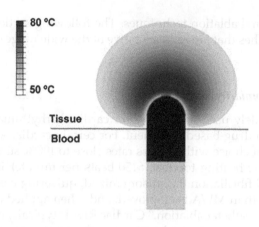

FIGURE 9.10
Computer simulation of tissue temperature profile after 1 min heating from cardiac RFA catheter shown in Figure 9.9. Temperatures above ~50°C create an ablation lesion that halts electrical conduction signals. Care is required to avoid blood clot formation around the active electrode that is in direct contact with blood.

9.3.5.3 Cosmetics

Narins and Narins [232] used an RF device to induce tightening of skin via uniform volumetric heating into deep dermis, producing, in effect, a "nonsurgical facelift." Twenty treatment areas in 17 patients were treated to evaluate the efficacy and safety of RF treatment to the brow and jowls. The technique was reported to produce gradual skin tightening in most patients with no adverse effects. Fitzpatrick et al. [233] studied 86 subjects who were evaluated for 6 months after treatment with an RF tissue-tightening device. A single treatment produced objective and subjective reductions in peri-orbital wrinkles and measurable changes in brow position. These changes were indicative of a thermally induced early tissue-tightening effect followed by additional tightening over a time course consistent with thermal wound healing response. Dover et al. reviewed 5,700 patient treatments of RF facial skin tightening with either single pass or multiple pass RF ablation [234]. They found improved response with the multiple pass approach with 92% maintaining agreeable skin tightening 6 months after treatment vs. 52% for single pass.

Sadick and Shaoul [235] treated 40 adult patients (skin phenotypes II–V) with varied facial and non-facial hair colors with a combination of laser and RF energy. Maximum hair reduction was observed at 6–8 weeks after each treatment. An average clearance of 75% was observed in all body locations at 18 months. No significant adverse sequelae were reported. They concluded that combined laser and RF energy with contact cooling is a safe and effective method of long-term hair reduction in patients of diversified skin type and hair color.

Chess [236] evaluated the use of combination laser (915 nm) and RF (1 MHz) energies for treatment of varicose veins (0.3–5.0 mm vessel diameters) in 35 sites in 25 patients. At 1 and 6 month follow-ups, ~77% of treatment sites exhibited 75–100% vessel clearance, and 90% had >50% vessel clearance. The authors concluded that the combination laser and RF system was effective and safe for treating leg veins, including telangiectases, venulectases, and reticular veins.

9.3.5.4 Miscellaneous Applications of RFA

Li et al. [237] evaluated the effect of RFA treatment of 22 patient's palates on speech, swallowing, taste, sleep, and snoring. After a mean follow-up of 14 months, no adverse effects were reported. While the success of RF volumetric reduction of the palate diminishes with time, the minimal invasiveness of RFA contributed to a high patient acceptance of retreatment and improvement after snoring relapse. Baba et al. [238] performed a meta-analysis of 20 studies that determined that temperature controlled RFA was clinically effective in reducing respiratory disturbance and sleepiness due to obstructive sleep apnea.

Hultcrantz and Ericsson [239] compared two techniques for pediatric tonsil surgery with respect to pain and postoperative morbidity. The two methods were partial tonsil resection with RFA vs. traditional tonsillectomy. They concluded that RF appears to be a safe and reliable method for tonsil surgery with much less postoperative morbidity than regular tonsillectomy.

Wanitphakdeedecha et al. [240] studied the efficacy and safety profile of RF and dynamic muscle activation technology for treatment of abdominal cellulite in 25 females. They found 92% of patients were satisfied with treatment outcome with average loss in circumference of 2.5 cm at 4-week follow-up.

An endoscopic radiofrequency procedure (Stretta) has been used for over a decade to treat recurrent gastroesophageal reflux disease (GERD). Fass et al. [241] conducted a systematic review and meta-analysis of 28 clinical studies with 2,468 patients treated with Stretta. He found that the RF procedure very significantly improves subjective and objective clinical endpoints in treatment of lower esophageal sphincter, and therefore should be considered as a viable alternative in the clinical management of GERD.

9.4 Concluding Remarks

While there are controversies concerning potential health effects of low-level EM field exposure, this chapter describes some of the many beneficial effects of EM energy at orders of magnitude higher field strengths. Diathermy has been used in rehabilitation medicine for more than half a century and millions of patients have benefited from moderate temperature treatments of muscle and ligament pain. Clinical investigations of moderate temperature hyperthermia and high-temperature thermal ablation treatments for cancer have clearly demonstrated the efficacy of controlled EM power deposition for a wide range of diseases. The literature includes extensive compilations of clinical use of therapeutic heating devices for cancer therapy as well as non-oncologic cosmetic procedures. Complex ongoing optimization of EM heating equipment and thermal dosimetry procedures to control treatment make heat delivery an art. Thus, interdisciplinary teamwork between medical, engineering, and biological sciences is vital to the continued expansion of successful medical applications of EM technology.

9.5 Acknowledgements

The authors would like to express appreciation to an extended list of contributors to the evolution of Hyperthermia and Thermal Ablation therapies. In particular, the authors would like to thank Mark Dewhirst and Maxim Itkin for providing valuable information on hyperthermia and RF ablation, and John McDougall (deceased) and Joe Elder for comments on the original text.

References

1. Lehmann, J., ed. *Therapeutic Heat and Cold*. 4th ed., Williams and Wilkens: Baltimore, MD, 1990.
2. Dewhirst, M.W., Stauffer, P.R., Das, S.K., Craciunescu, O.I. and Vujaskovic, Z., Hyperthermia in *Clinical Radiation Oncology*, Gunderson, L. and Tepper, J., Editors, Elsevier: Philladelphia, PA. pp. 381–98, 2016.
3. Sneed, P.K., Stauffer, P.R., Li, G., Sun, X. and Myerson, R., Hyperthermia in *Textbook of Radiation Oncology Third Edition*, Phillips, T., Hoppe, R. and Roach, M., Editors, Elsevier Saunders Co: Philadelphia, PA. pp. 1564–93, 2010.
4. Wust, P., Hildebrandt, B., Sreenivasa, G., Rau, B., Gellermann, J., Riess, H., Felix, R. and Schlag, P.M., Hyperthermia in combined treatment of cancer. *Lancet Oncol*. **3**(8): pp. 487–97, 2002.
5. Christensen, D.A. and Durney, C.H., Hyperthermia production for cancer therapy: A review of fundamentals and methods. *J Microw Power*. **16**: pp. 89–105, 1981.
6. Guy, A. and Chou, C., eds. Physical aspects of localized heating by radio frequency waves. in *Hyperthermia in Cancer Therapy*, Storm, K., Editor, G.K. Hall Publisher: Boston. 279, 1982.
7. Guy, A.W., Dosimetry associated with exposure to non-ionizing radiation: Very low frequency to microwaves. *Health Phys*. **53**(6): pp. 569–84, 1987.
8. Stauffer, P.R., Evolving technology for thermal therapy of cancer. *Int J Hyperthermia*. **21**(8): pp. 731–44, 2005.
9. Stauffer, P.R. and Paulides, M.M., Hyperthermia therapy for cancer, in *Comprehensive Biomedical Physics*, Brahme, A., Editor, Elsevier: Oxford. pp. 115–51, 2014.
10. van Rhoon, G.C., External electromagnetic methods and devices, in *Physics of Thermal Therapy: Fundamentals and Clinicial Applications*, Moros, E.G., Editor, Taylor and Francis: Boca Ratan, FL. pp. 139–58, 2013.
11. Stauffer, P.R., Diederich, C.J. and Seegenschmiedt, M.H., Interstitial heating technologies, in *Thermoradiotherapy and Thermochemotherapy: Volume 1, Biology, Physiology and Physics*, Seegenschmiedt, M.H., Fessenden, P. and Vernon, C.C., Editors, Springer-Verlag: Berlin, New York. pp. 279–320, 1995.
12. Huang, S.K., Radio-frequency catheter ablation of cardiac arrhythmias: Appraisal of an evolving therapeutic modality. *Am Heart J*. **118**(6): pp. 1317–23, 1989.
13. Langberg, J.J., Wonnell, T., Chin, M.C., Finkbeiner, W., Scheinman, M. and Stauffer, P., Catheter ablation of the atrioventricular junction using a helical microwave antenna: A novel means of coupling energy to the endocardium. *Pacing Clin Electrophysiol*. **14**(12): pp. 2105–13, 1991.
14. Ernst, S., Catheter ablation: General principles and advances. *Card Electrophysiol Clin*. **9**(2): pp. 311–17, 2017.
15. Friedman, M., Mikityansky, I., Kam, A., Libutti, S.K., Walther, M.M., Neeman, Z., Locklin, J.K. and Wood, B.J., Radiofrequency ablation of cancer. *Cardiovasc Intervent Radiol*. **27**(5): pp. 427–34, 2004.
16. Goldberg, S.N., Grassi, C.J., Cardella, J.F., Charboneau, J.W., Dodd, G.D., 3rd, Dupuy, D.E., Gervais, D.A., Gillams, A.R., Kane, R.A., Lee, F.T., Jr., et al., Image-guided tumor ablation: Standardization of terminology and reporting criteria. *J Vasc Interv Radiol*. **20**(7 Suppl): pp. S377–90, 2009.
17. Goldberg, S.N., Radiofrequency tumor ablation: Principles and techniques. *Eur J Ultrasound*. **13**(2): pp. 129–47, 2001.
18. Abbas, P.J., Tejani, V.D., Scheperle, R.A. and Brown, C.J., Using neural response telemetry to monitor physiological responses to acoustic stimulation in hybrid cochlear implant users. *Ear Hear*. **38**(4): pp. 409–25, 2017.
19. Garverick, S.L., Kane, M., Ko, W.H. and Maniglia, A.J., External unit for a semi-implantable middle ear hearing device. *Ear Nose Throat J*. **76**(6): pp. 397–401, 1997.
20. Scheffer, H.J., Vroomen, L.G., de Jong, M.C., Melenhorst, M.C., Zonderhuis, B.M., Daams, F., Vogel, J.A., Besselink, M.G., van Kuijk, C., Witvliet, J., et al., Ablation of locally advanced pancreatic cancer with percutaneous irreversible electroporation: Results of the phase I/II panfire study. *Radiology*. **282**(2): pp. 585–97, 2017.

21. Arunachalam, K., Maccarini, P., De Luca, V., Tognolatti, P., Bardati, F., Snow, B. and Stauffer, P., Detection of vesicoureteral reflux using microwave radiometry-system characterization with tissue phantoms. *IEEE Trans Biomed Eng.* **58**(6): pp. 1629–36, 2011.

22. Jacobsen, S., Stauffer, P.R. and Neuman, D.G., Dual-mode antenna design for microwave heating and noninvasive thermometry of superficial tissue disease. *IEEE Trans Biomed Eng.* **47**(11): pp. 1500–9, 2000.

23. Stauffer, P.R., Maccarini, P.F., Arunachalam, K., De Luca, V., Salahi, S., Boico, A., Klemetsen, O., Birkelund, Y., Jacobsen, S.K., Bardati, F., et al., Microwave radiometry for non-invasive detection of vesicoureteral reflux (vur) following bladder warming. *Proc SPIE.* **7901**: p. 79010V, 2011.

24. Stauffer, P.R., Snow, B.W., Rodrigues, D.B., Salahi, S., Oliveira, T.R., Reudink, D. and Maccarini, P.F., Non-invasive measurement of brain temperature with microwave radiometry: Demonstration in a head phantom and clinical case. *Neuroradiol J.* **27**(1): pp. 3–12, 2014.

25. Meaney, P.M., Geimer, S.D. and Paulsen, K.D., Two-step inversion with a logarithmic transformation for microwave breast imaging. *Med Phys.* 44(8):4239–4251–2017.

26. Meaney, P.M., Microwave imaging and emerging applications. *Int J Biomed Imaging.* **2012**: p. 252093, 2012.

27. Gabriel, C., Gabriel, S. and Corthout, E., The dielectric properties of biological tissues: I. Literature survey. *Phys Med Biol.* **41**(11): pp. 2231–49, 1996.

28. Gabriel, S., Lau, R.W. and Gabriel, C., The dielectric properties of biological tissues: II. Measurements in the frequency range 10 Hz to 20 GHz. *Phys Med Biol.* **41**(11): pp. 2251–69, 1996.

29. Gabriel, S., Lau, R.W. and Gabriel, C., The dielectric properties of biological tissues: III. Parametric models for the dielectric spectrum of tissues. *Phys Med Biol.* **41**(11): pp. 2271–93, 1996.

30. Johnson, C.C. and Guy, A.W., Nonionizing electromagnetic wave effects in biological materials and systems. *Proc IEEE.* **60**: pp. 692–718, 1972.

31. Ohguri, T., Imada, H., Yahara, K., Morioka, T., Nakano, K., Terashima, H. and Korogi, Y., Radiotherapy with 8-MHz radiofrequency-capacitive regional hyperthermia for stage III non-small-cell lung cancer: The radiofrequency-output power correlates with the intraesophageal temperature and clinical outcomes. *Int J Radiat Oncol Biol Phys.* **73**(1): pp. 128–35, 2009.

32. van Rhoon, G.C., van der Zee, J., Broekmeyer-Reurink, M.P., Visser, A.G. and Reinhold, H.S., Radiofrequency capacitive heating of deep-seated tumours using pre-cooling of the subcutaneous tissues: Results on thermometry in dutch patients. *Int J Hyperthermia.* **8**(6): pp. 843–54, 1992.

33. Crezee, J., Kaatee, R.S., van der Koijk, J.F. and Lagendijk, J.J., Spatial steering with quadruple electrodes in 27 MHz capacitively coupled interstitial hyperthermia. *Int J Hyperthermia.* **15**(2): pp. 145–56, 1999.

34. Solbiati, L., Livraghi, T., Goldberg, S.N., Ierace, T., Meloni, F., Dellanoce, M., Cova, L., Halpern, E.F. and Gazelle, G.S., Percutaneous radio-frequency ablation of hepatic metastases from colorectal cancer: Long-term results in 117 patients. *Radiology.* **221**(1): pp. 159–66, 2001.

35. Goldberg, S.N., Gazelle, G.S., Solbiati, L., Livraghi, T., Tanabe, K.K., Hahn, P.F. and Mueller, P.R., Ablation of liver tumors using percutaneous RF therapy. *AJR Am J Roentgenol.* **170**(4): pp. 1023–8, 1998.

36. Kumler, I., Parner, V.K., Tuxen, M.K., Skjoldbye, B., Bergenfeldt, M., Nelausen, K.M. and Nielsen, D.L., Clinical outcome of percutaneous RF-ablation of non-operable patients with liver metastasis from breast cancer. *Radiol Med.* **120**(6): pp. 536–41, 2015.

37. Stauffer, P.R., Diederich, C.J. and Pouliot, J., Thermal therapy for cancer, in *Brachytherapy Physics*, 2nd Edition, Joint AAPM/ABS Summer School, Med. Phys. Monograph No. 31, Thomadsen, B., Rivard, M. and Butler, W., Editors. pp. 901–32, 2005.

38. Pennes, H.H., Analysis of tissue and arterial blood temperatures in the resting human forearm. *J Appl Phys.* **1**: pp. 93–122, 1948.

39. Song, C.W., Choi, I.B., Nah, B.S., Sahu, S.K. and Osborn, J.L., Microvasculature and perfusion in normal tissues and tumors, in *Thermoradiotherapy and Thermochemotherapy: Volume 1, Biology, Physiology and Physics*, Seegenschmiedt, M.H., Fessenden, P. and Vernon, C.C., Editors, Springer-Verlag: Berlin, New York. pp. 139–56, 1995.

40. Song, C.W., Park, H. and Griffin, R.J., Improvement of tumor oxygenation by mild hyperthermia. *Radiat Res.* **155**(4): pp. 515–28, 2001.

41. Dewhirst, M.W., Vujaskovic, Z., Jones, E. and Thrall, D., Re-setting the biologic rationale for thermal therapy. See comment. *Int J Hyperthermia*. **21**(8): pp. 779–90, 2005.

42. Datta, N.R., Krishnan, S., Speiser, D.E., Neufeld, E., Kuster, N., Bodis, S. and Hofmann, H., Magnetic nanoparticle-induced hyperthermia with appropriate payloads: Paul ehrlich's "magic (nano)bullet" for cancer theranostics? *Cancer Treat Rev.* **50**: pp. 217–27, 2016.

43. Domingos-Pereira, S., Cesson, V., Chevalier, M.F., Derre, L., Jichlinski, P. and Nardelli-Haefliger, D., Preclinical efficacy and safety of the TY21A vaccine strain for intravesical immunotherapy of non-muscle-invasive bladder cancer. *Oncoimmunology.* **6**(1): p. e1265720, 2017.

44. Zhou, L., Zhang, M., Fu, Q., Li, J. and Sun, H., Targeted near infrared hyperthermia combined with immune stimulation for optimized therapeutic efficacy in thyroid cancer treatment. *Oncotarget.* **7**(6): pp. 6878–90, 2016.

45. Repasky, E.A., Evans, S.S. and Dewhirst, M.W., Temperature matters! And why it should matter to tumor immunologists. *Cancer Immunol Res.* **1**(4): pp. 210–6, 2013.

46. Dahl, O., Interaction of heat and drugs in vitro and in vivo, in *Thermoradiotherapy and Thermochemotherapy: Volume 1, Biology, Physiology and Physics*, Seegenschmiedt, M.H., Fessenden, P. and Vernon, C.C., Editors, Springer-Verlag: Berlin, New York. pp. 103–21, 1995.

47. Datta, N.R., Ordonez, S.G., Gaipl, U.S., Paulides, M.M., Crezee, H., Gellermann, J., Marder, D., Puric, E. and Bodis, S., Local hyperthermia combined with radiotherapy and/or chemotherapy: Recent advances and promises for the future. *Cancer Treat Rev.* **41**(9): pp. 742–53, 2015.

48. Hahn, G.M., Potential for therapy of drugs and hyperthermia. *Cancer Res.* **39**: pp. 2264–68, 1979.

49. Peeken, J.C., Vaupel, P. and Combs, S.E., Integrating hyperthermia into modern radiation oncology: What evidence is necessary? *Front Oncol.* **7**: p. 132, 2017.

50. Dewhirst, M.W., Using hyperthermia to augment drug delivery, in *Physics of Thermal Therapy: Fundamentals and Clinical Applications*, Moros, E.G., Editor, CRC Press: Boca Raton, FL. pp. 279–92, 2013.

51. Huang, Q., Hu, J.K., Lohr, F., Zhang, L., Braun, R., Lanzen, J., Little, J.B., Dewhirst, M.W. and Li, C.Y., Heat-induced gene expression as a novel targeted cancer gene therapy strategy. *Cancer Res.* **60**(13): pp. 3435–9, 2000.

52. Lee, Y.J., Lee, H. and Borrelli, M.J., Gene transfer into human prostate adenocarcinoma cells with an adenoviral vector: Hyperthermia enhances a double suicide gene expression, cytotoxicity and radiotoxicity. *Cancer Gene Ther.* **9**(3): pp. 267–74, 2002.

53. Li, G.C., He, F., Shao, X., Urano, M., Shen, L., Kim, D., Borrelli, M., Leibel, S.A., Gutin, P.H. and Ling, C.C., Adenovirus-mediated heat-activated antisense ku70 expression radiosensitizes tumor cells in vitro and in vivo. *Cancer Res.* **63**(12): pp. 3268–74, 2003.

54. Luo, J., Wu, X., Zhou, F., Zhou, Y., Huang, T., Liu, F., Han, G., Chen, L., Bai, W., Sun, J., et al., Radiofrequency hyperthermia promotes the therapeutic effects on chemotherapeutic-resistant breast cancer when combined with heat shock protein promoter-controlled HSV-TK gene therapy: Toward imaging-guided interventional gene therapy. *Oncotarget.* **7**(40): pp. 65042–51, 2016.

55. Kok, H.P., Gellermann, J., van den Berg, C.A., Stauffer, P.R., Hand, J.W. and Crezee, J., Thermal modelling using discrete vasculature for thermal therapy: A review. *Int J Hyperthermia*. **29**(4): pp. 336–45, 2013.

56. Paulides, M.M., Stauffer, P.R., Neufeld, E., Maccarini, P.F., Kyriakou, A., Canters, R.A., Diederich, C.J., Bakker, J.F. and Van Rhoon, G.C., Simulation techniques in hyperthermia treatment planning. *Int J Hyperthermia*. **29**(4): pp. 346–57, 2013.

57. Dewhirst, M.W., Viglianti, B.L., Lora-Michiels, M., Hanson, M. and Hoopes, P.J., Basic principles of thermal dosimetry and thermal thresholds for tissue damage from hyperthermia. *Int J Hyperthermia.* **19**(3): pp. 267–94, 2003.

58. Dewey, W.C., Arrhenius relationships from the molecule and cell to the clinic. *Int J Hyperthermia.* **25**(1): pp. 3–20, 2009.

59. Sapareto, S.A. and Dewey, W.C., Thermal dose determination in cancer therapy. *Int J Radiat Oncol Biol Phys.* **10**: pp. 787–800, 1984.

60. Cheung, A.Y. and Neyzari, A., Deep local hyperthermia for cancer therapy: External electromagnetic and ultrasound techniques. *Cancer Res. (Supplement).* **44**: pp. 4736s–44s, 1984.
61. Lee, E.R., Electromagnetic superficial heating technology, in *Thermoradiotherapy and thermochemotherapy*, Seegenschmiedt, M.H., Fessenden, P. and Vernon, C.C., Editors, Springer-Verlag: Berlin, Heidelberg. pp. 193–217, 1995.
62. Chou, C. and Ren, R., eds. Radiofrequency hyperthermia in cancer therapy. in *Biomedical Engineering Handbook*, 2nd ed. Vol. 1, Bronzino, J., Editor, CRC Press: Boca Raton. 93, 2000.
63. Chou, C.K., Evaluation of microwave hyperthermia applicators. *Bioelectromagnetics.* **13**(6): pp. 581–97, 1992.
64. Stauffer, P., Rodrigues, D., Sinahon, R., Sbarro, L., Beckhoff, V. and Hurwitz, M., Using a conformal waterbolus to adjust heating patterns of microwave waveguide applicators. in *Proceedings of SPIE. 2017*. San Francisco: SPIE Press, Bellingham WA, **100660**: pp, 100660N1–N15.
65. Gelvich, E.A. and Mazokhin, V.N., Resonance effects in applicator water boluses and their influence on SAR distribution patterns. *Int J Hyperthermia.* **16**(2): pp. 113–28, 2000.
66. Lee, E.R., Kapp, D.S., Lohrbach, A.W. and Sokol, J.L., Influence of water bolus temperature on measured skin surface and intradermal temperatures. *Int J Hyperthermia.* **10**(1): pp. 59–72, 1994.
67. Neuman, D.G., Stauffer, P.R., Jacobsen, S. and Rossetto, F., SAR pattern perturbations from resonance effects in water bolus layers used with superficial microwave hyperthermia applicators. *Int J Hyperthermia.* **18**(3): pp. 180–93, 2002.
68. Van der Gaag, M.L., De Bruijne, M., Samaras, T., Van der Zee, J. and Van Rhoon, G.C., Development of a guideline for the water bolus temperature in superficial hyperthermia. *Int J Hyperthermia.* **22**(8): pp. 637–56, 2006.
69. Crezee, J., Van Haaren, P.M., Westendorp, H., De Greef, M., Kok, H.P., Wiersma, J., Van Stam, G., Sijbrands, J., Zum Vorde Sive Vording, P., Van Dijk, J.D., et al., Improving locoregional hyperthermia delivery using the 3-D controlled AMC-8 phased array hyperthermia system: A preclinical study. *Int J Hyperthermia.* **25**(7): pp. 581–92, 2009.
70. Kok, H.P., de Greef, M., Wiersma, J., Bel, A. and Crezee, J., The impact of the waveguide aperture size of the 3d 70 MHz AMC-8 locoregional hyperthermia system on tumour coverage. *Phys Med Biol.* **55**(17): pp. 4899–916, 2010.
71. Turner, P.F., Regional hyperthermia with an annular phased array. *IEEE Trans Biomed Eng.* **31**: pp. 106–14, 1984.
72. Gellermann, J., Hildebrandt, B., Issels, R., Ganter, H., Wlodarczyk, W., Budach, V., Felix, R., Tunn, P.U., Reichardt, P. and Wust, P., Noninvasive magnetic resonance thermography of soft tissue sarcomas during regional hyperthermia: Correlation with response and direct thermometry. *Cancer.* **107**(6): pp. 1373–82, 2006.
73. Juang, T., Stauffer, P.R., Craciunescu, O.A., Maccarini, P.F., Yuan, Y., Das, S.K., Dewhirst, M.W., Inman, B.A. and Vujaskovic, Z., Thermal dosimetry characteristics of deep regional heating of non-muscle invasive bladder cancer. *Int J Hyperthermia.* 30(3):176–83 2014.
74. Van Rhoon, G.C., Van Der Heuvel, D.J., Ameziane, A., Rietveld, P.J., Volenec, K. and Van Der Zee, J., Characterization of the sar-distribution of the Sigma-60 applicator for regional hyperthermia using a schottky diode sheet. *Int J Hyperthermia.* **19**(6): pp. 642–54, 2003.
75. Hynynen, K., Roemer, R., Anhalt, D., Johnson, C., Xu, Z.X., Swindell, W. and Cetas, T., A scanned, focused, multiple transducer ultrasonic system for localized hyperthermia treatments. *Int J Hyperthermia.* **26**(1): pp. 1–11, 2010.
76. McDannold, N., Tempany, C., Jolesz, F. and Hynynen, K., Evaluation of referenceless thermometry in MRI-guided focused ultrasound surgery of uterine fibroids. *J Magn Reson Imaging.* **28**(4): pp. 1026–32, 2008.
77. Hand, J.W., Trembly, B.S. and Prior, M.V., Physics of interstitial hyperthermia: Radiofrequency and hot water tube techniques, in *Hyperthermia and Oncology, vol. 3*, Urano, M. and Douple, E., Editors, VSP: Zeist. pp. 99–134, 1991.
78. Handl-Zeller, L., ed. *Interstitial Hyperthermia*. Springer-Verlag: Wien, New York, 1992.

79. Strohbehn, J.W., Interstitial techniques for hyperthermia, in *Physics and Technology of Hyperthermia*, Field, S.B. and Franconi, C., Editors, Martinus Nijhoff Publishers: Dordrecht, Boston, Lancaster. pp. 211–40, 1987.
80. Chan, K.W., McDougall, J.A. and Chou, C.K., FDTD simulations of clini-therm applicators on inhomogeneous planar tissue models. *Int J Hyperthermia*. **11**(6): pp. 809–20, 1995.
81. Hand, J.W., Vernon, C.C., Prior, M.V. and Forse, G.R., Current sheet applicator arrays for superficial hyperthermia, in *Hyperthermic Oncology 1992, vol. 2*, Gerner, E. and Cetas, T., Editors, Arizona Board of Regents: Tucson. pp. 193–7, 1993.
82. Kok, H.P., De Greef, M., Correia, D., Vording, P.J., Van Stam, G., Gelvich, E.A., Bel, A. and Crezee, J., FDTD simulations to assess the performance of CFMA-434 applicators for superficial hyperthermia. *Int J Hyperthermia*. **25**(6): pp. 462–76, 2009.
83. Kok, P., Correia, D., De Greef, M., Van Stam, G., Bel, A. and Crezee, J., SAR deposition by curved CFMA-434 applicators for superficial hyperthermia: Measurements and simulations. *Int J Hyperthermia*. **26**(2): pp. 171–84, 2010.
84. Lee, E.R., Wilsey, T.R., Tarczy-Hornoch, P., Kapp, D.S., Fessenden, P., Lohrbach, A.W. and Prionas, S.D., Body conformable 915 MHz microstrip array applicators for large surface area hyperthermia. *IEEE Trans Biomed Eng*. **39**(5): pp. 470–83, 1992.
85. Lee, W.M., Gelvich, E.A., van der Baan, P., Mazokhin, V.N. and van Rhoon, G.C., Assessment of the performance characteristics of a prototype 12-element capacitive contact flexible microstrip applicator (CFMA-12) for superficial hyperthermia. *Int J Hyperthermia*. **20**(6): pp. 607–24, 2004.
86. Stauffer, P.R., Maccarini, P., Arunachalam, K., Craciunescu, O., Diederich, C., Juang, T., Rossetto, F., Schlorff, J., Milligan, A., Hsu, J., et al., Conformal microwave array (CMA) applicators for hyperthermia of diffuse chest wall recurrence. *Int J Hyperthermia*. **26**(7): pp. 686–98, 2010.
87. van Rhoon, G.C., Rietveld, P.J. and van der Zee, J., A 433 MHz lucite cone waveguide applicator for superficial hyperthermia. *Int J Hyperthermia*. **14**(1): pp. 13–27, 1998.
88. Samulski, T.V., Grant, W.J., Oleson, J.R., Leopold, K.A., Dewhirst, M.W., Vallario, P. and Blivin, J., Clinical experience with a multi-element ultrasonic hyperthermia system: Analysis of treatment temperatures. *Int J Hyperthermia*. **6**(5): pp. 909–22, 1990.
89. Underwood, H.R., Burdette, E.C., Ocheltree, K.B. and Magin, R.L., A multi-element ultrasonic hyperthermia applicator with independent element control. *Int J Hyperthermia*. **3**: pp. 257–67, 1987.
90. Hiraoka, M., Nishimura, Y., Nagata, Y., Mitsumori, M., Okuno, Y., Li, P.Y., Takahashi, M., Masunaga, S., Akuta, K., Koish, M., et al., Clinical results of thermoradiotherapy for soft tissue tumours. *Int J Hyperthermia*. **11**(3): pp. 365–77, 1995.
91. Lee, C.K., Song, C.W., Rhee, J.G., Foy, J.A. and Levitt, S.H., Clinical experience using 8 MHz radiofrequency capacitive hyperthermia in combination with radiotherapy: Results of a phase I/II study. *Int J Radiat Oncol Biol Phys*. **32**(3): pp. 733–45, 1995.
92. Notter, M., Piazena, H. and Vaupel, P., Hypofractionated re-irradiation of large-sized recurrent breast cancer with thermography-controlled, contact-free water-filtered infra-red-A hyperthermia: A retrospective study of 73 patients. *Int J Hyperthermia*. 2016 Sep 28:1-10. [Epub ahead of print], pp. 1–10, 2016.
93. Hiraoka, M., Jo, S., Akuta, K., Nishimura, Y., Takahashi, M. and Abe, M., Radiofrequency capacitive hyperthermia for deep-seated tumors. I. Studies on thermometry. *Cancer*. **60**(1): pp. 121–27, 1987.
94. Kikuchi, M., Amemiya, Y., Egawa, S., Onoyama, Y., Kato, H., Kanai, H., Saito, Y., Tsukiyama, I., Hiraoka, M., Mizushina, S., et al., Guide to the use of hyperthermic equipment. 1. Capacitively-coupled heating. *Int J Hyperthermia*. **9**(2): pp. 187–203, 1993.
95. Mochiki, E., Shioya, M., Sakurai, H., Andoh, H., Ohno, T., Aihara, R., Asao, T. and Kuwano, H., Feasibility study of postoperative intraperitoneal hyperthermochemotherapy by radiofrequency capacitive heating system for advanced gastric cancer with peritoneal seeding. *Int J Hyperthermia*. **23**(6): pp. 493–500, 2007.
96. Sahinbas, H., Rosch, M. and Demiray, M., Temperature measurements in a capacitive system of deep loco-regional hyperthermia. *Electromagn Biol Med*. **36**(3): pp. 248–58, 2017.

97. Astrahan, M.A. and Norman, A., A localized current field hyperthermia system for use with 192-iridium interstitial implants. *Med Phys.* **9**(3): pp. 419–24, 1982.
98. Lagendijk, J.J.W., Visser, A.G., Kaatee, R.S.J.P., Crezee, J., van der Koijk, J.F., de Bree, J., Kotte, A.N.T.J., Kanis, A.P., Kroeze, H., Levendag, P.C., et al., Interstitial hyperthermia & treatment planning: The 27 MHz multi-electrode current source method. *Nucletron-Odelft Activity Report No.6.* pp. 83–90, 1995.
99. Visser, A.G., Deurloo, I.K.K., Levendag, P.C., Ruifrok, A.C.C., Cornet, B. and van Rhoon, G.C., An interstitial hyperthermia system at 27 MHz. *Int JHyperthermia.* **5**: pp. 265–276, 1989.
100. Vora, N., Forell, B., Joseph, C., Lipsett, J. and Archambeau, J., Interstitial implant with interstitial hyperthermia. *Cancer.* **50**(11): pp. 2518–23, 1982.
101. Oleson, J.R., Hyperthermia by magnetic induction: I. Physical characteristics of the technique. *Int J Radiat Oncol Biol Phys.* **8**: pp. 1747–56, 1982.
102. Oleson, J.R., A review of magnetic induction methods for hyperthermic treatment of cancer. *IEEE Trans Biomed Eng.* **31**(1): pp. 91–97, 1984.
103. Storm, F.K., Baker, H.W., Scanlon, E.F., Plenk, H.P., Meadows, P.M., Cohen, S.C., Olson, C.E., Thompson, J., Khandekar, J.D., Roe, D., et al., Magnetic induction hyperthermia: Results of a 5-year multi-institutional national cooperative trial in advanced cancer patients. *Cancer.* **55**: pp. 2677–87, 1985.
104. Johannsen, M., Thiesen, B., Wust, P. and Jordan, A., Magnetic nanoparticle hyperthermia for prostate cancer. *Int J Hyperthermia.* **26**(8): pp. 790–5, 2010.
105. Mack, C.F., Stea, B., Kittelson, J.M., Shimm, D.S., Sneed, P.K., Phillips, T.L., Swift, P.S., Luk, K., Stauffer, P.R., Chan, K.W., et al., Interstitial thermoradiotherapy with ferromagnetic implants for locally advanced and recurrent neoplasms. *Int J Radiat Oncol Biol Phys.* **27**: pp. 109–15, 1993.
106. Maier-Hauff, K., Ulrich, F., Nestler, D., Niehoff, H., Wust, P., Thiesen, B., Orawa, H., Budach, V. and Jordan, A., Efficacy and safety of intratumoral thermotherapy using magnetic iron-oxide nanoparticles combined with external beam radiotherapy on patients with recurrent glioblastoma multiforme. *J Neurooncol.* **103**(2): pp. 317–24, 2011.
107. Stauffer, P.R., Cetas, T.C. and Jones, R.C., Magnetic induction heating of ferromagnetic implants for inducing localized hyperthermia in deep-seated tumors. *IEEE Trans Biomed Eng.* **31**(2): pp. 235–51, 1984.
108. Stea, B., Kittelson, J., Cassady, J.R., Hamilton, A., Guthkelch, N., Lulu, B., Obbens, E., Rossman, K., Shapiro, W., Shetter, A., et al., Treatment of malignant gliomas with interstitial irradiation and hyperthermia. *Int J Radiat Oncol Biol Phys.* **24**(4): pp. 657–67, 1992.
109. Turner, P.F. and Kumar, L., Computer solution for applicator heating patterns. *Natl Cancer Inst Monogr.* **61**: pp. 521–23, 1982.
110. Gellermann, J., Wlodarczyk, W., Ganter, H., Nadobny, J., Fahling, H., Seebass, M., Felix, R. and Wust, P., A practical approach to thermography in a hyperthermia/magnetic resonance hybrid system: Validation in a heterogeneous phantom. *Int J Radiat Oncol Biol Phys.* **61**(1): pp. 267–77, 2005.
111. Gellermann, J., Wlodarczyk, W., Feussner, A., Fahling, H., Nadobny, J., Hildebrandt, B., Felix, R. and Wust, P., Methods and potentials of magnetic resonance imaging for monitoring radio-frequency hyperthermia in a hybrid system. *Int J Hyperthermia.* **21**(6): pp. 497–513, 2005.
112. Hand, J.W., Biophysics and technology of electromagnetic hyperthermia, in *Methods of External Hyperthermia Heating*, Gautherie, M., Editor, Springer-Verlag: Berlin, Heidelberg. pp. 1–60, 1990.
113. Myerson, R.J., Moros, E.G., Diederich, C.J., Haemmerich, D., Hurwitz, M.D., Hsu, I.C., McGough, R.J., Nau, W.H., Straube, W.L., Turner, P.F., et al., Components of a hyperthermia clinic: Recommendations for staffing, equipment, and treatment monitoring. *Int J Hyperthermia.* **30**(1): pp. 1–5, 2014.
114. Bruggmoser, G., Bauchowitz, S., Canters, R., Crezee, H., Ehmann, M., Gellermann, J., Lamprecht, U., Lomax, N., Messmer, M.B., Ott, O., et al., Quality assurance for clinical studies in regional deep hyperthermia. *Strahlenther Onkol.* **187**(10): pp. 605–10, 2011.
115. Muller, J., Hartmann, J. and Bert, C., Infrared camera based thermometry for quality assurance of superficial hyperthermia applicators. *Phys Med Biol.* **61**(7): pp. 2646–64, 2016.

116. Trefna, H.D., Crezee, H., Schmidt, M., Marder, D., Lamprecht, U., Ehmann, M., Hartmann, J., Nadobny, J., Gellermann, J., van Holthe, N., et al., Quality assurance guidelines for superficial hyperthermia clinical trials: I. Clinical requirements. *Int J Hyperthermia.* **33**(4): pp. 471–482, 2017. DOI: 10.1080/02656736.2016.1277791.

117. Bruggmoser, G., Some aspects of quality management in deep regional hyperthermia. *Int J Hyperthermia.* **28**(6): pp. 562–9, 2012.

118. Dobšíček-Trefná, H., Crezee, J., Schmidt, M., Marder, D., Lamprecht, U., Ehmann, M., Nadobny, J., Hartmann, J., Lomax, N., Abdel-Rahman, S., et al., Quality assurance guidelines for superficial hyperthermia clinical trials: II. Technical requirements for heating devices. *Strahlenther Onkol.* **193**(5): pp. 351–66, 2017.

119. Dewhirst, M.W., Phillips, T.L., Samulski, T.V., Stauffer, P., Shrivastava, P., Paliwal, B., Pajak, T., Gillim, M., Sapozink, M., Myerson, R., et al., RTOG quality assurance guidelines for clinical trials using hyperthermia. *Int J Radiat Oncol Biol Phys.* **18**(5): pp. 1249–59, 1990.

120. Emami, B., Stauffer, P., Dewhirst, M.W., Prionas, S., Ryan, T., Corry, P., Herman, T., Kapp, D.S., Myerson, R.J., Samulski, T., et al., RTOG quality assurance guidelines for interstitial hyperthermia. *Int J Radiat Oncol Biol Phys.* **20**: pp. 1117–24, 1991.

121. Hand, J.W., Lagendijk, J.J.W., Andersen, J.B. and Bolomey, J.C., Quality assurance guidelines for ESHO protocols. *Int J Hyperthermia.* **5**(4): pp. 421–28, 1989.

122. Lagendijk, J.J.W., van Rhoon, G.C., Hornsleth, S.N., Wust, P., De Leeuw, A.C.C., Schneider, C.J., van der Zee, J., van Heek-Romanowski, R., Rahman, S.A. and Gromoll, C., ESHO quality assurance guidelines for regional hyperthermia. *Int J Hyperthermia.* **14**(2): pp. 125–33, 1998.

123. Sapozink, M.D., Corry, P.M., Kapp, D.S., Myerson, R.J., Dewhirst, M.W., Emami, B., Herman, T., Prionas, S., Ryan, T., Samulski, T., et al., RTOG quality assurance guidelines for clinical trials using hyperthermia for deep-seated malignancy. *Int J Radiat Oncol Biol Phys.* **20**(5): pp. 1109–15, 1991.

124. Schneider, C.J., van Dijk, J.D., De Leeuw, A.A., Wust, P. and Baumhoer, W., Quality assurance in various radiative hyperthermia systems applying a phantom with LED matrix. *Int J Hyperthermia.* **10**(5): pp. 733–47, 1994.

125. Shrivastava, P., Luk, K., Oleson, J., Dewhirst, M., Pajak, T., Paliwal, B., Perez, C., Sapareto, S., Saylor, T. and Steeves, R., Hyperthermia quality assurance guidelines. *Int J Radiat Oncol Biol Phys.* **16**(3): pp. 571–87, 1989.

126. Hjertaker, B.T., Froystein, T. and Schem, B.C., A thermometry system for quality assurance and documentation of whole body hyperthermia procedures. *Int J Hyperthermia.* **21**(1): pp. 45–55, 2005.

127. Hornsleth, S.N., Frydendal, L., Mella, O., Dahl, O. and Raskmark, P., Quality assurance for radiofrequency regional hyperthermia. *Int J Hyperthermia.* **13**(2): pp. 169–85, 1997.

128. Samaras, T., van Rhoon, G.C. and Sahalos, J.N., Theoretical investigation of measurement procedures for the quality assurance of superficial hyperthermia applicators. *Int J Hyperthermia.* **18**(5): pp. 416–25, 2002.

129. Visser, A.G. and van Rhoon, G.C., Technical and clinical quality assurance, in *Thermoradiotherapy and Thermochemotherapy: Volume 1 Biology, Physiology, and Physics*, Seegenschmiedt, M.H., Fessenden, P. and Vernon, C.C., Editors, Springer-Verlag: Berlin, Heidelberg, NY. pp. 453–72, 1995.

130. Neufeld, E., Paulides, M.M., van Rhoon, G.C. and Kuster, N., Numerical modeling for simulation and treatment planning of thermal therapy, in *Physics of Thermal Therapy: Fundamentals and Clinical Applications*, Moros, E.G., Editor, CRC Press: Boca Raton, FL. pp. 119–38, 2013.

131. Datta, N.R., Rogers, S., Ordonez, S.G., Puric, E. and Bodis, S., Hyperthermia and radiotherapy in the management of head and neck cancers: A systematic review and meta-analysis. *Int J Hyperthermia.* **32**(1): pp. 31–40, 2016.

132. Datta, N.R., Puric, E., Klingbiel, D., Gomez, S. and Bodis, S., Hyperthermia and radiation therapy in locoregional recurrent breast cancers: A systematic review and meta-analysis. *Int J Radiat Oncol Biol Phys.* **94**(5): pp. 1073–87, 2016.

133. Vernon, C.C., Hand, J.W., Field, S.B., Machin, D., Whaley, J.B., van der Zee, J., van Putten, W.L.J., van Rhoon, G.C., van Dijk, J.D.P., Gonzalez-Gonzalez, D., et al., Radiotherapy with or without hyperthermia in the treatment of superficial localized breast cancer: Results from five randomized controlled trials. *Int J Radiat Oncol Biol Phys.* **35**(4): pp. 731–44, 1996.

134. Notter, M., Piazena, H. and Vaupel, P., Hypofractionated re-irradiation of large-sized recurrent breast cancer with thermography-controlled, contact-free water-filtered infra-red-A hyperthermia: A retrospective study of 73 patients. *Int J Hyperthermia.* **33**(2): pp. 227–36, 2017.

135. Datta, N.R., Rogers, S., Klingbiel, D., Gomez, S., Puric, E. and Bodis, S., Hyperthermia and radiotherapy with or without chemotherapy in locally advanced cervical cancer: A systematic review with conventional and network meta-analyses. *Int J Hyperthermia.* **32**(7): pp. 809–21, 2016.

136. Chen, H.W. and Jei, J.W.L., A randomized trial of hyperthermoradiochemotherapy for uterine cervix. *Chin J Oncol.* **24**: pp. 249–51, 1997.

137. Franckena, M., Stalpers, L.J., Koper, P.C., Wiggenraad, R.G., Hoogenraad, W.J., van Dijk, J.D., Warlam-Rodenhuis, C.C., Jobsen, J.J., van Rhoon, G.C. and van der Zee, J., Long-term improvement in treatment outcome after radiotherapy and hyperthermia in locoregionally advanced cervix cancer: An update of the dutch deep hyperthermia trial. *Int J Radiat Oncol Biol Phys.* **70**(4): pp. 1176–82, 2008.

138. Hua, Y., Ma, S., Fu, Z., Hu, Q., Wang, L. and Piao, Y., Intracavity hyperthermia in nasopharyngeal cancer: A phase III clinical study. *Int J Hyperthermia.* **27**(2): pp. 180–6, 2011.

139. Kang, M., Liu, W.Q., Qin, Y.T., Wei, Z.X. and Wang, R.S., Long-term efficacy of microwave hyperthermia combined with chemoradiotherapy in treatment of nasopharyngeal carcinoma with cervical lymph node metastases. *Asian Pac J Cancer Prev.* **14**(12): pp. 7395–400, 2013.

140. Zhao, C., Chen, J., Yu, B. and Chen, X., Improvement in quality of life in patients with nasopharyngeal carcinoma treated with non-invasive extracorporeal radiofrequency in combination with chemoradiotherapy. *Int J Radiat Biol.* **90**(10): pp. 853–8, 2014.

141. De Haas-Kock, D.F.M., Buijsen, J., Pijls-Johannesma, M., Lutgens, L., Lammering, G., van Mastrigt, G.A.P.G., De Ruysscher, D.K.M., Lambin, P. and van der Zee, J., Concomitant hyperthermia and radiation therapy for treating locally advanced rectal cancer. *Cochrane Database Syst Rev.* (3): p. CD006269, 2009.

142. Schroeder, C., Gani, C., Lamprecht, U., von Weyhern, C.H., Weinmann, M., Bamberg, M. and Berger, B., Pathological complete response and sphincter-sparing surgery after neoadjuvant radiochemotherapy with regional hyperthermia for locally advanced rectal cancer compared with radiochemotherapy alone. *Int J Hyperthermia.* **28**(8): pp. 707–14, 2012.

143. Perez, C.A., Pajak, T., Emami, B., Hornback, N.B., Tupchong, L. and Rubin, P., Randomized phase III study comparing irradiation and hyperthermia with irradiation alone in superficial measurable tumors. Final report by the radiation therapy oncology group. *Am J Clin Oncol.* **14**(2): pp. 133–41, 1991.

144. Waterman, F.M., Dewhirst, M.W., Fessenden, P., Samulski, T.V., Stauffer, P., Emami, B., Corry, P., Prionas, S.D., Sapozink, M., Herman, T., et al., RTOG quality assurance guidelines for clinical trials using hyperthermia administered by ultrasound. *Int J Radiat Oncol Biol Phys.* **20**(5): pp. 1099–107, 1991.

145. Overgaard, J., Gonzalez Gonzalez, D., Hulshof, M.C., Arcangeli, G., Dahl, O., Mella, O. and Bentzen, S.M., Hyperthermia as an adjuvant to radiation therapy of recurrent or metastatic malignant melanoma. A multicentre randomized trial by the european society for hyperthermic oncology. *Int J Hyperthermia.* **12**(1): pp. 3–20, 1996.

146. Jones, E.L., Oleson, J.R., Prosnitz, L.R., Samulski, T.V., Vujaskovic, Z., Yu, D.H., Sanders, L.L. and Dewhirst, M.W., Randomized trial of hyperthermia and radiation for superficial tumors. *J Clin Oncol.* **23**(13): pp. 3079–85, 2005.

147. Overgaard, J., Gonzalez Gonzalez, D., Hulshof, M.C.C.M., Arcangeli, G., Dahl, O., Mella, O. and Bentzen, S.M., Randomised trial of hyperthermia as adjuvant to radiotherapy for recurrent or metastatic malignant melanoma. *Lancet.* **345**: pp. 540–43, 1995.

148. Crezee, H. and Inman, B.A., The use of hyperthermia in the treatment of bladder cancer. *Int J Hyperthermia.* **32**(4): pp. 349–50, 2016.

149. Masunaga, S.I., Hiraoka, M., Akuta, K., Nishimura, Y., Nagata, Y., Jo, S., Takahashi, M., Abe, M., Terachi, T., Oishi, K., et al., Phase I/II trial of preoperative thermoradiotherapy in the treatment of urinary bladder cancer. *Int J Hyperthermia.* **10**(1): pp. 31–40, 1994.

150. van der Zee, J., Gonzalez Gonzalez, D., van Rhoon, G.C., van Dijk, J.D., van Putten, W.L. and Hart, A.A., Comparison of radiotherapy alone with radiotherapy plus hyperthermia in locally advanced pelvic tumours: A prospective, randomised, multicentre trial. Dutch deep hyperthermia group. *Lancet.* **355**(9210): pp. 1119–25, 2000.

151. Wittlinger, M., Rodel, C.M., Weiss, C., Krause, S.F., Kuhn, R., Fietkau, R., Sauer, R. and Ott, O.J., Quadrimodal treatment of high-risk T1 and T2 bladder cancer: Transurethral tumor resection followed by concurrent radiochemotherapy and regional deep hyperthermia. *Radiother Oncol.* **93**(2): pp. 358–63, 2009.

152. Colombo, R., Da Pozzo, L.F., Salonia, A., Rigatti, P., Leib, Z., Baniel, J., Caldarera, E. and Pavone-Macaluso, M., Multicentric study comparing intravesical chemotherapy alone and with local microwave hyperthermia for prophylaxis of recurrence of superficial transitional cell carcinoma. *J Clin Oncol.* **21**(23): pp. 4270–6, 2003.

153. Schrier, B.P., Hollander, M.P., van Rhijn, B.W., Kiemeney, L.A. and Witjes, J.A., Prognosis of muscle-invasive bladder cancer: Difference between primary and progressive tumours and implications for therapy. *Eur Urol.* **45**(3): pp. 292–6, 2004.

154. Colombo, R., Salonia, A., Leib, Z., Pavone-Macaluso, M. and Engelstein, D., Long-term outcomes of a randomized controlled trial comparing thermochemotherapy with mitomycin-c alone as adjuvant treatment for non-muscle-invasive bladder cancer (NMIBC). *BJU Int.* **107**(6): pp. 912–8, 2011.

155. Sugimachi, K., Kitamura, K., Baba, K., Ikebe, M., Morita, M., Matsuda, H. and Kuwano, H., Hyperthermia combined with chemotherapy and irradiation for patients with carcinoma of the oesophagus—a prospective randomized trial. *Int J Hyperthermia.* **8**(3): pp. 289–95, 1992.

156. Sugimachi, K., Kuwano, H., Ide, H., Toge, T., Saku, M. and Oshiumi, Y., Chemotherapy combined with or without hyperthermia for patients with oesophageal carcinoma: A prospective randomized trial. *Int J Hyperthermia.* **10**(4): pp. 485–93, 1994.

157. Wang, J., Li, D. and Chen, N., Intracavitary microwave hyperthermia combined with external irradiation in the treatment of esophageal cancer. *Zhonghua Zhong Liu Za Zhi.* **18**(1): pp. 51–4, 1996.

158. Kuwano, H., Sumiyoshi, K., Watanabe, M., Sadanaga, N., Nozoe, T., Yasuda, M. and Sugimachi, K., Preoperative hyperthermia combined with chemotherapy and irradiation for the treatment of patients with esophageal carcinoma. *Tumori.* **81**(1): pp. 18–22, 1995.

159. Nakajima, M., Kato, H., Sakai, M., Sano, A., Miyazaki, T., Sohda, M., Inose, T., Tanaka, N., Suzuki, S., Masuda, N., et al., Planned esophagectomy after neoadjuvant hyperthermochemoradiotherapy using weekly low-dose docetaxel and hyperthermia for advanced esophageal carcinomas. *Hepato-Gastroenterology.* **62**(140): pp. 887–91, 2015.

160. Sheng, L., Ji, Y., Wu, Q. and Du, X., Regional hyperthermia combined with radiotherapy for esophageal squamous cell carcinoma with supraclavicular lymph node metastasis. *Oncotarget.* **8**(3): pp. 5339–48, 2017.

161. Karasawa, K., Muta, N., Nakagawa, K., Hasezawa, K., Terahara, A., Onogi, Y., Sakata, K., Aoki, Y., Sasaki, Y. and Akanuma, A., Thermoradiotherapy in the treatment of locally advanced non-small cell lung cancer. *Int J Radiat Oncol Biol Phys.* **30**: pp. 1171–77, 1994.

162. Sakurai, H., Hayakawa, K., Mitsuhashi, N., Tamaki, Y., Nakayama, Y., Kurosaki, H., Nasu, S., Ishikawa, H., Saitoh, J.I., Akimoto, T., et al., Effect of hyperthermia combined with external radiation therapy in primary non-small cell lung cancer with direct bony invasion. *Int J Hyperthermia.* **18**(5): pp. 472–83, 2002.

163. Mitsumori, M., Zeng, Z.F., Oliynychenko, P., Park, J.H., Choi, I.B., Tatsuzaki, H., Tanaka, Y. and Hiraoka, M., Regional hyperthermia combined with radiotherapy for locally advanced non-small cell lung cancers: A multi-institutional prospective randomized trial of the international atomic energy agency. *Int J Clin Oncol.* **12**(3): pp. 192–8, 2007.

164. Shen, H., Li, X.D., Wu, C.P., Yin, Y.M., Wang, R.S. and Shu, Y.Q., The regimen of gemcitabine and cisplatin combined with radio frequency hyperthermia for advanced non-small cell lung cancer: A phase II study. *Int J Hyperthermia*. 27(1): pp. 27–32, 2011.

165. Wang, Y.Y., Lin, S.X., Yang, G.Q., Liu, H.C., Sun, D.N. and Wang, Y.S., Clinical efficacy of cyberknife combined with chemotherapy and hyperthermia for advanced non-small cell lung cancer. *Mol Clin Oncol*. 1(3): pp. 527–30, 2013.

166. Tilly, W., Gellermann, J., Graf, R., Hildebrandt, B., Weissbach, L., Budach, V., Felix, R. and Wust, P., Regional hyperthermia in conjunction with definitive radiotherapy against recurrent or locally advanced prostate cancer T3 PN0 M0. *Strahlenther Onkol*. 181(1): pp. 35–41, 2005.

167. Maluta, S., Dall'Oglio, S., Romano, M., Marciai, N., Pioli, F., Giri, M.G., Benecchi, P.L., Comunale, L. and Porcaro, A.B., Conformal radiotherapy plus local hyperthermia in patients affected by locally advanced high risk prostate cancer: Preliminary results of a prospective phase ii study. *Int J Hyperthermia*. 23(5): pp. 451–6, 2007.

168. Issels, R.D., Lindner, L.H., Verweij, J., Wust, P., Reichardt, P., Schem, B.C., Abdel-Rahman, S., Daugaard, S., Salat, C., Wendtner, C.M., et al., Neo-adjuvant chemotherapy alone or with regional hyperthermia for localised high-risk soft-tissue sarcoma: A randomised phase 3 multicentre study. *Lancet Oncol*. 11(6):561-70 2010.

169. de Jong, M.A., Oldenborg, S., Bing Oei, S., Griesdoorn, V., Kolff, M.W., Koning, C.C. and van Tienhoven, G., Reirradiation and hyperthermia for radiation-associated sarcoma. *Cancer*. 118(1): pp. 180–7, 2012.

170. Eckert, F., Gani, C., Kluba, T., Mayer, F., Kopp, H.G., Zips, D., Bamberg, M. and Muller, A.C., Effect of concurrent chemotherapy and hyperthermia on outcome of preoperative radiotherapy of high-risk soft tissue sarcomas. *Strahlenther Onkol*. 189(6): pp. 482–5, 2013.

171. Sneed, P.K., Stauffer, P.R., McDermott, M.W., Diederich, C.J., Lamborn, K.R., Prados, M.D., Chang, S., Weaver, K.A., Spry, L., Malec, M.K., et al., Survival benefit of hyperthermia in a prospective randomized trial of brachytherapy boost +/- hyperthermia for glioblastoma multiforme. *Int J Radiat Oncol Biol Phys*. 40(2): pp. 287–95, 1998.

172. Stea, B., Rossman, K., Kittelson, J., Shetter, A., Hamilton, A. and Cassady, J.R., Interstitial irradiation versus interstitial thermoradiotherapy for supratentorial malignant gliomas: A comparative survival analysis. *Int J Radiat Oncol Biol Phys*. 30(3): pp. 591–600, 1994.

173. van der Horst, A., Versteijne, E., Besselink, M.G.H., Daams, J.G., Bulle, E.B., Bijlsma, M.F., Wilmink, J.W., van Delden, O.M., van Hooft, J.E., Franken, N.A.P., et al., The clinical benefit of hyperthermia in pancreatic cancer: A systematic review. *Int J Hyperthermia*. Nov 23:1-11 [Epub ahead of print] pp. 1–11, 2017. DOI: 10.1080/02656736.2017.1401126.

174. Dewhirst, M.W., Connor, W.G. and Sim, D.A., Preliminary results of a phase III trial of spontaneous animal tumors to heat and/or radiation: Early normal tissue response and tumor volume influence on initial response. *Int J Radiat Oncol Biol Phys*. 8(11): pp. 1951–61, 1982.

175. Dewhirst, M.W., Sim, D.A., Sapareto, S. and Connor, W.G., Importance of minimum tumor temperature in determining early and long-term responses of spontaneous canine and feline tumors to heat and radiation. *Cancer Res*. 44: pp. 43–50, 1984.

176. Kapp, D.S. and Cox, R.S., Cumulative minutes of isoeffective hyperthermia with T90=43°C is the treatment parameter most predictive for outcome in patients with metastatic adenocarcinoma of the breast and single tumor nodules per treatment field. *Int J Radiat Oncol Biol Phys*. 27(Suppl 1): pp. 315–6, 1993.

177. Kapp, D.S. and Cox, R.S., Thermal treatment parameters are most predictive of outcome in patients with single tumor nodules per treatment field in recurrent adencarcinoma of the breast. *Int J Radiat Oncol Biol Phys*. 33: pp. 887–99, 1995.

178. Leopold, K.A., Dewhirst, M.W., Samulski, T.V., Dodge, R.K., George, S.L., Blivin, J.L., Prosnitz, L.R. and Oleson, J.R., Cumulative minutes with T90 greater than tempindex is predictive of response of superficial malignancies to hyperthermia and radiation. *Int J Radiat Oncol Biol Phys*. 25: pp. 841–47, 1993.

179. Oleson, J.R., Samulski, T.V., Leopold, K.A., Clegg, S.T., Dewhirst, M.W., Dodge, R.K. and George, S.L., Sensitivity of hyperthermia trial outcomes to temperature and time: Implications for thermal goals of treatment. *Int J Radiat Oncol Biol Phys*. **25**: pp. 289–297, 1993.

180. Reddy, G., Dreher, M.R., Rossmann, C., Wood, B.J. and Haemmerich, D., Cytotoxicity of hepatocellular carcinoma cells to hyperthermic and ablative temperature exposures: In vitro studies and mathematical modelling. *Int J Hyperthermia*. **29**(4): pp. 318–23, 2013.

181. Knudsen, M., Riishede, A., Lucke, A., Gelineck, J., Keller, J. and Baad-Hansen, T., Computed tomography-guided radiofrequency ablation is a safe and effective treatment of osteoid osteoma located outside the spine. *Dan Med J*. **62**(5) pii: A5059: 2015.

182. Selli, C., Scott, C.A., Garbagnati, F., De Antoni, P., Moro, U., Crisci, A. and Rossi, S., Transurethral radiofrequency thermal ablation of prostatic tissue: A feasibility study in humans. *Urology*. **57**(1): pp. 78–82, 2001.

183. Ahmed, M., Brace, C.L., Lee, F.T., Jr. and Goldberg, S.N., Principles of and advances in percutaneous ablation. *Radiology*. **258**(2): pp. 351–69, 2011.

184. Rasmussen, L.H., Lawaetz, M., Bjoern, L., Vennits, B., Blemings, A. and Eklof, B., Randomized clinical trial comparing endovenous laser ablation, radiofrequency ablation, foam sclerotherapy and surgical stripping for great saphenous varicose veins. *Br J Surg*. **98**(8): pp. 1079–87, 2011.

185. van Boxem, K., van Eerd, M., Brinkhuizen, T., Patijn, J., van Kleef, M. and van Zundert, J., Radiofrequency and pulsed radiofrequency treatment of chronic pain syndromes: The available evidence. *Pain Pract*. **8**(5): pp. 385–93, 2008.

186. Goldberg, S.N., Gazelle, G.S., Solbiati, L., Livraghi, T., Tanabe, K.K., Hahn, P.F. and Mueller, P.R., Ablation of liver tumors using percutaneous RF therapy. *AJR. Am J Roentgenol*. **170**(4): pp. 1023–8, 1998.

187. Rossi, S., Di Stasi, M., Buscarini, E., Quaretti, P., Garbagnati, F., Squassante, L., Paties, C.T., Silverman, D.E. and Buscarini, L., Percutaneous RF interstitial thermal ablation in the treatment of hepatic cancer. *AJR. Am J Roentgenol*. **167**(3): pp. 759–68, 1996.

188. Cooper, J. and Gimpelson, R.J., Summary of safety and effectiveness data from FDA: A valuable source of information on the performance of global endometrial ablation devices. *J Reprod Med*. **49**(4): pp. 267–73, 2004.

189. Markovic, J.N. and Shortell, C.K., Update on radiofrequency ablation. *Perspect Vasc Surg Endovasc Ther*. **21**(2): pp. 82–90, 2009.

190. Rossmann, C. and Haemmerich, D., Review of temperature dependence of thermal properties, dielectric properties, and perfusion of biological tissues at hyperthermic and ablation temperatures. *Crit Rev Biomed Eng*. **42**(6): pp. 467–92, 2014.

191. Haemmerich, D., Staelin, S.T., Tungjitkusolmun, S., Mahvi, D.M. and Webster, J.G., In-vivo conductivity of hepatic tumors. *Physiol Meas*. **24**(2): pp. 251–60, 2003.

192. Tsai, J.Z., Will, J.A., Hubbard-Van Stelle, S., Cao, H., Tungjitkusolmun, S., Choy, Y.B., Haemmerich, D., Vorperian, V.R. and Webster, J.G., In-vivo measurement of swine myocardial resistivity. *IEEE Trans Biomed Eng*. **49**(5): pp. 472–83, 2002.

193. Gabriel, S., Lau, R.W. and Gabriel, C., The dielectric properties of biological tissues: Ii. Measurements in the frequency range 10 Hz to 20 GHz. *Phys Med Biol*. **41**(11): pp. 2251–69, 1996.

194. Pop, M., Molckovsky, A., Chin, L., Kolios, M.C., Jewett, M.A. and Sherar, M.D., Changes in dielectric properties at 460 kHz of kidney and fat during heating: Importance for radiofrequency thermal therapy. *Phys Med Biol*. **48**(15): pp. 2509–25, 2003.

195. Gabriel, C., Gabriel, S. and Corthout, E., The dielectric properties of biological tissues: I. Literature survey. *Phys Med Biol*. **41**(11): pp. 2231–49, 1996.

196. Ryan, T.P. and Brace, C.L., Interstitial microwave treatment for cancer: Historical basis and current techniques in antenna design and performance. *Int J Hyperthermia*. **33**(1): pp. 3–14, 2017.

197. King, R., Trembly, B. and Strohbehn, J., The electromagnetic field of an insulated antenna in a conducting or dielectric medium. *IEEE Trans Microw Theory Tech*. **31**: pp. 574–83, 1983.

198. Turner, P., Interstitial equal-phased arrays for EM hyperthermia. *IEEE Trans Microw Theory Tech*. **34**: pp. 572–7, 1986.

199. Satoh, T., Stauffer, P.R. and Fike, J.R., Thermal distribution studies of helical coil microwave antennas for interstitial hyperthermia. *Int J Radiat Oncol Biol Phys.* **15**(5): pp. 1209–18, 1988.
200. Satoh, T. and Stauffer, P.R., Implantable helical coil microwave antenna for interstitial hyperthermia. *Int J Hyperthermia.* **4**(5): pp. 497–512, 1988.
201. Lee, D.J., O'Neill, M.J., Lam, K.S., Rostock, R. and Lam, W.C., A new design of microwave interstitial applicators for hyperthermia with improved treatment volume. *Int J Radiat Oncol Biol Phys.* **12**(11): pp. 2003–8, 1986.
202. Ryan, T.P., Mechling, J.A. and Strohbehn, J.W., Absorbed power deposition for various insertion depths for 915 MHz interstitial dipole antenna arrays: Experiment versus theory. *Int J Radiat Oncol Biol Phys.* **19**(2): pp. 377–87, 1990.
203. Hurter, W., Reinbold, F. and Lorenz, W., A dipole antenna for interstitial microwave hyperthermia. *IEEE Trans Microw Theory Tech.* **39**: pp. 1048–54, 1991.
204. Schepps, J.L. and Foster, K.R., The UHF and microwave dielectric properties of normal and tumour tissues: Variation in dielectric properties with tissue water content. *Phys Med Biol.* **25**(6): pp. 1149–59, 1980.
205. Schwan, H.P. and Piersol, G.M., The absorption of electromagnetic energy in body tissues; a review and critical analysis. *Am J Phys Med.* **34**(3): pp. 425–48; concl, 1955.
206. Pillai, K., Akhter, J., Chua, T.C., Shehata, M., Alzahrani, N., Al-Alem, I. and Morris, D.L., Heat sink effect on tumor ablation characteristics as observed in monopolar radiofrequency, bipolar radiofrequency, and microwave, using ex vivo calf liver model. *Medicine (Baltimore).* **94**(9): p. e580, 2015.
207. Brace, C.L., Radiofrequency and microwave ablation of the liver, lung, kidney, and bone: What are the differences? *Curr Probl Diagn Radiol.* **38**(3): pp. 135–43, 2009.
208. Goldberg, S.N., Solbiati, L., Hahn, P.F., Cosman, E., Conrad, J.E., Fogle, R. and Gazelle, G.S., Large-volume tissue ablation with radio frequency by using a clustered, internally cooled electrode technique: Laboratory and clinical experience in liver metastases. *Radiology.* **209**(2): pp. 371–80, 1998.
209. Haemmerich, D., Chachati, L., Wright, A.S., Mahvi, D.M., Lee, F.T., Jr. and Webster, J.G., Hepatic radiofrequency ablation with internally cooled probes: Effect of coolant temperature on lesion size. *IEEE Trans Biomed Eng.* **50**(4): pp. 493–500, 2003.
210. Bowles, B.J., Machi, J., Limm, W.M., Severino, R., Oishi, A.J., Furumoto, N.L., Wong, L.L. and Oishi, R.H., Safety and efficacy of radiofrequency thermal ablation in advanced liver tumors. *Arch Surg.* **136**(8): pp. 864–9, 2001.
211. Breen, D.J. and Lencioni, R., Image-guided ablation of primary liver and renal tumours. *Nat Rev Clin Oncol.* **12**(3): pp. 175–86, 2015.
212. Decadt, B. and Siriwardena, A.K., Radiofrequency ablation of liver tumours: Systematic review. *Lancet Oncol.* **5**(9): pp. 550–60, 2004.
213. McGahan, J.P., Browning, P.D., Brock, J.M. and Tesluk, H., Hepatic ablation using radiofrequency electrocautery. *Invest Radiol.* **25**(3): pp. 267–70, 1990.
214. Curley, S.A., Izzo, F., Delrio, P., Ellis, L.M., Granchi, J., Vallone, P., Fiore, F., Pignata, S., Daniele, B. and Cremona, F., Radiofrequency ablation of unresectable primary and metastatic hepatic malignancies: Results in 123 patients. *Ann Surg.* **230**(1): pp. 1–8, 1999.
215. Solbiati, L., Percutaneous ultrasound-guided radio frequency ablation of HCC and liver metastases: Results and long-term 7-year follow-up. *Ultrasound Med Biol.* **29**(5 Suppl): p. S48, 2003.
216. Meloni, M.F., Chiang, J., Laeseke, P.F., Dietrich, C.F., Sannino, A., Solbiati, M., Nocerino, E., Brace, C.L. and Lee, F.T., Jr., Microwave ablation in primary and secondary liver tumours: Technical and clinical approaches. *Int J Hyperthermia.* **33**(1): pp. 15–24, 2017.
217. Livraghi, T., Solbiati, L., Meloni, M.F., Gazelle, G.S., Halpern, E.F. and Goldberg, S.N., Treatment of focal liver tumors with percutaneous radio-frequency ablation: Complications encountered in a multicenter study. *Radiology.* **226**(2): pp. 441–51, 2003.
218. Venkatesan, A.M., Wood, B.J. and Gervais, D.A., Percutaneous ablation in the kidney. *Radiology.* **261**(2): pp. 375–91, 2011.

219. Pinto, C.H., Taminiau, A.H., Vanderschueren, G.M., Hogendoorn, P.C., Bloem, J.L. and Obermann, W.R., Technical considerations in ct-guided radiofrequency thermal ablation of osteoid osteoma: Tricks of the trade. *AJR Am J Roentgenol.* **179**(6): pp. 1633–42, 2002.

220. Lindner, N.J., Ozaki, T., Roedl, R., Gosheger, G., Winkelmann, W. and Wortler, K., Percutaneous radiofrequency ablation in osteoid osteoma. *J Bone Joint Surg Br.* **83**(3): pp. 391–6, 2001.

221. Vanderschueren, G.M., Taminiau, A.H., Obermann, W.R. and Bloem, J.L., Osteoid osteoma: Clinical results with thermocoagulation. *Radiology.* **224**(1): pp. 82–6, 2002.

222. Lanza, E., Thouvenin, Y., Viala, P., Sconfienza, L.M., Poretti, D., Cornalba, G., Sardanelli, F. and Cyteval, C., Osteoid osteoma treated by percutaneous thermal ablation: When do we fail? A systematic review and guidelines for future reporting. *Cardiovasc Intervent Radiol.* **37**(6): pp. 1530–9, 2014.

223. Dupuy, D.E., Liu, D., Hartfeil, D., Hanna, L., Blume, J.D., Ahrar, K., Lopez, R., Safran, H. and DiPetrillo, T., Percutaneous radiofrequency ablation of painful osseous metastases: A multi-center american college of radiology imaging network trial. *Cancer.* **116**(4): pp. 989–97, 2010.

224. Dupuy, D.E., DiPetrillo, T., Gandhi, S., Ready, N., Ng, T., Donat, W. and Mayo-Smith, W.W., Radiofrequency ablation followed by conventional radiotherapy for medically inoperable stage i non-small cell lung cancer. *Chest.* **129**(3): pp. 738–45, 2006.

225. Crocetti, L. and Lencioni, R., Radiofrequency ablation of pulmonary tumors. *Eur J Radiol.* **75**(1): pp. 23–7, 2010.

226. Sidoff, L. and Dupuy, D.E., Clinical experiences with microwave thermal ablation of lung malignancies. *Int J Hyperthermia.* **33**(1): pp. 25–33, 2017.

227. Jeffrey, S.S., Birdwell, R.L., Ikeda, D.M., Daniel, B.L., Nowels, K.W., Dirbas, F.M. and Griffey, S.M., Radiofrequency ablation of breast cancer: First report of an emerging technology. *Arch Surg.* **134**(10): pp. 1064–8, 1999.

228. Ito, T., Oura, S., Nagamine, S., Takahashi, M., Yamamoto, N., Yamamichi, N., Earashi, M., Doihara, H., Imoto, S., Mitsuyama, S., et al., Radiofrequency ablation of breast cancer: A retro-spective study. *Clin Breast Cancer.*18(4): e495-e500 2017.

229. Uppot, R.N. and Gervais, D.A., Imaging-guided adrenal tumor ablation. *AJR Am J Roentgenol.* **200**(6): pp. 1226–33, 2013.

230. Wood, B.J., Abraham, J., Hvizda, J.L., Alexander, H.R. and Fojo, T., Radiofrequency ablation of adrenal tumors and adrenocortical carcinoma metastases. *Cancer.* **97**(3): pp. 554–60, 2003.

231. Kanpolat, Y., Savas, A., Bekar, A. and Berk, C., Percutaneous controlled radiofrequency tri-geminal rhizotomy for the treatment of idiopathic trigeminal neuralgia: 25-year experience with 1,600 patients. *Neurosurgery.* **48**(3): pp. 524–32; discussion 532–4, 2001.

232. Narins, D.J. and Narins, R.S., Non-surgical radiofrequency facelift. *J Drugs Dermatol.* **2**(5): pp. 495–500, 2003.

233. Fitzpatrick, R., Geronemus, R., Goldberg, D., Kaminer, M., Kilmer, S. and Ruiz-Esparza, J., Multicenter study of noninvasive radiofrequency for periorbital tissue tightening. *Lasers Surg Med.* **33**(4): pp. 232–42, 2003.

234. Dover, J.S. and Zelickson, B., Results of a survey of 5,700 patient monopolar radiofrequency facial skin tightening treatments: Assessment of a low-energy multiple-pass technique leading to a clinical end point algorithm. *Dermatol Surg.* **33**(8): pp. 900–7, 2007.

235. Sadick, N.S. and Shaoul, J., Hair removal using a combination of conducted radiofrequency and optical energies--an 18-month follow-up. *J Cosmet Laser Ther.* **6**(1): pp. 21–6, 2004.

236. Chess, C., Prospective study on combination diode laser and radiofrequency energies (ELOS) for the treatment of leg veins. *J Cosmet Laser Ther.* **6**(2): pp. 86–90, 2004.

237. Li, K.K., Powell, N.B., Riley, R.W., Troell, R.J. and Guilleminault, C., Radiofrequency volumet-ric reduction of the palate: An extended follow-up study. *Otolaryngol Head Neck Surg.* **122**(3): pp. 410–4, 2000.

238. Baba, R.Y., Mohan, A., Metta, V.V. and Mador, M.J., Temperature controlled radiofrequency ablation at different sites for treatment of obstructive sleep apnea syndrome: A systematic review and meta-analysis. *Sleep Breath.* **19**(3): pp. 891–910, 2015.

239. Hultcrantz, E. and Ericsson, E., Pediatric tonsillotomy with the radiofrequency technique: Less morbidity and pain. *Laryngoscope.* **114**(5): pp. 871–7, 2004.
240. Wanitphakdeedecha, R., Iamphonrat, T., Thanomkitti, K., Lektrakul, N. and Manuskiatti, W., Treatment of abdominal cellulite and circumference reduction with radiofrequency and dynamic muscle activation. *J Cosmet Laser Ther.* **17**(5): pp. 246–51, 2015.
241. Fass, R., Cahn, F., Scotti, D.J. and Gregory, D.A., Systematic review and meta-analysis of controlled and prospective cohort efficacy studies of endoscopic radiofrequency for treatment of gastroesophageal reflux disease. *Surg Endosc.* 31 (12): 4865–4882 2017.

10

Transcranial Magnetic and Electric Stimulation

Shoogo Ueno and Masaki Sekino

University of Tokyo

Tsukasa Shigemitsu

Central Research Institute of Electric Power Industry

CONTENTS

10.1 Introduction

Transcranial magnetic stimulation (TMS) is a technique to stimulate the human brain transcranially by pulsed magnetic fields generated by a coil positioned outside the head. The pulsed magnetic fields induce electric fields in the brain, and the induced electric fields stimulate the brain. Stimulation of human brain by TMS with a round coil was reported by Barker et al. (1985). The success of the human brain stimulation by TMS made a strong impact on the scientific community. By TMS with a round coil, however, it was difficult to stimulate a localized area of the brain. A method of localized brain stimulation by TMS with a figure-eight coil was proposed by Ueno et al. (1988), and stimulation of the human motor cortex within a 5 mm resolution was successfully realized (Ueno et al., 1989). The functional map of the human motor cortex was obtained in a 5 mm resolution by this method (Ueno et al., 1990). TMS with a figure-eight coil is now used worldwide in cognitive brain research and clinical medicine.

For therapeutic applications of magnetic brain stimulation, rapid-rate transcranial magnetic stimulation or repetitive TMS (rTMS) with a series of repetitive pulses at several or several tens of hertz is used, for example, as an alternative approach to induce seizure for the treatment of depression in place of electroconvulsive therapy (ECT) (Fitzgerald and Daskalakis, 2012; Georg and Wasserman, 1994). This approach could allow selective stimulation of brain sites that are involved in depression, thus reducing side effects such as memory deficits due to electrical disruption of function in unrelated sites (Chandos et al., 1996). The technique of rTMS has promising potential applications not only for the treatment of depression but also for Parkinson's disease, dementia, and other brain diseases, as well as for reduction of intractable pain and rehabilitation or recovery process of an injured brain after a stroke (Ueno, 2012; Ueno and Sekino, 2015).

From the viewpoint of a therapeutic application of rTMS for neurological disorders, a number of animal studies testing the basic mechanisms of rTMS-induced alternations of neurotrophic factors, gene expression, and changes in plasticity have been conducted. The experimental results obtained by Fujiki and Steward (1997) and by other groups (Funamizu et al., 2005; Müller et al., 2000; Ogiue-Ikeda et al., 2003a,b, 2005; Ueno and Fujiki., 2007) suggest that there is strong evidence that the expression of certain genes such as the immediate early gene, astrocyte-specific glial fibrillary acidic protein (GFAP) messenger ribonucleic acid (mRNA), and brain-derived neurotrophic factor (BDNF) are altered in response to rTMS. This indicates that the measurable effects of rTMS reach the cellular and molecular levels.

Risk and safety aspects of rTMS with pulse trains of high frequencies need to be investigated (Karlström et al., 2006; Lin, 2016; Pascual-Leone et al., 2002; Wassermann, 1998). Shigemitsu and Ueno (2017) reviewed issues of biological effects and safety aspects of the electromagnetic fields (EMFs) related to rTMS and magnetic resonance imaging (MRI) as a diagnostic technique.

Transcranial electrical stimulation (TES) has a longer history compared with TMS. One of the typical examples is electroconvulsive therapy (ECT). The ECT is a technique to stimulate the human brain electrically using two electrodes put on the surface of the head in order to induce convulsive seizures in a patient for the treatment of depression and other mental and brain diseases.

In both TMS and ECT, it is important to estimate the current densities in and around the targeted areas, and for the treatment planning, it is essential to obtain three-dimensional spatial distributions of the induced or injected currents in the brain. Comparison of current distributions in ECT and TMS is studied by Sekino and Ueno (2002, 2004).

Another example of TES is transcranial direct current stimulation (tDCS). The tDCS is a rather new technique to stimulate the human brain transcranially by weak DC (direct current) electric currents for the treatment of brain disorders.

In this chapter, principles and applications of transcranial magnetic and electric stimulation are introduced. First, electrical and mathematical bases are described. Second, principles and important applications of TMS are introduced. Third, comparison of TMS and ECT is studied. Fourth, recent advances in therapeutic applications of transcranial magnetic and electric stimulation of the human brain are reviewed. Finally, safety aspects and guidelines of the TMS and TES are discussed.

10.2 Physical Bases

10.2.1 Principles of TMS

10.2.1.1 Basic Principles

Basic principle of magnetic stimulation of the brain is based on electromagnetic induction which Michael Faraday (1791–1867) discovered in 1831. When a coil positioned on the surface of the head is driven by transient electric currents, time-varying magnetic fields are generated by the coil. The time-varying magnetic fields penetrate into the brain without attenuation in the intensity of magnetic fields as the scalp is "transparent" for magnetic fields. The time-varying magnetic fields induce electric fields in the brain by the Faraday's law. The electric fields are described by electric currents, called eddy currents, which flow in the brain in the manner of closed loop. These electric fields or electric currents stimulate the nervous system in the brain when the stimulating condition exceeds the threshold of nerve excitation.

The magnetic stimulation is understood as an electric stimulation mediated by magnetic fields because the resulting biological effects originate from the induced electric fields. Considering that the magnetic permeabilities of biological tissues are nearly equal to that of free space, electric properties of biological tissues play important roles in biological effects of alternating and pulsed magnetic fields. At low frequencies below tens of kilohertz, depolarization of excitable membrane is the dominant mechanism of biological effects, and thermal effects are negligible in many cases.

Inducing electric fields specifically in the target region of the brain enables us to activate neurons in this region. Figures 10.1 and 10.2(a) show stimulations of the primary motor cortex. The stimulation causes a contraction of the corresponding muscles.

Magnetic field is generated as a pulse with durations usually shorter than 1 ms. Typical waveforms are a monophasic pulse consisting of one positive peak and biphasic pulses consisting of a pair of positive and negative peaks. The intensity of magnetic field generated from the coil is proportional to the coil current.

TMS is now widely used for diagnostics, therapies, and basic studies of brain function. In addition to the brain, the spinal root, the diaphragm, and the heart can also be magnetically stimulated. Applications of magnetic stimulations to artificial respiration and defibrillation have been explored.

10.2.1.2 Stimulator Coils

Circular coils have been used since TMS was invented. As the simplest structure among various types of coils, the circular coils are still widely used today. As shown in Figure 10.2(b), the coil conductors are wound up circularly in this coil. The electric fields

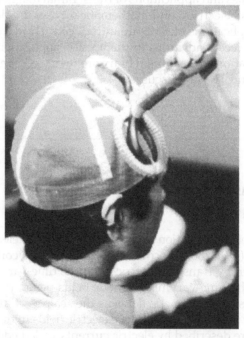

FIGURE 10.1
Transcranial magnetic stimulation (TMS) of the primary motor cortex.

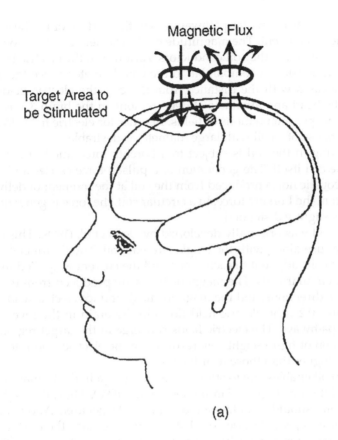

(a)

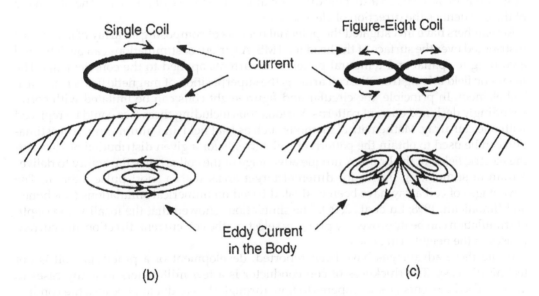

FIGURE 10.2
(a) Localized stimulation of the brain using TMS. (b) Eddy current induced by a circular coil. (c) Eddy current induced by a figure-eight coil.

generated in the brain form circular pathways along the surface of the head in the direction opposite to the coil current. The magnitude of electric field is zero below the center of the coil, and is highest below the coil conductors. As a result, the electric fields distribute in an area whose dimension is comparable to the coil diameter. Since the magnitude of magnetic field decreases with the distance from the coil, the electric fields are highest at the surface of the head and attenuate at deep regions in the brain. Coils with smaller diameters exhibit steeper attenuations of fields. In order for electric fields to reach deeper regions in the brain, use of a coil with large diameter is desirable.

The current flowing in the coil is subject to a Lorentz force due to the magnetic field generated from the coil itself. The generation of a pulsed force causes a vibration of coil conductors. The acoustic noise produced from the coil at the moment of delivering stimulation originates from the Lorentz force. In a circular coil, the force is generated outwardly so that the coil gets slightly distended.

The figure-eight coil was originally developed by Ueno et al. (1988). This coil is now in widespread clinical use along with the single circular coil. The figure-eight coil consists of a pair of circular coils adjacent to each other, and the current is applied in the opposite directions to these circular coils. The magnetic fields are produced from the two circular coils in the opposite directions, and the magnetic fields induce electric fields in the brain. As shown in Figure 10.2©, the electric field flows in the brain in the reversed direction, forming two loop pathways. The electric fields converge in the target region in the brain below the intersection of figure-eight coil, resulting in the electric field intensity approximately three times higher than those near the target.

The figure-eight coil enables one to stimulate a target area in the human cerebral cortex with a spatial resolution as high as 5 mm (Ueno et al., 1990). Thus, this coil is extremely effective when stimuli should be delivered to a specific target area. Another advantage of this coil is the ability to provide a vectorial stimulation because the electric fields in the target area are induced in a specific direction along the surface of the head. The placement of the coil defines the direction of electric field.

Researchers have investigated the potential benefits of composing an array of small coils distributed over the surface of the head for TMS. A variety of stimulations can be delivered according to spatial and temporal patterns of currents applied to the coil elements. The magnetic field arising from the coil array is the superposition of magnetic fields from each coil element. In principle, the circular and figure-eight coils can be imitated with correspondingly designed current patterns. Various coils including these two could be replaced with one coil array. Mathematical methods such as lead field and minimum-norm estimation can be used to obtain the pattern of coil currents for a given distribution of stimulating electric fields in the brain. A unique advantage of the coil array is the ability to deliver a train of stimulating pulses for different target areas with a short pulse interval. The advantages of coil array have been evaluated based on numerical simulations (Ruohonen and Ilmoniemi, 1998; Lu et al., 2009). The simulations showed that the focality and depth of stimulation can be improved by properly selecting the coil current direction and current phases in the neighboring coils.

While these advantages have been reported, development of a prototype coil is not technically easy. The thickness of coil conductor is a few millimeters in many cases to allow pulsed currents of kiloamperes to flow through the conductor. Because the conductor should be wound in multiple turns, miniaturization of element coil is limited. When driving currents are applied to multiple coils for imitating a large coil, adjacent coils may have currents in the opposite directions. Such currents do not contribute to the generation of magnetic fields but cause ohmic loss and decreased efficiency. In addition, the coil array requires much larger driving circuits and cables compared with the single coils. The research and development of coil array will be carried out considering the balance of its unique advantages and technical challenges.

10.2.1.3 Driving Circuit

The driving circuit for magnetic stimulation supplies pulsed electric currents to the stimulator coil. Figure 10.3(a, b) shows simplified circuit diagrams for generating monophasic and biphasic pulses, respectively. The circuit is composed of a power supply, a high voltage generator, a stimulator coil, a capacitor, and a semiconductor switch. The power supply circuit generates DC voltages from the AC input. The high voltage generator outputs voltages of kilovolts for charging the capacitor. The resistance limits the current for charging the capacitor. The circuit of storing electric charges in the capacitor and then discharging for providing currents to the coil enables the generation of strong current from relatively small equipment. When the thyristor is turned on after the positive charging of capacitor, electric current begins to flow in the coil. Here, the circuit is equivalent to the coil L and capacitor C connected serially. Sinusoidal current flows in these elements with the pulse width T given by the following equation:

$$T = 2\pi\sqrt{LC} \tag{10.1}$$

After turning on the thyristor, the current gradually increases and reaches the maximum at the moment of the charge in capacitor reducing to zero. In the biphasic circuit of Figure 10.3(b), the current subsequently begin to decrease, and the capacitor is negatively charged. When the current reduces to zero, the negative capacitor voltage reaches the minimum. Then, the current takes the same time course with the reversed polarity. The diode that is connected parallel to the thyristor in the opposite direction allows the reverse current to flow. When the coil current reduces to zero again, the capacitor is positively charged. The circuit is deactivated at the moment because the thyristor is turned off. The capacitor voltage ideally recovers to the level before the pulse generation. In actual circuits, however, voltage drop occurs because of the resistance in coil and capacitor. The capacitor is charged

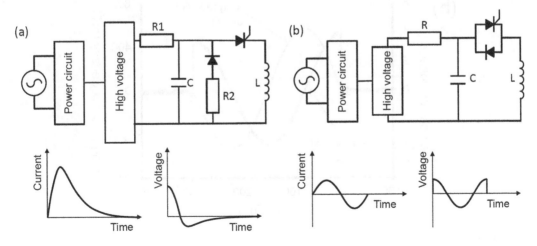

FIGURE 10.3
Circuit diagrams for generating (a) monophasic pulse and (b) biphasic pulse.

again before subsequent pulse generation so that the voltage recovers to the initial value. The repetition rate of pulse generation is controlled by the internal unit, allowing the circuit to generate single pulse and repeated pulses with rates ranging typically from 1 to 20 Hz.

The circuit elements such as capacitor and thyristor have maximum rated powers. The circuit can be substantially downsized if one uses single pulse only (Epstein, 2008; De Sauvage et al., 2010). Pulse generations with high repetition rates require relatively large elements. Some of the repetitive pulse generator is equipped with multiple capacitors.

10.2.1.4 Measurement of Pulsed Field

Magnetic fields for stimulation are generated typically with intensities of approximately 1 T and pulse widths of hundreds of microseconds. A search coil is suitable for measuring such magnetic fields. The search coil is fabricated winding a lead wire several times with a diameter of a few millimeters. When the magnetic field at the location of search coil varies with time, a voltage is induced in the search coil because of electromagnetic induction. The instantaneous induced voltage is proportional to the time rate of change in magnetic field intensity. The induced voltage of search coil reflects the magnetic field component parallel to the winding axis of search coil. Figure 10.4(a) shows a

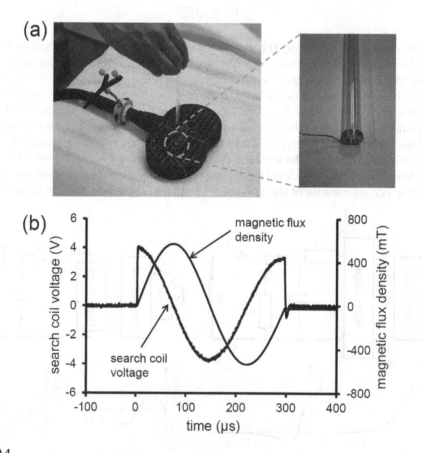

FIGURE 10.4

(a) A homemade search coil for measuring magnetic fields generated from the stimulating coil. (b) Measured search coil voltage and estimation of magnetic field intensity.

measurement of magnetic field using a search coil (Ueno and Sekino, 2015). The search coil is attached to the stimulator coil with its axis perpendicular to the winding plane of the stimulator coil, and the search coil measures the magnetic field component of this axis. The induced voltage is recorded using an oscilloscope. The following formula gives the induced voltage V:

$$V = \pi a^2 N \frac{dB}{dt} \tag{10.2}$$

where B is the generated magnetic field, a and N are the respective radius and number of turns of the search coil. The integral of voltage with respect to time gives the estimation of magnetic field intensity

$$B = \frac{1}{\pi a^2 N} \int_0^t V(\tau) d\tau \tag{10.3}$$

Figure 10.4(b) shows the waveforms of measured voltage and estimated magnetic field intensity.

The magnetic field generated from the coil is proportional to the current flowing in the stimulator coil. The current of the stimulator coil can be measured using a commercialized current transformer. The current transformer should be selected considering current magnitudes of kiloamperes. The output of current transformer is also recorded using the oscilloscope.

10.2.2 Numerical Analysis of Electromagnetic Fields

The finite element method (FEM) is a numerical framework for solving partial differential equations. The method originally evolved in the field of structural mechanics. The basic principle is based on the variation method. First, a functional is derived so that a first-order minute error in the field distribution gives a resulting influence in only second order. Then, the volume for analysis is divided into meshes. Tetrahedral or hexahedral elements are usually used for a simple generation of meshes and flexible modeling of curving surfaces. The use of tetrahedral elements enables extremely flexible generation of meshes according to the target of calculation. Due to this characteristic, the mesh density can be increased locally at locations where the field steeply varies or the target object has complex geometry. Various algorithms for automatically generating meshes have been investigated. After the generation of meshes, the nodes are assigned on the sides or on the vertexes of each element, and an expansion of field equation is derived in terms of unknown parameters on the nodes. Substitution of this equation into the functional gives an expansion of functional with the unknown parameters. Due to the variation principle, this expression takes an extremal value with respect to a minimal variation of the unknown parameters. The differential of the expression by the unknown parameters is equal to zero. Doing this calculation for the all unknown parameters gives a simultaneous linear equation for the unknown parameters. Numerical analyses lead to the solution for the unknown parameters.

The scalar potential finite difference (SPFD) method is widely used for calculating induced electric fields in biological bodies. The target body is modeled with voxels, and the equation of electromagnetic field is solved with electric scalar potentials at the nodes contained as unknown parameters. For using this method, the skin depth should be much larger than the dimension of calculated body, and the secondary magnetic field arising from induced current should be much smaller than the primary current. These conditions are satisfied in typical electromagnetic fields in TMS. The following equation is obtained by combining Faraday's law, current continuity equation, and Ohm's law, and discretizing the equation about the node 0:

$$\sum_{n=1}^{6} s_n \phi_n - \left(\sum_{n=1}^{6} s_n \right) \phi_0 = j\omega \sum_{n=1}^{6} (-1)^n s_n l_n A_{0n} \tag{10.4}$$

where ϕ_n is the electric scalar potential at the node n, A_{0n} is the external magnetic vector potential parallel to the side n of the voxel connecting the nodes 0 and n, l_n is the length of side n, and s_n is the conductance of side n given by

$$s_n = \bar{\sigma}_n a_n / l_n \tag{10.5}$$

Here, a_n is the area of face perpendicular to the side n, and σ_n is the mean conductivity of 4 voxels sharing the node n.

For calculating the electric field in the voxel, first, a system of equations is constructed from Equation (10.4) with the electric scalar potentials ϕ_n included as unknown parameters and for all nodes having finite conductivities. The electric scalar potential is obtained by solving the system of equations using sparse matrix methods such as successive overrelaxation. Then, the electric fields on the sides of voxel are calculated from magnetic vector potentials and electric scalar potentials. The electric field of voxel is obtained for x, y, and z components as the average of electric fields on the four sides.

10.2.3 Electric Properties of Living Tissues

10.2.3.1 Debye Model of Dielectric Properties and Cole-Cole Plot

A material's permittivity and conductivity generally depend on the frequency of an applied field, and this phenomenon is called dispersion. Because biological tissues have multiple mechanisms for electric conduction, such as the drift of ions and the rotation of polar molecules, tissues exhibit relatively complicated dispersion. Debye's equation of complex permittivity is widely accepted as a model of dispersion:

$$\varepsilon^*(\omega) = \varepsilon_\infty + \frac{\varepsilon_0 - \varepsilon_\infty}{1 + i\omega\tau} \tag{10.6}$$

where τ is the relaxation time and where ε_0 and ε_∞ indicate the respective permittivities at sufficiently low and high frequencies (compared with $1/\tau$). With ω ranging from 0 to ∞, a plot of Equation (10.6) on a complex plane produces a semicircle, as shown in Figure 10.5, which is called a Cole-Cole plot.

10.2.3.2 Frequency Characteristics of Tissues

There are multiple sources of dielectric polarization in a tissue, such as charges on cell membranes and polar molecules (including water), and these polarizations have different

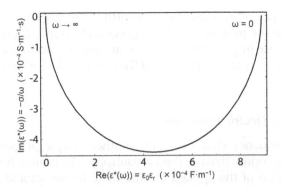

FIGURE 10.5
Representative Cole-Cole plot of a material.

relaxation times. With four relaxation times, an extended version of Equation (10.6) is used for modeling the tissue's complex permittivity:

$$\varepsilon^*(\omega) = \varepsilon_\infty + \sum_{m=1}^{4} \frac{\Delta\varepsilon_m}{1+(i\omega\tau_m)^{1-\alpha_m}} + \frac{\sigma_i}{j\omega\varepsilon_0} \qquad (10.7)$$

where $\Delta\varepsilon_m$ indicates the drop in permittivity for a frequency range across $\omega = 1/\tau_m$, which corresponds to each relaxation time τ_m; σ_i indicates the ionic conductivity. The above empirically defined equation is well fitted to the measured complex permittivities in a broad frequency range, from 10 Hz to 100 GHz (Gabriel et al., 1996). Figure 10.6 shows the

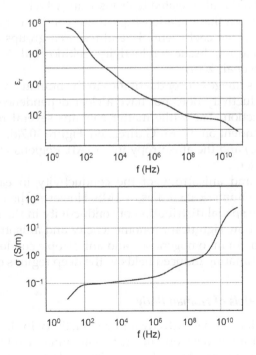

FIGURE 10.6
Frequency characteristics of electric permittivity ε_r and conductivity σ of gray matter.

frequency characteristics of gray matter's permittivity and conductivity, obtained by fitting Equation (10.7) to the measured values (Ueno and Sekino, 2015). An increase in frequency causes a decrease in permittivity and an increase in conductivity. A Cole-Cole plot of a tissue differs from a semicircle because of the tissue's relatively complicated frequency characteristics.

10.2.3.3 Anisotropy of Electric Properties

In addition to the frequency characteristics, another unique property of biological tissues' permittivity and conductivity is their anisotropy. The permittivity and conductivity depend on the direction of the applied electric field. In nerves and muscles, cells form fibrous microscopic structures, and the cells align in a specific direction. Because the cell membranes hinder ions' ability to pass through the membranes, ions easily move in the direction of fibers but are mostly unable to move orthogonally. Consequently, conductivity exhibits higher values in the direction of fibrous structures. Because of cell membranes' resistance, low-frequency currents flow mainly through extracellular spaces. Furthermore, because of surface charges on cell membranes, a tissue's effective permittivity becomes high when an electric field is applied in the direction perpendicular to the cell membrane. In a measurement of the conductivity of the cerebral cortex, the conductivity varied by a factor of 1.7, depending on the measurement direction (Hoeltzell et al., 1979). The anisotropies originating from the membrane structures become prominent when considerable quantities of ions oscillating in an AC field collide with membranes. These anisotropies become negligibly small at frequencies higher than a megahertz.

Conductivity depends on the viscosity of extracellular fluid because the balance between the electrostatic force and viscous drag governs an ion's drift velocity. The diffusion coefficient of extracellular fluid is also related to its viscosity, which is described by the Stokes-Einstein equation. Based on these relationships, tissue conductivity can be obtained from extracellular fluid's diffusion coefficient. Several research groups have reported the use of diffusion MRI for mapping tissue conductivity (Sekino et al., 2003; Sekino et al., 2005; Sekino et al., 2009; Tuch et al., 2001).

Figure 10.7(a–c) shows images of conductivities in the human brain (Sekino et al., 2005). The gray matter's conductivity does not have a clear dependence on the MPG (Mortin Probing Gradient) direction. The white matter contains several regions where conductivities are highly dependent on the MPG direction. Figure 10.7(d, e) shows images of the mean conductivity (MC) and the anisotropy index (AI). Regions with high AI values are found in the white matter.

The inhomogeneity and anisotropy of the conductivity in each tissue is not normally considered in the numerical studies of TMS. However, the results of induced field analyses depend on the spatial distribution of conductivity in the models. The results of conductivity imaging show significant inhomogeneity and anisotropy in the white matter. Therefore, the use of an inhomogeneous and anisotropic conductivity model is desirable, particularly for estimating induced fields in the deep regions of the brain.

10.2.3.4 Numerical Models of Human Body

Modeling the distributions of permittivity and conductivity in the body is an important endeavor. Several institutions develop and distribute numerical human models without charge for noncommercial users (Nagaoka et al., 2004; Christ et al., 2010). A few software developers provide numerical human models specifically for use with their software.

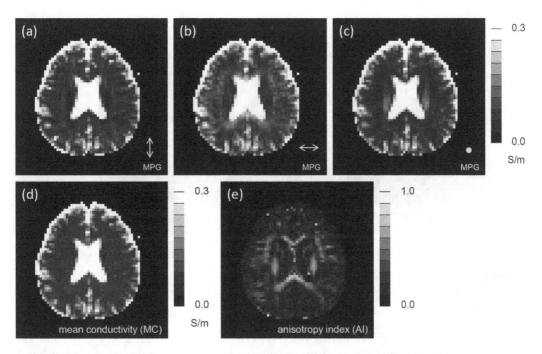

FIGURE 10.7
Conductivity imaging of the human brain using diffusion MRI. (a–c) Images of the estimated conductivities in the anterior-posterior, right-left, and superior-inferior directions, respectively. (d, e) Images of the mean conductivity and anisotropy index.

These models are built by segmenting an anatomical dataset (obtained from MRI, CT, or dissected slices of a cadaver) into tens of tissues. Each voxel in the dataset has a labeling number to indicate a particular tissue type, such as bone or muscle. A model's typical spatial resolution is 1 mm. Because there is no method to automatically segment the entire body, building a model necessitates extensive manual procedures that require significant effort and time. These models can be used for various purposes, such as electric and magnetic stimulations, microwave hyperthermia, and electromagnetic fields in MRI systems.

The National Institute of Information and Communications Technology (NICT), Japan, develops and distributes numerical human models (Nagaoka et al., 2004). This group provides standard male and female models with average body sizes. These models were built by segmenting a 3D MRI dataset into 51 different tissues with a spatial resolution of 2 mm. The models can be deformed to assume a variety of postures.

The above models relate each voxel in the dataset to a tissue type. Other databases should be utilized to ascertain permittivity and conductivity values of different tissues. The values are estimated for a target frequency using Equation (10.7). Because typical models of the human body consist of cubic voxels, the model has immediate applicability to simulation methods that use cubic cells, such as the scalar-potential finite-difference method and the impedance method. The FEM is also available. Figure 10.8 shows the numerical analysis of eddy current using the standard human head model (Sekino and Ueno, 2004).

Analyses of induced electric field distributions in TMS have been carried out using simplified models consisting of concentric spheres or the realistic human head models. The use of simplified spherical model is effective because of a lower amount of calculation,

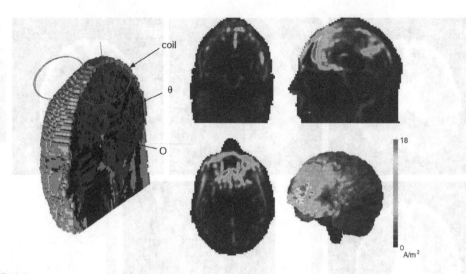

FIGURE 10.8
Numerical model of the human brain and calculated distributions of eddy currents in the brain induced by TMS with a figure-eight coil.

especially for theoretically evaluating the coil performance depending on coil design. The realistic human head model providing precise anatomy of the brain, on the other hand, is valuable for estimating the electric field that is not able to be measured experimentally. The results of analyses using the realistic model reveal the influence of complex brain geometries such as gyrus and sulcus on the induced electric fields.

In TMS, the resting motor threshold and therapeutic effect have individual variations. Difference in electric field according to the shape of the brain may underlie this individual variation. The geometry of standard head model is different from that of individual subjects, and it has been difficult to investigate the individual variation using the standard model. For understanding the origin of individual variation, the brain model should be generated individually and perform analyses of electric fields.

In some recent studies, numerical models based on individual brain shapes have been generated and used for analyses (Opitz et al., 2013). The aim was to show the individual variation in electric fields and to investigate the correlation with motor evoked potentials (MEPs). The individual numerical models are generated from the MRI of subjects.

10.3 Techniques and Applications of TMS

10.3.1 Localized Stimulation Using a Figure-Eight Coil

Figure 10.2 shows principle of localized stimulation of the human brain by using a figure-eight coil. Basic principle is to concentrate induced eddy currents in the target area by a pair of time-varying magnetic fields. A pair of coils is positioned outside the head so that time-varying magnetic fields pass though the head in opposite directions around the target. The induced currents are merged in the target area. The convergence of eddy currents acts to raise the current densities in the target area, where depolarization of neural tissues in the brain can be caused.

Since the concentrated eddy currents beneath the intersection of the figure-eight coil flow in a direction parallel to the tangent of both circular coils, vectorial stimulation can be achieved. The neural fibers can be excited easily when the fibers are stimulated by the eddy currents that flow parallel to the nerve fibers.

Figure 10.9 shows that the intensity of the eddy current density in the target increases as the diameter of figure-eight coils becomes larger (Ueno and Sekino, 2015). The maximum eddy current density induced by the 100 mm coil was twice as high as that of the 40 mm coil. The maximum eddy current density was observed on the surface of the target for all the coils. The magnetic fields attenuate with the distance from the coil. The above-mentioned two characteristics of figure-eight coil, both the intensity of eddy current density and the penetration depth can be adjusted by varying the diameters.

Magnetic stimulation of the human motor cortex related to the hand area is achieved in this method of TMS with a figure-eight coil. Figure 10.10 shows MEPs measured at the thenar muscles of the left hand responded by the stimulation of point A in the motor cortex in the right hemisphere (Ueno et al., 1990). When we stimulate point B, C, B', and C' 5 mm away from point A, we observe no MEP signals from the thenar muscles. This means that we successfully stimulated a motor cortex within a 5 mm resolution.

10.3.2 Functional Mapping by TMS with a Figure-Eight Coil

Figure 10.11 shows functional distribution of the human motor cortex related to the hand and foot areas (Ueno et al., 1990). Magnetic brain stimulation was carried out at all grid points of the meshed region on the surface of the head. The distance between the neighboring grid points is 5 mm. The arrow shows current directions for neural excitation. An optimal direction of stimulating currents for neural excitation exists in each functional area in the cortex.

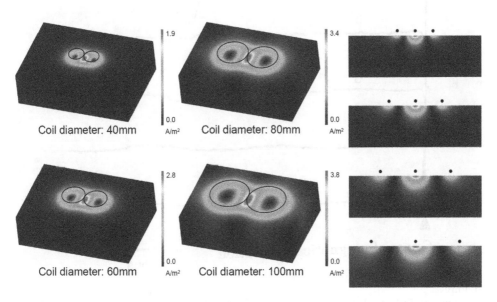

FIGURE 10.9
Distributions of eddy currents in a conductive cuboid induced by figure-eight coils with different diameters. Large diameter leads to broad and deep distributions of eddy currents.

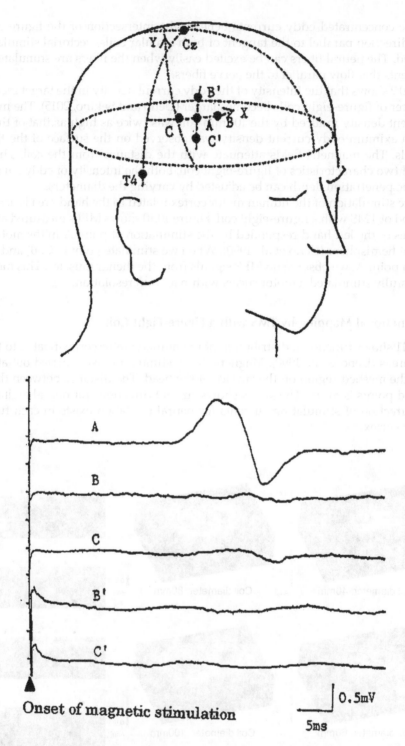

FIGURE 10.10

Motor responses to TMS. A: Thenar point stimulation. B: Stimulation at a point 5 mm posterior to the thenar point. C: Stimulation at a point 5 mm anterior to the thenar point. B′: Stimulation at a point 5 mm above the thenar point. C′: Stimulation at a point 5 mm lower from the thenar point.

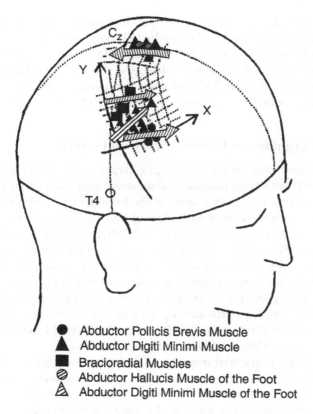

FIGURE 10.11
Functional distribution of the human motor cortex related to the hand and foot areas. The arrows show current directions for neural excitation. The distance between grid points is 5 mm.

The existence of orientation of current vectors for neural excitation in the brain may be partially understood by the anatomical structures of the neural tissues in the brain. In other words, it may be possible to estimate both functional and anatomical organization of the neural networks from the mapping of these current vectors for neural excitation. The integrated studies using both TMS and magnetic resonance diffusion tensor magnetic resonance imaging (DTI) may reveal more detailed mechanisms for dynamic neural connectivity and networks in the brain.

A coil navigation system is used for precisely positioning the stimulator coil above the targeted area. Reflective spheres are fixed on the stimulator coil and on the patient as markers. An infrared binocular camera observes these reflective spheres, which enables the system to estimate the position and orientation of the markers. The system enables us to see the position of stimulator coil relative to the head in real time. The binocular camera achieves submillimeter accuracy in estimating the position of markers. Introducing such a navigation system enables us to precisely and quickly place the stimulator coil above the target position. This is particularly valuable for highly localized stimulations using figure-eight coils.

Functional mapping of the brain is applied also for neurosurgery (Ueno and Fujiki, 2007). Identifications of the motor and language areas before the surgery are important for the prevention of damages to these areas.

There are other techniques available for functional mapping of the brain. For example, identification of the motor area can be conducted using fMRI, and identification of the language area can be conducted with the Wada test. However, the accuracy of the identification using fMRI has not yet been established, and the Wada test has a problem of invasiveness. The identification using TMS is totally noninvasive, and TMS can be performed even in an operating room. For these reasons, TMS is useful for surgical planning.

10.3.3 Studies of Cognition and Memory/Retrieval Processes

TMS enables spatiotemporal controls of brain activities, with both excitation and disturbance. By virtue of this feature, neuroscientists developed the virtual lesion approach in which TMS causes a transient disturbance in the brain function. Brain function is generally realized through interactions of multiple regions of the brain. For instance, in the processes of visual perceptions such as visual search, letter recognition, and face recognition, giving TMS to a specific part of the brain causes a reduction in the performance of visual perception in some cases. These findings indicate that the stimulated area is necessary for the realization of visual perception. The influences of TMS on visual perception have been investigated with precisely controlled locations and timings for administering virtual lesions. This methodology provides a powerful tool for investigating the mechanism of spatiotemporal information processing in the brain. Virtual lesion facilitates the accumulation of knowledge on the localization of brain function.

Episodic memory is a sequential memory related to memorable things, which contains time, place, and emotion of the memories. It is a kind of long-term memory, and is sometimes related to personal experiences, or social occurrences. It is generally recognized that the prefrontal area has a role in generation of episodic memories, but there are still different hypotheses about the localization of the detailed function in the prefrontal area.

Epstein et al. (2002) carried out a study to reveal this localization. As shown in Figure 10.12, ten Japanese subjects underwent sequential visual stimuli, which contained 18 sets of Kanji words and abstract patterns, and TMS pulses were delivered between the visual stimulations. The TMS coil was placed at the left dorsolateral prefrontal cortex (DLPFC), the right DLPFC, the cranial vertex, and off the head. After the set of stimuli, the subjects took a test for checking the memory correctness of the pair of Kanji and abstract patterns. The subjects had less correct responses with the right DLPFC stimulation, compared with the stimulations on other areas. This result indicates that the right DLPFC has a role in generating the episodic memory. As in this example, TMS can elucidate the mechanisms of higher brain function.

10.3.4 Hippocampus and rTMS (Repetitive TMS)

10.3.4.1 Effects of TMS on Long-Term Potentiation (LTP)

Long-term potentiation (LTP) is a long-lasting increase in the efficacy of synaptic transmission resulting from a high frequency stimulation (Bliss et al., 1973). LTP in the hippocampus is thought to be a typical model of synaptic plasticity related to learning and memory. The most commonly used protocol for LTP induction is an electric stimulation to hippocampus slices. Electric stimulation to the hippocampus slices, typically to the Schaffer collaterals, generates excitatory postsynaptic potentials (EPSPs) in the postsynaptic CA1 cells. If the Schaffer collaterals are stimulated only two or three times per minute, the magnitude of the evoked EPSP in the CA1 neurons remains constant. However, a brief, high-frequency

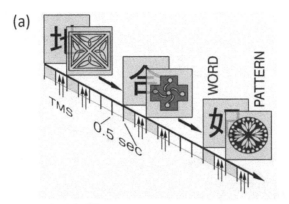

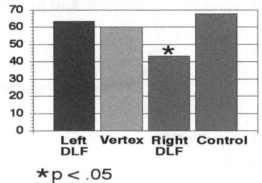

(b) **Percentage of Correct Responses by TMS Stimulation Site**

*p < .05

FIGURE 10.12

(a) Timeline (left to right) for presentation of Kanji words and abstract patterns. Pulses of TMS are indicated by paired vertical arrows. (b) Overall percent correct for subsequent recall of paired associates according to site of TMS. The comparison of interest is between the left and right DLPFC, with an active TMS control at the vertex. The asterisk indicates P < 0.05 for right versus left DLPFC.

train of stimuli to the same neurons causes LTP, which is evident as a long-lasting increase in EPSP magnitude, as shown in Figure 10.13(a) (Ogiue-Ikeda et al., 2003a,b). This high-frequency electric stimulation of a neuron is called tetanus stimulation.

Ogiue-Ikeda et al. (2003a,b) investigated the effects of rTMS on rat hippocampus, focusing on changes in LTP after rTMS. The authors first investigated the influence of rTMS on field excitatory postsynaptic potentials (fEPSP) after applying tetanus stimulation to the rat hippocampus. The rats were magnetically stimulated by a round coil positioned over the head. The peak magnetic fields were set to 0.50 T (lower than motor threshold) and 1.25 T (above motor threshold) at the center of the coil. The rats received 10 s trains of 25 pulses/s with a 1 s intertrain interval, four times per day for 7 days. After magnetic stimulation for 7 days, hippocampus slices were prepared and fEPSPs were recorded from the dendrites of CA1 pyramidal cells by stimulating Schaffer collaterals. There was no significant difference between the LTP of the 0.50 T stimulated and sham control groups. The LTP of the 1.25 T stimulated group, however, was inhibited compared with the LTP of the sham control group, suggesting that the synaptic plasticity in the hippocampus was impaired by strong TMS, as shown in Figure 10.13(c).

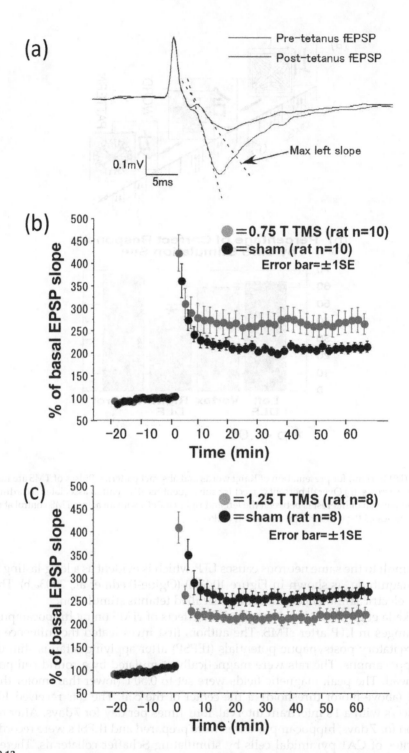

FIGURE 10.13
(a) Basic mechanisms of LTP. The plots show the changes in field EPSP (fEPSP) after LTP induction stimuli (tetanus stimulation). (b, c) Changes in LTP at rat hippocampus slices after rTMS: LTPs of 0.75 T stimulated and sham control groups and LTPs of 1.25 T stimulated and sham control groups.

The authors also demonstrated the same rTMS experiment to examine the dependency on the field intensity. Rats were magnetically stimulated for 7 days with the condition described above, but the peak magnetic fields at the center of the coil were modified as 0.75 and 1.00 T. LTP enhancement was observed only in the 0.75 T rTMS group, as shown in Figure 10.13(b), while no change was observed in the 1.00 T rTMS group. These results suggest that the effect of rTMS on LTP depends on the stimulus intensity.

10.3.4.2 Ischemic Tolerance of Hippocampus

A mild exposure to cerebral ischemia confers transient tolerance to a subsequent ischemic challenge in the brain. This phenomenon of ischemic tolerance has been confirmed in various animal models of forebrain ischemia and focal cerebral ischemia. On the contrary, CA1 pyramidal neurons in the hippocampus are highly vulnerable to cerebral ischemia (Ogiue-Ikeda et al., 2005). Brief periods (minutes) of severe ischemia cause neuronal degeneration in the CA1 region 3–7 days after the ischemia by apoptosis (Kirino et al., 1982). Recent studies have focused on applying electric stimulation to the brain via electrodes to potentially reduce ischemic symptoms (Glickstein et al., 2001). However, the invasiveness of electric stimulation (for example, surgery and anesthetization) reduces its feasibility as a treatment.

Instead of invasive electric stimulation, Ogiue-Ikeda et al. (2005) investigated the acquisition of ischemic tolerance in the rat hippocampus using rTMS. Based on the authors' previous studies about rTMS effects on hippocampus LTP (Ogiue-Ikeda et al., 2003a,b), the stimulus intensity was set at 0.75 T. The rats received 0.75 T rTMS of 1,000 pulses/day for 7 days. The fEPSPs were measured in the hippocampal CA1. After rTMS treatment, the hippocampus slices were exposed to ischemic conditions to examine the influence of rTMS on ischemic tolerance. LTP was induced in the animals. The LTP of the stimulated group was enhanced compared with the LTP of the sham control group in each ischemic condition (Figure 10.14), suggesting that rTMS has the potential to protect hippocampal function from ischemia.

10.3.4.3 Protection of Hippocampal CA3 Cells

Parkinson's disease (PD) is a neurodegenerative brain disorder that occurs when neurons in the substantia nigra die or become impaired. Normally, these cells produce dopamine. Dopamine allows smooth, coordinated function of the body's muscles; therefore, less dopamine leads the patient less ability to regulate their movements and emotions.

In recent years, some clinical studies of single or rTMS for PD have been performed. A pioneering study has been published by Pascual-Leone et al. (1994). In the report, effects of 5 Hz rTMS on several neurological parameters such as choice reaction time (cRT), movement time (MT), and error rate (ER) in a serial reaction-time task were investigated in six medicated patients with PD and 10 age-matched normal controls. In normal subjects, subthreshold 5 Hz rTMS did not significantly change cRT, slightly shortened MT, but increased ER. In the patients, rTMS significantly shortened cRT and MT without affecting ER. The authors mentioned that the repetitive, subthreshold motor cortex stimulation can improve performance in patients with PD and could be useful therapeutically.

In animal experiments, Funamizu et al. (2005) demonstrated that rTMS showed protecting effects on the lesioned rats by administering a neurotoxin MPTP (1-methyl-4-phenyl-1,2,3,6-tetrahydropyridine. Forty 8 h before rTMS treatment, MPTP was injected into the rats to induce specific damages in dopaminergic neurons. Subsequently, the rats received

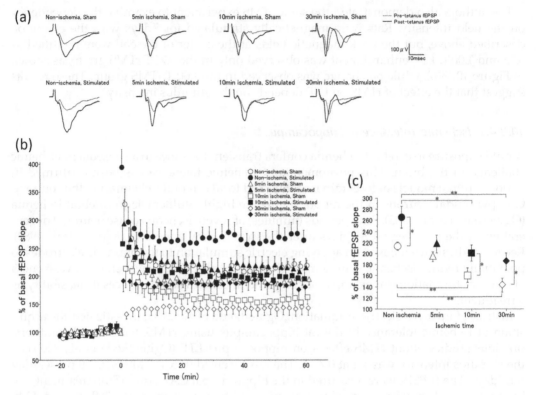

FIGURE 10.14
Effects of rTMS on ischemic tolerance of hippocampus. (a) Examples of pre-tetanus and post-tetanus fEPSPs after each ischemic condition. (b) LTP in the stimulated and sham control groups in each ischemic condition. (c) Average value of the maintenance phases of LTP (ranging from 10 min after tetanus stimulation to 60 min).

1.25 T rTMS. rTMS effects were examined by histological studies at substantia nigra which contains a high population of dopaminergic neurons and checking the behavioral parameters (functional observational battery-hunched posture score). The functional observational battery-hunched posture score for the MPTP-rTMS group was significantly lower and the number of rearing events was higher compared with the MPTP-sham group. These behavioral parameters revert to control levels. The double-labeling immunofluorescence experiments using tyrosine hydroxylase as the dopaminergic marker and NeuN as specific neuronal marker showed that the number of surviving dopamine neurons in the MPTP-sham rats were significantly reduced compared with that of the substantia nigra pars compacta in the undamaged rats while the number of those neurons of MPTP-rTMS group was significantly larger than the MPTP-sham group (Figure 10.15) (Funamizu et al., 2005). These results suggested that rTMS treatment reactivates the dopaminergic system in lesion rats.

10.3.5 TMS Treatment at Home

Current magnetic stimulators are only operated by doctors and are available only at large hospitals. Therefore, only a limited number of patients are able to be treated by rTMS. Moreover the effect of rTMS is temporary and the brain must be treated at fixed intervals—every day, if possible. The development of inexpensive, compact, and energy

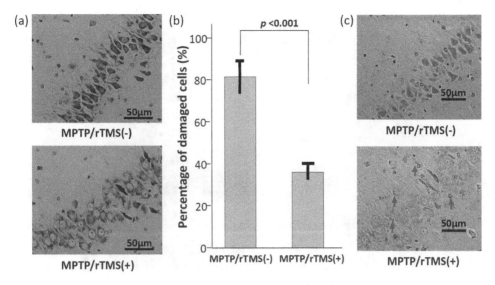

FIGURE 10.15
Effects of rTMS on MPTP-treated rats. The application of TMS reaulted in a decrease of damaged cells in substantia nigra.

efficient magnetic stimulators that can be installed at a patient's home is necessary to generalize magnetic stimulation treatment.

Researchers have sought to find a method to increase the efficiency of electromagnetic coils to induce magnetic stimulators operate at low powers. Though a variety of coils have been proposed previously, these coil designs have mainly aimed at controlling the region and depth of stimulation, rather than the application of magnetic fields at low driving currents. To attain this objective, several papers have been published on how to increase efficiency of coil by changing its shape. Sekino et al. (2015) shifted the center of the inner peripheral circle of each coil toward the middle of the figure-eight coil to enhance the concentration of electric field directly under the center of the figure-eight coil, as shown in Figure 10.16. This coil design had an increased efficiency of 22% and decreased heat generation in proportion to the square of the current.

On the other hand, researchers have aimed to compensate the loss of robustness to locational error arising from the high locality of the induced electric field by adequately increasing the range where electric field deploys. In one approach, Yamamoto et al. (2015) proposed a bowl-shaped coil. They increased the uniformity of the induced electric field in the brain by arranging conductor along surface of head. Additionally, the intensity and range of induced electric coil is adjustable by changing the density and coverage of the conductor.

To make magnetic stimulators inexpensive, researchers have focused on improving the coil navigation system. In the conventional method, the stimulator coil is placed above the target point using an infrared binocular camera. Unfortunately, this system is not suited to home treatment because of its large size and cost. Accordingly, a compact and inexpensive positioning system has been developed (Okada et al., 2012). In this new system, glass with an attached magnetic sensor has been developed. This system made it possible to not only decide the position of the coil with higher accuracy by 5 mm but also decrease the size of the whole positioning system.

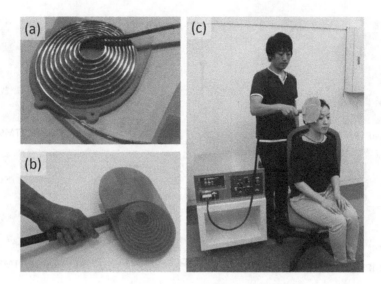

FIGURE 10.16
(a) Formation of an eccentric spiral coil on a plastic insulator case. (b) Finished eccentric coil equipped with a grip and a lead cable. Coil conductors are observed through a 1mm thick insulator. (c) A prototype magnetic stimulator system for home treatment.

10.4 The Therapeutic and Rehabilitation Applications of TMS and TES

The previous sections described the fundamental issues for the basic concept of electromagnetic induction, principle and the operation of TMS, and the outline of the transcranial electric stimulation (TES) and the electroconvulsive therapy (ECT).

In ancient Egypt and ancient Greece, torpedo electric fish were used commonly for the treatment of migraine and epilepsy. In the late 18th century, Giovanni Aldini, the nephew of Luigi Galvani, and later professor of experimental physics at the University of Bologna, used electrical stimulation in human patients to improve melancholy (Parent, 2004, Rowbottom and Susskind, 1984). In 1870, Julius Edward Hitzig, German neuropsychiatrist, with Gustav Theodor Fritsch, professor at the University of Berlin, began electrophysiological studies of brain and applied electrical stimulation to the localization of primary motor cortex (Rowbottom and Susskind, 1984). These historical facts give the development of transcranial electrical stimulation (TES). TES can be divided into two major forms: anodal and cathodal transcranial direct current stimulation (anodal tDCS and cathodal tDCS).

In 1831, Michael Faraday discovered the principles of electromagnetic induction. This principle of induction led to the possibility of using magnetic fields to generate currents. This principle is behind the inductive brain stimulation with eddy currents. In 1896, using noninvasive stimulation of the brain with time-varying magnetic fields, Jaques-Arsène d'Arsonval, professor of the College de France, has reported a phenomenon called magnetophosphene. This phenomenon is the visual sensation induced in human brain.

In the 1980s, noninvasive stimulation method induced a new tool in its modern form. Barker, the University of Sheffield, demonstrated that by placing the stimulating coil on the human head, the neurons in the head are activated (Barker et al., 1985, 1987). They used short pulses of time-varying magnetic field to induce the electrical currents in the brain.

They demonstrated conduction of nerve impulses from motor cortex stimulates contractions in the hand. Ueno introduced a method to stimulate a local region of the head by a figure-eight-coil (Ueno et al., 1988), and they succeeded in stimulating the human cortex in a 5 mm resolution (Ueno et al., 1990). Since then, this transcranial magnetic stimulation (TMS) has become popular technique in the research of brain activity because of its easy use as noninvasive stimulation tool.

Now, TMS is an effective method for medical diagnosis, particular in studying the function of the human brain. This method is based on the principles of electromagnetic induction in the brain, using time-varying magnetic field. The important development for therapeutic applications of magnetic brain stimulation is rTMS with trains of stimuli. The rTMS uses repetitive magnetic pulses at 1–50 Hz.

On 15 April 1938, the use of electrical stimulus treatment in epilepsy and in mental illness was introduced by two Italian physicians, Ugo Cerlett and Lucio Bini (Rowbottom and Susskind, 1984). Since then, this electrical treatment has been used as ECT for clinical practice. This newly developed ECT spread rapidly through Europe and North America in the 1950s and 1960s. In 1976, ECT was cleared by the FDA for the treatment of depression as a "pre-amendment device." ECT has been used to treat a variety of psychiatric disorders: depression (unipolar and bipolar), schizophrenia, bipolar manic (and mixed) states, catatonia, and schizoaffective disorder. The waveforms for ECT are high current, approximately 800 mA, with trains (AC or pulsed bursts) lasting 1–6 s/cycle. The electrodes are placed either unilaterally or bilaterally on the cranium (Guleyupoglu et al., 2013).

Depending on mainly the waveform of current, there are three methods of TES: tDCS, transcranial alternating current stimulation (tACS), and a special form of tACS, transcranial random noise stimulation. These technologies are considered well tolerated and operated (Kadosh, 2014). tDCS uses a DC in two forms depending on the direction of applied current: anodal tDCS and cathodal tDCS. Here, we mention the basics of tDCS because tDCS is widely used among the TES techniques.

10.4.1 Transcranial Magnetic Stimulation (TMS)

Transcranial magnetic stimulation (TMS) is a noninvasive stimulation technique. TMS is referred to as repetitive transcranial magnetic stimulation (rTMS) when TMS pulses are applied as a periodic repeating pattern.

Over the past decades, rTMS has become tools in therapeutic application. Defining by frequency of stimulation, there are two rTMS treatments: low-frequency rTMS and high-frequency rTMS. Low-frequency rTMS refers to 1 Hz or less- and high-frequency rTMS is stimulation at frequencies from 5 to 20 Hz.

The therapeutic and rehabilitation applications of TMS (rTMS) have been mainly studied for brain diseases, such as depression, Parkinson's disease (PD), Alzheimer's disease (AD), stroke, and pain. This section reviews the therapeutic and rehabilitation applications of TMS, particularly, in the context of depression, pain, stroke, PD, and AD.

10.4.1.1 rTMS for Pain

Chronic pain can be neuropathic and non-neuropathic. Neuropathic pain (NP) is one type of refractory chronic pain. It originates from a lesion or disease of somatosensory systems. Non-NP is due to an excess of nociception secondary to inflammation or tissue lesion, or is psychogenic (Lefaucheur et al., 2014). To treat chronic pain syndromes, Tsubokawa et al. (1991) described, in 1991, first clinical experience using epidural motor cortex stimulation

(MCS) with surgically implanted electrodes. They attempted to treat drug-resistant neuropathic pain (NP). They show the production of long-term analgesia in patients with chronic neuropathic pain. Because MCS requires an invasive implantation of electrodes, as a candidate for the treatment of chronic pain, rTMS has been proposed to reproduce the analgesic effects of MCS.

According to several reports, high-frequency (5 Hz) rTMS of motor cortex (M1) can have pain-relieving effects in NP patients. To confirm these results, Hosomi et al. (2013), as a randomized, double-blind, sham-controlled, crossover study at 7 centers, assessed the safety and efficacy of a daily 10-session (500 pulse/session) of high-frequency rTMS targeting M1 in 70 patients with NP and with a follow-up of 17 days. The short-term pain relief was assessed using a visual analog scale (VAS). The short-term change in the short form of the McGill pain questionnaire (SF-MPQ) was assessed. The rTMS showed significant short-term improvements in VAS and SF-MPQ scores. In conclusion, their findings demonstrate that daily high-frequency rTMS of M1 is tolerable and transiently provides modest pain relief in NP patients.

Based on evidence-based guidelines, a group of European experts recommended that the treatment of high-frequency rTMS of M1 be accepted as a Level A recommendation for the truly significant analgesic effect in patients with NP (Lefaucheur et al., 2014).

10.4.1.2 rTMS for PD

Parkinson's disease (PD) is a progressive neurodegenerative disorder characterized by resting tremor, bradykinesia, rigidity, gait disorder, and postural instability (Chou et al., 2015). The incidence of PD rises with age, affecting approximately 1% of the population older than 60 years and approximately 4% of those older than 80 tears. The prevalence of PD worldwide is expected to more than double by 2030 (Chou et al., 2015).

Using low-frequency (5 Hz) rTMS of motor cortex, Pascual-Leone et al. (1994) published a pioneering study in six medicated patients with PD. Effects of low-frequency 5 Hz rTMS on several neurological parameters such as cRT, MT, and ER in a serial reaction-time task were investigated. In normal subjects, subthreshold rTMS did not significantly change cRT, shortened MT, but increased ER. In patients, rTMS shortened significantly cRT and MT without affecting ER. Finally, they mentioned that repetitive, subthreshold motor cortex stimulation can improve performance in patient with PD and could be useful therapeutically.

To investigate rTMS in the treatment of motor symptoms in PD, using randomized, double blind, sham-controlled study, Benninger et al. (2012) studied safety and efficacy of 50 Hz rTMS of the motor cortices in 8 sessions over 2 weeks, a session/day for 4 consecutive days/week. 50 Hz rTMS was applied to both primary motor cortices (M1) in each session. They investigated 26 patients aged 40–80 years with mild to moderate PD: 13 received 50 Hz rTMS and 13 sham. They used 90 mm circular coil, connected to a Magstim-Rapid magnetic stimulator (Whitland, UK), placed at the optimal position for motor-evoked potentials (MEPs) in abductor pollicis brevis (APB) on each side. Assessment of safety and clinical efficacy over a 1-month period included time tests of gait and bradykinesia, the Unified Parkinson's Disease Rating Scale (UPDRS). rTMS did not improve gait, bradykinesia, global and motor UPDRS, and lengthened the cortical silent period. In conclusion, 50 Hz rTMS of the motor cortices appears safe, but fails to improve motor performance and functional status in PD.

Maruo and colleagues investigated the efficacy of 3 consecutive days of high-frequency rTMS over the MI foot area on motor symptoms in 21 patients with PD using a randomized, double blind cross-over trial (Maruo et al., 2013). Motor effects were evaluated using the Unified Parkinson's Disease Rating Scale part III (UPDRS-III), the self-assessment motor score, the VAS, the 10 m walking test, and finger tapping. High-frequency rTMS improved significantly the UPDRS-III, VAS, the walking test, and finger tapping measurement. In contrast, no significant improvement was observed in depression and apathy scales. Consecutive days of rTMS did not significantly increase the improvement in motor symptoms. As a randomized, double-blind, placebo-controlled study, Makkos et al. (2016) also evaluated the impact of bilateral M1 rTMS on depression in PD. 56 patients with PD and mild-to-moderate depression participated in this study. High-frequency rTMS was applied over the primary motor cortex bilaterally for 10 days. This study demonstrates the beneficial effects of high-frequency bilateral M1 rTMS on depression and health-related quality of life in PD.

rTMS has been investigated as a potential therapy. During the past two decades, the use of rTMS in PD has been examined which the effectiveness of rTMS have yielded mixed results. This is possibly due to the lack of statistical power and the variation in treatment protocols. By reviewing the literature for the researches with rTMS in PD, the meta-analysis was conducted to evaluate the effectiveness of rTMS in the treatment of PD (Chou et al., 2015; Chung and Mak., 2016; Shukla et al., 2016; VonLoh et al., 2013; Zanjani et al., 2015). The pooled evidence from the meta-analysis suggests that rTMS improves motor symptoms for patients with PD.

10.4.1.3 rTMS for Depression

The use of rTMS to treat depression is one of the most promising applications of non-invasive brain stimulation. For patients who have no response to anti-depressant medication, the rTMS was first approved for clinical application by the US Food and Drug Administration (FDA) as a treatment for major depression patients in 2008. This Guideline for rTMS was updated in 2011 (FDA, 2011).

Current evidence is that major depression is associated with prefrontal cortex asymmetry (Lin, 2016). The efficiency of rTMS treatment for depression is related to high-frequency simulation of the left dorsolateral prefrontal cortex (DLPFC). However, the effect of rTMS in healthy subjects is still unclear. Moulier et al. (2016) determined the impact of ten sessions of high-frequency (10 Hz) rTMS with Magstim Super Rapid stimulator applied to the DLPFC on mood and emotion recognition in healthy subjects (right-handed volunteers aged 18–65 years old). The TMS coil was positioned on the left DLPFC through neuronavigation. This study was conducted as a two-arm double-blind randomized trial. Twenty healthy right-handed subjects with aged between 18 and 65 years old were randomly assigned to an active rTMS-treated group (n = 10) or a sham-treated group (n = 10). The delivery parameters were as follows: twenty-five 8 s trains of 10 Hz; 30 s intertrain intervals; 2,000 pulses/session. In total, 10 rTMS sessions were programmed every workday for 2 weeks. In conclusion, this study did not show any deleterious effect on mood and emotion recognition of 10 rTMS sessions applied on DLPFC in healthy subjects. Compared to sham-treated group, the active rTMS-treated group presented a significant improvement in their adaptation to daily life.

O'Reardon et al. (2007) conducted first randomized, controlled trial study at 23 sites (29 in the US, 2 in Australia and 1 in Canada). In this study, patients with a DSM-IV diagnosis of Major depressive disorder (MDD) were antidepressant medication free. The aim of this study was to test whether TMS over the left dorsolateral prefrontal cortex (DLPFC) is effective and safe in the acute treatment of MDD. The study consists of three phases: a

1 week no treatment; a 4–6 week randomized, controlled acute treatment phase of daily treatment with TMS or sham; and a 3 weeks taper phase during which patients started of antidepressant medication. Then 6 months to examine the durability of TMS's acute effects was followed. 301 medication-free patients aged 18–70 years old were randomized to active (n = 155) and sham (n = 146). Treatment parameters were 120% magnetic field intensity, motor threshold (MT), at a repetition rate, 10 Hz frequency, train duration of 4 s, intertrain interval of 26 s and 75 trains/session. A treatment session lasted for 37.5 min for a total of 3000 pulses. Active TMS was significantly superior to sham TMS on the Montgomery-Asberg Depression Rating Scale (MADRS) at 4 weeks. In conclusion, TMS was effective in treating major depression with minimal side effects. It offers clinicians a novel alternative for the treatment of this disorder.

Levkovitz and colleagues also conducted a double-blind randomized placebo-controlled multicenter trial at 20 sites (13 in the US, 4 in Israel, 2 in Germany and 1 in Canada) (Levkovitz et al., 2015). The aim of this study was to investigate the efficacy and safety of Hesel-coil (H-coil) deep TMS applied daily in patients. The patients with 22–68 years old were antidepressant medication free with a DSM-IV diagnosis of MDD. Patients had either failed one to four antidepressant trials or not tolerated two antidepressant treatments. Patients were randomly assigned to either active deep TMS (n = 212) or sham (n = 181). The left DLPFC was chosen as the treatment target site by placing the coil. The acute treatment phase was 5 days/week for 4 weeks. During the maintenance phase, patients were treated twice a week for 12 weeks. Treatment parameters were 120% MT, 18 Hz frequency, train duration of 2 s, intertrain interval of 20 s and 55 trains in each session for total of 1980 pulses over 20 min. Primary and secondary efficacy endpoints at 5 week were the change in the Hamilton Depression Rating Scale (HDRS-21) score and response/remission rates at 5 weeks. Deep TMS induced 6.39-point improvement in HDRS-21 scores and a 3.28 point improvement was observed in sham treatment-group. Response rates were 38.4% for deep TMS versus 21.4% for sham treatment. Remission rates were 32.6% for deep TMS versus 14.6% for sham treatment.

10.4.1.4 rTMS for Stroke

Lim et al. (2014) investigated the effect of LF rTMS on post-stroke dysphagia and compared the results with that of two other protocols. Two other therapies were the conventional dysphagia therapy (CDT) and neuromuscular electrical stimulation (NMES). 47 patients were randomly assigned to three groups; the mean age of the CDT group was 62.5 ± 8.2 years old, in the rTMS group, the mean age was 59.8 ± 11.8 years old and in the NMES group, the mean age was 66.3 ± 15.4 years old. rTMS was performed at 100% resting motor threshold with 1 Hz for 20 min/session (total 1,200 pulses a day), 5 days/ week for 2 weeks. In NMES group, electrical stimulation was applied to the anterior neck for 30 min/session (5 days/week for 2 weeks). Dysphagia may cause serious complications such as aspiration pneumonia, dehydration, malnutrition, even death. The investigators evaluated the functional dysphagia scale (FDS), pharyngeal transit time (PTT), the penetration-aspiration scale (PAS), and the American Speech-Language Hearing Association National Outcomes Measurement System (ASHA NOMS) swallowing scale. The results demonstrated that both rTMS and NMES induced the early recovery of the swallowing function for liquid in stroke patients, but no difference was observed between two methods.

Li et al. (2015) identified the literature published until June 2014 by performing a search of electronic databases. Then, they investigated the efficacy and safety of low-frequency rTMS (LF rTMS) in post-stroke aphasia through reviewing systematically and meta-analysis of randomized controlled trials (RCTs). After a total of 879 articles, 4 RCTs with a total of 132 patients were included in the meta-analysis. Checking the efficacy and safety of LF rTMS in post-stroke aphasia via systematic review and meta-analysis showed that LF rTMS was beneficial for post-stroke patients with regard to naming and changes in brain excitability. The finding obtained from meta-analysis indicates that LF rTMS is a relative safe and effective treatment for naming.

The use of rTMS after stroke has two therapeutic goals: (1) to promote functional recovery by modulating synaptic mechanisms and "priming" neuronal circuitry for learning/LTP, and (2) to restore abnormal cortical excitability of the affected or non-affected hemispheres (Tang et al., 2015). From animal studies, rTMS does alter cortical excitability and promote plasticity with a beneficial impact on behavior. It also suggested rTMS may induce neuro-protection (Tang et al., 2015).

From 1988 to 2012, for stroke patients with limb motor deficit, there are only 141 publications of the effects of rTMS and 132 for tDCS (Klomjai et al., 2015). From Cochrane review, 19 RCTs with 588 patients for the effects of rTMS and 18 RCTs with 450 patients for the effect of tDCS were found. rTMS and tDCS contribute to physiological and pathophysiological studies in motor control. The increasing number of studies leads to the possible therapeutic use of both rTMS and tDCS to improve motor recovery after stroke.

10.4.2 Transcranial Direct Current Stimulation

In 1998, Priori and colleagues described first the human motor cortex excitability by a weak direct current (DC) applied to the scalp (Priori et al., 1998). 15 healthy right-handed volunteers aged 25–43 years participated in the study. The investigators placed a pair of electrodes: one stimulating electrode over the left motor cortex (7 cm lateral to the vertex), and the other under the chin. The range of current, 0.075–0.5 mA was below conscious cutaneous sensory threshold. A weak (less than 0.5 mA, 7 s) anodal scalp DC depressed significantly the excitability of the human motor cortex. They mentioned that this may lead to the application of weak scalp DC in therapy, possibly in disorders associated with abnormal motor cortical excitability.

In 2000, Nitsche and Paulus (2000) first demonstrated changes in motor cortex excitability by the application of weak tDCS in healthy humans. A total of 53 healthy subjects was used. They recorded MEPs 50 ms before the end of a 4 s phase of either cathodal or anodal motor cortical current stimulation at 1 mA. MEP amplitudes were increase after 5 min of anodal tDCS applied to the motor cortex. They were decreased after cathodal tDCS application. This tDCS application was painless and modulated cortical excitability. In contrast to modulatory effects of rTMS, modulatory effects of tDCS depend on current direction (Edwardson et al., 2013). In conclusion, tDCS appears to be a promising tool for clinical neuroplasticity research.

As noninvasive therapies of electric stimulation, the applications of tDCS were reviewed. Anodal tDCS leads to depolarization and cathodal tDCS hyperpolarization. The duration of stimulation is 10–20 min with a peak current of a 1–2 mA (Guleyupoglu et al., 2013).

Flöel (2014) reviewed the use of tDCS in patients with mild cognitive impairment, AD, movement disorders, epilepsy, and post-stroke rehabilitation of motor and cognitive deficits. Lefaucheur (2016) presented a comprehensive overview of the raw data of the clinical effect of tDCS in patients, as a guide to researchers.

10.4.2.1 tDCS for Depression

Two double-blind, sham-controlled trials using left prefrontal anodal tDCS reported positive results in major depression (MD) (Boggio et al., 2008; Fregni et al., 2006). Fregni et al., reported the improvement of Hamilton Depression Rating Scale (HAMD) scores after 5 sessions, 20 min, of anodal tDCS at 1 mA. Boggio et al., reported similar results. They enrolled 40 patients with MD, randomly divided into three groups: active anodal tDCS over the left DLPFC, active anodal tDCS over the occipital cortex, and sham tDCS. They applied 2 mA with treatment of 20 min/day for 10 days and found that the improvement of HDRS scores in DLPFC tDCS treated group. Subsequently, as a double-blind, sham-controlled trial, Loo et al. (2010) used 40 patients with severe MD, randomly assigned to active anodal tDCS and sham groups. Anodal tDCS stimulation was applied over the left DLPFC. Stimulation was given at 1 mA for 20 min. The measure of mood evaluation was the Montgomery-Asberg Depression Rating Score (MADRS). Overall depression scores improved significantly over tDCS treatment, but there was no between-group difference in the five session, sham-controlled phase. In the Fregni et al., study, tDCS was given at 1 mA for 20 min. Compared to the Fregni et al., study, Loo et al., did not show any difference between active anodal tDCS and sham tDCS. The response to active anodal tDCS over ten treatment sessions is comparable to that reported by Boggio et al. These discussions indicate that further study may demonstrate a difference between active tDCS and sham tDCS. It is recommended that the efficacy of tDCS in MD be further evaluated over a longer treatment period.

Here, we introduce two review papers focusing on meta-analysis of randomized, double-blind and sham-controlled trials (RCTs) of tDCS in major depression (MD) (Berlim et al., 2013) and addressing the efficacy, safety and tolerability of TDCS in the treatment of depression (Meron et al., 2015). Berlim et al., searched the literature published from 1998 through July 2012. Their meta-analysis was carried out for 6 RCTs with 200 patients with MD. No significant difference was found between active tDCS and sham tDCS in terms of both response and remission rates. This meta-analysis shows that the clinical utility of tDCS as treatment for MD remains unclear. Meron et al. (2015) also carried out meta-analysis of 10 RCTs comparing active tDCS to sham tDCS, with 393 patients with major depressive episodes in the context of unipolar or bipolar disorders. tDCS may be efficacious for treatment of MD. From both meta-analyses, it is suggestive that including larger samples, future studies over longer treatment periods are needed.

10.4.2.2 tDCS for PD

Parkinson's disease (PD) is a neurodegenerative disorder that includes motor symptoms such as tremor, postural instability, rigidity, bradykinesia. In a double-blind, randomized, sham-controlled study, Benninger et al. (2010) investigated whether anodal tDCS of the motor and prefrontal cortices improves gait and bradykinesia in 25 patients with PD (13 receiving tDCS and 12 sham). tDCS was applied in 8 sessions within 2-1/2 weeks when patients were receiving dopaminergic medication. In the anodal tDCS-treatment group, the motor area and prefrontal area were stimulated at 2 mA for 20 min. The follow-up evaluations were performed 24 h, 1 month, and 3 month after the last tDCS intervention session. Evaluations include gait (the time to walk 10 m), bradykinesia, on subjective perception on health and well-being, visuomotor speed, and procedural learning. The motor tests and the Unified Parkinson's Disease Rating Scale (UPDRS) were assessed while patients were on and off medication. Gait improved after tDCS, walking time decreased significantly with tDCS, bradykinesia decreased significantly with tDCS. This effect persists for longer than 3 months. No differences were found for changes in the UPDRS, reaction time, visuomotor speed, procedural learning, mood, and well-being between tDCS and sham interventions. Benninger et al., concluded that tDCS of the motor and prefrontal cortices may have a therapeutic potential in PD, but better stimulation is needed.

Fregni et al. (2006) measured the impact of tDCS on cortical excitability in patients with PD. After anodal tDCS and cathodal tDCS over motor cortex (M1), MEPs were measured and correlated with improvement in motor function. These results showed that after anodal tDCS stimulation, the increase of MEP amplitudes. In contrast, cathodal tDCS decreased MEP amplitudes. Changes in MEP tended to correlate with motor improvements measured by the UPDRS-III. It suggested that an enhancement of cortical excitability after stimulation in patients with PD.

In order to provide an overview of the effects if tDCS on neurophysiological and behavioral outcome measures in PD patients, Broeder et al. (2015) reviewed systematically the literature published throughout the last ten years. They indentified ten studies for review after examining the research strategy and the implementation of inclusion and exclusion criteria. After reviewing ten studies, they discussed the effects of tDCS on neurophysiological parameters, motor skills and cognitive functioning. Results confirmed that tDCS applied to motor cortex had significant results on motor function, and to a lesser extent on cognitive test. The physiological mechanism underlying the long-term effects of tDCS on cortical excitability in the PD brain is still unclear.

10.4.2.3 tDCS for AD

Alzheimer disease (AD) is a cause of dementia. Memory disturbances appear, affecting the ability to learn and retrieve information and later causing impairments in recognition memory and attention (Ferrucci et al., 2008). Ferrucci et al., evaluated the cognitive effect of tDCS (anodal, cathodal, and sham stimulation) over the temporoparietal (TP) areas in three sessions in ten elderly patients (75.2±7.3 years old) with mild probable AD. In each session, recognition memory and visual attention were tested before and 30 min after tDCS at 1.5 mA for 15 min. After anodal tDCS, accuracy of the word recognition memory task increased, whereas after cathodal tDCS memory performance worsened and after sham tDCS it remained unchanged. This shows that the improvement is polarity specific. tDCS left the visual attention-reaction times unchanged. Anodal tDCS increases the excitability of the motor cortex, which leads probably to improve function in TP areas. Anodal tDCS presumably benefits memory performance.

Boggio et al. (2009) investigated the impact of anodal tDCS on visual recognition memory (VRM), working memory (WM), and selective attention in ten patients aged 70–92 years with mild probable AD. Patients received three sessions of anodal tDCS (left dorsolateral prefrontal cortex, left temporal cortex) and sham stimulation with an intensity of 2 mA for 30 min. The main finding was that tDCS to the DLPFC enhanced performance on VRM, compared with sham stimulation. The investigators emphasized that this is the first trial showing that tDCS can enhance a component of recognition memory.

10.4.2.4 tDCS for Stroke

Numerous studies have reported the beneficial effect of cortical stimulation in improving motor recovery in patients after stroke. In the first double blind sham-controlled crossover study, Hummel et al. (2005) desired to test the hypothesis that noninvasive stimulation of the motor cortex could improve motor function in the paretic hand of patients with stroke. Six patients with a history of a single ischemic cerebral infarct aged 38–84 years participated in the study. Current of 1 mA remained on for 20 min in the tDCS session and for up to 30 s in the sham session. Hand function was measured using the Jebsen–Taylor hand function test (JTT). The investigators demonstrated an improvement of JTT, a set of hand functions that mimic activities of daily living (ADL), after a single session of anodal tDCS stimulation. This effect was not seen with sham. Further, in the same experimental design, Hummel et al. (2006) tested the effects of tDCS on pinch force (PF) and simple reaction time (RT) tasks in patients with chronic stroke. Eleven patients (57.0±16.0 years) with a history of a single mostly subcortical ischemic cerebral infarct participated. Anodal tDCS was delivered for 20 min in the tDCS session and for up to 30 s in the sham session. Anodal tDCS shortened RT and improved PF in the paretic hand. tDCS of $M1_{affected\ hemisphere}$ can modulate performance of motor tasks.

Hesse and colleagues examined the safety and methodology of using tDCS with robot-assisted arm training (AT), to inform planning a larger RCT (Hesse et al., 2007, 2011). As a pilot study, ten patients with averaged age 63.3 years, after an ischemic stroke 4–8 weeks and no history of epilepsy, participated. Eight patients had with cortical lesion and two patients with subcortical lesions. All had severe arm paresis. They received 30 20 min sessions of AT over 6 weeks. 1.5 mA tDCS was applied during the first 7 min. The anodal tDCS was applied over the lesioned hemisphere and the cathodal tDCS above the contralateral orbit. Arm and language impairment were assessed with the Fugl–Meyer motor score and the Aachener Aphasie test. Arm function of three patients improved significantly. In the seven patients with cortical lesions, arm function changed little. As a result of this combination of tDCS with robot-assisted bilateral arm therapy, these procedures are safer and the improvement of motor performance in patients with subcortical mesion was found. The number of patients was small and the protocol did not include a sham group. So, these positive results led to further double-blind randomized sham-controlled multicenter trial (Hesse et al., 2011). This study included three conditions; anodal tDCS, cathodal tDCS and sham with robot-assisted therapy. 96 patients with ischemic supratentorial lesion of 3–8 week's duration were included in this study. There were no significant changes between the 3 groups following intervention. No difference in motor or daily living changes after anodal tDCS, cathodal tDCS, and sham tDCS at the end of the intervention and three months after 2 mA, 20 min, 30 sessions. In conclusion, neither anodal nor cathodal tDCS enhanced the effect of bilateral AT.

Yun et al. (2015) investigated simply whether tDCS can improve cognition in stroke patients. 45 stroke patients (20 males and 25 females with average age 62.7 years) with cognitive dysfunction were included in this study using prospective, double-blind, randomized case-control trials. The treatment groups were three: (1) anodal tDCS of the left anterior temporal lobe, (2) anodal tDCS of the right anterior temporal lobe, and (3) sham stimulation. tDCS was delivered for 30 min at 2 mA, five times/week, for a total of three weeks. The evaluation of cognitive impairment was based on a computerized neuropsychological test (CNT), Korean mini-mental state examination (K-MMSE). The Korean version of the Modified Barthel Index (K-MBI) was used to assess ADL functionality. There was significant improvement in the verbal learning test on the CNT in the left anodal tDCS group. The investigators mentioned that tDCS can successfully be used as a treatment modality for patients with cognitive dysfunction after stroke.

Baker et al. (2010) determined if anodal tDCS would improve naming accuracy in stroke patients with aphasia (PWA) when applied to the scalp overlying the left frontal cortex ten patients with chronic stroke-induced aphasia, received 5 days of anodal tDCS (1 mA;

20 min) and 5 days of sham tDCS while performing a computerized anomia treatment. These results suggest that anodal tDCS over the left frontal cortex can lead to enhanced naming accuracy in PWA and further investigation involving greater number of patients is needed to confirm the effect revealed in this pilot study.

10.5 Biological, Health Effects, and Safety Aspects of Electromagnetic Fields Related to TMS/TES

Transcranial magnetic (TMS) and electric stimulation (tDCS) use an electromagnetic field (EMF) generated in the body. The biological effects of the TMS and tDCS are mediated through the electromagnetic field. Therefore, a clear understanding of the biological effects of electromagnetic fields related to TMS/tDCS techniques is necessary (Peterchev et al., 2012).

This section describes basic issues of biological effects, risk, and safety related to TMS. In the TMS technique, a pulse-shaped time-varying magnetic field is used to induce the electric field in the brain that activates the neurons. TMS is characterized by the diameter and shape of the coil, such as round and figure-eight, and the amplitude, wave and duration of the applied pulse-shaped time-varying magnetic field. Although the operation of TMS necessitates the time-varying magnetic field, understanding of biological and health effects of time-varying magnetic fields associated with TMS is still unknown. In clinical and therapeutic application of TMS, the interaction of the magnetic field with human body is very important for the operation.

Here, the biological and health effects of the magnetic field associated with the operation of TMS are reviewed briefly. As well as the short description of the safety issues, the guideline is given. This guideline provides a consideration of human health risk for both patients and medical staff. Finally, we summarize in conclusion remarks on the biological and health issues related to the operation of TMS.

There are many reports about EMF-related effects in synaptic plasticity. Balassa et al. (2013) determined the effects of a long-term extremely low-frequency magnetic field (ELF-MF) (50 Hz, 0.5 and 3 mT) on synaptic functions in the developing brain in rats. Rats were chronically exposed to ELF-MF during two critical periods of brain development, at the embryonic stage (second gestation week) and the early postnatal age (newborns for 7 days). Excitability and plasticity of neocortical and hippocampal areas were tested on both brain slices. The basic excitability of hippocampal slices was increased at both embryonic and early postnatal age stages. There was a significant decrease in the efficacy of long-term potentiation (LTP) in neocortex, but not in hippocampal slices. The treatment at the early postnatal age stage had no significant effect on plasticity phenomena. In conclusion, EMF-MF has significant effects on basic neuronal functions and synaptic plasticity in brain slice originating from rats exposed either in fetal or in newborn period.

10.5.1 Effects of the Time-Varying Magnetic Fields on Biological Systems

The time-varying magnetic field serves for the spatial localization in the image reconstruction process in MRI technique. In TMS technique, by placing a figure-eight-coil or round coil on the head over the region of particular interest, the time-varying magnetic field acts as to induce electric current due to Faraday's induction law.

Using a wide variety of experimental models, many studies have investigated the biological effects of time-varying magnetic fields (IARC, 2002; ICNIRP, 2003b, 2009b; NIEHS, 1998; WHO, 2007).

The coupling between the time-varying magnetic field and the body has been summarized by the World Health Organization (WHO, 2007). For magnetic fields, the permeability of tissue is the same as that of air, so the field in tissues is the same as the external field. Human and animal bodies do not significantly perturb the field distribution. Key features of dosimetry for exposure of human and animal to low time-varying magnetic fields include:

- for a given magnetic field strength and orientation, higher electric fields are induced in the bodies of larger subject because the possible conduction loops are larger;
- the induced electric field and current depend on the orientation of the external magnetic field to the body. Generally induced fields in the body are greatest when the field is aligned from the front of the back of the body, but for some organs the highest values are for different field alignments;
- the weakest electric fields are induced by a magnetic field oriented along the principal body axis;
- the distribution of the induced electric field is affected by the conductivity of the various organs and tissues.

As already mentioned above, the time-varying magnetic field induces electric currents in the body by the Faraday's law of induction, in the patient during MRI and TMS examination. The induction stimulates nerves and muscles. The nerve stimulation may cause discomfort. Electric fields may also be induced by movement in static magnetic field.

After the review and the evaluation of low frequency electric and magnetic fields for the carcinogenicity, IARC classified power frequency magnetic fields as possibly carcinogenic to humans (Group 2B). This classification was strongly influenced by epidemiological studies, which have observed increased risks of childhood leukemia at magnetic field greater than 0.3–0.4 µT (IARC, 2002).

Although epidemiological studies in children shows an increased risk of childhood leukemia exposed to power frequency magnetic field, there is a lack of supporting evidence for such effect from animal studies and/or in vitro studies. In addition, there is no plausible mechanism.

Due to the absence of plausible mechanism and no induction of cancer in animals study, the expert reports have not concluded that there is no causal relationship between the magnetic field exposure and the risk of childhood leukemia (SCENIHR, 2009, 2013, 2015).

There have been many epidemiological studies of people exposed to power frequency magnetic fields in home and work place. However, there are not enough epidemiological studies on cancer risks among patients or medical staffs undergoing MRI and TMS examinations.

10.5.2 Biological Effects of the Time-Varying Magnetic Fields Related to TMS/TES

As described briefly in the previous section, the TMS and TES as noninvasive treatments have been used for neuropsychiatric disorders. Although the two noninvasive tools are widely used, the mechanisms underlying the efficacy of these treatments remain essentially unexplained.

There are no enough experimental studies on the biological effects of the TMS-related magnetic field. Experiments with animals have sought to provide information on the molecular mechanism of action of rTMS. The effects of rTMS in rodents are greatly dependent on (1) frequency and field intensity of the stimulation, (2) the acute or chronic mode of treatment, (3) the total number of pulses, (4) the shape and dimension of coils, and (5) the state of the animals, anesthetized or awake (Rajan et al., 2017).

Ueyama et al. (2011) examined chronic rTMS effects on hippocampal neurogenesis in rats. Using a 70 mm figure-of-eight coil (Magstim Super Rapid), they set the stimulating parameters to 20 Hz and 70% of rTMS device's maximum power. They administered bromodeoxyuridine (BrdU) and 1,000 pulses of rTMs daily for 14 consecutive days. Rats were divided into two groups: control group (n = 5) and rTMS-treatment group (n = 5). The coil was placed horizontally over the scalp and aligned parallel with the body of the rat. rTMS treatments did not induce seizures. Cell proliferation in the dentate gyrus was examined. The results show that in the rTMS-treated group, BrdU-positive cells were significantly increased, which suggest that hippocampal neurogenesis might be involved in the antidepressant effects of chronic rTMS.

In order to understand the neurobiological mechanisms of underlying transcranial brain stimulation, animal exposure experiments have been carried out over past two decades. There are review papers published in recent years describing the underlying mechanisms of the effects of noninvasive brain stimulation such as TMS and tDCS techniques (Chervyakov et al., 2015; Cirillo et al., 2017; Cullen and Young, 2016; Lisanby et al., 2000).

Numerous studies have been carried out in trying to understand the action of TMS/tDCS (Tang et al., 2015; Jackson et al., 2016). Tang et al., presented the summary of *in vitro* and *in vivo* studies and preclinical models of Parkinson's disease, depression, and stroke. Through this review, they suggest that basic research can contribute to the understanding of how rTMS induced plasticity can be modulated.

Focusing on the neurobiological findings of *in vivo* and *in vitro* studies of the effects of TMS and tDCS, particularly on the changes of synaptic plasticity, we will review and summarize the findings of animal experimental studies. They cover the effects observed on second messenger, induction of immediate early genes, gene expression, neurotransmitter release, neurotrophic factor, neuroendocrine system, oxidative stress, and so on. They offer to deepen the understanding of the basic processes underlying cellular and molecular mechanisms in human studies. Below, we summarize the main findings of exposure experiments with animal model in different topics.

10.5.2.1 Effect of TMS on Neurobiological System

Using anesthetized and awake rats, Gersner et al. (2011) evaluated and compared the long-term effects of high-frequency (20 Hz) and low-frequency (1 Hz) rTMS on the markers of neuroplasticity such as brain-derived neurotrophic factor (BDNF) and GluR1 subunit of AMPA receptor. Then, they assessed whether the long-term effects depend on spontaneous neural activity, by comparing the neurochemical alterations induced by rTMS in anesthetized and awake rats. rTMS was administered daily for 10 days during a 2-week period, and brains were removed 3 days after the last stimulation to measure lasting effects on markers for neuroplasticity. Levels of BDNF, GluR1, and phosphorylated GluR1 were assessed in the hippocampus, prelimbic cortex, and striatum. They found that high-frequency rTMS increased neuroplasticity markers in awake rats, while decreasing them in anesthetized rats. Low-frequency rTMS did not induce significant long-term effects on these markers in both anesthetized and awake rats. This study gives the importance of spontaneous neural activity during rTMS and high-frequency rTMS can induce long-lasting effects on BDNF and GluR1.

10.5.2.1.1 Effects of rTMS on Gene Expression

Etiévant et al. (2015) examined whether high-frequency (15 Hz) rTMS with a small figure-eight coil (inner diameter 2.5 cm; outer diameter 5 cm) applied for five consecutive days over the frontal cortex of awake mice (male and female C57BL/6JWT) can induce changes of protein expression and chromatin organization similar to those resulting from chronic drug treatment. Stimulation consisted of three trains of 150 pulses at 15 Hz with an interval of 0.5 s, a total of 450 pulses. The coil was placed flat on the scalp over the frontal cortex. The results indicate that rTMS induces prolonged changes in the expression of proteins such as cyclin-dependent kinase 5 (CDK5) and the postsynaptic density protein 95 (PSD-95). Both proteins are involved in modulating synaptic plasticity. These modifications were associated with changes of histone acetylation (HA). So, rTMS can induce long-lasting epigenetic changes of gene expression from a modulation of HA.

10.5.2.1.2 Effects of rTMS on Neurotransmission

Using microdialysis in anesthetized adult male Wistar rats, Keck et al. (2000a) monitored the intrahypothalamic release of arginine vasopressin (AVP) and amino acids (glutamate, glutamine, aspartate, swerine, arginine, taurine, γ-aminobutyric acid) and the intrahippocampal release of monoamines (dopamine, noradrenaline, serotonin) and their metabolites (homovanillic acid, 3,4-dihydroxyphenylacetic acid, 5-hydroxyindoleacetic acid) after the treatment of acute high-frequency (20 Hz) TMS (20 trains of 2.5 s). In response to rTMS, a continuous reduction in AVP release of up to 50% within the hypothalamic paraventricular nucleus was observed. Within this nucleus, the release of taurine, aspartate and serine were selectively stimulated by rTMS. In addition, in the dorsal hippocampus the extracellular concentration of dopamine was elevated in response to rTMS. They concluded this was the first *in vivo* evidence that acute rTMS of frontal brain regions has a differentiated modulatory effect on neurotransmitters/neuromodulator systems in distinct brain areas.

Kanno et al. (2003) clarified the effects of acute high-frequency (25 Hz) 1 T rTMS treatment on extracellular serotonin (5-HT) concentrations in the rat prefrontal cortex (PFC) by using *in vivo* microdialysis methods. A magnetic stimulator (AAA-10723; Nihon Kohden, Tokyo) with a figure-eight-shaped coil (AAA-15062, Nihon Kohden) was used for the acute rTMS. This treatment consisted of 500 stimuli with 60% of maximum output resulting from 20 trains at 25 Hz for 1 s with 1 min intervals. This results show that acute rTMS treatment of the frontal brain in rats, eliminated the increase in 5-HT levels induced by the sham treatment in the rat PFC, and is related to the serotonergic neuronal system in the rat PFC. This may have therapeutic implications for emotional disorders.

rTMS in the human brain can lead to long-lasting changes in cortical excitability. The cellular and molecular mechanisms underlying rTMS-induced plasticity remain unclear. Lenz et al. (2015) examined the high-frequency (10 Hz) rTMS-induced plasticity of excitatory postsynapses using mouse entorhino-hippocampal slice cultures. By employing whole-cell patch-clamp recording of CA1 pyramidal neurons, they found evidence for a preferential potentiation of excitatory synapses on proximal dendrites of CA1 neurons (2–4 h after stimulation). The rMS induced activation of voltage-gated sodium channels, L-type voltage-gated calcium channels, and N-methyl-D-aspartate receptors (NMDAr). From these results, they propose a cellular model for the preferential strengthening of excitatory synapses on proximal dendrites after rMS *in vitro*. This is based on a cooperative effect of synaptic glutamatergic transmission and postsynaptic depolarization.

It has been proposed that long-term potentiation (LTP)/long-term depression (LTD)-like plasticity of excitatory synapses underly rTMS effects on cortical excitability. However, less attention has been paid to rTMS-induced changes in inhibitory neurotransmission. As series of experiments, Lenz et al. (2016) studied the plasticity of inhibitory neurotransmission on CA1 pyramidal neurons employed high-frequency (10 Hz) rTMS of mouse entorphino-hippocampal slice cultures. The rMS induced Ca^{2+}-dependent reduction in GABAergic synaptic strength (2–4 h after stimulation). This high-frequency rMS acts on dendritic, but not somatic inhibition. The reduction in clustered gephyrin is detected in CA1 stratum radiatum of rTMS-treated anaesthetized mice. Lenz et al., proposed that rMS acts on network excitability and connectivity through the induction of coordinated Ca^{2+}-mediated changes of specific subsets of excitatory and inhibitory synapses on principal neurons.

In order to understand rTMS-induced neural plasticity at the cellular level, Vlachos et al. (2012) established an *in vitro* model of rTMS using mouse organotypic entorhino-hippocampal slice culture. Using this *in vitro* model of rTMS, they assessed functional and structural properties of excitatory synapses in mature hippocampal CA1 pyramidal neurons (Vlachos et al., 2012). Entorhino-hippocampal slice cultures were prepared at postnatal days 4–5 from C57BL/6J × Balb/cJ or Thy1-GFP mice. Cultures were stimulated using a Magstim Rapid magnetic stimulator with high frequency (10 Hz), nine trains of 100 pulses with an intertrain interval of 30 s. rMS induces a long-lasting increase in glutamatergic synaptic strength, which is accompanied by structural remodeling of dendritic spines, are shown judging from whole-cell patch-clamp recording, immunohistochemistry, and time-lapse techniques. The effects of rMS on spine sixe were predominantly seen in small spines. In addition, this study showed that rMS-induced postsynaptic changes depend on the NMDA receptor-mediated accumulation of GluA1-containing AMPA receptors. In conclusion, these results provide first experimental evidence that rMS induces coordinated functional and structural plasticity of excitatory postsynapses. This is consistent with a long-term potentiation (LTP) of synaptic transmission.

10.5.2.1.3 *Effects of rTMS on Neurotrophic Factors*

Three reports about the effects of rTMS on neuroplasticity using animal models are introduced. Gersner et al. (2011) evaluated and compared the long-term effects of high-frequency (20 Hz) and low-frequency (1 Hz) rTMS on the markers of neuroplasticity such as brain-derived neurotrophic factor (BDNF) and GluR1 subunit AMPA receptor. Then, they assessed whether these effects depend on spontaneous neural activity, by comparing the neurochemical alterations induced by rTMS in 32 anesthetized and 32 awake male Sprague-Dawley rats. Ten daily sessions of both rTMS were administered over the rat brain, and brains were removed 3 days after the last stimulation to measure lasting effects on markers for neuroplasticity. rTMS stimulation was applied using a small circular coil (inner diameter, 2.5 cm; outer diameter, 5 cm) at 60% of maximum output of a Rapid² stimulator. The coil was placed over the rat's head to allow maximal stimulation over frontal cortex. Levels of BDNF, GluR1, and phosphorylated GluR1 were assessed in the hippocampus, prelimbic cortex, and striatum. BDNF is a member of the neurotrophin family and is abundant in the adult brain. It was found that high-frequency stimulation induced profound effect on the markers of neuroplasticity. Markers were increased in awaken rats and decreased in anesthetized animals. In contrast, low-frequency stimulation did not induce significant long-term effects on these markers in either state. This study highlights the importance of spontaneous neural activity during rTMS administration and demonstrates that high-frequency rTMS can induce long-lasting effects on BDNF and GluR1, which may underlie the clinical benefits of this treatment in neuroplasticity-related disorders.

In same approach, Müller et al. (2000) investigated the effects of long-term rTMS on the expression of BDNF, cholecystokinin (CCK), and neuropeptide tyrosine (NPY) mRNA in rat brain. They examined the effects of TMS on the expression of both BDNF mRNA and protein as well as of the neuroactive peptides CCK and NPY mRNA in distinct area of the rat brain. The rats were treated with high-frequency (20 Hz) 4 T rTMS with round shaped coil (inner diameter 6 mm; outer diameter 57 mm) with 150 stimuli/day resulting from three trains at a rate of 20 Hz for 2.5 s. A significant increase was found in BDNF mRNA in the hippocampal areas CA3 and CA3c in the granule cell layer, as well as in the parietal and piriform cortex. A significant increase in CCK mRNA was observed in all brain regions. NPY mRNA expression was not altered. In conclusion, BDNF may contribute to the neuroprotective effects of rTMS. Further, the rTMS-induced changes in BDNF and CCK expression are similar to those reported after antidepressant drug treatment and electroconvulsive seizures.

The evidence shows that the disruption of hippocampal neurotrophins secretion leads to memory deficits in Alzheimer's disease (AD) animal model. The AD animal models have been proposed. In the proposal, the pathological features include deposits of amyloid-βpeptide (Aβ) and neurofibrillary tangles (NFTs) which characterize AD brain. Aβ oligomers (main components: $A\beta_{1-40}$ and $A\beta_{1-42}$) are the typical endogenous neurotoxic substances. Tan et al. (2013) investigated whether low-frequency (1 Hz) 0.4 T rTMS can regulate endogenous neurotrophins contents and rescue spatial memory deficits. rTMS treatment with 9 cm diameter round coil was used. The pattern of one session rTMS consisted of 20 burst trains, each train with 20 pulses at 1 Hz with 10 s intertrain intervals, in total 400 stimuli and pulse width was 70 μs. They considered that rats with spatial memory deficits identified by Morris water maze test were a suitable $A\beta_{1-42}$-induced toxicity rat model. Further, they reported that severe deficits in long-term potentiation (LTP) and spatial memory were observed in an $A\beta_{1-42}$-induced toxicity rat model. In conclusion, neurotrophins (nerve growth factor (NGF) and BDNF) and NMDA-receptor levels were decreased in $A\beta_{1-42}$-induced toxicity rat model. The rTMS reversed markedly the decrease in neurotrophins contents. This rTMS-induced increment of neurotrophins upregulated hippocampal NMDA-receptor expression. The rTMS rescued deficits in LTP and spatial memory of rats with $A\beta_{1-42}$-induced toxicity model. These results indicate that low-frequency rTMS increases hippocampal neurotrophins and NMDA-receptor contents in $A\beta_{1-42}$-induced toxicity model rats. This helps to enhance hippocampal LTP and reverse $A\beta_{1-42}$-mdiated memory deficits.

10.5.2.1.4 Effects of rTMS on Neuroendocrine System

There are several reports of the effect of rTMS on neuroendocrine system in rats. Here, we present the results of two reports (Hedges et al., 2002; Keck et al., 2000b).

To test the hypothesis that TMS may alter the hypothalamic-pituitary-adrenal (HPA) axis, Hedges et al. (2002) evaluated the effects of short-term TMS on corticosterone and testosterone in adult male rats immediately and after 3, 6, 9, 12, 24, and 48 h recovery periods following a single TMS and effects on prolactin over a 2 h recovery period after a one-time TMS application. 84 Sprague-Dawley (SD) rats were randomly divided into seven groups. In each group, one half of the rats received TMS and one half was sham-treated. TMS was administered via Magnetism Rapid Magnetic Stimulator (Magnetism Company Limited, Wales, UK) through a 5 cm, figure-eight coil for rats at 15 Hz and 80% power for 3 s. The

TMS was applied by placing the rat into a flat-bottomed Plexiglas tube. Following the TMS and sham application, trunk blood of rat was obtained via decapitation. TMS had no effects on plasma testosterone at any of the times over 48 h. There were no significant differences in prolactin concentrations between TMS and sham treatments. TMS rats displayed significantly lower corticosterone concentrations at 6 and 24 h after a single application. From this study, the results show that TMS (1) alters the HPS stress axis and (2) provides time-course data for the implications of the hormonal mechanisms. This mechanism may be involved in the actions of TMS.

Keck et al. (2000b) investigated the effects of rTMS on brain functions in adult male rats. The rats were treated with daily high-frequency (20 Hz), 4 T rTMS administration (three trains of 20 Hz; 2.5 s) for 8 weeks from 4 weeks on. This experiment was designed to investigate the effects of chronic rTMS on the behavioral performance of rats in various tests that are known to have the potential to activate the HPA system. In this study, the forced swim test was chosen to assess acute stress, and to assess anxiety-related behavior, the elevated plus-maze and social interaction were chosen. The elevated plus-maze test is one of the most widely used nonconditioned animal models of anxiety (Kanno et al., 2003; Pellow et al., 1985). The release patterns of corticotropin (ACTH) and corticosterone were monitored for characterization of the activity of the HAP system. In the forced swim test, treated rats showed a more active stress coping strategy than the control rats. This was accompanied by a significantly attenuated stress-induced elevation of plasma ACTH concentrations. No changes were found in the anxiety-related behavior of the rats. Chronic rTMS treatment of frontal brain regions in rats resulted in a change in coping strategy that was accompanied by an attenuated neuroendocrine stress response in rats.

10.5.2.1.5 Effects of rTMS on Oxidative Response and Cell Death

The immediate early gene expression in rat brain was compared between high-frequency (25 Hz) 2 T rTMS and electroconvulsive stimulation (ECS) (Ji et al., 1998). The rTMS was administered to awake rats by using a round coil (5 cm diameter). The coil was held above the rat's head at close proximity to the site of stimulation at the orbit level. ECS was applied as follows: car clip electrodes connected to an ECT stimulator (unit 7801, Ugo Basile, Varese, Italy) were used on awake male adult rats. To induce maximal convulsive seizures, 1 s stimulation at 100 Hz, 5 ms pulse width, 90 mA electric current were chosen. Results were that ECS induces a rapid increase of *c-fos* mRNA expression through the brain in the hippocampus and neocortex. On the other hand, a single rTMS application produces a more discrete stimulation of *c-fos* mRNA expression. Most notably, rTMS results in strongly increased *c-fos* expression, predominately in the paraventricular nucleus of the thalamus (PVT) and specific cortical regions, and moderate expression in regions controlling circadian rhythms. ECS induces strong activation of *c-fos* expression in all cortical regions and hippocampus, but weaker activation in the PVT and suprachiasmatic nucleus (SCN).

Using a vascular dementia (VaD) rat model, Yang et al. (2015) determined whether low-frequency (1 Hz) 0.5 T rTMS protects pyramidal cell from apoptosis and promotes hippocampal synaptic plasticity. In this study, learning and memory were evaluated via Morris water maze (MWM), and the ultrastructure of hippocampal CA1 neurons was examined by electron microscopy. Hippocampal synaptic plasticity was assessed by long-term potentiation (LTP). The expression of *N*-methyl-D-aspartic acid receptor 1 (NMDAR1), Bcl-2, and Bax proteins was assessed by Western plot. Bcl-2 promotes cell survival and Bax promotes cell death. LTP is considered essential for cognition and the synaptic plasticity is the cellular basis for memory formation and cognition. Yang et al., applied rTMS for 600 s daily for 10 days during a 2-week period. Rats treated with rTMS had reduced escape latencies, increased swimming time and significantly less synaptic structure damage. The results show that rTMS improves learning and memory, protects the synapse, and increases synaptic plasticity in VaD model rats. In conclusion, increased Bcl-2 expression—upregulation—and reduced Bax expression—downregulation—may be a novel protective mechanism of rTMS treatment for VaD.

Using a rat spinal cord injury (SCI)-induced pain model, Kim et al. (2013) studied the effectiveness of high-frequency (25 Hz) 0.2 T rTMS and the relationship between the modulation of pain and the changes of neuroglial expression. In order to clarify this, the attenuation of microglial and astroglial activations in the spinal cord below injuries by rTMS was investigated in relation to the modulation of pain after SCI. A round type coil (7 cm diameter) of biphasic current waveform was positioned around the bregma at 1 cm from the skull of the SD rats. The parameters of stimulation were as follows: biphasic current waveform, 370 μs, 0.2 T, 25 Hz repetition rate, 3 s on/off cycle for 20 min. The stimulations were applied 5 days/week for 8 weeks from the 4th day after SCI. Elevated expressions of Iba1 and glial fibrillary acidic protein (GFAP), the markers of microglial and astrocyte, were observed in dorsal and ventral horns respectively at the L4 and L5 levels in SCI rats. In SCI rats treated with rTMS, these expressions were significantly reduced by about 30%. This study suggests that the attenuation of activation is related to pain modulation after SCI.

10.5.2.2 Effects of tDCS on Neurobiological System

tDCS can be used to induce changes in cortical excitability by passing a weak constant current of about 1–2 mA to the brain through the paired saline-filled electrodes placed on the scalp above cortical area. The constant DC may be passed for 5–20 min.

Here, focusing on the neurobiological system, recently obtained experimental results from *in vitro* and *in vivo* studies are discussed briefly. This is essential and the first step for a full understanding of the neurobiological effects of tDCS.

10.5.2.2.1 Effects of tDCS on Neural System

Although tDCS is a noninvasive brain stimulation to modulate cortical excitability, which cellular compartments mediate changes in cortical excitability remains unaddressed. Cellular compartments include somas, dendrites, axons and their terminals. They note that increased/decreased excitability under the anode/cathode electrode is nominally associated with membrane depolarization/hyperpolarization. Using rat cortical brain slices (motor cortex), Rahman et al. (2013) considered the acute effects of DCS on excitatory synaptic efficacy. Cortical brain slices were prepared from male young adult Wistar rats aged 3–6 weeks. These results suggest that somatic polarization together with axon terminal polarization may be important for synaptic pathway-specific modulation of DCS. In conclusion, synaptic efficacy occurs at somata and axon terminals during acute DCS. This efficacy depends on the direction of cortical current flow. This underlies modulation of neuronal excitability during tDCS.

Jiang et al. (2012) investigated the effects of tDCS on hemichannel pannexin-1 (PX1) in cortical neurons and neural plasticity in the early stage of cerebral ischemia. It is suggested that ischemia may induce opening of the hemichannel pannexin-1, which leads to the increase of membrane permeability and ionic dysregulation. The opening of the hemichannel pannexin-1 leads to changes in neuron excitability and intercellular communication after ischemic injury. Anodal and cathodal tDCS were applied for 30 min each day starting on day 1 after stroke. tDCS parameters were set to a frequency of 10 Hz and current intensity of 0.1 mA. Adult male Sprague-Dawley rats received tDCS daily and were killed on the 3rd, 7th, and 14th days after tDCS application. Density of denditic spines (DS) and PX1 mRNA expression were compared among groups. Motor function was assessed using the beam walking test. This study showed that daily anodal tDCS application to the ipsilesional cortex and daily cathodal tDCS application to the contralesional cortex for 30 min after cerebral infarction increased significantly the density of dendritic spines of cortical neurons on day 3, 7, and 14 after stroke. An increase of PX1 mRNA expression on days 3, 7, and 14 was induced. In addition, tDCS did not decrease the upregulated PX1 mRNA expression after stroke on day 3. tDCS increased the DS density after stroke. This indicates that the application of tDC may promote neural plasticity after stroke.

A tDCS-induced LTP in mouse motor cortex and a polarity-specific modulation of LTP induction in the rat hippocampus has been demonstrated. A link between DCS and synaptic plasticity has been established by experimental studies using an animal model. Ranieri et al. (2012) evaluated the effects of anodal and cathodal DCS on rat brain slice on long-term potentiation (LTP). To do this, they investigated the effects of anodal and cathodal DCS on Male Wistar rat coronal hippocampal slices on LTP and evaluated the mechanism underlying the observed effects of DCS on synaptic plasticity. And then, they explored the effect of DCS on the expression of two immediate early genes, *c-fos* and *zif268*. DCS was applied to the brain slice through two Ag-AgCl electrodes with 9 mm diameter submerged in artificial cerebrospinal fluid (aCSF) and connected to two poles of the DC stimulator. From this stimulator, a current 200–250 μA was delivered for 20 min. The expression of *zif268* protein in the cornus ammonis (CA) region was increased in a subregion-specific manner after the application of both anodal and cathodal DCS. And in the CA and in dentate gyrus regions of hippocampal, the increase of *c-fos* protein expression was less pronounced. Brain-derived neurotrophic factor (BDNF) expression was found to be reduced in cathodal DCS stimulated slices. In conclusion, DCS modulates LTP induction in a polarity-specific manner and affects gene expression.

There are few reports on the effects of noninvasive brain stimulation on glial cells. The glial cells are active participants in brain function and maintain homeostasis, modulate neurotransmission, and control blood flow to regions of brain activity (Barres, 2008). Among glial cells, astrocytes respond to neuronal activity and are the most numerous cell type in the brain. The activity of astrocytes may contribute to LTP by activating postsynaptic membrane. Microglial cells also play important roles in synaptic plasticity. Ruohonen and Karhu (2012) explored the possibility that tDCS of the brain affects glial cells. As a theoretical calculation, cable theory is used to estimate transmembrane potentials in neurons and glial cells. Based on the simplified cable theory, tDCS may affect the transmembrane of glial cells and the balance of neurotransmitters. This gives the possibility that tDCS could manipulate glial cell because glial cells are active participants in brain function.

10.5.2.2.2 *Effects of tDCS on Neurotransmission*

Tanaka et al. (2013) investigated whether the application of cathodal and anodal tDCS affects extracellular dopamine (DA) and serotonin (5-HT) levels in the rat striatum. Cathodal and anodal tDCS was applied for 10 min with a current of 800 μA; the current density was 32.0 A/m^2 from an electrode attached on the skin of the scalp (STG1002; Multi Channel Systems, Germany). Using in vivo microdialysis, the changes of extracellular dopamine level in the basal ganglia induced by tDCS was measured. This method measures directly dopamine level via a probe inserted into a target brain region. Dialysis samples were collected every 10 min until at least 4,000 min after the stimulation. Following the application of cathodal tDCS foe 10 min, extracellular dopamine levels increased for more than

400 min. There were no significant changes in extracellular serotonin levels. In conclusion, cathodal tDCS applied to frontal cortex but not anodal tDCS increased DA release in the dorsal striatum, 5-HT release was not affected. This suggests that tDCS has a direct and/or indirect effect on the dopaminergic system in the subcortical area.

10.5.2.2.3 Effects of tDCS on Oxidative Response and Cell Death

Pikhovych et al. (2016) studied the effect of multisession tDCS on microglia activation and neurogenesis, endogenous neural stem cells, in the mouse brain. Twenty male 10–12 weeks old C57BL/6JRj mice were randomly divided into five different groups. At each group, mice were received 10 days of anodal- and cathodal-tDCS with different currents of 250 or 500 μA. The fifth was the control (no tDCS) group. Mice received 10 days of tDCS. tDCS was applied continuously for 15 min using a constant current stimulator (CX-6650, Schneider Electronics, Gleichen, Germany). The anesthetized mouse was connected to the stimulator via a silver-coated electrode. Mice were euthanized by decapitation 2 days after the last tDCS session. Frozen brains were cut into coronal sections of 10 μm. Activated microglia in the cerebral cortex and neuroblasts generated in the subventricular zone were assessed. Both anodal and cathodal tDCS induced neurogenesis from the subventricular zone. This data suggests that tDCS elicits its action through immunomodulation and neurogenesis and the effects of tDCS may be animal- and polarity-specific.

The effect of multisession tDCS in the rat brain *in vivo* has been studied (Rueger et al., 2012). Adult Wistar rats were divided into either anodal or cathodal stimulation for either 5 or 10 consecutive days (500 μA, 15 min) with a constant current stimulator (CX-6650, Schneider Electronics, Gleichen, Germany). Inflammatory and regenerative processes with tDCS have been demonstrated to occur in the absence of cortical lesion after 5 and 10 consecutive days of multi-session tDCS. Both anodal and cathodal tDCS induced an innate immune response with early upregulation of Iba1-positive activated microglia. Only cathodal tDCS increased the number of endogenous neural stem cells (NSC) in the stimulated cortex. tDCS attracts cells inflicted in reparative and regenerative responses in the stimulated site. This data suggests that tDCS in human stroke patients might elicit NSC activation and modulate neuroinflammation.

10.5.3 The Evaluation of Magnetic Field Exposure during the Operation of TMS

During the TMS treatment, the subjects/patients and medical staffs are exposed to pulsed magnetic fields. The evaluations of exposure of these persons during the TMS treatment will be given briefly. TMS uses a pulsed magnetic field that induces electric currents in the neurons of the brain to cause de-polarization of hyper-polarization. In use of TMS, the magnetic field strength of TMS coils falls off so rapidly with distance from the surface of the stimulating coil. However, the magnetic field spills over to medical staffs. The safety analysis is rarely addressed for medical staffs (Karlström et al., 2006; Møllerløkken et al., 2017).

10.5.3.1 Magnetic Field Exposure for Subjects and Patients

A single session of TMS (rTMS) does not carry the risk of significant pulsed magnetic field exposure since the total time is too short (Loo et al., 2008; Rossi et al., 2009). Given a TMS pulse duration of 250 μs, a typical treatment course of rTMS as used in psychiatric disorder application (e.g., 10 Hz, 20×5 s trains, 20 sessions) yields about 5 s of total exposure (Loo et al., 2008). It is unclear whether the high-intensity, pulsed stimulation involved TMS has the same biological implications as the chronic, low-intensity public and occupational exposures (Loo et al., 2008). The prospective studies would be desirable because of no clear effects of long-term exposure to subjects and patients during the operation of TMS (rTMS).

10.5.3.2 Magnetic Field Exposure for Medical Staffs

Similar to the subjects and patients, safety considerations during the operation of TMS (rTMS) are rarely addressed for medical staffs exposed to pulsed magnetic field. It is judicious for TMS (rTMS) medical staffs to position themselves within the room as far away from the stimulating coil as practical (Rossi et al., 2009).

The Swedish research group investigated the effects of pulsed magnetic field on the medical staffs during the treatment with TMS/rTMS (Karlström et al., 2006). The TMS/rTMS system used in this study was MegPro unit with a magnetic coil transducer model MC-B70 (Medtronic). The principles of localized TMS magnetic stimulation are summarized and the risk and level of occupational field exposure of the medical staffs is analyzed with reference to ICNIRP guidelines for pulsed magnetic fields below 100 kHz in ICNIRP (2003a). Measurements and analysis of the occupational exposure of the medical staffs to pulsed magnetic field, working with the TMS/rTMS system, are presented. In this conclusion, workers exposure limits for the pulsed magnetic field are at a distance of about 70 cm from the surface of the stimulating coil. The medical staffs can be exposed to magnetic field levels exceeding both EMF Directive 2013/35/EU and ICNIRP guidelines. It is recommended that unnecessary exposure is limited. In the case of TMS, medical staff should not work at a distance of less than 70 cm from the transducer (Karlström et al., 2006). Medical staff exposure can be reduced relatively easily by mounting the coil on a mechanically arm close to the patients (Karlström et al., 2006; Stamm, 2014).

Møllerløkken et al. (2017) from Norway investigated the exposure of the medical staff working with the MagVenture TMS/rTMS system with a figure-eight coil and no presence of the patient, through measurements of pulsed magnetic field at varying distances from the emitting coil and different power setting (94–127 A/s), in relation to the occupational exposure limits given by the EMF Directive 2013/35/EU. In addition, their aim was to find the potential hazard zone surrounding the TMS unit. Fourteen measurements were done which displayed exposures exceeding the given guidelines up to a distance of 40 cm from the stimulating coil. The study shows that the exposure of the medical staffs in this type of treatment may exceed the given guidelines for occupational exposure. This necessitates good routines in information and treatment procedures to avoid this exposure.

Bottauscio et al. (2014, 2016) calculated the electric current densities induced inside a human head model based on a voxel dataset (Virtual Family, Duke mode) by TMS and investigated the exposure experienced by the staff executing TMS. They propose a shielding system composed of an aluminum half cylinder placed around the stimulating coil. The analysis used the Duke anatomical model (Virtual Family) to represent the nursing staff and calculated with a finite-element approach. Their calculation shows operator exposure exceeds the basic restrictions suggested by the guidelines of the ICNIRP, when the distance from the coil decreases below 64 cm, and the minimal distance is reduced to 38 cm by the conductive shield. In addition, the medical staff exposure reduces when the stimulating coil is above the operator's head, while it worsens as the position of the coil descends at the height of shoulders and chest. For TMS, worker exposure can be reduced easily by mounting coil close to the patient. Zucca et al. (2017) show the introduction of the passive shield around the TMS coils does not affect the diagnostic and/or therapeutic treatment. The presence of a passive conductive shield reduces the exposure levels on the operator's side. In this study, they developed, using of the Duke anatomical model of the

Virtual Family dataset, models of patient head, and the operator body. Two commercially available stimulators (with a circular spiral coil and a figure-of-eight shaped coil) were considered in order to quantify the effectiveness of passive shield.

These observations and calculations make necessary further research to confirm the safety operation of TMS and to determine the limiting distance to the stimulating coil.

10.5.4 Guidelines and Safety Consideration Related to TMS

The International Commission on Non-Ionizing Radiation Protection (ICNIRP) published two guidelines, which are for static magnetic field and for low frequency electromagnetic fields (up to 100 kHz) (ICNIRP, 2009a, 2010, 2014). Using these guidelines, the European Parliament proposed the EMF Directive.

This EMF Directive 2013/35/EU addresses all known biophysical effects and indirect effects caused by electromagnetic fields (up to 300 GHz) in order not only to ensure the health and safety of each worker on an individual basis, but also to create a minimum basis of protection for all workers in the European Union (European Parliament and Council, 2013).

The EMF Directive 2013/35/EU gives exposure limit values (ELVs): health effect ELVs and sensory effect ELVs and action levels (ALs), which are aimed to prevent adverse health effects. In the Directive 2013/35/EU, it is stated that it is necessary to introduce measures protecting workers from the risks associated with electromagnetic fields, owing to their effects on the health and safety of workers.

The advantage of TMS use is noninvasiveness. It has the possibility to stimulate localized small brain areas. This indicates that the risk and safety assessment are needed for the use of TMS. Historically, Wassermann (1998) reported in the review of TMS, the known potential adverse effects of rTMS such as seizure induction, effects on cognition, effects on mood, transient effects on hormones, transient effect on lymphocytes, transient auditory threshold shift, pain and headache, burns from scalp electrodes, psychological consequences of induced seizure, based on a Workshop discussion held in June 1996.

10.5.4.1 Time-Varying Electromagnetic Fields

The TMS and rTMS high-intensity, fast magnetic pulses induce a rapid polarization of the nerve cells though the induction of eddy current in targeted area. This means that safety guidelines have been discussed for avoiding excitation of the central nervous system (ICNIRP, 1998, 2010; WHO, 2007).

The ICNIRP published guideline for limiting exposure to time-varying electric and magnetic field in the frequencies range between 1 Hz and 100 kHz (see Tables 2–4 in ICNIRP 2010, 2014). This guideline has two separate guidances for occupational exposure and for the public. Occupational exposure refers to healthy adults exposed to time-varying electric and magnetic fields from 1 Hz to 10 MHz at their workplaces. This guideline was based on established evidence of the acute effects for protection from the nervous system effects. The then established adverse effects include perception of surface electric charge, direct stimulation of nerve and muscle tissues and induction of retinal phosphenes. Based on the ICNIRP guidelines, the European Parliament introduced its Directive.

Basic restrictions for human exposure to time-varying electric and magnetic fields in the frequencies range between 1 Hz and 10 MHz are shown (see Table 2 in ICNIRP 2010, 2014). Basic restrictions are specified in term of the induced electric field strength to prevent nervous system response including peripheral (PNS) and central nerve stimulation (CNS) and the induction of magnetophosphenes.

Reference levels are obtained from the basic restrictions by mathematical modeling (see Table 4 in ICNIRP (2010, 2014). Because of the physical quantities, the induced electric field (V/m) and specific absorption rate (SAR) in the body cannot be measured directly, the reference levels up to 10 MHz are set using of the strength of incident electric and magnetic fields (unperturbed values) in the ICNIRP guideline (ICNIRP, 2010). According to the guideline, occupational exposure below the reference levels assures that the basic restrictions are not exceeded.

Guidelines for TMS (rTMS) have not been established. The present understanding is that TMS appear to be safe a technique in the case of using of current safety guidelines (Groppa et al., 2012; Loo et al., 2008; O'Reardon et al., 2007; Perera et al., 2016; Rossi et al., 2009; VonLoh et al., 2013; Wassermann, 1998).

Exposure to TMS is extremely short compared with environmental sources such as electrical appliances. The field strength produced by TMS is an approximately 2 T, and this field strength is nearly similar to the static magnetic field strength produced by clinically used MRI systems. The difference between MRI and TMS is the total exposure time. The total exposure time during the TMS procedure is extremely short.

Loo et al. (2008) pointed out that long-term exposure effects of subjects and experimenters to the high-intensity pulsed magnetic fields involved in TMS are yet unknown. However, there is no evidence of adverse effects from magnetic field exposure during TMS. The extensive review on TMS study has been published by the TMS study group.

10.5.4.2 Safety Guidelines of TMS in Therapeutic Applications

The report of TMS safety study group, on behalf of the International Federation of Clinical Neurophysiology (IFCN), provided updated-detailed guidelines, which cover issues of risk and safety of the use of TMS in clinical practice and research (Rossi et al., 2009). The report addressed the undesired effects and risks of emerging TMS interventions, the applications of TMS in patients with implanted electrodes in the central nervous system, and safety aspects of TMS in neuroimaging environments. In their report, they recommended limits of stimulation parameters and other important precautions, monitoring of subjects, expertise of the rTMS team, and ethical issues.

Based on the report of IFCN, Groppa et al. (2012) described how TMS can be used diagnostically to detect an impairment of central motor conduction in corticospinal or corticobulbar pathways. Then they lay out the general principles that apply to a standardized clinical examination with single-pulse TMS. In total, they give a practical guide to diagnostic TMS. Including a practical guide, their guidelines cover the practical aspects of TMS in a clinical setting. They discussed the technical and physiological aspects of TMS that are relevant for its diagnostic use. To this purpose, they published an updated version of a 15 item standard questionnaire for the screening of every candidate before TMS investigations (Rossi et al., 2011). The article published by IFCN provides safety and ethical guidelines for the clinical use of TMS. It is mentioned that they pay no attention to human health problems from exposure to pulsed magnetic fields utilized in TMS and MRI.

Generally speaking, as the technologies advance, MRI can be routinely used for diagnosis in many hospitals and TMS can be used fundamentally for brain research and therapeutic applications. TMS has been developed significantly and gradually for neurological diseases and mental illnesses in recent years. However, there has not been enough research for health effects from the magnetic field exposure during TMS (Wassermann et al., 1996, 1998; Wassermann and Zimmermann, 2012).

Our scientific understanding of the physical and biological effects of electromagnetic fields has been gradually improved from much research. These studies provide valuable insight into the fundamental mechanisms of the electromagnetic fields associated with MRI/TMS. Since the introduction of MRI as a diagnostic technique, the patients, MRI staffs, and other workers exposed to electromagnetic field generated during MRI diagnostic scan has increased. A need is gradually grown regarding the understanding of the health effects related to MRI and TMS and maintaining the safety of the patients and the medical staff. However, the overall health risk assessment of the magnetic field associated with the MRI/TMS examinations is incomplete due to the lack of enough scientific understanding.

Now, the EMF Directive 2013/35/EU laid down the minimum safety requirements regarding the exposure of workers to risks arising from electromagnetic fields (European Parliament and Council, 2013). And this EMF Directive came into force on 1 July 2016. The goal of this EMF Directive includes generally the protection of the health and safety of workers and the creation of a minimum basis of protection for worker. This EMF Directive 2013/35/EU was officially adopted to protect against effect of occupational exposure to electromagnetic field in the frequency range up to 300 GHz during work based on the recommendations of the ICNIRP.

Stam (2014) pointed out that the high action levels for magnetic fields in the EMF Directive on workers exposed to magnetic fields can be exceeded at workplaces near medical equipment of MRI and TMS, etc.

The EMF Directive contains three derogations from its exposure limit requirements: no application of the exposure limits in relation to the use of MRI scanner, military activities, and limited derogations for industrial activities.

Taking this EMF Directive 2013/35/EU into consideration, the European Commission published the practical guide entitled "Non-binding guide to good practice for implementation of EMF Directive 2013/35/EU on electromagnetic fields" (European Commission, 2015). This practical guide has three volumes and was published before the Directive came into effect. The practical guide, volume 1, gives advice on carrying out risk assessment. Volume 2 presents twelve case studies. Volume 3 assists for carrying out an initial assessment of the risks from electromagnetic fields in workplace. This practical guide is very useful for workers, employer, and regulatory authorities.

ICNIRP published statements on diagnostic devices using nonionizing radiation (ICNIRP, 2017). This statement (1) reviews the range of diagnostic nonionizing radiation (NIR) devices (including MRI and rTMS) currently used in clinical settings, (2) documents the relevant regulations and policies covering patients and health care workers, (3) reviews the evidence around potential health risks to patients and health care workers exposed to diagnostic NIR, and (4) identifies situations of high NIR exposure from diagnostic devices in which patients or health care workers might not be adequately protected by current regulations. This document introduces the guidelines or regulations for protection of patients and workers and the National and international organizations responsible for regulations. For safety use of diagnostic devices with MRI and TMS, this document gives the useful information.

10.5.4.3 Safety Aspects of the TMS and TES in Therapeutic Applications

Evidence-based guidelines on the therapeutic uses of rTMS and tDCS issued by a group of European experts of the European Chapter of the International Federation of Clinical Neurophysiology are presented (Lefaucheur et al., 2014, 2017).

In order to establish the evidence-based guidelines of rTMS, the expert group of Europe was commissioned. This group evaluated the evidence from numerous published papers up until March 2014, which include pain, movement disorders such as PD, stroke, amyotrophic lateral sclerosis, multiple sclerosis, epilepsy, consciousness disorders, tinnitus, depression, anxiety disorders, obsessive-compulsive disorder, schizophrenia, craving/addiction, and conversion (Lefaucheur et al., 2014). From evaluations of this group, there is a sufficient body of evidence for acceptance of Level A recommendation (definite efficacy) for the analgesic effect of high-frequency rTMS of the primary motor cortex (M1) contralateral to the pain and the antidepressant effect of high-frequency rTMS of the left dorsolateral prefrontal cortex (DLPFC). The proposed of Level B recommendation (probable efficacy) is for the antidepressant effect of low-frequency rTMS of the right DLPFC, high-frequency rTMS of the left DLPFC for the negative symptoms of schizophrenia and low-frequency rTMS of contralesional M1 in chronic motor stroke. A Level C recommendation (possible efficacy) includes low-frequency rTMS of the left TP cortex in tinnitus and auditory hallucinations. The group mentioned that it remains to be determined how to optimize rTMS protocols and techniques to give them relevance in routine clinical practice. This group highlights that (1) numerous studies have shown that rTMS produced significant clinical effects in patients with various neurological and psychiatric disorders, and (2) Level A or B evidence supports an efficacy of rTMS protocols in depression, pain, motor stroke, and schizophrenia.

In addition to the earlier evidence-based guidelines for rTMS, the same group opened the evidence-based guidelines of tDCS after the evaluation of numerous published papers up until September 2016 (Lefaucheur et al., 2017). The group gathered knowledge about the state of the art of the therapeutic use of tDCS, which include PD, other movement disorders, AD, tinnitus, depression, schizophrenia, and craving/addiction. From evaluations of this group, current evidence did not allow making any recommendation of Level A (definite efficacy) for any indication. The recommendations of Level B (probable efficacy) are proposed for (1) anodal tDCS of the left primary motor cortex (M1) (with right orbitofrontal cathode) in fibromyalgia, (2) anodal tDCS of the left dorosolateral prefrontal cortex (DLPFC) (with right orbitofrontal cathode) in major depressive episode without drug resistance, and (3) anodal tDCS of the right DLPFC (with left DLPFC cathode) in addiction/craving. A Level C recommendation (possible efficacy) is proposed for anodal tDCS of the left M1 (or contralateral to pain side, with right orbitofrontal cathode) in chronic lower limb neuropathic pain secondary to spinal cord lesion. This group commented that it remains to be clarified whether the probable or possible therapeutic effects of tDCS are clinically meaningful and how to optimally perform tDCS in a therapeutic setting. In summary, this group highlights (1) Level B evidence (probable efficacy) was found for fibromyalgia, depression, and craving, and (2) the therapeutic relevance of tDCS needs to be further explored in these and other indication.

Antal et al. (2017) updated the safety of low-intensity TES including tDCS based on available published research and clinical data in animal models and in human studies through the end of 2016. Here, low-intensity TES is defined as electric current intensities <4 mA, a total stimulation duration of up to 60 min/day, and electrode size between 1 and 100 cm^2 with frequencies between 0 and 10 kHz. Based on the overview of published papers, they discussed safety aspects of the stimulation and recent regulatory issues.

TMS technique appeared in its modern form in 1985 and became a technical success. MRI is a technical success for diagnosis, and now MRI scanners are in many hospitals. Thus, both MRI and TMS are noninvasive and effective technologies for diagnostic and rehabilitation uses. Both technologies are based on the utilization of electromagnetic fields. As

MRI and TMS technologies advance, there is a growing need for understanding the health effects of MRI and TMS for maintaining the safety of the patients and medical staffs. This means that the safety use of MRI and TMS should be harmonized with the understanding of biological and health effects of the electromagnetic fields utilized in both technologies.

In future, the study of personnel working should be conducted to investigate the health effects of exposure to the electromagnetic fields. It would also ensure a safe working environment for the medical staff in line with National and International guidelines and the EMF Directive 2013/35/EU. Such fruitful research and understanding of TMS and TES (tDCS) will improve their ability as therapeutic potentials, both by answering the questions of the health effect and to treat diseases.

10.6 New Horizons

Through the principles and applications of transcranial magnetic and electric stimulation we discussed in this chapter, the field of human brain stimulation has opened new horizons in brain research and medical applications. The area of transcranial magnetic and electric stimulation is an interdisciplinary field mostly related to bioelectromagnetics and bioengineering where magnetics, electrical engineering, physics, biology, and medicine overlap.

Here, as concluding remarks, we discuss the recent advances in transcranial magnetic stimulation and transcranial electric stimulation to envision new horizons in the interdisciplinary fields.

10.6.1 Deep Brain Stimulation for Therapeutic Application

A method of deep brain stimulation (DBS) with implanted electrodes has been used for the treatments of brain dysfunctions. As reviewed by Kringelbach et al (2007), the DBS has brought good news for patients who are afflicted with, for example, unbearable chronic pain, resistant movement, and affective disorders including major depression. Although DBS is a powerful tool, it is an invasive method to insert and implant electrodes inside the deeper part of the brain.

If an alternative noninvasive method for deep brain stimulation is introduced, new horizons will be opened in this area. The transcranial magnetic stimulation (TMS) is a promising potential tool for the realization of deep brain stimulation. In researching deep TMS (dTMS), several attempts have been reported. There are several coil configurations potentially suitable for dTMS; double cone, H-coil, and Halo coils.

The double cone coil (Lontis et al., 2006; Roth et al., 2002; Ugawa et al., 1995) operates on the same principle as the figure-eight coil configuration where a pair of opposing directed time-varying magnetic fields around a target increase induced electric fields in the targeted areas (Ueno et al., 1988). The two circular coils have a fixed angle between them, and their diameter is larger than that of the figure-eight coil. The double-cone coil induces a greater electric field intensity to stimulate the deeper brain regions compared with other coils. However, the surrounding large areas in the brain are also stimulated. In other words, the focality, i.e., the degree in focalization or degree in focusing, is poor, and undesirable areas are also simultaneously stimulated by the double-cone coil system.

Another coil configuration for dTMS is called the H-coil (Roth et al., 2007; Zangen et al., 2005). The H-coils have complex winding patterns based on numerical calculations of three-dimensional brain phantom models to achieve effective stimulation of deep brain structures and are used for the treatment of a variety of psychiatric and neurological disorders. Although the H-coils are used for clinical applications, nontargeted areas of the brain are also stimulated.

A family of dTMS coil designs called the Halo coil was proposed to increase the induced electric fields at depth in the brain (Crowther et al., 2011). The Halo coil system is composed of a small coil on the top of the head and a large circular coil around the head, called Halo-circular assembly (HCA) coil.

Computational studies were carried out in order to evaluate the focality of these three types of coil configurations (Lu and Ueno, 2013, 2015, 2017). Three-dimensional distributions of the induced electric fields in realistic head models by dTMS coils were calculated by an impedance method, and the results were compared with that of a standard figure-eight coil (Ueno et al., 1988, 1990). Simulation results show that double cone and H-coils have deep field penetration at the expense of higher and wider spread induced electric fields in superficial cortical regions. The double cone and HCA coils have better ability to stimulate deep brain subregions compared to that of the H-coil. In the meantime, both double cone and HCA coils increase the risk for optical nerve excitation (Lu and Ueno, 2017).

In order to reduce the risk for optical nerve stimulation and increase focality in deep brain stimulation, another new coil configuration system was proposed (Lu and Ueno, 2015). The proposed system is composed of a Halo coil and two circular coils (HTC coil). For the HTC coil with currents flowing in opposite direction in the neighboring coils, over-threshold electric fields can be produced in deep brain regions, while the subthreshold fields are produced in superficial cortical areas. The HTC coil with varied coil parameters and different injected currents provides a flexible way for deep brain stimulation with better ratio of deep region field relative to field at the shallow areas.

A series of the simulation studies suggest that although the dTMS coils offer a new tool with potential for both research and clinical applications for psychiatric and neurological disorders associated with dysfunctions of deep brain regions, the selection of the most suitable coil settings for a specific clinical application should be based on a balanced evaluation between stimulation depth and focality (Lu and Ueno, 2017). Further studies are needed for better focality in deep TMS.

The studies on TMS and reward circuits in the brain are important and interesting for the understanding of the neuronal connectivity in the brain as well as for the potential treatments of dysfunctions such as depression and PD. For example, Wassermann's group have studied reward-related activity in the human motor cortex (Kapogiannis et al., 2008), modulation of corticospinal excitability by reward (Mooshagian et al., 2015), reward processing abnormalities in Parkinson disease (Kapogiannis et al., 2011), and so on. The study concludes that TMS of the human primary motor cortex M1 may be useful as a quantitative measure of reward-related activity (Kapogiannis et al., 2008).

As we discussed in Section 10.4, it seems that rTMS, tDCS, and other brain stimulation techniques are promising for treatments of depression and other psychiatric disorders (Fitzgerald and Daskalakis, 2012; Fitzgerald et al., 2013).

In 2011, Fitzgerald reviewed the current state of development and application of a wide range of brain stimulation approaches in the treatment of disorders (Fitzgerald, 2011). The brain stimulation methods that he reviewed include vagus nerve stimulation, rTMS, tDCS, ECT, and magnetic seizure therapy. The review concludes that it appears likely that the range of psychiatric treatments available for patients will grow over the coming years to progressively include a number of novel brain stimulation techniques.

In 2013, Enticott et al. (2013) examined a double-blind, randomized trial of deep rTMS for autism spectrum disorder and came to the following conclusion: Deep rTMS to bilateral dorsomedial PFC yielded a reduction in social relating impairment and socially related anxiety.

Further studies are needed in the area of deep TMS.

10.6.2 Combination of TMS/tDCS with DTI and EEG

Dynamic brain electrical activities elicited by TMS have been studied by the combinations of TMS with diffusion tensor imaging (DTI), TMS with electroencephalographic (EEG) measurements, TMS with functional magnetic resonance imaging (fMRI), and so on.

The invention of DTI and *in vivo* fiber tractography (Basser et al., 1994, 2000) contribute to the studies on DTI-based neural trajectories in TMS. De Geeter and her coworkers (2012) studied a DTI-based model for TMS and effective electric fields along realistic neural trajectories for modeling the stimulation mechanisms of TMS. Based on their model, De Geeter et al. (2015) focused on the stimulation of the hand area of the left primary motor cortex, M1, with a figure-eight coil (Ueno et al., 1988, 1990) to get deeper insights on the stimulation mechanisms. The studies using DTI and TMS are useful to visualize exciting fronts and neural trajectories and also to improve and integrate the early proposed models of nerve excitation elicited by magnetic stimulation (Basser et al., 1992; Hyodo and Ueno, 1996; Liu and Ueno, 2000; Lu et al., 2008; Nagarajan et al., 1993; Roth and Basser, 1990; Ueno et al., 1991).

EEG measurements just after the onset of brain stimulation by TMS are important to study dynamic neuronal connectivity in the brain in a high temporal (msec) and high spatial (mm) resolution. Ilmoniemi et al. (1997) successfully measured neuronal electrical responses to magnetic stimulation. The combination of TMS with simultaneous EEG has enabled us to study dynamic intra- and interhemispheric interactions, cortical inhibitory processes, cortical plasticity and oscillations, and so on (Ilmoniemi and Dubravko, 2010; Ilmoniemi and Dubravko, 2010; Iramina et al., 2002, 2003; Iwahashi et al., 2009; Maki and Ilmoniemi, (2010); Torii et al., 2012; Marshall et al., 2015; Raij et al., 2008).

The combination of TMS with fMRI or DTI is also interesting and important. In the severe electromagnetic noise environment caused by TMS, it is rather difficult to combine TMS with simultaneous fMRI or DTI, but data of fMRI and DTI are used for studying the effects of TMS on the changes in functional organization of the brain. For example, Fox et al. (2012) reviewed studies on the measuring and manipulating brain connectivity with resting state functional connectivity MRI (fcMRI) and TMS, classifying many publications into three general network properties; anatomical connectivity, functional connectivity, and response to perturbation/stimulation. TMS is a useful noninvasive method to assess brain connectivity in human subjects noninvasively for controlled, individualized neuronal network modulation.

Transcranial magnetic stimulation and transcranial electric stimulation are thus leading medicine and biology into new horizons through their novel applications of electricity, electromagnetism, and computational electromagnetism. With the increasing integration of medicine and engineering, transcranial magnetic and electric stimulation accelerates neuroscience and medicine related to brain research and treatments. Studies of safety aspects and guidelines in this field should be consistently continued.

Acknowledgments

The authors thank Drs. T. Tashiro, T. Matsuda, M. Fujiki, K. Iramina, O. Hiwaki, A. Hyodo, R. Liu, M. Ogiue-Ikeda, H. Funamizu, T. Maeno, C. M. Epstein, S. Sekino-Yamguchi, M. Lu, Y. Saitoh, S. Nakasono, K. Yamazaki, and other coworkers for their valuable cooperation and support for the studies this chapter.

References

Antal, A., Alekseichuk, I., Bikson, M., Brockmöller, J., Brunoni, A.R., Chen, R., Cohen, L.G., Dowthwaite, G., Ellrich, J., Flöel, A., Fregni, F., George, M.S., Hamilton, R., Haueisen, J., Herrmann, C.S., Hummel, F.C., Lefaucheur, J.P., Liebetanz, D., Loo, C.K., McCaig, C.D., Miniussi, C., Miranda, P.C., Moliadze, V., Nitsche, M.A., Nowak, R., Padberg, F., Pascual-Leone, A., Poppendieck, W., Priori, A., Rossi, S., Rossini, P.M., Rothwell, J., Rueger, M.A., Ruffini, G., Schellhorn, K., Siebner, H.R., Ugawa, Y., Wexler, A., Ziemann, U., Hallett, M., and Paulus, W. 2017. Low intensity transcranial electric stimulation: Safety, ethical, legal regulatory and application guidelines. *Clinical Neurophysiology*, 128, 1774–1809.

Baker, J.M., Rorden, C., and Fridriksson, J. 2010. Using transcranial direct-current stimulation to treat stroke patients with aphasia. *Stroke*, 41, 1229–1236.

Balassa, T., Varró, P., Elek, S., Drozdovsky, O., Szemersxzky, R., Világi, I., and Bárdos, G. 2013. Changes in synaptic efficacy in rat brain slices following extremely low-frequency magnetic field exposure at embryonic and early postnatal age. *International Journal of Developmental Neuroscience*, 31, 724–730.

Barker, A.T., Jalinous, R., and Freeston, I.L. 1985. Non-invasive magnetic stimulation of human motor cortex. *Lancet*, 325, 1106–1107.

Barker, A.T., Freeston, I.L., Jalinous, R., and Jarrat, J.A. 1987. Magnetic stimulation of the human brain and peripheral nervous system: An introduction and the results of an initial clinical evaluation. *Neurosurgery*, 20, 100–109.

Barres, B.A. 2008. The mystery and magic of glia: A perspective on their roles in health and disease. *Neuron*, 60, 430–440.

Basser, P.J., Wijesinghe, R. S., and Roth, B.J. 1992. The activating function for magnetic stimulation derived from a three-dimensional volume conductor model, *IEEE Transactions on Biomedical Engineering*, 39, 1207–1211.

Basser, P.J., Mattiello, J., and Le Bihan, D. 1994. Estimation of the effective self-diffusion tensor from the NMR spin echo. *Journal of Magnetic Resonance, B* 103, 247–254.

Basser, P.J., Pajevic, S., Pierpaoli, C., Duda, J., and Aldroubi, A. 2000. In vivo fiber tractography using DT-MRI data. *Magnetic Resonance in Medicine*, 44, 625–632.

Benninger, D.H., Lomarev, M., Lopez, G., Wassermann, E.M., Li, X., Considine, E., and Hallett, M. 2010. Transcranial direct current stimulation for the treatment of Parkinson's disease. *Journal of Neurology, Neurosurgery and Psychiatry*, 81, 1105–1111.

Benninger, D.H., Iseki, K., Kranick, S., Luckenbaugh, D.A., Houdayer, E., and Hallett, M. 2012. Controlled study of 50Hz repetitive transcranial magnetic stimulation for the treatment of Parkinson's disease. *Neurorehabilitation and Neural Repair*, 26, 1096–1105.

Berlim, M.T., Van den Eynde, F., and Daskalakis, Z.J. 2013. Clinical utility of transcranial direct current stimulaiton (tDCS) for treating major depression: A systematic review and meta-analysis of randomized, double-blind and sham-controlled trials. *Journal of Psychiatric Research*, 47, 1–7.

Bliss, T.V.P. and Lomo, T. 1973. Long-lasting potentiation of synaptic transmission in the dentate area of the anaesthetized rabbit following stimulation of the perforant path. *The Journal of Physiology*, 232, 357–74.

Boggio, P.S., Rigonatti, S.P., Ribeiro, R.B., Myczlowski, M.L., Nitsche, M.A., Pascual-Leone, A., and Fregni, F. 2008. A randomized, double-blind clinical trial on the efficacy of cortical direct current stimulation for the treatment of major depression. *International Journal of Neuropsychopharmacology*, 11, 249–254.

Boggio, P.S., Khoury, L.P., Mazrtins, D.C., Martins, O.E., deMacedo, E.C., and Fregni, F. 2009. Temporal cortex direct current stimulation nhances performance on a visual recognition memory task in Alzheimer disease. *J Neurology Neurosurgery and Psychiatry*, 80, 444–447.

Bottauscio, O., Chiampi, M., Zilberti, L., and Zucca, M. 2014. Evaluation of electromagnetic phenomena induced by transcranial magnetic stimulation. *IEEE Transactions on Magnetics*, 50, 1033–1036.

Bottauscio, O., Zucca, M., Chiampi, M., and Ziberti, L. 2016. Evaluation of the electric field induced in transcranial magnetic stimulation operators. *IEEE Transactions on Magnetics*, 52, ID.5000204.

Broeder, S., Nackaerts, E., Heremans, E., Vervoort, G., Meesen, R., Verheyden, G., and Nieuboer, A. 2015. Transcranial direct current stimulation in Parkinson's disease: Neurophysiological mechanisms and behavioral effects. *Neuroscience & Biobehavioral Reviews*. 57, 105–117.

Chandos, B., Khan, A., Lai, H., and Lin, J.C. 1996. The application of electromagnetic energy to the treatment of neurological and psychiatric diseases. In Ueno, S. (Ed.) *Biological Effects of Magnetic and Electromagnetic Fields*. Plenum Press, New York and London: pp. 161–169.

Chervyakov, A.V., Chernyavsky, A.Yu., Sinitsyn, D.O., and Piradov, M.A. 2015. Possible mechanisms underlying the therapeutic effects of transcranial magnetic stimulation. *Frontiers in Human Neuroscience*, 9, 303.

Christ, A., Kainz, W., Hahn, E.G., Honegger, K., Zefferer, M., Neufeld, E., Rascher, W., Janka, R., Bautz, W., Chen, J., Kiefer, B., Schmitt, P., Hollenbach, H.P., Shen, J., Oberle, M., Szczerba, D., Kam, A., Guag, J.W., and Kuster, N. 2010. The virtual family – development of surface-based anatomical models of two adults and two children for dosimetric simulations. *Physics in Medicine and Biology*, 55, 23–38.

Chou, Y.H., Hickey, P.T., Sundman, M., Song, A.W., and Chen, N.K. 2015. Effects of repetitive transcranial magnetic stimulation disease: A systematic review and meta-analysis. *JAMA Neurology*, 72, 432–440.

Chung, C.L., and Mak, M.K. 2016. Effect of repetitive transcranial magnetic stimulation on physical function and motor signs in Parkinson's disease: A systematic review and meta-analysis. *Brain Stimulation*, 9, 475–487.

Cirillo, G., Di Pino, G., Capone, F., Ranieri, F., Florio, I., Todisco, V., Tedeschi, G., Funke, K., and Di Lazzaro, V. 2017. Neurobiological after-effects of non-invasive brain stimulation. *Brain Stimulation*, 10, 1–18.

Crowther, L.J., Marketos, P., Williams, P.I., Melikhov, Y., and Jiles, D.C. 2011. Transcranial magnetic stimulation: Improved coil design for deep brain investigation. *Journal of Applied physics*, 109, 07B314.

Cullen, C.L., and Young, K.M. 2016. How does transcranial magnetic stimulation influence glial cells in the central nervous system? *Frontiers in Neural Circuits*, 10, 26.

De Geeter, N., Crevecoeur, G., Dupre, L., Van Hecke, W., and Leemans, A. 2012. A DTI-based model for TMS using the independent impedance method with frequency-dependent tissue parameters. *Physics in Medicine and Biology*, 57, 2169–2188.

De Geeter, N., Crevecoeur, G., Leemans, A., and Dupre, L. 2015. Effective electric fields along realistic DTI-based neural trajectories for modeling the stimulation mechanisms of TMS. *Physics in Medicine and Biology*, 60, 453–471.

De Sauvage, R.C., Beuter, A., Lagroye, I., and Veyret, B. 2010. Design and construction of a portable transcranial magnetic stimulation (TMS) apparatus for migraine treatment. *Journal of Medical Devices*, 4, 015002-1–6.

Edwardson, M.A., Lucas, T.H., Carey, J.R., and Fetz, E.E. 2013. New modalities of brain stimulation for stroke rehabilitation. *Experimental Brain Research*, 224, 335–358.

Enticott, P.G., Fitzgibbon, B.M., Kennedy, H.A., Arnold, S.L., Elliot, D., Peachey, A., Zangen, A., and Fitzgerald, P.B. 2013. Double-blind, randomized trial of deep repetitive transcranial magnetic stimulation (rTMS) for autism spectrum disorder. *Brain Stimulation*, 6, 1–6.

Epstein, C.M., Sekino, M., Yamaguchi, K., Kamiya, S., and Ueno, S. 2002. Asymmetries of prefrontal cortex in human episodic memory: Effects of transcranial magnetic stimulation on learning abstract patterns. *Neuroscience Letters*, 320, 5–8.

Epstein, C.M. 2008. A six-pound battery-powered portable transcranial magnetic stimulator. *Brain Stimulation*, 1, 128–130.

Etiévant, A., Manta, S., Latapy, C., Maqgno, L.A., Fecteau, S., and Beaulieu, J.M. 2015. Repetitive transcranial magnetic stimulation induces long-lasting changes in protein expression and histone acetylation. *Scientific Reports*, 5, 16873.

European Parliament and Council. 2013. Directive 2013/35/EU of the European Parliament and of the Council of 29 June 2013 on the minimum health and safety requirements regarding the exposure of workers to the *Neurology* risks arising from physical agents (electromagnetic fields) (20th individual Directive within the meaning of Article 16(1) of Directive 89/391/EEC) and repealing Directive 2004/40/EC. *Official Journal of the European Union*, 56, 1–21, L179.

European Commission. 2015. *Non-Binding Guide to Good Practice for Implementing Directive 2013/35/EU Electromagnetic Fields*. Vol. 1: Practical Guide, Vol. 2: Case Studies and Vol. 3: Specific Guide for SMEs. Directorate-General for Employment, Social Affairs and Inclusion. Publication Office of the European Union, Luxembourg.

FDA. 2011. *Guidance for Industry and Food and Drug Administration Staff-ClassII Special Controls Guidance Document: Repetitive Transcranial Magnetic Stimulation (rTMS) Systems*. FDA, Bethesda MD. www.fda.gov/RegulatoryInformation/Guidance/ucm265269.htm.

Ferrucci, R., Mameli, F., Guidi, I., Mrakic Sposta, S., Vergari, M., Marceglia, S., Cogiamanian, F., Barbieri, S., Scarpini, E., and Priori, A. 2008. Transcranial direct current stimulation improves recognition memory in Alzheimer disease. *Neurology*, 71, 493–498.

Fitzgerald, P.B. 2011. The emerging use of brain stimulation treatments for psychiatric disorders. *Australian and New Zealand Journal of Psychiatry*, 45, 923–938.

Fitzgerald, P.B., and Daskalakis, Z.J. 2012. A practical guide to the use of repetitive transcranial magnetic stimulation in the treatment of depression. *Brain Stimulation*, 5: 287–296.

Fitzgerald, P.J., Hoy, K.E., Singh, A., Gunewardene, R., Slack, C., Ibrahim, S., Hall, P.J., and Daskalakis, Z.J. 2013. Equivalent beneficial effects of unilateral and bilateral prefrontal cortex transcranial magnetic stimulation in a large randomized trial in treatment-resistant major depression. *International Journal of Neuropsychopharmacology*, 16, 1975–1984.

Flöel, A. 2014. tDCS-enhanced motor and cognitive function in neurological disease. *Neuroimage*, 85, 934–947.

Fox, M.D., Halko, M.A., Eldaief, M.C., and Pascual-Leone, A. 2012. Measuring and manipulating brain connectivity with resting state functional connectivity magnetic resonance imaging (fcMRI) and transcranial magnetic stimulation (TMS). *Neuroimaging*, 62, 2232–2243.

Fregni, F., Boggio, P.S., Santos, M.C., Lima, M., Vieira, A.L., Rigonatti, S.P., Silva, M.T., Barbosa, E.R., Nitsche, M.A., and Pascual-Leone, A. 2006. Noninvasive cortical stimulation with transcranial direct current stimulation in Parkinson's disease. *Movement Disorders*, 21, 1693–1702.

Fujiki, M., and Stewart, O. 1997. High frequency transcranial magnetic stimulation for protection against delayed neuronal death induced by transient ischemica. *Journal of Neurosurgery*, 99, 1063–1069.

Funamizu, H., Ogiue-Ikeda, M., Mukai, H., Kawato, S., and Ueno, S. 2005. Acute repetitive transcranial magnetic stimulation reactivates dopaminergic system in lesion rats. *Neuroscience Letters*, 383, 77–81.

Gabriel, C., Gabriel, S., and Corthout, E. 1996. The dielectric properties of biological tissues: I. Literature survey. *Physics in Medicine and Biology*, 41, 2231–2249.

Gabriel, S., Lau, R.W., and Gabriel, C. 1996. The dielectric properties of biological tissues: II. Measurements in the frequency range 10 Hz to 20 GHz. *Physics in Medicine and Biology*, 41, 2251–2269.

Georg, M.S., and Wassermann, E.M. 1994. Rapid-rate transcranial magnetic stimulation and ECT. *Convulsive Therapy*, 10, 251–254.

Gersner, R., Kravetz, E., Feil, J., Pell, G., and Zangen, A. 2011. Long-term effects of repetitive transcranial magnetic stimulation on markers for neuroplasticity: Differential outcomes in anesthetized and awake animals. *Journal of Neuroscience*, 31, 7521–7526.

Glickstein, S.B., Ilch, C.P., Reis, D.J., and Golanov, E.V. 2001. Stimulation of the subthalamic vasodilator area and fastigial nucleus independently protects the brain against focal ischemia. *Brain Research*, 912, 47–59.

Groppa, S., Oliviero, A., Eisen, A., Quartarone, A., Cohen, L.G., Mall, V., Kaelin-Lang, A., Mima, T., Rossi, S., Thickbroom, G.W., Rosini, P.M., Ziemann, U., Valls-Solé, J., and Siebner, H.R. 2012. A practical guide to diagnostic transcranial magnetic stimulation: Report of an IFCN Committee. *Clinical Neurophysiology*, 123, 858–882.

Guleyupoglu, B., Schestatsky, P., Edwards, D., Fregni, F., and Bikson, M. 2013. Classification of methods in transcranial electrical stimulation (tES) and evolving strategy from historical approaches to contemporary innovations. *Journal of Neuroscience Methods*, 219, 297–311.

Hedges, D.W., Salyer, D.L., Higginbotham, B.J., Lund, T.D., Hellewell, J.L., Ferguson, D., and Lephant, E.D. 2002. Transcranial magnetic stimulation (TMS) effects on testosterone, prolactin, and corticosterone in adult male rats. *Biological Psychiatry*, 51, 417–421.

Hesse, S., Wener, C., Schonhardt, E.M., Bardeleben, A., Jenrich, W., and Kirker, S.G.B. 2007. Combined transcranial direct current stimulation and robot-assisted arm training in subacute stroke patients: A pilot study. *Restorative Neurology and Neuroscience*, 25, 9–15.

Hesse, S., Waldner, A., Mehrholz, J., Tomelleri, C., Pohl, M., and Werner, C. 2011. Combined transcranial direct current stimulation and robot-assisted arm training in subacute stroke patients: An exploratory, randomized multicenter trial. *Neurorehabilitation and Neural Repair*, 25, 838–846.

Hoeltzell, P.B., and Dykes, R.W. 1979. Conductivity in the somatosensory cortex of the cat – evidence for cortical anisotropy. *Brain Research*, 177, 61–82.

Hosomi, K., Shomokawa, T., Ikoma, K., Nakamura, Y., Sugiyama, K., et al., 2013. Daily repetitive transcranial magnetic stimulation of primary motor cortex for neuropathic pain: A randomized, multicenter, double-blind, crossover, sham-controlled trial. *Pain*, 154, 1065–1072.

Hummel, F.C., Celnik, P., Giraux, P., Flöel, A., Wu, W.H., Gerloff, C., and Cohen, L.G. 2005. Effects of non-invasive cortical stimulation on skilled motor function in chronic stroke. *Brain*, 128, 490–499.

Hummel, F.C., Voller, B., Celnik, P., Flöel, A., Giraux, P., Gerloff, C., and Cohen, L.G. 2006. Effects of brain polarization on reaction times and pinch force in chronic stroke. *BMC Neuroscience*, 7, 73.

Hyodo, A., and Ueno, S. 1996. Nerve excitation model for localized magnetic stimulation of finite neuronal structures. *IEEE Transactions on Magnetics*, 32, 5112–5114.

IARC. 2002. *Non-Ionizing Radiation. Part 1: Static and Extremely Low Frequency (ELF) Electric and Magnetic Fields*. IARC Monographs on the Evaluation of Carcinogenic Risks to Humans, Volume 80. International Agency for Research Cancer, Lyon.

ICNIRP. 1998. Guidelines for limiting exposure to time-varying electric, magnetic, and electromagnetic fields (up to 300 GHz). *Health Physics*, 74, 494–522.

ICNIRP. 2003a. Guidelines on determining compliance of exposure to pulsed and complex non-sinusoidal waveforms below 100 kHz with ICNIRP guidelines. *Health Physics*, 84, 383–387.

ICNIRP. 2003b. *Exposure to Static and Low Frequency Electromagnetic Fields, Biological Effects and Health Consequences (0–100 kHz)*. Matthes, R., McKinlay, A.F., Bernhardt, J.H., Vecchia, O., Veyret, B. (Eds.) ICNIRP, Oberschleissheim.

ICNIRP. 2009a. Guidelines on limits to exposure from static magnetic fields. *Health Physics*, 96, 504–514.

ICNIRP. 2009b. *Exposure to High Frequency Electromagnetic Fields, Biological Effects and Health Consequences (100 kHz–300 GHz). Review of the Scientific Evidence and Health Consequences*. ICNIRP, Oberschleissheim.

ICNIRP. 2010. Guidelines on limiting exposure to time-varying electric, magnetic and electromagnetic fields (up to 100 kHz). *Heath Physics*, 99, 818–836. (Erratum, 2011). 100, 112.

ICNIRP. 2014. Guidelines for limiting exposure to electric field induced by movement of the human body in a static magnetic fields and by time-varying magnetic field below 1Hz. *Health Physics*, 106, 418–425.

ICNIRP. 2017. ICNIRP statement on diagnostic devices using non-ionizing radiation: Existing regulations and potential health risks. *Health Physics*, 112, 305–321.

Ilmoniemi, R.J., Virtanen, J., Karhu, J., Aronen, H.J., Naatanen, R., and Katila, T. 1997. Neuronal responses to magnetic stimulation reveal cortical reactivity and connectivity. *Neuroreport*, 8, 3537–3540.

Ilmoniemi, R.J., and Dubravko, K. 2010. Methodology for combined TMS and EEG. *Brain Topography*, 22, 233–248.

Iramina, K., Maeno, T., Kowatari, Y., and Ueno, S. 2002. Effects of transcranial magnetic stimulation on EEG activity. *IEEE Transactions on Magnetics*, 38, 3347–3349.

Iramina, K., Maeno, T., Nonaka, Y., and Ueno, S. 2003. Measurement of evoked electroencephalography induced by transcranial magnetic stimulation. *Journal of Applied Physics*, 93, 6718–6720.

Iwahashi, M., Koyama, Y., Hyodo, A., Hayami, T., Ueno, S., and Iramina, K. 2009. Measurements of evoked electroencephalograph by transcranial magnetic stimulation applied to motor cortex and posterior parietal cortex. *Journal of Applied Physics*, 105, 07B321.

Jackson, M.P., Rahman, A., Lafon, B., Kronberg, G., Ling, D., Parra, L.C., and Bikson, M. 2016. Animal models of transcranial direct current stimulation: Methods and mechanisms. *Clinical Neurophysiology*, 127, 3425–3454.

Ji, R.R., Schlaepfer, T., Aizenman, C.D., Epstein, C.M., Qiu, D., Huang, J.C., and Rupp, F. 1998. Repetitive transcranial magnetic stimulation activates specific regions in rat brain. *Proceedings of the National Academy of Sciences of the USA*, 95, 15635–15640.

Jiang, T., Xu, R.X., Zhang, A.W., Di, W., Xiao, Z.J., Miao, J.Y., Luo, N., and Fang, Y.N. 2012. Effects of transcranial direct current stimulation on hemichannel pannexin-1 and neural plasticity in rat model of cerebral infarction. *Neuroscience*, 226, 421–426.

Kadosh, R.S. 2014. *The Stimulated Brain: Cognitive Enhancement Using Non-Invasive Brain Simulation.* Academic Press, Elsevier, Cambridge.

Kanno, M., Matsumoto, M., Togashi, H., Yoshioka, M., and Mano, Y. 2003. Effects of acute repetitive transcranial magnetic stimulation on extracellular serotonin concentration in the rat prefrontal cortex. *Journal of Pharmacological Sciences*, 93, 451–457.

Kapogiannis, D., Campion, P., Grafman, J., and Wassermann, E.M. 2008. Reward-related activity in the human motor cortex. *European Journal of Neuroscience*, 27, 31–37.

Kapogiannis, D., Mooshagian, E., Campion, P., Grafman, J., Zimmermann, T.J., Ladt, K.C., and Wassermann, E.M. 2011. Reward processing abnormalities in Parkinson's disease. *Movement Disorders*, 26, 1451–1457.

Karlström, E.F., Lundström, R., Stensson, O., and Mild, K.H. 2006. Therapeutic staff exposure to magnetic field pulses during TMS/rTMS treatments. *Bioelectromagnetics*, 27, 156–158.

Keck, M.E., Sillaber, I., Ebner, K., Welt, T., Toschi, N., Kaehler, S.T., Singewald, N., Philippu, A., Elbel, G.K., Wotjak, C.T., Holsber, F., Landgraf, R., and Engelmann, M. 2000a. Acute transcranial magnetic stimulation of frontal brain regions selectively modulates the release of vasopressin, biogenic amines and amino acids in the rat brain. *European Journal of Neuroscience*, 12, 3713–3720.

Keck, M.E., Engelmann, M., Muller, M.B., Henninger, M.S., Hermann, B., Rupprecht, R., Neumann, I.D., Toschi, N., Landgraf, R., and Post, A. 2000b. Repetitive transcranial magnetic stimulation induces active coping strategies and attenuates the neuroendocrine stress response in rats. *Journal of Psychiatric Research*, 34, 265–276.

Kim, J.Y., Choi, G.S., Cho, Y.W., Cho, H., Hwang, S.J., and Ahn, S.H. 2013. Attenuation of spinal cord injury-induced astroglial and microglial activation by repetitive transcranial magnetic stimulation in rats. *Journal of Korean Medical Science*, 28, 295–299.

Kirino, T. 1982. Delayed neuronal death in the gerbil hippocampus following ischemia. *Brain Research*, 239, 57–69.

Klomjai, W., Lackmy-Vallée, A., Roche, N., Pradat-Diehl, P., and Marchand-Pauvert, V. 2015. Repetitive transcranial magnetic stimulation and transcranial direct current stimulation in motor rehabilitation after stroke: An update. *Annals of Physical and Rehabilitation Medicine*, 58, 220–224.

Kringelbach, M.L., Jenkinson, N., Owen, S.L.F., and Aziz, T.Z. 2007. Translational principles of deep brain stimulation. *Nature Reviews Neuroscience*, 8, 623–635.

Lefaucheur, J.P., Andre-Obadia, N., Antal, A., Ayache, S.S., Baeken, C., Benninger, D.H., Cantello, R.M., Cincotta, M., de Carvalho, M., De Ridder, D., Devanne, H., et al., 2014. Evidence-based guidelines in the therapeutic use of repetitive transcranial magnetic stimulation (TMS). *Clinical Neurophysiology*, 125, 2150–2206.

Lefaucheur, J.P. 2016. A comprehensive database of published tDCS clinical trials (2005–2016). *Clinical Neurophysiology*, 46, 319–398.

Lefaucheur, J.P., Antal, A., Ayache, S.S., Benninger, D.H., Brunelin, J., Cogiamanian, F., Cotelli, M., De Ridder, D., Ferrucci, R., Langguth, B., Marangolo, P., Mylius, V., Nitsche, M.A., Padberg, F., Palm, U., Poulet, E., Priori, A., Rossi, S., Schecklmann, M., Vanneste, S., Ziemann, U., Garcia-Larra, L., and Paulus, W. 2017. Evidence-based guidelines in the therapeutic use of transcranial direct current stimulation (tDCS). *Clinical Neurophysiology*, 128, 56–92.

Lenz, M., Platschek, S., Priesemann, V., Becker, D., Willems, L.M., Ziemann, U., Deller, T., Müller-Dahlhaus, F., Jedlicka, P., and Vlachos, A. 2015. Repetitive magnetic stimulation induces plasticity of excitatory postsynapses on proximal dendrites of cultured mouse CA1 pyramidal neurons. *Brain Structure and Function*, 220, 3323–3337.

Lenz, M., Galanis, C., Müller-Dahlhaus, F., Opitz, A., Wierenga, C.J., Szabö, G., Ziemann, U., Deller, T., Funke, K., and Vlachos, A. 2016. Repetitive magnetic stimulation induces plasticity of inhibitory synapses. *Nature Communications*, 7, 10020.

Levkovitz, Y., Isserles, M., Padberg, F., Lisanby, S.H., Bystritsky, A., Xia, G., Tendler, A., Daskalakis, Z.J., Winston, J.L., Dannon, P., Hafez, H.M., Reti, I.M., Morazles, O.G., Schlaepfer, T.E., Hollander, E., Berman, J.A., Husain, M.M., Sofer, U., Stein, A., Adler, S., Deutsch, L., Deutsch, F., Roth, Y., George, M.S., and Zangen, A. 2015. Efficacy and safety of deep transcranial magnetic stimulation for major depression: A prospective multicenter randomized controlled trial. *World Psychiatry*, 14, 64–73.

Li, Y., Qu, Y., Yuan, M., and Du, T. 2015. Low-frequency repetitive transcranial magnetic stimulation for patients with aphasia after stroke: A meta-analysis. *Journal of Rehabilitation Medicine*, 47, 675–681.

Lim, K.B., Lee, H.J., Yoo, J., and Kwon, Y.G. 2014. Effect of low-frequency rTMS and NMES on subacute unilateral hemispheric stroke with dysphagia. *Annals of Rehabilitation Medicine*, 38, 592–602.

Lin, J.C. 2016. Minimally invasive transcranial magnetic stimulation (TMS) treatment for major depression. *The Radio Science Bulletin*, 357, 57–59.

Lisanby, S.H., Luber, B., Perera, T., and Sackeim, H.A. 2000. Transcranial magnetic stimulation: Applications in basic neuroscience and neuropsychopharmacology. *International Journal of Neuropsychopharmacology*, 3, 259–273.

Liu, R., and Ueno, S. 2000. Calculating the activating function of nerve excitation in inhomogeneous volume conductor during magnetic stimulation using finite element method. *IEEE Transactions on Magnetics*, 36, 1796–1799.

Lontis, E.R., Voigt, M., and Struijk, J.J. 2006. Focality assessment in transcranial magnetic stimulation with double and cone coils. *Journal of Clinical Neurophysiology*, 23, 462–471.

Loo, C.K., McFarquhar, T.F., and Mitchell, P.B. 2008. A review of the safety of repetitive transcranial magnetic stimulation as a clinical treatment for depression. *International Journal of Neuropsychopharmacology*, 11, 131–147.

Loo, C.K., Sachev, P., Martin, D., Pigot, M., Alonzo, A., Malhi, G.S., Lagopoulos, J., and Mitchell, P. 2010. A double-blind, sham-controlled trial of transcranial direct current stimulation for the treatment of depression. *International Journal of Neuropsychopharmacology*, 13, 61–69.

Lu, M., Ueno, S., Thorlin, T., and Persson, M. 2008. Calculating the activating function in the human brain by transcranial magnetic stimulation. *IEEE Transactions on Magnetics*, 44, 1438–1441.

Lu, M., Ueno, S., Thorlin, T., and Persson, M. 2009. Calculating the current density and electric field in human head by multichannel transcranial magnetic stimulation. *IEEE Transactions on Magnetics*, 45, 1662–1665.

Lu, M., and Ueno, S. 2013. Calculating the electric fields in the human brain by deep transcranial magnetic stimulation. *Proceedings of the IEEE Engineering in Medicine and Biology Society*, 376–379.

Lu, M., and Ueno, S. 2015. Computational study toward deep transcranial magnetic stimulation using coaxial circular coils. *IEEE Transactions on Biomedical Engineering*, 62, 2911–2919.

Lu, M., and Ueno, S. 2017. Comparison of the induced fields using different coil configurations during deep transcranial magnetic stimulation. *PLoS One*, 12, e0178422.

Maki, H., and Ilmoniemi, R.J. 2010. EEG oscillations and magnetically evoked motor potentials reflect motor system excitability in overlapping neuronal populations. *Clinical Neurophysiology*, 121, 492–501.

Makkos, A., Pal, E., Aschermann, Z., Janszky, J., Balazs, E., Takacs, K., Karadi, K., Komoly, S., and Kovacs, N. 2016. High-frequency repetitive transcranial magnetic stimulation can improve depression in Parkinson's disease: A randomized, double-bland, placebo-controlled study. *Neuropsychobiology*, 73, 169–177.

Marshall, T.R., O'Shea, J., Jensen, O., and Bergmann, T.O. 2015. Frontal eye fields control attentional modulation of alpha and gamma oscillations in contralateral occipitoparietal cortex. *Journal of Neuroscience*, 35, 1–10.

Maruo, T., Hosomi, K., Shimokawa, T., Kishima, H., Oshino, S., Morris, S., Kageyama, Y., Yokoe, M., Yoshimine, T., and Saitoh, Y. 2013. High-frequency repetitive transcranial magnetic stimulation over the primary foot motor area in Parkinson's disease. *Brain Stimulation*, 6, 884–891.

Meron, D., Hedger, N., Garner, M., and Baldwin, D.S. 2015. Transcranial direct current stimulation (tDCS) in the treatment of depression: Systematic review and meta-analysis of efficacy and tolerability. *Neuroscience & Biobehavioral Reviews*, 57, 46–62.

Møllerløkken, O.J., Stavang, H., and Mild, K.H. 2017. Staff exposure to pulsed magnetic fields during depression treatment with transcranial magnetic stimulation. *International Journal of Occupational Safety and Ergonomics*, S23, 139–142.

Mooshagian, E., Keisler, A., Zimmermann, T., Schweickert, J.M., and Wassermann, E.M. 2015. Modulation of corticospinal excitability by reward depends on task framing. *Neuropsychologia*, 68, 31–37.

Moulier, V., Gaudeau-Bosma, C., Isaac, C., Allard, A.C., Bouaziz, N., Sidhoumi, D., Braha-Zeitoun, S., Benadhira, R., Thomas, F., and Januel, D. 2016. Effect of repetitive transcranial magnetic stimulation on mood in healthy subjects. *Socioaffective Neuroscience & Psychology*, 6, 29672.

Müller, M.B., Toschi, N., Kresse, A.E., Post, A., and Keck, M.E. 2000. Long-term repetitive transcranial magnetic stimulation increases the expression of brain-derived neurotrophic factor and cholecystokinin mRNA, but not neuropeptide tyrosine mRNA in specific areas of rat brain. *Neuropsychopharmacology*, 23, 205–215.

Nagaoka, T., Watanabe, S., Sakurai, K., Kunieda, E., Watanabe, S., Taki, M., and Yamanaka, Y. 2004. Development of realistic high-resolution whole-body voxel models of Japanese adult males and females of average height and weight, and application of models to radio-frequency electromagnetic-field dosimetry. *Physics in Medicine and Biology*, 49, 1–15.

Nagarajan, S.S., Durand, M., and Warman, E.N. 1993. Effects of induced electric fields on finite neuronal structures: A simulation study. *IEEE Transactions on Biomedical Engineering*, 40, 1175–1188.

NIEHS. 1998. *Assessment of Health Effects from Exposure to Power-Line Frequency Electric and Magnetic Fields*. Portier, C.J. and Wolfe, M.S. (Eds.) (NIH Publ.No.98–3981). NIEHS, Research Triangle Park, NC.

Nitsche, M.A., and Paulus, W. 2000. Excitability changes induced in the human motor cortex by weak transcranial direct current stimulation. *The Journal of Physiology*, 527(Pt 3), 633–639.

Ogiue-Ikeda, M., Kawato, S., and Ueno, S. 2003a. The effect of repetitive transcranial magnetic stimulation on long-term potentiation in rat hippocampus depends on stimulation intensity. *Brain Research*, 993, 222–226.

Ogiue-Ikeda, M., Kawato, S., and Ueno, S. 2003b. The effect of transcranial magnetic stimulation on long-term potentiation in rat hippocampus. *IEEE Transactions on Magnetics*, 39, 3390–3392.

Ogiue-Ikeda, M., Kawato, S., and Ueno, S. 2005. Acquisition of ischemic tolerance by repetitive transcranial magnetic stimulation in the rat hippocampus. *Brain Research*, 1037, 7–11.

Okada, A., Nishikawa, A., Fukushima, T., Taniguchi, K., Miyazaki, F., Sekino, M., Yasumuro, Y., Matsuzaki, T., Hosomi, K., and Saitoh, Y. 2012. Magnetic navigation system for home use of repetitive transcranial magnetic stimulation (rTMS). *Proceedings, ICME International Conference on Complex Medical Engineering*, 112–118.

Opitz, A., Legon, W., Rowlands, A., Bickel, W.K., Paulus, W., amd Tyler, W.J. 2013. Physiological observations validate finite element models for estimating subject-specific electric field distributions induced by transcranial magnetic stimulation of the human motor cortex. *Neuroimage*, 81, 253–264.

O'Reardon, J.P., Solvason, H.B., Janiacak, P.G., Sampson, S., Isenberg, K.E., Nahas, Z., McDonld, W.M., Avery, D., Fitzgerald, P.B., Loo, C., Demitrack, M.A., George, M.S., and Sackeim, H.A. 2007. Efficay and safety of transcranial magnetic stimulation in the acute treatment of major depression: A multisite randomized controlled trial. *Biological Psychiatry*, 62, 1208–1216.

Parent, A. 2004. Giovanni Aldini: From animal electricity to human brain stimulation. *Canadian Journal of Neurological Sciences*, 31, 576–584.

Pascual-Leone, A., Valls-Sole, J., Brasil-Neto, J.P., Cammarota, A., Grafman, J., and Hallett, M. 1994. Akinesia in Parkinson's disease. II. Effects of subthreshold repetitive transcranial motor cortex stimulation. *Neurology*, 44, 892–898.

Pascual-Leone, A., Davey, N., Rothwell, J., Wassermann, E.M., and Puri, B.K. 2002. *Handbook of Transcranial Magnetic Stimulation*. Hodder Arnold, London.

Pellow, S., Chopin, P., File, S.E., and Briley, M. 1985. Validation of open: Close arm entries in an elevated plus-maze as a measure of anxiety in the rat. *Journal of Neuroscience Methods*, 14, 149–167.

Perera, T., George, M.S., Grammer, G., Janicak, P.G., Pascual-Leone, A., and Wirecki, T.S. 2016. The clinical TMS society consensus review and treatment recommendations for TMS therapy for major depressive disorder. *Brain Stimulation*, 9, 336–346.

Peterchev, A.V., Wagner, T.A., Miranda, P.C., Nitsche, M.A., Paulus, W., Lisanby, S.H., Pascual-Leone, A., and Bikson, M. 2012. Fundamentals of transcranial electric and magnetic stimulation dose: Definition, selection, and reporting practices. *Brain Stimulation*, 5, 435–453.

Pikhovych, A., Stolberg, N.P., Flitsch, L.J., Walter, H.L., Graf, R., Fink, G.R., Schroeter, M., and Rueger, M.A. 2016. Transcranial direct current stimulation modulates neurogenesis and microglia activation in the mouse brain. *Stem Cells International*, ID 2715196.

Priori, A., Berardelli, A., Rona, A., Accornero, N., and Manfredi, M. 1998. Polarization of the human motor cortex through the scalp. *NeuroReport*, 9, 2257–2260.

Rahman, A., Reato, D., Arlotti, M., Gasca, F., Datta, A., Parra, L.C., and Bikson, M. 2013. Cellular effects of acute direct current stimulation: Somatic and synaptic terminal effects. *Journal of Physiology*, 591, 2563–2578.

Raij, T., Karhu, J., Kicic, D., Lioumis, P., Julkunen, P., Lin, F.H., Ahveninen, J., Ilmoniemi, R.J., Makela, J.P., Hamalainen, M., Rosen, B.H., and Belliveau, J.W. 2008. Parallel input makes the brain run faster. *NeuroImage*, 40, 1792–1797.

Rajan, T.S., Ghilardi, M.M., Wang, H.Y., Mazzon, E., Bramanti, P., Restivo, D., and Quartarone, A. 2017. Mechansim of action for rTMS: A working hypothesis based on animal studies. *Frontiers in Physiology*, 8, 457.

Ranieri, F., Podda, M.V., Riccardi, E., Frisullo, G., Dileone, M., Profice, P., Pilato, F., Di Lazzaro, V., and Grassi, C. 2012. Modulation of LTP at rat hippocampal CA3-CA1 synapses by direct current stimulation. *Journal of Neurophysiology*, 107, 1868–1880.

Rossi, S., Hallett, M., Rossini, P.M., Pascual-Leone, A., and the Safety of TMS Consensus Group. 2009. Safety, ethical considerations, and application guidelines for the use of transcranial magnetic stimulation in clinical practice and research. *Clinical Neurophysiology*, 120, 2008–2039.

Rossi, S., Hallett, M., Rossini, P.M., and Pascual-Leone, A. 2011. Screening questionnaire before TMS: An update. *Clinical Neurophysiology*, 122, 1686.

Roth, Y., Zangen, A., and Hallett, M. 2002. A coil design for transcranial magnetic stimulation of deep brain regions. *Journal of Clinical Neurophysiology*, 19, 361–370.

Roth, Y., Amir, A., Levkovitz, Y., and Zangen, A. 2007. Three-dimensional distributions of the electric fields induced in the brain by transcranial magnetic stimulation using figure-8 and deep H-coils. *Journal of Clinical Neurophysiology*, 24, 31–38.

Roth, B.J., and Basser, P.J. 1990. A model of the stimulation of a nerve fiber by electromagnetic induction. *IEEE Transactions on Biomedical Engineering*, 37, 588–597.

Rowbottom, M., and Susskind, C. 1984. *Electricity and Medicine-History of Their Interaction*. San Francisco Press, San Francisco, CA.

Rueger, M.A., Keuters, M.H., Walberer, M., Braun, R., Klein, R., Sparing, R., Fink, G.R., Graf, R., and Schroeter, M. 2012. Multisession transcranial direct current stimulation (tDCS) elicits inflammatory and regenerative processes in the rat brain. *PLoS One*, 7, e43776.

Ruohonen, J., and Ilmoniemi, R.J. 1998. Focusing and targeting of magnetic brain stimulation using multiple coils. *Medical & Biological Engineering & Computing*, 36, 297–301.

Ruohonen, J., and Karhu, J. 2012. tDCS possibly stimulates glial cells. *Clinical Neurophysiology*, 123, 2006–2009.

Scientific Commission on Emerging and Newly Identified Health Risks (SCENIHR). 2009. *Health Effects of Exposure to EMF*. European Commission, Brussels.

Scientific Commission on Emerging and Newly Identified Health Risks (SCENIHR). 2013. *Preliminary Opinion on Potential Health Effects of Exposure to Electromagnetic Fields (EMF)*. European Commission, Brussels.

Scientific Commission on Emerging and Newly Identified Health Risks (SCENIHR). 2015. *Preliminary Opinion on Potential Health Effects of Exposure to Electromagnetic Fields (EMF)*. European Commission, Brussels.

Sekino, M., and Ueno, S. 2002. Comparison of current distributions in electroconvulsive therapy and transcranial magnetic stimulation. *Journal of Applied Physics*, 91, 8730–8732.

Sekino, M., Yamaguchi, K., Iriguchi, N., and Ueno, S. 2003. Conductivity tensor imaging of the brain using diffusion-weighted magnetic resonance imaging. *Journal of Applied Physics*, 93, 6730–6732.

Sekino, M., and Ueno, S. 2004. FEM based determination of optimum current distribution in transcranial magnetic stimulation as an alternative to electroconvulsive therapy. *IEEE Transactions on Magnetics*, 42, 3575–3577.

Sekino, M., Inoue, Y., and Ueno, S. 2005. Magnetic resonance imaging of electrical conductivity in the human brain. *IEEE Transactions on Magnetics*, 41, 4203–4205.

Sekino, M., Ohsaki, H., Yamaguchi-Sekino, S., Iriguchi, N., and Ueno, S. 2009. Low-frequency conductivity tensor of rat brain tissues inferred from diffusion MRI. *Bioelectromagnetics*, 30, 489–499.

Sekino, M., Ohsaki, H., Takiyama, Y., Yamamoto, K., Matsuzaki, T., Yasumuro, Y., Nishikawa, A., Maruo, T., Hosomi, K., and Saitoh, Y. 2015. Eccentric figure-eight coils for transcranial magnetic stimulation. *Bioelectromagnetics*, 36. 55–65.

Shigemitsu, T., and Ueno, S. 2017. Biological and health effects of electromagnetic fields related to the operation of MRI/TMS. *Spin*, 7, 1–17.

Shukla, A.W., Shuster, J.J., Chung, J.W., Vaillancourt, D.E., Patten, C., Ostrem, J., and Okun, M.S. 2016. Repetitive transcranial magnetic stimulation (rTMS) therapy in Parkinson's disease: A meta-analysis. *PM R*, 8, 356–366.

Stamm, R. 2014. The revised electromagnetic fields directive and worker exposure in environments with high magnetic flux densities. *Annals of Occupational Hygiene*, 58, 529–541.

Tan, T., Xie, J., Liu, T., Chen, X., Zheng, X., Tong, Z., and Tian, X. 2013. Low-frequency (1 Hz) repetitive transcranial magnetic stimulation (rTMS) reverses Aβ (1–42)-mediated memory deficits in rats. *Experimental Gerontology*, 48, 786–794.

Tanaka, T., Takano, Y., Tanaka, S., Hironaka, N., Kobayashi, K., Hanakawa, T., Watanabe, K., and Honda, M. 2013. Transcranial direct-current stimulation increases extracellular dopamine levels in the rat striatum. *Frontiers in Systems Neuroscience*, 7, 6.

Tang, A., Thickbroom, G., and Rodger, J. 2015. Repetitive transcranial magnetic stimulation of the brain: Mechanisms from animal and experimental models. *The Neuroscientist*, 1–13.

Torii, T., Sato, A., Nakahara, Y., Iwahashi, M., Itoh, Y., and Iramina, K. 2012. Frequency-dependent effects of repetitive transcranial magnetic stimulation on the human brain. *Neuroreport*, 19, 1065–1070.

Tsubokawa, T., Katayama, Y., Yamamoto, T., Hirayama, T., and Koyama, S. 1991. Chronic motor cortex stimulation for treatment of central pain. *Acta Neurochirurgica Supplement*, 52, 137–139.

Tuch, D.S., Wedeen, V.J., Dale, A.M., George, J.S., and Belliveau, J.W. 2001. Conductivity tensor mapping of the human brain using diffusion tensor MRI. *Proceedings of the National Academy of Sciences of USA*, 98, 11697–11701.

Ueno, S., Tashiro, T., and Harada, K. 1988. Localized stimulation of neural tissue in the brain by means of a paired configuration of time-varying electric fields. *Journal of Applied Physics*, 64, 5862–5864.

Ueno, S., Matsuda, T., Fujiki, M., and Hori, S. 1989. Localized stimulation of the human motor cortex by means of pair of opposing magnetic fields. *Digest of International Magnetics Conference*, Washington, D.C.: GD–10.

Ueno, S., Matsuda, T., and Fujiki, M. 1990. Functional mapping of the human cortex obtained by focal and vectorial magnetic stimulation of the brain. *IEEE Transactions on Magnetics*, 26, 1539–1544.

Ueno, S., Matsuda, T., and Hiwaki, O. 1991. Estimation of structures of neural fibers in the human brain by vectorial magnetic stimulation. *IEEE Transactions on Magnetics*, 27, 5387–5389.

Ueno, S., and Fujiki, M. 2007. Magnetic stimulation. In Andra, W. and Nowak, H. (Eds.) *Magnetism in Medicine A Handbook Second Completely Revised and Enlarged Edition*. Wiley-VHC, Weinheim: pp. 511–528.

Ueno, S. 2012. Studies on magnetism and bioelectromagnetics for 45 years: From magnetic analog memory to human brain stimulation and imaging. *Bioelectromagnetics*, 33, 3–22.

Ueno, S., and Sekino, M. 2015. *Biomagnetics: Principles and Applications of Biomagnetic Stimulation and Imaging*. CRC Press, Taylor and Francis Group, Boca Raton, London, New York.

Ueyama, E., Ukai, S., Ogawa, A., Yamamoto, M., Kawaguchi, S., Ishi, R., and Shinosaki, K. 2011. Chronic repetitive transcranial magnetic stimulation increases hippocampal neurogenesis in rats. *Psychiatry and Clinical Neurosciences*, 65, 77–81.

Ugawa, Y., Uesaka, Y., Teran, Y., Hanajima, R., and Kanazawa, I. 1995. Magnetic stimulation over the cerebellum in humans. *Annals Neurology*, 37, 703–713.

Vlachos, A., Müller-Dahhaus, F., Rosskopp, J., Lenz, M., Ziemann, U., and Deller, T. 2012. Repetitive magnetic stimulation induces functional and structural plasticity of excitatory postsynapses in mouse organotypic hippocampal slice cultures. *Journal of Neuroscience*, 32, 17514–17523.

VonLoh, M., Chen, R., and Kluger, B. 2013. Safety of transcranial magnetic stimulation in Parkinson's disease: A review of the literature. *Parkinsonism and Related Disorders*, 19, 573–585.

WHO. 2007. *Extremely Low Frequency Fields*. Environmental Health Criteria 238. World Health Organization, Geneva.

Wassermann, E.M., Grafman, J., Berry, C., Hollnagel, C., Eild, K., Clark, K., and Hallett, M. 1996. Use and safety of a new repetitive transcranial magnetic stimulator. *Electroencephalography Clinical Neurophysiology*, 101, 412–417.

Wassermann, E.M. 1998. Risk and safety of repetitive transcranial magnetic stimulation: Report and recommendations from the International Workshop on the safety of repetitive transcranial magnetic stimulation June 5–7, 1996. *Electroencephalography Clinical Neurophysiology*, 108, 1–16.

Wassermann, E.M., and Zimmermann, T. 2012. Transcranial magnetic brain stimulation: Therapeutic promises and scientific gaps. *Pharmacology and Therapeutics*, 133, 98–107.

Yamamoto, K., Suyama, M., Takiyama, Y., Kim, D., Saitoh, Y., and Sekino, M. 2015. Characteristics of bowl-shaped coils for transcranial magnetic stimulation. *Journal of Applied Physics*, 117, 17A318.

Yang, H.Y., Liu, Y., Xie, J.C., Liu, N.N., and Tian, X. 2015. Effects of repetitive transcranial magnetic stimulation on synaptic plasticity and apoptosis in vascular dementia rats. *Behavioural Brain Research*, 281, 149–155.

Yun, G.J., Chun, M.H., and Kim, B.R. 2015. The effects of transcranial direct-current stimulation on cognition in stroke patients. *Journal of Stroke*, 17, 354–358.

Zangen, A., Roth, Y., Voller, B., and Hallett, M. 2005. Transcranial magnetic stimulation of deep brain regions; evidence for efficacy of the H-coil. *Clinical Neurophysiology*, 116, 775–779.

Zanjani, A., Zakzanis, K.K., Daskalakis, Z.J., and Chen, R. 2015. Repetitive transcranial magnetic stimulation of the primary motor cortex in the treatment of motor signs in Parkinson's disease: A quantitative review of the literature. *Movement Disorders*, 30, 750–758.

Zucca, M., Bottauscio, C., Chiampi, M., and Zilberti, L. 2017. Operator safety and field focality in aluminium shielded transcranial magnetic stimulation. *IEEE Transactions on Magnetics*, 53(11), DOI:10.1109/TMAG.2017.2709402.

11

Computational Modeling of Transepithelial Endogenous Electric Signals

Somen Baidya and Ahmed M. Hassan
University of Missouri-Kansas City

Min Zhao
University of California, Davis

CONTENTS

11.1 Introduction

Natural wound healing is a highly complicated process that consists of several timed stages of cell signaling, migration, and proliferation. It is difficult to divide the wound healing process into distinct phases since several of these phases overlap. However, there is a general consensus that wound healing can be subdivided into four major phases [1–3].

1. *Hemostasis*: Hemostasis is the natural response of the body to inhibit the continuous flow of blood through the wound. This phase is initiated within the very first few moments of injury and it includes the adhesion and coagulation of *platelets*

around the wound site to create a primary seal to prevent further blood loss [4,5]. *Platelets* also release some major signaling proteins like *cytokines, chemokines*, and hormones to initiate the following phase of inflammation [6].

2. *Inflammation*: Inflammation is the stage in which the response of the immune system is initiated by protecting against foreign objects such as bacteria, debris, and dead cells at the wound site [6,7]. During the inflammation phase, the permeability of the capillaries at the wound site increases, which results in the leak of blood plasma and white blood cells into the surrounding tissue. The first type of white blood cells encountered is *neutrophils*, which engulf and digest the contaminants [7]. This process is medically defined as *phagocytosis*. Soon after the *neutrophils* die off, another type of white blood cell, *monocytes* migrate from the bloodstream to the wound and mature to form *macrophages*, which further continue the process of *phagocytosis* [8]. *Macrophages* also play a pivotal role in initiating the third phase of proliferation by releasing several growth factors [6,7].

3. *Proliferation*: The proliferation phase is a combination of several overlapping phases of *granulation tissue* formation, *angiogenesis*, and *reepithelization* [9]. The *cytokines* secreted by *macrophages* attract granulation tissue, which contain a particular cell type, *fibroblasts* [10]. *Fibroblasts* secret strong fibrous material named *collagen* that provides strength and texture to the granulation tissue. New capillaries are also formed in the granulation tissue as a part of the *angiogenesis* phase [6,7]. Concurrently, the endothelial cells proliferate and cover the top bed of the wound during the reepithelization phase [10]. *Fibroblast* cells transform into *myofibroblast*, which contracts the wound edges to draw them together [7].

4. *Remodeling*: During the remodeling phase, a stronger *collagen* material replaces the original *collagen* material via a process that is known as *collagenases* [11]. The wound contraction continues for several weeks until the natural cell death, *apoptosis*, of the scar tissue [12]. This phase may take several weeks up to 2 years [13].

While the wound healing mechanism consists of a complex combination of several overlapping events in a precise order, it is also prone to interruptions in any of its stages. An interruption in one of the stages may lead to a nonhealing or a *chronic wound*, which is defined as a wound that fails to heal through in an orderly and timely manner [14]. According to the Wound Healing Foundation, approximately 6.5 million patients suffer from chronic wounds, which are wounds that heal in an abnormal or a longer than usual manner [15]. The annual economic impact of these chronic wounds is estimated to be $39 billion, which indicates to the importance of finding an effective treatment modality to accelerate the healing of chronic wounds [15]. It is important to emphasize that many factors contribute to wound healing such as antibiotic-resistant biofilm, blood circulation, and chemical stimulus from growth factors [16]. For example, several experiments have demonstrated the significant relationship between the oxygen supply to the wound center and new capillary development [17]. Other studies focused on the effect of the mechanical forces in the wound's environment on its healing rate [18]. In this chapter, we are concentrating on investigating the role of electrical signals, whether they are naturally generated or applied externally, as one of the promising approaches for accelerating the healing of chronic wounds [3,19,20].

A voltage or a potential difference, similar to a battery, exists across the epithelial layers lining the body's inner cavities and the outer skin surface [1,19,21]. This voltage difference is typically termed the transepithelial potential (TEP) and it is created by the continuous pumping of the positive sodium ions (Na^+) from the external medium to the stroma, under the epithelial layer, and the pumping of the negative chloride ions (Cl^-) in the opposite direction [1,19,21]. Tight junctions between the cells keep the ions segregated and maintain the TEP. In an intact skin with no wounds, the stroma is at a higher potential than the external fluid by an amount equal to this TEP. Figure 11.1 shows the epithelial layer covering the cornea of the eye and the external fluid, which in this case, is the tear film. The corneal epithelium is only one of the many kinds of epithelial tissues, but it can be used as an excellent and practical model for TEP in many other body sites [1,19,21]. When a wound is created, a short circuit is established across the TEP and a field is created which drives electric currents laterally toward the wound [1,19,21]. The wound-induced electric currents have a considerable effect on all four phases of wound healing [3]. In the *hemostasis* phase, the wound current increases the blood flow toward the wound center [3] and provides an antibacterial shield against the growth of multiple bacterial organisms [22]. In the *proliferative* phase, the wound currents govern membrane transport and collagen matrix organization [3]. The main contribution of the wound currents is observed during the remodeling phase by enabling cell migration and proliferation [3].

Several *in vitro* studies were performed on the different cell types involved in wound healing to investigate their response to endogenous electric field [23–31]. For example, *macrophages* typically migrate toward the anode whereas *monocytes* migrate toward the cathode under external electrical excitation of the same order of magnitude as the naturally generated fields (5 mV/mm) [23]. The phagocytic behavior of *macrophages* was also observed to increase toward specific targets under electrical stimuli [23]. *Fibroblast* cells, which are mainly active in the *proliferation* phase, have also been reported to show directional migration when exposed to electric fields [25–28]. Cohen et al. demonstrated that electric fields can control the migration trajectories of a monolayer epithelial sheet [29]. Cathodal migration of epidermal stem cells (EpSCs) under an electric field of 50–400 mv/mm was reported in [30]. The same direction of migration was also reported in the case of human corneal epithelial cells under 150 mV/mm electrical excitation [31].

Researchers also revealed that the *angiogenesis* process (formation of new capillaries in the granulation tissue) is upregulated in the presence of small direct current (DC) electric field due to the increase in the number of angiogenic proteins and endothelial growth factors [32,33]. The endogenous electric field was also found to have *bacteriostatic* effect

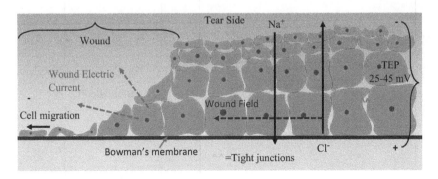

FIGURE 11.1
Bioelectrical signals created by a wound in the skin (adapted from [19]).

by intervening bacterial proliferation [34,35]. Figure 11.2 summarizes the wound healing aspects affected by electrical stimulation (adapted from [7]).

These *in vitro* studies provide substantial evidence of the effect of endogenous electric field on the natural wound healing process, which has encouraged researchers to test the use of external electrical stimulation as another potential modality to improve chronic wound cases *in vivo*. Although the electrical stimulation (ES) parameters can vary significantly from one study to the other, can be typically classified into three major categories: (i) direct current (DC), (ii) alternating current (AC), and (iii) pulsed current (PC) (Figure 11.3) [3]. DC is the unidirectional flow of charged particle generally lasting for 1 ms to 1 s [36]. DC stimulus closely mimics the endogenous wound current spatially and temporally but it has the drawback of increased skin temperature, which can irritate the nearby healthy tissues [37]. For this reason, some studies used low-intensity direct current (LIDC) to improve the side effects of the electric stimulus [3]. In AC stimulus, the charged particles periodically reverse their directions as shown in Figure 11.3. PC uses pulses with either a unidirectional (monophasic) or bidirectional (biphasic) flow of electrons or ions whose waveform can be symmetric or asymmetric based on the application as shown in Figure 11.3.

All the reported clinical trials incorporate some form of ES similar to one of the three categories in Figure 11.3. However, different modalities have been developed based on the

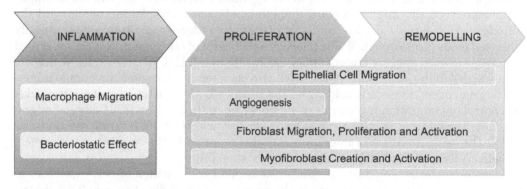

FIGURE 11.2
Wound-healing stages affected by ES [7].

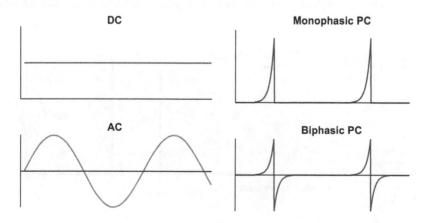

FIGURE 11.3
Temporal depiction of different electrical stimulation modalities [7].

target site of ES (i.e., tissue or nerves) and how the ES characteristics (e.g., frequency, voltage, etc.) are varied during the treatment duration. Some of the commonly reported ES modalities are Transcutaneous Electric Nerve Stimulation (TENS), Frequency Rhythmic Electrical Modulation System (FREMS), Biofeedback ES, and Bioelectric Dressing. TENS is a PC ES that employs low frequency, biphasic pulses transmitted through electrodes at the skin of the wound site [38]. Initially, TENS was employed to stimulate nerves for pain reduction by stimulating peripheral nerves, but it was also found to affect wound healing because of its resultant increase in blood perfusion rate [3]. FREMS is a noninvasive technique, which employs a specific sequence of weak PC with rapid variations in pulse frequency and distribution [39]. In FREMS, the pulse duration, frequency, voltage, and the treatment length is automatically tuned based on the patients' conditions [39]. Biofeedback ES is a stimulation modality that uses feedback from the skin impedance to modulate the applied PC [40]. The Bioelectric dressing is a special kind of medical dressing that activates its polarized characteristics in the presence of a wound [41]. The goal of the dressing is to emulate the endogenous wound currents by sustaining a local voltage around the wound site [41].

The previously described ES modalities have been tested *in vivo* in multiple studies [3,7,42,43]. One study by Talebi on 39 guinea pigs demonstrated that wound healing depended on the direction of the ES applied [43]. Two experiments were performed, in the first case the anode was placed at the wound site and in the second case the cathode was placed at the wound site. The second electrode was placed far from the wound. Both cases were compared to a Control group with identical electrode placement but with no ES applied. When the anode was placed at the wound site, it led to a faster wound healing rate than the cathodal stimulation [43]. A detailed review of the effect of ES on animal wound healing is presented in [7,42]. The main conclusions of these reviews are that externally applied ES may expedite the wound healing process by directional migration, cell proliferation, collagen deposition, or increased blood flow, but it does not necessarily have an effect on cross-linking and alignment of collagen during the remodeling phase of the wound healing process.

Similarly, ES has been tested in several *in vivo* studies involving wounds in humans. A summary of exogenous ES application in human chronic wound cases and its effectivity is enlisted in Table 11.1 [3,7]. The existing literature on external ES application on human cases is categorized mainly based on the common ES modalities previously described in [3,7].

As shown in Table 11.1, the parameters administered in the different modalities varied significantly based on each study design. The majority of the studies were only focusing on the short-term effects of their proposed ES modality and the duration of the studies extended from 3 to 12 weeks. The conclusion drawn from these studies is that, irrespective of the stimulation routine, ES has a general tendency to increase the wound-healing rate and reduce the associated pain. However, to the best of our knowledge, no technique is capable of predicting the optimum electrical stimulation routine that can effectively improve chronic wound healing for all cases. Therefore, there is a strong need for an optimized standard ES therapy that will irrevocably reduce wound area, accelerate the healing of the wound, reduce pain, and minimize scarring [3]. Before such an optimized stimulation can be developed, a quantitative understanding of the effect of endogenous current on wound healing is needed. That is, many of the pathways by which electric signals accelerate wound healings are still not fully quantified. If these pathways are understood, we can efficiently propose electrical stimulation techniques to target them. Moreover, the temporal and spatial patterns of the endogenous wound generated electric signals needs also to be quantified with respect to the wound stage, size, and shape. Only by the knowledge of the spatial and temporal patterns of these naturally generated wound electric

TABLE 11.1

A Summary of the Reported Effects of Different ES Modalities on Wound Healing [3,7]

Type of Wound	Type of ES	No. of Patients		Parameters	Duration	No. of Cases with Improved Wound Healing and/or Reduced Pain
		Treatment	Control			
Pulsed Current						
Chronic dermal ulcer	Monophasic pulsed vs. sham	26	24	29.2 V, 29.2 mA, 132 μs pulse	30 min twice for 4 weeks	66% WAR vs. sham 33%
Pressure ulcer	High voltage pulsed vs. sham	45	15	100–175 V, 50 μs pulse, 120 Hz	45–120 min daily for 5 weeks	Significant WAR compared to control
Pressure ulcer	Monophasic pulsed	61	NA	128 pps, 35 mA	30 min twice daily	4 cases of complete healing
Leg/Foot ulcer	High-voltage pulsed vs. sham	50	51	50–200V, 50–100 μs pulse, 100 Hz	0.5–1 h daily for 20–90 days	3 cases of accelerated wound healing and WAR
Leg/Foot ulcer	High-voltage pulsed vs. sham	96	47	50–150 V, 100 μs, 100 Hz	50 min stimulation for 6 time or 8 h daily	2 increased wound healing case and WAR
Diabetic ischemic wound	High-voltage pulsed	38	NA	140–360 V, 90–100 μs	45–60 min session for 14–16 weeks	6 improved healing
Direct Current						
Pressure ulcer	LIDC	78	59	300–600 μA	8 weeks	6 cases of complete wound closure and WAR
Foot/Leg ulcer	LIDC	62	15	300–500 μA	45–120 min, 3–5 days a week for 5–8 weeks	5 cases of improved healing
Ischemic ulcer	LIDC vs. sham	6	6	Not stated	Until healed	1 LIDC group healed twice as fast as control
Biofeedback ES						
Acute biopsy wound	Biofeedback	79	79	0.004 mA, 20–80 V, 60 Hz	2 weeks to until full recovery	6 cases of improved scar symptom with increased angiogenic response

(Continued)

TABLE 11.1 (*Continued*)

A Summary of the Reported Effects of Different ES Modalities on Wound Healing [3,7]

Type of Wound	Type of ES	No. of Patients Treatment	No. of Patients Control	Parameters	Duration	No. of Cases with Improved Wound Healing and/or Reduced Pain
FREMS						
Foot/Leg ulcer	FREMS vs. Control	66	59	0–300 V, 1–1000 Hz, 10–40 μs, 100–170 μA	40 min daily, 5 days a week for 3 weeks to full recovery	Significant WAR reported
Venous ulcers	FREMS vs. control	10	10	Not stated	5 days a week for 3 weeks	1 Reduced pain and area of ulcers
TENS						
Diabetic leg venous ulcer	TENS vs. Placebo	24	27	80 Hz, 1 ms pulse width	2 times a day for 84 Days	10 full recovery as compared to 4 in case of placebo, WAR
Healthy volunteers	TENS	31	NA	High frequency: 110 Hz, 200 μs Low frequency: 4 Hz, 200 μs	15 min	1 Local increase in blood flow
Blister wound	TENS	9	NA	High frequency: 100 Hz. Low frequency: 2 Hz	45 min	2 Stimulated perfusion
Bioelectric dressings						
Skin graft donor sites	Bioelectric dressing	13	NA	2–10 mV, 0.6–0.7 V, 10 μA	1 month	4 cases

In the entries above, pps stands for pulses per seconds; WAR refers to Wound Area Reduction; LIDC refers to Low-Intensity Direct Current, and Sham or Placebo represent the control group where patients did the same procedure as the active treatment without actually having the ES.

signals, can we develop external techniques to enhance them at all times and all locations in the vicinity of the wound. However, experimental measurements can only access a limited number of spatial and temporal positions without disturbing the wound itself. Therefore, there is a strong need for an accurate computational model that can generate a detailed spatial and temporal map of these electric signals in the vicinity of different kinds of wounds. This computational model should be accurately calibrated from experimental measurements and it needs to be validated by being capable of generating new outcomes that can be validated using alternative experiments.

In this chapter, we will introduce the reader to some of the latest research in the field of the mathematical and computational modeling of endogenous TEP. Most of the reported literature focuses on modeling an intact epithelium and, therefore, this will be the main emphasis of this chapter. However, at the end of the chapter, we will also review some modeling techniques that have the potential to simulate realistic wound-induced electric signals. Therefore, the main goal of this chapter is to introduce a methodology that can help a beginner start building their own computational model for the endogenous electrical signals generated by a wound in any epithelial system. We believe that only by developing accurate wound healing models, will we be able to understand the effect of endogenous current in the wound healing process in more details and propose a generalized external stimulation routine that can alleviate the economic and social burden of chronic wound cases.

This chapter is organized as follows. In Section 11.2, we summarize the main concepts of developing a mathematical model of the intact epithelium TEP. We demonstrate the discussed methodology by implementing one example of an intact system with a TEP. In Section 11.3, we discuss several methodologies that have the potential to accurately model the electric signals induced by healing epithelial wounds.

11.2 Mathematical Modeling of Intact Epithelium

11.2.1 Fundamental Equations

At the coarsest level, epithelial tissue can be modeled by three basic compartments: apical, basolateral, and cellular as shown in Figure 11.4. The TEP is a generated by the movement of ions across these compartments. In this representation, all of the cells in Figure 11.1 are grouped into one compartment termed the cellular compartment with the side in contact with the external fluid termed the apical membrane and the other side termed as the basolateral membrane. The transport in all of the intercellular spacing in Figure 11.1 is then also combined into the paracellular transport in Figure 11.4. The mechanism behind this ion transport may be due to simple electrodiffusion forces through ion-specific channels or it might involve a complex mechanism such as in the case of active transport and cotransport where multiple ions are grouped together while moving from one epithelial compartment to the other. The transport of one ionic species is strongly coupled to the transport of other ionic species. Therefore, an accurate mathematical model of any kind of TEP requires considering all the transport systems associated with the ionic species in that specific system.

Depending on the location and type of the epithelial tissue, the nature and the properties of the transport system associated with each ion species may vary significantly. However, all epithelial models are based on the conservation of mass and electroneutrality in all epithelium compartments [44]. Another common assumption is that the bathing solution,

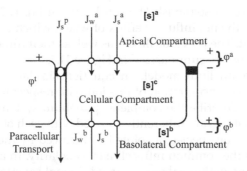

FIGURE 11.4
Schematic representation of the general epithelial model. Superscript "a" stands for apical compartment, "b" stands for basolateral compartment, "p" stands for paracellular transport and "c" stands for cellular compartment [44]. The arrowheads denote direction of positive flux J. The "+" and "−" symbols denote the orientation of membrane potential (for example, a positive ϕ_t means apical compartment is positive with respect to the basolateral compartment).

in contact with the apical side of the epithelium layer, is assumed infinite in volume such that trans-epithelial ion transports do not alter ion concentrations in the bathing solution [44]. For an intact epithelium layer, a common approximation is to merge all the cells compromising the epithelium layer into a single *cell* compartment that exchanges ions with the apical and basolateral compartments.

Based on the previous assumptions, a set of differential equations is typically developed to describe the temporal variations of volume and ion concentrations of the cellular compartment. These differential equations describe the solute and water fluxes across each of the epithelial compartments as functions of electrochemical gradients, membrane transport parameters, and kinetic descriptions of the active transport and cotransport channels. Therefore, these equations are typically described as *electrokinetic* models. Figure 11.4 illustrates the simplest form of an epithelial transport system that is comprised of a single ion or a single solute. The parameters $[s]^a$, $[s]^b$, $[s]^c$ denote the concentration of the solute $[s]$ in the apical, basolateral, and cellular compartments, respectively. To maintain the osmolarity of the cellular compartment, each membrane acts as a semipermeable membrane for water fluxes allowing water to cross compartments to maintain osmotic equilibrium. Conservation of cellular water yields an equation that describes the temporal variation in the cell's volume as a function of water fluxes (Eq. 11.1) [44]:

$$\frac{dV}{dt} = A^a J_w^a + A^b J_w^b; \tag{11.1}$$

where A^a and A^b are the areas of the apical and basolateral membrane (m²), J_w^a and J_w^b [m³/(s m²)] are the respective apical and basolateral water fluxes. For each ion concentration in the cellular compartment, the concentration also varies temporally according to the following relation (Eq. 11.2) [44]:

$$V\frac{d[s]^c}{dt} = A^a J_s^a - A^b J_s^b - [s]^c \left(A^a J_w^a + A^b J_w^b \right); \tag{11.2}$$

where V is the volume of the intracellular compartment in m³, J_s^a [mol/(s m²)] is the influx of ion s across apical membrane, and J_s^b [mol/(s m²)] is an efflux, and $[s]^c$ (mol/m³) is the intracellular concentration of solute [s]. The third term in Eq. 11.2 reflects the change in the concentration due to the net influx or efflux of water, which can dilute or concentrate the cellular compartment. The previous fluxes, as well as their directions into or out of the intracellular compartment, are summarized in Figure 11.4.

For each ion in the epithelium model, an equation similar to Eq. 11.2 is needed to describe the change in the concentration of this ion with respect to time. Therefore, $N + 1$ equations are needed to describe the complete epithelium system, one for each ion and one for water. These equations are inherently coupled with each other such that change in the concentration of each ion species or solute is influenced by the common intracellular concentration as well as the common intracellular osmolarity. In addition, if the solute is composed of charged ions with a valance z_s, an additional constraint of electroneutrality must be imposed. To enforce electroneutrality, the summation of the concentrations of all ions, weighted by their positive or negative valences, should equal zero. The membrane currents can be derived from the summation of apical and basolateral fluxes for a system of two or more ion species (Eq. 11.3) [44]:

$$I_a = FA^a \sum_s z_s J_s^a \tag{11.3a}$$

$$I_b = FA^b \sum_s z_s J_s^b \tag{11.3b}$$

where F is Faraday's constant. Cellular electroneutrality constraints are imposed by ensuring the current entering the cell across the apical membrane (I_a) is equal to the current leaving the cellular compartment across the basolateral membrane (I_b) [i.e., $I_a = I_b$]. The influx or efflux for each solute across a membrane is a direct function of the membrane potential. The mathematical model of a certain epithelial system can, therefore, be summarized into finding the membrane potential at each time instant that ensures that the electroneutrality constraint is met. The following subsections, will discuss the ions typically involved in the TEP, the nature of the fluxes, and the relationship between the fluxes and the membrane potential.

11.2.1.1 Passive Transport

Passive solute flux across all membranes is assumed to occur by electrodiffusion through ion-specific channels in each membrane. These fluxes are termed passive since no energy is consumed by the cell to generate this flux. However, this flux is generated due to diffusion forces, from regions of high ion concentration to regions of lower ion concentration, or due to drift forces, caused by the electric fields generated between regions of high voltage to regions of lower voltage [21]. Passive transport of ions is typically described by the Goldman–Hodgkin–Katz (GHK) equation (Eq. 11.4) (see Appendix a for the derivation):

$$J_s^x = P_s z_s U_X \frac{\left([s]_1 - [s]_2 e^{-z_s U_X}\right)}{1 - e^{-z_s U_X}} \tag{11.4}$$

where J_s^X is defined as the flux of solute [s] through membrane X, $[s]_1$ and $[s]_2$ are the solute concentration in compartments 1 and 2 on either sides of the membrane. The parameter P_s is the permeability of solute s through membrane X. To facilitate the analysis of the equations, it is common in the literature to use dimensionless potential/voltage instead of the actual potential/voltage in Volts. The dimensionless potential is achieved by normalizing the original potential by a constant $\dfrac{RT}{F}$ (i.e. $U_X = \dfrac{\phi_X RT}{F}$). Here R is the universal gas constant and T is the temperature of the system.

11.2.1.2 Active Transport

In passive transport, ions move from regions of high concentration to regions of lower concentration. Similarly, positive ions move in the same direction as the incident electric field, whereas negative ions move in the opposite direction. However, in some cases, ions can move in the opposite direction of the electric field or from regions of low concentration to regions of higher concentration. This process is called active transport because it involves ion pumps that consume energy in the form of adenosine tri-phosphate (ATP). The main active pump which is present in the majority of cells is the 3Na$^+$/2K$^+$ ATPase pump that uses hydrolysis to pump three Sodium (Na$^+$) ions out of the cell and two potassium (K$^+$) ions into the cell. This is performed against the concentration gradient since typically the extracellular medium contains more Na$^+$ and fewer K$^+$ ions than the intracellular medium. Driving Na$^+$ out of the cell in the opposite direction of the concentration gradient facilitates transport of several proteins, glucose, and other nutrients into the cell [2,45,46].

In epithelial tissue, the 3Na$^+$/2K$^+$ ATPase pumps are concentrated in the basolateral membrane (see Figure 11.5) of an epithelial system and are absent from the apical membrane. The most commonly used equation to describe the flux of the 3Na$^+$/2K$^+$ ATPase is given by (Eq. 11.5) [45,46]

$$J^b_{Na} = J_{Na,max} \left[\frac{\left[Na^+ \right]_c}{\left[Na^+ \right]_c + K^{Na}} \right]^3 \left[\frac{\left[K^+ \right]_b}{\left[K^+ \right]_b + K^{K}} \right]^2 \left(a \cdot U_b + b \right) \tag{11.5a}$$

$$J^b_K = J_{K,max} \left[\frac{\left[Na^+ \right]_c}{\left[Na^+ \right]_c + K^{Na}} \right]^3 \left[\frac{\left[K^+ \right]_b}{\left[K^+ \right]_b + K^{K}} \right]^2 \left(a \cdot U_b + b \right) \tag{11.5b}$$

where $J_{Na,max}$ and $J_{K,max}$ are the maximum turnover rates of the Na$^+$ and K$^+$ fluxes, respectively, due to the 3Na$^+$/2K$^+$ ATPase pump. The value of the parameter $J_{K,max}$ is typically

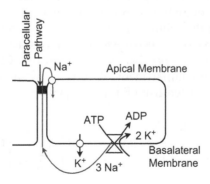

FIGURE 11.5
An epithelial monolayer illustrating the Na$^+$ channels on apical membrane and 3Na$^+$/2K$^+$ ATPase pump in the basolateral membrane. Because of the localized distribution of ions a loop current (blue arrow) is produced to maintain overall system electroneutrality [2].

two-thirds of the value of the parameter $J_{Na,max}$ since the $3Na^+/2K^+$ ATPase pump moves three Na^+ ions out of the cellular compartment for every two K^+ ions its pumps in. The term $(a. U_b + b)$ is described as the potential dependent factor since the pump is not electroneutral. Values of K^{Na} and K^K are defined as saturation constants for the intracellular Na^+ and basolateral K^+ ions. The values of the parameters a, b, K^{Na}, and K^K vary based on the type of the epithelium tissue. Another form of the $3Na^+/2K^+$ ATPase pump kinetics that has been also reported in several other models is depicted in Eq. 11.6 below [45]:

$$J_{3Na^+/2K^+} = J_{Na^+/K^+\ pump,max} \left[\frac{\left[Na^+ \right]_c}{\left[Na^+ \right]_c + K_{int,Na}^{pump}\left(1 + \frac{\left[K^+ \right]_c}{K_{int,K}^{pump}} \right)} \right]^3 \left[\frac{\left[K^+ \right]_b}{\left[K^+ \right]_b + K_{ext,K}^{pump}\left(1 + \frac{\left[Na^+ \right]_b}{K_{ext,Na}^{pump}} \right)} \right]^2$$

(11.6)

In Eq. 11.6, Na^+ and K^+ fluxes are independent of the potential difference between the compartments. The $3Na^+/2K^+$ ATPase pumps one extra positive ion outside of the cellular compartment than what it pumps inside the cell, in effect maintaining a higher concentration of Na^+ ions and a lower concentration of K^+ ions in the cellular compartment [2]. Also, it has a general effect of making the cellular compartment more negative in potential than the extracellular basolateral compartment [2].

11.2.1.3 Cotransport

Cotransport channels are associated with many kinds of epithelial tissues. Cotransport is a process that does not require ATPase activity rather it utilizes the movement of one ion down the concentration gradient to transport other solutes into or out of the cell [47]. Transport of solutes in this case is performed by one protein or by a protein complex. Any cotransport system that allows transportation of two or solutes in the same direction, either inward or outward through the cell membrane is referred as *symport* [47], whereas two solutes transported through the membrane in the opposite direction (i.e., one going in, the other one going out of the cellular compartment) via a cotransport system is defined as *antiport* [47]. One example of *symport* system is the $Na^+/K^+/2Cl^-$ pump located in basolateral membrane which pumps one Na^+, one K^+, and two Cl^- ions from the basolateral compartment to the cellular compartment (all ions in the same direction). The respective cotransport flux can be calculated from Eq. 11.7 as [45]

$$J_{Na^+/K^+/2Cl^-} = J_{Na^+/K^+/2Cl^-,max} \left(\frac{\left[Na^+ \right]_b}{\left[Na^+ \right]_b + K_{Na}} \frac{\left[K^+ \right]_b}{\left[K^+ \right]_b + K_K} \frac{\left[Cl^- \right]_b}{\left[Cl^- \right]_b + K_{Cl,1}} \frac{\left[Cl^- \right]_b}{\left[Cl^- \right]_b + K_{Cl,2}} \right.$$

$$\left. - \frac{\left[Na^+ \right]_c}{\left[Na^+ \right]_c + K_{Na}} \frac{\left[K^+ \right]_c}{\left[K^+ \right]_c + K_K} \frac{\left[Cl^- \right]_c}{\left[Cl^- \right]_c + K_{Cl,1}} \frac{\left[Cl^- \right]_c}{\left[Cl^- \right]_c + K_{Cl,2}} \right)$$

(11.7)

Where $J_{Na^+/K^+/2Cl^-}$ is the maximum turnover rate of the cotransporter and K_{Na}, K_K, and K_{Cl1}, K_{Cl2} are the saturation constants of Na^+, K^+, and Cl^-, respectively.

11.2.2 Electrokinetic Models in Different Epithelial Tissues

In this section, we will summarize some of the salient differences between the reported in electrokinetic models of different types of epithelial tissues from different organs reported in the literature (i.e., airway, nasal, corneal, conjunctival, renal, etc.) [48–58]. In most of the reported models, the epithelium tissue is modeled using the three basic compartments: apical, basolateral, and cellular as previously described. In some cases, the apical compartment may be referred as mucosal and basolateral compartment is referred as serosal depending on the epithelial system. The permeability coefficients of some of the most common active and passive channel present in the apical/basolateral membranes of different epithelium tissue are reported in different studies [45,46,48–58]. All the passive electrodiffusion channels employ the GHK equation to calculate the respective ion fluxes. Similarly, the permeability coefficients for paracellular transports of several epithelial systems can be found listed in [45,46,48–58]. The variations in the modeling parameters generate transepithelial potentials that vary over in a wide range from a couple of millivolts to tens of millivolts to simulate different tissue locations [45,48–58]. For example, a TEP of $\approx -50\,mV$ was reported in Bronchial Epithelia in [55] and a TEP of $\approx -8\,mV$ was reported in Human Airway Epithelia in [48].

11.2.3 Algorithm

The evaluation of the model involves integrating Eqs. 11.1 and 11.2 from an initial time ($t_{initial}$) to a final time (t_{final}) using appropriate numerical methods for the solution of ordinary differential equations [59]. The detailed steps of the computation are as follows:

1. Transport parameters, initial conditions $t_{initial}$, t_{final}, and Δt are specified. The simulation begins with setting the independent variable to $t_{initial}$.

2. Membrane potentials are calculated using the algorithm shown in Figures 11.6 and 11.7.

3. Solute and water fluxes are computed using the membrane potentials and respective flux equations (Eqs. 11.4–11.7).

4. The state equations Eqs. 11.1 and 11.2 are evaluated and integrated numerically to $t + \Delta t$. The simplest form of numerical integration formula can be implemented by using forward Euler method [60]. For example, cell volume of an epithelial system according to Eq. 11.1 at time $t + \Delta t$ will follow $V_{t+\Delta t} = V_t + \left(A^a J_w^a + A^b J_w^b\right)\Delta t$. This solution algorithm is an explicit method, which requires careful selection of Δt to ensure stability [59].

5. Terminate calculation if $t + \Delta t \geq t_{final}$. Otherwise, jump to step 2 and repeat the whole process.

During the computation of Step 4, the membrane potentials must be updated with the imposed constraint of electroneutrality. There are two separate algorithms for calculating the membrane potentials, based on whether we are simulating the short circuit condition,

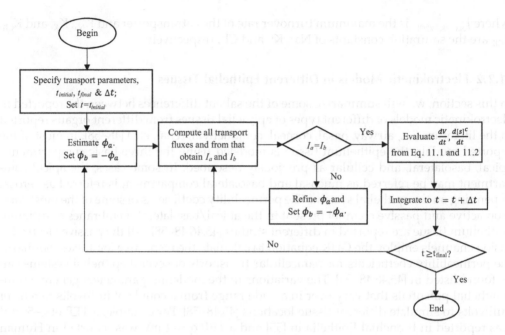

FIGURE 11.6
Flowchart showing the sequential computational steps involved in modeling epithelial systems under voltage-clamp condition [44]. Circle denotes begin or end; square boxes denotes mathematical operation; diamonds denotes decision. After each time step, one can record the interested values as per requirements i.e., ion concentration, potential, etc.

termed voltage clamp or the open circuit condition, termed the current clamp. The two different simulation configurations can be described as follows.

11.2.3.1 Voltage Clamp (Short Circuit) Case

This simulation resembles the voltage-clamp experimental setup where the transepithelial voltage is ϕ_t is maintained at a constant value and the transepithelial current, I_t, is measured. The most widely used value for the clamped ϕ_t is zero which results in the short circuit current, i.e., $I_t = I_{sc}$. In general, the trans-epithelial current I_t is composed of two components: (i) the para-cellular current I_p and (ii) the apical/basolateral current I_a/I_b. To maintain the electroneutrality of the cellular compartment $I_a = I_b$. For a short-circuit condition, computation of I_a and I_b requires either the apical potential ϕ_a or the basolateral potential ϕ_b, since the transepithelial potential ϕ_t is already fixed at a known value. The calculation of either ϕ_a or ϕ_b one will lead to determination of the other since $\phi_t = \phi_a + \phi_b = 0$. The procedure involves (i) taking an initial guess for ϕ_a, (ii) calculating $\phi_b = \phi_t - \phi_a$, and (iii) calculating I_a and I_b using the values of ϕ_a and ϕ_b; check whether $I_a = I_b$ (iv) repeat the whole iteration until $I_a = I_b$ is met. Therefore, the analytical solution of this problem is intractable, which is why we have to implement a numerical procedure based on the Newton–Raphson method (see details in Appendix b) [61]. According to the Newton–Raphson method, an updated approximation of the potential ϕ_a' can be achieved from the predecessor value of ϕ_a as follows, $\phi_a' = \phi_a - \dfrac{f(\phi_a)}{f'(\phi_a)}$, where $f(\phi_a)$ in this case is formulated using the equation $I_a = I_b$. The complete algorithm of the voltage clamp configuration is depicted in Figure 11.6.

11.2.3.2 *Current Clamp (Open Circuit) Case*

In the case of the current clamp setup, the transepithelial I_t current is held constant at a predefined value, typically $I_t = 0$, and the resulting transepithelial potential ϕ_t is measured/ calculated. Since the paracellular pathways have small but nonzero permeability values, I_p must exists in a manner that $I_a + I_p = I_t$ and $I_a = I_b$ to maintain the overall electroneutrality of apical and basolateral chambers. In other words, for open-circuit condition, there will be a loop current which flow across the transcellular pathways and complete the loop back via paracellular pathway. In this case, we need to simultaneously estimate ϕ_a or ϕ_b using a similar Newton–Raphson numerical method [61] as discussed in the previous section. The overall procedure for current clamp case is depicted in Figure 11.7.

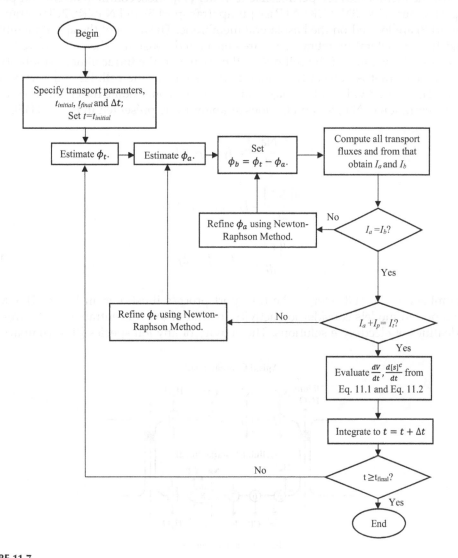

FIGURE 11.7

Flowchart showing the sequential computational steps involved in modeling epithelial systems under current-clamp condition [44]. The major difference of this algorithm in comparison to the voltage clamp condition is the added checkpoint of $I_a + I_b = I_t$. In current clamp setup, we have to estimate both ϕ_t and ϕ_a.

11.2.4 Implementation

To further clarify the previous equations, the results of the electrokinetic model developed in [45] are recreated. In this model, the ion transport systems of human respiratory airway epithelia are simulated. The model includes three compartments (apical, basolateral, and cellular) separated by two membranes (apical and basolateral) as depicted in Figure 11.8. The membrane between the apical and cellular compartments is referred to as the apical membrane, which is generally permeable to Na$^+$, K$^+$, and Cl$^-$ ions. The basolateral membrane, between the cellular and basolateral compartments, allows diffusion of only K$^+$ and Cl$^-$ ions. There also exists a paracellular pathway, which allows ionic diffusion of all ions between the apical and basolateral compartment without crossing the cellular compartment. All the membranes are permissible to water [45]. Most common active and passive transport systems like 3Na$^+$/2K$^+$ ATPase pump (transport 5) and Na$^+$/K$^+$/2Cl$^-$ cotransport (transport 8) are located on the basolateral membrane. The areas of the apical membrane, A^a, and the basolateral membrane, A^b, are considered constant. Therefore, to reflect the variations in the volume of the cell due to the change in the intracellular osmolarity, the only parameter that is subject to change is the height of the cellular compartment H_c. Equation 11.2 is subdivided into 3 major equations to accommodate the change in intracellular concentration of Na$^+$, K$^+$, and Cl$^-$ ions as analytically presented in Eq. 11.8 [45]:

$$\frac{d\left[\mathrm{Na^+}\right]}{dt} = J_1 - 3J_5 + J_8 \tag{11.8a}$$

$$\frac{d\left[\mathrm{K^+}\right]}{dt} = J_2 + 2J_5 - J_7 + J_8 \tag{11.8b}$$

$$\frac{d\left[\mathrm{Cl^-}\right]}{dt} = J_3 - J_6 + 2J_8 \tag{11.8c}$$

The numbers in Eq. 11.8 refer to the transport process illustrated in Figure 11.8. Many of the reported models consider ion activity instead of ion concentrations to address the non-idealities of electrolyte solutions. The activity of any ion species [s] in compartment

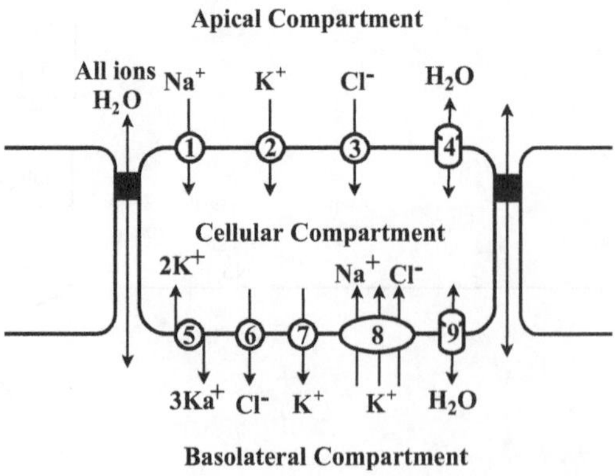

FIGURE 11.8
Schematic representation of airway epithelial model [45]. The paracellular pathway permits all ion species. Transport 4 and 9 accounts for the water flux inside or outside of the cellular compartment.

x is defined by the relationship, $a_s^x = \gamma_x[s]_x$, where γ_x is the nondimensional constant that depends on electrolyte chemical composition, concentration and temperature [62]. For this study, activity coefficient $\gamma_x = 0.76$ was considered for both intracellular and extracellular solution [62]. Equation 11.1 was modified in the following form for a cellular compartment with a constant surface area:

$$\frac{dH_c}{dt} = V_{H_2O}\left[P_{H_2O}^a\left(Osm_c - Osm_a\right) + P_{H_2O}^b\left(Osm_c - Osm_b\right)\right] \tag{11.9}$$

where, $P_{H_2O}^a$ and $P_{H_2O}^b$ are the water permeabilities of the apical and basolateral membranes, respectively, and V_{H_2O} is the molar volume of water. Osm denotes the osmolarity of any compartment x, defined by the relationship $Osm_x = \mu_x \sum [s]_x$, where μ_x is the osmotic coefficient (for this study 0.93 [62]).

From our previous description, the transport fluxes of electrodiffusion will follow the GHK equation. The active and cotransport flux equations were adjusted for the specific airway epithelial system. The transport equations used in this study are as follows (Eq. 11.10) [45]:

$$J_1 = P_{Na}^a U_a \frac{\left(a_{Na}^a - a_{Na}^c e^{-U_a}\right)}{1 - e^{-U_a}} \tag{11.10a}$$

$$J_2 = P_K^a U_a \frac{\left(a_K^a - a_K^c e^{-U_a}\right)}{1 - e^{-U_a}} \tag{11.10b}$$

$$J_3 = -P_{Cl}^a U_a \frac{\left(a_{Cl}^a - a_{Cl}^c e^{-U_a}\right)}{1 - e^{U_a}} \tag{11.10c}$$

$$J_4 = P_{H_2O}^a\left(Osm_c - Osm_a\right) \tag{11.10d}$$

$$J_5 = J_{Na^+/K^+ \, pump,max}\left[\frac{[Na^+]_c}{[Na^+]_c + K_{int,Na}^{pump}\left(1 + \frac{[K^+]_c}{K_{int,K}^{pump}}\right)}\right]^3\left[\frac{[K^+]_b}{[K^+]_b + K_{ext,K}^{pump}\left(1 + \frac{[Na^+]_b}{K_{ext,Na}^{pump}}\right)}\right]^2 \tag{11.10e}$$

$$J_6 = -P_{Cl}^b U_b \frac{\left(a_{Cl}^c - a_{Cl}^b e^{-U_b}\right)}{1 - e^{U_b}} \tag{11.10f}$$

$$J_7 = P_K^b U_b \frac{\left(a_K^c - a_K^b e^{-U_b}\right)}{1 - e^{-U_b}} \tag{11.10g}$$

$$J_8 = J_{\text{Na}^+/\text{K}^+/2\text{Cl}^-,\text{max}} \left(\frac{\left[\text{Na}^+\right]_b}{\left[\text{Na}^+\right]_b + K_{\text{Na}}} \frac{\left[\text{K}^+\right]_b}{\left[\text{K}^+\right]_b + K_{\text{K}}} \frac{\left[\text{Cl}^-\right]_b}{\left[\text{Cl}^-\right]_b + K_{\text{Cl},1}} \frac{\left[\text{Cl}^-\right]_b}{\left[\text{Cl}^-\right]_b + K_{\text{Cl},2}} \right.$$

$$\left. - \frac{\left[\text{Na}^+\right]_c}{\left[\text{Na}^+\right]_c + K_{\text{Na}}} \frac{\left[\text{K}^+\right]_c}{\left[\text{K}^+\right]_c + K_{\text{K}}} \frac{\left[\text{Cl}^-\right]_c}{\left[\text{Cl}^-\right]_c + K_{\text{Cl},1}} \frac{\left[\text{Cl}^-\right]_c}{\left[\text{Cl}^-\right]_c + K_{\text{Cl},2}} \right) \tag{11.10h}$$

$$J_9 = P_{\text{H}_2\text{O}}^b (Osm_c - Osm_b) \tag{11.10i}$$

$$J_{\text{Na}}^p = P_{\text{Na}}^p U_t \frac{\left(a_{\text{Na}}^a - a_{\text{Na}}^b e^{-U_t}\right)}{1 - e^{-U_t}} \tag{11.10j}$$

$$J_{\text{Cl}}^p = -P_{\text{Cl}}^p U_t \frac{\left(a_{\text{Cl}}^a - a_{\text{Cl}}^b e^{U_t}\right)}{1 - e^{U_t}} \tag{11.10k}$$

P_{Na}^a, P_{K}^a, and P_{Cl}^a denote the permeability coefficient of Na$^+$, K$^+$, and Cl$^-$ ions, respectively, for the passive diffusion channels on apical membrane, while the permeability coefficients for K$^+$ and Cl$^-$ ion diffusion channels on basolateral membrane are denoted by P_{K}^b and P_{Cl}^b, respectively. P_{Na}^p and P_{Cl}^p denote the permeability coefficient of Na$^+$ and Cl$^-$ paracellular diffusion, respectively. $P_{\text{H}_2\text{O}}^a$ and $P_{\text{H}_2\text{O}}^b$ define the water permeability at the apical and basolateral membranes, respectively, whereas Osm_a, Osm_b, and Osm_c stand for the osmolarity of the apical, basolateral, and cellular compartments, respectively. The parameter U_x denotes the dimensionless potential, normalized by $\frac{RT}{F}$ (i.e. $U_x = \frac{\phi_x RT}{F}$). The potential for the cellular compartment is considered as reference. Keeping in mind the sign convention of Figure 11.4 (i.e., $\phi_a = \phi_a - \phi_c$ and $\phi_b = \phi_c - \phi_b$), the apical potential will be positive and the basolateral potential will be negative at steady state, as a consequence transepithelial potential is denoted as $\phi_t = \phi_b + \phi_a$. Equation 11.10i–Eq. 11.10k defines the paracellular fluxes of ions, which are also electrodiffusion transport systems, dependent on ϕ_t/U_t since paracellular transport channels involve ionic diffusion from basolateral to apical compartment without going through the cellular compartment. The associated transport properties at steady state are listed in Table 11.2 with appropriate units [45].

Using the transport flux equations and parameters, the ionic currents through each compartment can be calculated by summing over all the ionic fluxes in the respective compartment while also considering the direction of flux and valance of the respective ions (i.e., vector sum). The 3Na$^+$/2K$^+$ ATPase pump is an electrogenic pump, pumping three positive ions (Na$^+$) out of the cellular compartment while pumping two positive ions (K$^+$) inside the cellular compartment. Therefore, the 3Na$^+$/2K$^+$ ATPase pump will have a net positive ion directed out of the cellular compartment to the basolateral compartment. The Na$^+$/K$^+$/2Cl$^-$ cotransport process (transport 8) is an ion-neutral pump. Therefore, it will not contribute to the basolateral current as well as the water fluxes. All the other flux equations will combine to give rise to the apical, basolateral, paracellular currents I_a, I_b, and I_p (Eq. 11.11).

$$I_a = F(J_1 + J_2 - J_3) \tag{11.11a}$$

$$I_b = F(J_5 + J_7 - J_3) \tag{11.11b}$$

TABLE 11.2

Model Parameters Used to Develop the Airway Epithelia TEP Model [45]

Parameter	Description	Value	Reference
F	Faraday constant	96485 C/mol	
R	Universal gas constant	8.314 J/(mol·K)	
T	Temperature	310 K	
V_{H_2O}	Water molar volume	1.814×10^{-5} m^3/mol	
$[Na^+]_a = [Na^+]_b$	KBr (potassium bromide) solution	140 mM	[63]
$[K^+]_a = [K^+]_b$	KBr (potassium bromide) solution	5.2 mM	[63]
$[Cl^-]_a = [Cl^-]_b$	KBr (potassium bromide) solution	119.6 mM	[63]
$[Na^+]_c$	Intracellular Na$^+$ concentration	30.526 mM	[45]
$[K^+]_c$	Intracellular K$^+$ concentration	105.526 mM	[45]
$[Cl^-]_c$	Intracellular Cl$^-$ concentration	60.526 mM	[45]
$P_{Na^+}^a$	Apical Na$^+$ permeability	1.66×10^{-8} m/s	[45]
$P_{K^+}^a$	Apical K$^+$ permeability	0.26×10^{-8} m/s	[45]
$P_{Cl^-}^a$	Apical Cl$^-$ permeability	4.3×10^{-8} m/s	[45]
$J_{Na^+/K^+pump,max}$	Maximum pump flux	3.8×10^{-6} mol/m^2·s	[48]
$J_{Na^+/K^+/2Cl^-,max}$	Maximum cotransport flux	3.9×10^{-6} mol/m^2·s	[64]
$P_{K^+}^b$	Basolateral Na$^+$ permeability	7.9×10^{-8} m/s	[45]
$P_{Cl^-}^b$	Basolateral Cl$^-$ permeability	1.8×10^{-8} m/s	[45]
$P_{Na^+}^p$	Paracellular Na$^+$ permeability	3×10^{-8} m/s	[45]
$P_{Cl^-}^p$	Paracellular Cl$^-$ permeability	3×10^{-8} m/s	[45]
$P_{H_2O}^a$	Apical water permeability	240 µm/s	[65]
$P_{H_2O}^b$	Basolateral water permeability	24 µm/s	[65]
$\gamma_a = \gamma_b = \gamma_c$	Activity coefficients	0.76	[62]
$\mu_a = \mu_b = \mu_c$	Osmotic coefficients	0.93	[62]
$K_{int,Na}^{pump}$	3Na$^+$/2K$^+$ ATPase pump kinetics	1.3 mM	[64]
$K_{int,K}^{pump}$	3Na$^+$/2K$^+$ ATPase pump kinetics	12 mM	[64]
$K_{ext,Na}^{pump}$	3Na$^+$/2K$^+$ ATPase pump kinetics	32 mM	[64]
$K_{ext,K}^{pump}$	3Na$^+$/2K$^+$ ATPase pump kinetics	0.14 mM	[64]
K_{Na}	Na$^+$/K$^+$/2Cl$^-$ cotransporter kinetics	105 mM	[48]
K_K	Na$^+$/K$^+$/2Cl$^-$ cotransporter kinetics	1.22 mM	[48]
$K_{Cl,1}$	Na$^+$/K$^+$/2Cl$^-$ cotransporter kinetics	103 mM	[48]
$K_{Cl,2}$	Na$^+$/K$^+$/2Cl$^-$ cotransporter kinetics	23.9 mM	[48]

The associated transport equations are as described in Eq. 11.10.

$$I_p = F\left(J_{Na^+}^p + J_{Cl^-}^p \right) \qquad (11.11c)$$

By definition, the apical current is positive when positive ions are flowing from the apical to the cellular compartment and the basolateral current is positive when the flow of positive ions is from the cellular to the basolateral compartment. Similarly, paracellular current is considered in the direction of apical to basolateral compartment. To impose the second fundamental constraint on any epithelial model, which is the constraint of electroneutrality, I_a, I_b, and I_p must follow $I_a = I_b$ in case of short circuit condition and $I_a = I_b = -I_p$ in case of open circuit condition as depicted in Figures 11.6 and 11.7.

11.2.5 Results

In this section, similar results to those reported in [45] are presented using the previously described algorithm. For simplicity, we neglected the transient change in osmolality and hence the changes in the cell height in the following results.

The measurement setup was done under the open circuit or current-clamp condition. In Figures 11.9 and 11.10, we show the steady-state prediction of the model up to 10 min after the simulation starts. Ouabain, an enzyme that inhibits the $3Na^+/2K^+$ ATPase pump, is applied after 10 min from reaching steady state. The $3Na^+/2K^+$ ATPase pump is the major contributor to the TEP buildup as well as the build-up of the high concentration of K^+ and the low concentration of Na^+ in the cellular compartment. After the pump is deactivated by Ouabain (*in silico* this is implemented by switching the value of P_5 from its steady-state value to), intracellular Na^+ concentration increases, as shown in Figure 11.9a, since no transport system is pumping Na^+ out of the cellular compartment. Similarly, the K^+ concentration decreases in the cellular compartment as shown in Figure 11.9b. Figure 11.9c shows that the cellular Cl^- concentration increases slightly, but the change is overall negligible with respect to the changes in the other ions in Figure 11.9a,b. The epithelial chamber will eventually lose its TEP voltage as shown in the plot of ϕ_t in Figure 11.9d.

Since the performed simulation is under open circuit condition, the apical, basolateral, and paracellular will have the following relationship $I_a = I_b = -I_p = I_{eq}$. After the application of Ouabain, we can see a significant decrease in the transepithelial current I_{eq} as shown in Figure 11.10a. As previously discussed, the $3Na^+/2K^+$ ATPase pump has a major contribution to the transepithelial potential buildup. After inhibition of the pump

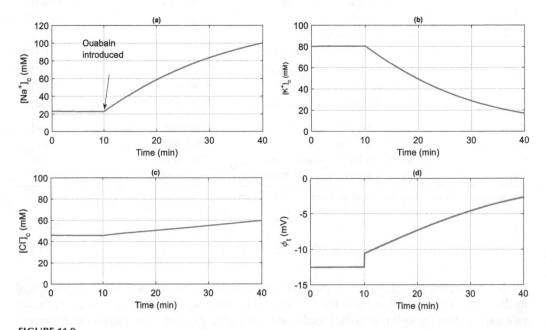

FIGURE 11.9
The variation of the intracellular concentration (a) Sodium Na^+, (b) potassium K^+, (c) Chloride Cl^-, and (d) the variation in the TEP (transepithelial potential) due to application of Ouabain after 10 min from reaching steady state.

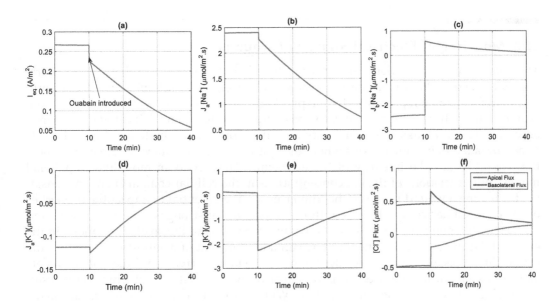

FIGURE 11.10
Effect of Ouabain application at 10 min on (a) Apical/Basolateral/Paracellular current ($I_{eq} = I_a = I_b = -I_p$), (b) Apical Na$^+$ Flux (J_1), (c) basolateral Na$^+$ flux (J_8-3J_5), (d) Apical K$^+$ Flux (J_2), (e) Basolateral K$^+$ flux ($2J_5 - J_7 + J_8$) (f) chloride Cl$^-$ flux through the apical (J_3) and basolateral membane ($2J_7 - J_6$).

by applying Ouabain, the potential diminishes (see Figure 11.9d) consecutively leading the transepithelial current to decrease as shown in Figure 11.10a. Figure 11.10b–f depicts the effect of Ouabain on the Na$^+$, K$^+$, and Cl$^-$ fluxes in apical and basolateral membrane. As the Na$^+$ concentration in the cellular compartment increases as shown in Figure 11.9a, the Na$^+$ diffusion flux ($J_1 = J_a[Na^+]$) from the apical to the cellular compartment will decrease as shown in Figure 11.10b. Figure 11.10c shows the vector sum of the Na$^+$ flux across the basolateral membrane (i.e., $J_{Na+/K+/2Cl-} - J_{3Na+/2K+}$). Before the introduction of Ouabain (before 10 min), $J_{3Na+/2K+}$ component was prominent leading to overall Na$^+$ efflux (out of the cellular compartment). After Ouabain is administered, the direction of the overall Na$^+$ flux switches to become from the cellular compartment to the basolateral compartment (influx) through the Na$^+$/K$^+$/2Cl$^-$ cotransport. However, this Na$^+$ is still much lower than the Na$^+$ flux before Ouabain was administered. The apical and basolateral K$^+$ flux is depicted in Figure 11.10d,e, respectively. The apical K$^+$ flux is due to the passive electrodiffusion from the cellular to the apical compartment before Ouabain is administered. Therefore, the apical K$^+$ is flux is an efflux and therefore, it will have a negative sign as can be visualized from Figure 11.10d. As Ouabain is administered, the cellular K$^+$ concentration decreases leading to a decrease in the apical K$^+$ efflux. Basolateral K$^+$ remains as an outward flux from the cellular compartment even after Ouabain introduction indicating that the passive diffusion K$^+$ transports dominates the influx contribution of the Na$^+$/K$^+$/2Cl$^-$ cotransporter (see Figure 11.10e). The apical and basolateral Cl$^-$ fluxes are depicted in Figure 11.10f, summarizing the equal but opposite effect of Cl$^-$ ion in the transepithelial potential buildup. Although, after several minutes of Ouabain introduction, the overall Cl$^-$ flux becomes influx, contributing to increased Cl$^-$ concentration in the cellular compartment as shown by adding the two components in Figure 11.10f.

11.3 Modeling of Electrical Signals of Wounds

The intact epithelium models are developed based on the assumption that ion concentration in the extracellular medium is constant. Moreover, the intact epithelium is uniform and therefore can be represented by the previously described coarse-grained model consisting of only three compartments: (i) apical, (ii) basolateral, and (iii) cellular. The presence of a wound breaks this uniformity and, therefore, the computational model needs to be upgraded to include regions where the epithelium layer is intact and regions where the wound breaks the integrity of the epithelium layer. Also, in most intact epithelial models, only variations of the ion concentrations in the cellular compartment are considered. Creating a wound in the epithelium layer has the potential to impact the properties of the extracellular compartments with the impact being strongest near the wound and weakest at the points furthest from the wound. Considering the spatial variations in the extracellular ion concentrations will have an added impact of axial diffusion within the extracellular space. Therefore, besides having three ionic currents in three compartments (apical, basolateral, and paracellular), we will also have an axial current which is the result of variable extracellular ion concentration. Without the presence of any external electrical excitation, ionic movement in the extracellular flux will be theoretically governed by Nernst-Planck electrodiffusion equation (Eq. 11.A6) [66–69]. Axial transport of all ions will combine with the radial fluxes due to different transport mechanisms in the apical and basolateral membrane to form the endogenous electric currents in the case of an epithelial wound. In the following subsections, three models, which address the non-uniformity caused by wounds are discussed.

11.3.1 Axon Model

One of the first mathematical model developed for such an injury, which incorporates the axial as well as the radial diffusion fluxes, is the model of a wounded or an injured axon reported in [70]. In this study, the variations in the extracellular ion concentrations were demonstrated in the case of a transected axon. The one-dimensional Nernst-Planck electrodiffusion equation was adopted to describe the axial flow of ions in the extracellular space. The electrical influence of the electrodiffusion equation was the consequence of distributed electric charge in the extracellular fluid. The spatially varying electric field was modeled as a "liquid junction potential," a potential that arises from the difference in mobility or concentration gradient between the ions according to the following Eq. 11.12 (p denotes the ion species considered) [70]:

$$E^{lj} = \frac{RT}{F} \left(\frac{\sum_p z_p D_p \frac{\partial [p]}{\partial z}}{\sum_p z_p^2 D_p [p]} \right) \tag{11.12}$$

The overall axial current density will be then the summation of all ion fluxes due to extracellular diffusion process (i.e., $J\left(\frac{A}{m^2}\right) = F \sum_p z_p j_p$. From the definition of Ohm's law, the overall current density can be rewritten as a product of conductivity and electric field

$\left(\text{i.e., } J\left(\dfrac{A}{m^2}\right) = \sigma\left(E - E^{lj}\right)\right)$. Equating the combined electrodiffusion equation and ohm's law equivalent, the analytical formula of conductivity can be derived as Eq. 11.13 [70]:

$$\sigma = \frac{F^2}{RT} \sum_p z_p^2 D_p [p]$$

(11.13)

The relationships to determine the axial current density were then combined with the inter-compartmental ion fluxes to calculate the combined effect of variation in extracellular ion concentration. The temporal variation of the ion concentration will obey the continuity equations (Eq. 11.14) [70]:

$$\frac{\partial [p]_i}{\partial t} = -\frac{\partial j_p^{\text{int}}}{\partial z} - \frac{2\pi r_i}{S_i} j_p^{\text{mem}}$$

(11.14a)

$$\frac{\partial [p]_e}{\partial t} = -\frac{\partial j_p^{\text{ext}}}{\partial z} - \frac{2\pi r_i}{S_e} j_p^{\text{mem}}$$

(11.14b)

where, $[p]_e$ and $[p]_i$ is the intracellular and extracellular ion concentrations of ion species $[p]$, j_p^{int}, $\partial j_p^{\text{ext}}$, and j_p^{mem} are the ion fluxes of ion species $[p]$ in the intracellular and extracellular medium and through the membrane. S_i and S_e are the intracellular and extracellular cross-sectional areas considering the geometry of the axon is cylindrical in shape having an inner and outer radius of r_i and r_e. In the next step, the membrane potentials are updated based on the modified concentrations. The overall procedure can be demonstrated by the flowchart shown in Figure 11.11.

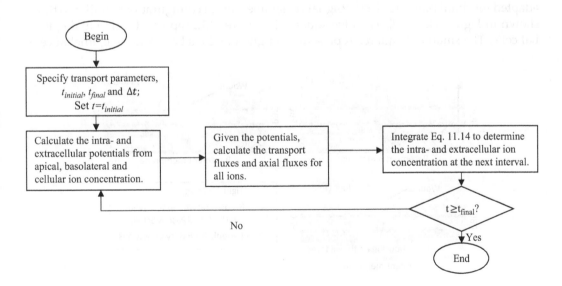

FIGURE 11.11
Flowchart showing the sequential computational steps involved in simulating endogenous wound current in the axon model.

11.3.2 Diffusion Drift Model

Recently, a two-dimensional model of the bioelectrical signals generated by growing breast tumors has been developed [66–68]. The model was based on the diffusion-drift model to effectively simulate the forces that drive the bioelectrical signals of dividing cancerous cells. The essence of the diffusion-drift model is the Poisson, Nernst-Planck, and Continuity equations [66–68]. The solution of these equations provides the spatial and the temporal variations of the concentration of each ion and the voltage in the system. However, these equations are highly nonlinear and coupled, and therefore, there are no closed form solutions to these equations for the realistic configuration of a healing wound. Therefore, to solve these equations, they need to be discretized both spatially in the x and y directions of the 2D domain and temporally in time (t). Differential equations with spatial and temporal variations are typically solved using one of two discretizations: (i) explicit temporal discretization and (ii) implicit temporal discretization. In explicit discretization, the electric potential is updated at every time step as a direct function of the ion concentrations at the previous time step. The implementation of the explicit discretization is simple but requires extremely small time steps to make the simulation stable. Implicit temporal discretization is unconditionally stable and, therefore, will allow significantly larger time steps than explicit discretization [66–68]. Implicit discretization in time provides stability at the expense of high implementation complexity since it requires the setup and solution of multiple large systems of equations, one for the potential and one for each ion considered [66–68]. Therefore, for slowly varying electric signals, similar to those exhibited in growing tumors and healing wounds, implicit discretization is typically preferred [66–68]. In addition to proposing implicit discretization for the time derivative, non-uniform spatial finite difference discretizations was implemented due to the large discrepancy in the dimensions of the cells and the intercellular spacing [66–68].

The bioelectrical signals generated by healing wounds are similar to those generated by breast tumors since both of them are slowly varying and caused by a disruption in the nominal charged ion distributions. Therefore, the diffusion-drift model was recently adapted for simulating the electric signals of simple wound configurations similar to those shown in Figure 11.12 [69]. The blue squares in Figure 11.12 represent individual epithelial cells. The small red squares represent the tight junctions between the epithelial cells

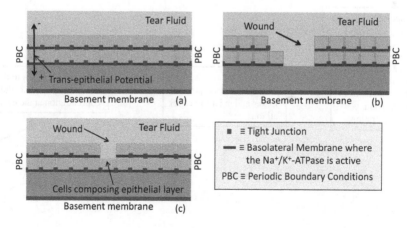

FIGURE 11.12
(a) Diffusion-Drift model of anof an intact epithelium, (b) deep and large wound configuration where 5 cells were removed due to an injury, and (c) a small wound configuration due to the removal of a single cell [69].

that help maintain the TEP. Periodic boundary conditions are employed to terminate the computational domain, and they should be placed significantly far from the wound center to approximately simulate the electric signals of a single wound [66–68]. Since the baso-lateral side is abundantly supplied by the blood vessels below, constant voltage and ion concentrations was assumed at the bottom boundary of the computational domain. The top boundary of the computational domain was assigned a Neumann boundary condition that the electric currents cannot penetrate. Figure 11.12a shows an intact epithelium layer, which will be used to generate the resting TEP before the wound is created. Figure 11.12b,c shows the creating of wounds by the removal of a different number of cells. Simple wound configurations were studied using this model and the model is currently being updated to account for more realistic wound configuration [69].

11.3.3 BioElectric Tissue Simulation Engine (BETSE)

Allen Discovery Center at Tufts University has developed a multi-physics simulator tool based on finite volume method to predict bioelectric patterns and their spatiotemporal dynamics by modeling the ion channel and gap junction activities [71]. There are a plethora of simulation tools available to model the nerve conduction which is an instantaneous phe-nomenon [72]. However, modeling bioelectrical signaling during a much slower process like wound healing requires modeling the ionic concentrations as spatially and temporally varying quantities. The group at Tufts University modeled their platform to keep track of ion concentrations and ion fluxes in space and time. The net charge distribution inside and outside of the cell then can be determined from the ion concentrations. Using these net charges, one can calculate the intracellular and extracellular voltage. The resulting change in voltage will affect the ion fluxes and from the net flux of ion, one can determine the endogenous current at a given time. The title of the environment is self-explanatory: BioElectric Tissue Simulation Engine (BETSE) [71].

The package uses an irregular Voronoi diagram-based cell grid (Figure 11.13), embedded within a square environmental grid. To include heterogeneity of tissue-like structures, the model allows the user to assign each cell with its unique cellular features like volume and cell membrane properties. Passive transport of solutes is derived from Nernst-Planck electrodiffusion equation. BETSE incorporates three distinct pathways for passive solute transport: (1) transmembrane, transport between intracellular and extracellular spaces through cell membrane; (2) intercellular, transport between adjacent cells through gap junctions; and (3) extracellular, ionic diffusion in the extracellular space due to concentra-tion gradient. Active ion fluxes will follow the same transport kinetics are discussed in our intact epithelium model. Changes in concentration will follow the continuity equation (Eq. 11.15) [71]:

$$\frac{\partial [s]_i}{\partial t} = -\nabla J_i^{\text{total}}$$

(11.15)

where $[s]_i$ is the concentration of ion species $[i]$ and J_i^{total} is the total flux of ion i. The net charge at each time step is then calculated from the summation of all ion concentrations. $p = \sum_i F z_i [s]_i$. The resultant potential will then follow the Poisson equation (Eq. 11.16) [71]:

$$\nabla^2 \phi = -\frac{F}{\varepsilon} \sum_i z_i [s]_i$$

(11.16)

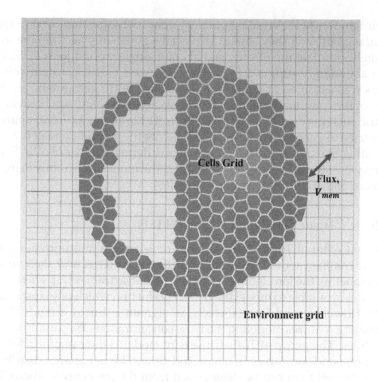

FIGURE 11.13
Schematic grid representation of the irregular Vornoi-based cell grid in a regular square environment to simulate heterogenous tissue structure (adapted from [71]).

where ϕ is the internal potential of the cell, which can be used to produce the corrected current density for the system.

In summary, several models have been developed to calculate the electric signals of intact epithelium layers. However, only preliminary modeling studies have been performed to simulate the electric signals generated by a wound. As these models are completed, we believe that they will shed light on the impact of electric signals on the wound healing process allowing the optimization of external ES as an effective treatment modality for wound healing acceleration.

Appendix

a GHK Equation

To ensure the proper functionality of a cell, which is the building block of any living organism, it is vital to maintain a specific concentration gradient between the intracellular and extracellular matrices. This concentration gradient is maintained by the controlled transport of different ions in or out of the cell. Two passive physical forces regulate the transport of a charged ion through the cell's membrane: (i) diffusion forces caused by concentration gradients and (ii) drift forces caused by electric fields generated due to voltage gradients.

i. Diffusion is defined as the net movement of ions, atoms, or molecules from a region of high concentration to a region of lower concentration. For the two concentration profiles depicted in Figure 11.A1, the ion flux or the rate of flow of the ion should be greater in the case of Figure 11.A1a, where the concentration of the ion [s] has a steeper gradient, than in the case of Figure 11.A1b. Moreover, the direction of the ion flux J is in the direction of decreasing ion concentration as shown in Figure 11.A1. Therefore, in a one-dimensional domain, the flux, J will be proportional to the negative of the derivative of [s] with respect to the spatial variable x. Introducing a proportionality constant D_s, the flux J can be expressed as

$$J = -D_s \frac{d[s]}{dx} \tag{11.A1}$$

ii. Drift motion is due to the force exerted on a charged particle in an electric field. To describe this, we start with the force that a unit charge experiences due to an electric field:

$$F = qE = \frac{d(mv)}{dt} = \frac{mv_d}{\tau} \tag{11.A2}$$

where F is the force, q is the unit charge, E is the electric field, v_d is the drift velocity of the charged particle, and τ is the time between two consecutive collisions of the charge particle. Ignoring collision acceleration or deceleration, we can simplify Eq. 11.A2 as [73]

$$v_d = \frac{qE\tau}{m} \tag{11.A3}$$

The mobility μ of a charge q can be expressed as $\mu = \frac{q\tau}{m}$; so that the drift velocity is $v_d = \mu E$ which simply states that in the presence of a spatially uniform electric field, the charge will move with a fixed velocity known as the drift velocity, which is proportional to the charge and inversely proportional to the mass of the charge. Note the current density associated with the flow of a charged solute within an electric field can be expressed as [73]

$$J = v_d z_s [s] = \mu E z_s [s] = -\mu z_s [s] \nabla \phi \tag{11.A4}$$

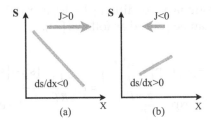

FIGURE 11.A1
Spatial distribution of a single ion species concentration [s]. J denoting the direction of the ion flux due to concentration gradient [73]. As per Eq. 11.A1, the ion flux is inversely proportional to the concentration gradient (hence larger arrow in case of (a)).

By definition, the electric field E can be related to the voltage ϕ as $E = -\nabla\phi$. The relation between ionic mobility μ and diffusion constant D_s is given by Einstein relationship: $D_s = \dfrac{\mu RT}{F}$ [73]. Therefore, the final relation of solute flux due to drift is [73]

$$J = -D_s \frac{z_s F}{RT}[s]\nabla\phi \tag{11.A5}$$

When the effects of the concentration gradient and the voltage gradient are combined, we get the total solute flux in a solution historically known as the *Nernst-Planck* equation [73]:

$$J = -D_s\left(\nabla[s] + \frac{z_s F}{RT}[s]\nabla\phi\right) \tag{11.A6}$$

Consider a setup where a semipermeable membrane of thickness L separates two solutions of solute $[s]$ and the potential difference across the membrane is V (i.e., $\dfrac{d\phi}{dx} = -\dfrac{V}{L}$). Let us assume, on the left of the membrane, the inside, the concentration $[s] = [s]_i$ and on the right of the membrane, the outside, the concentration $[s] = [s]_e$. At steady state and with no production of ions, the *Nernst-Planck* equation can be expressed as the one-dimensional relation [73]:

$$J = -D_s\left(\frac{d[s]}{dx} + \frac{z_s F}{RT}[s]\frac{d\phi}{dx}\right)$$

$$\Rightarrow J = -D_s\left(\frac{d[s]}{dx} - \frac{z_s F}{RT}[s]\frac{V}{L}\right)$$

$$\Rightarrow \frac{d[s]}{dx} - \frac{z_s FV}{RTL}[s] + \frac{J}{D_s} = 0 \tag{11.A7}$$

Equation 11.A7 is an ordinary differential equation for the concentration $[s]$, which can be integrated to yield [73]

$$\exp\left(-\frac{z_s VFx}{RTL}\right)[s] = \frac{JRTL}{D_s z_s VF}\left[\exp\left(-\frac{z_s VFx}{RTL}\right) - 1\right] + [s]_i \tag{11.A8}$$

Equation 11.A8 used the boundary condition $[s] = [s]_i$ at $x = 0$. By substituting $x = L$ and $[s] = [s]_e$ the GHK equation can be proved as follows [73]:

$$J = \frac{D_s}{L}\frac{z_s FV}{RT}\frac{[s]_i - [s]_e \exp\left(-\dfrac{z_s VF}{RT}\right)}{1 - \exp\left(-\dfrac{z_s VF}{RT}\right)} = P_s \frac{z_s FV}{RT}\frac{[s]_i - [s]_e \exp\left(-\dfrac{z_s VF}{RT}\right)}{1 - \exp\left(-\dfrac{z_s VF}{RT}\right)} \tag{11.A9}$$

where $P_s = \dfrac{D_s}{L}$ is defined as the permeability of ion $[s]$ through the semipermeable membrane that separates the two solutions.

b Newton-Raphson Method

The Newton-Raphson method [61] is a method for finding solutions to a real-valued function. For example, let us have a function $f(x)$ having x as an independent variable. The procedure starts with an initial guess x_0 that is reasonably close to the real root. A better approximation x_1 is then derived from the function value and its derivative at point $x = x_0$ (Eq. 11.A10). The procedure is repeated iteratively according to Eq. 11.A11 until sufficient accuracy is obtained as follows [61]:

$$x_1 = x_0 - \frac{f(x_0)}{f'(x_0)} \tag{11.A10}$$

$$x_{n+1} = x_n - \frac{f(x_n)}{f'(x_n)} \tag{11.A11}$$

References

1. C. Martin-Granados and C. D. McCaig, "Harnessing the electric spark of life to cure skin wounds," *Advances in wound care*, vol. 3, no. 2, pp. 127–138, 2014.
2. R. Nuccitelli, "A role for endogenous electric fields in wound healing," *Current topics in developmental biology*, vol. 58, pp. 1–26, 2003.
3. S. Ud-Din and A. Bayat, "Electrical stimulation and cutaneous wound healing: a review of clinical evidence," *Healthcare*, vol. 2, no. 4, pp. 445–467, 2014.
4. H. Rasche, "Haemostasis and thrombosis: an overview," *European Heart Journal Supplements*, vol. 3, no. Supplement Q, pp. Q3–Q7, 2001.
5. H. H. Versteeg, J. W. Heemskerk, M. Levi and P. H. Reitsma, "New fundamentals in hemostasis," *Physiological reviews*, vol. 93, no. 1, pp. 327–358, 2013.
6. A. C. d. O. Gonzalez, T. F. Costa, Z. d. A. Andrade and A. R. A. P. Medrado, "Wound healing-a literature review," *Anais Brasileiros de Dermatologia*, vol. 91, no. 5, pp. 614–620, 2016.
7. J. Hunckler and A. de Mel, "A current affair: electrotherapy in wound healing," *Journal of multidisciplinary healthcare*, vol. 10, p. 179, 2017.
8. C. T. Ambrose, "The Osler slide, a demonstration of phagocytosis from 1876: reports of phagocytosis before Metchnikoff's 1880 paper," *Cellular immunology*, vol. 240, no. 1, pp. 1–4, 2006.
9. H. Y. Chang, J. B. Sneddon, A. A. Alizadeh, R. Sood, R. B. West, K. Montgomery, J.-T. Chi, M. Van De Rijn, D. Botstein and P. O. Brown, "Gene expression signature of fibroblast serum response predicts human cancer progression: similarities between tumors and wounds," *PLoS Biology*, vol. 2, no. 2, p. e7, 2004.
10. K. S. Midwood, L. V. Williams and J. E. Schwarzbauer, "Tissue repair and the dynamics of the extracellular matrix," *The International Journal of Biochemistry & Cell Biology*, vol. 36, no. 6, pp. 1031–1037, 2004.
11. K. N. Riley and I. M. Herman, "Collagenase promotes the cellular responses to injury and wound healing in vivo," *Journal of Burns and Wounds*, 4, pp. 112–124, 2005.
12. D. R. Green, *Means to an End: Apoptosis and Other Cell Death Mechanisms*, Cold Spring Harbor, NY: Cold Spring Harbor Laboratory Press, 2011.
13. D. Nguyen, D. Orgill and G. Murphy, "The pathophysiologic basis for wound healing and cutaneous regeneration," In Orgill DP and Blanco C, (Eds.) *Biomaterials for Treating Skin Loss*. Cambridge: Woodhead Publishing Ltd. pp. 25–57, 2009.
14. G. S. Lazarus, "Definitions and guidelines for assessment of wounds and evaluation of healing," *Archives of Dermatology*, vol. 130, no. 4, p. 489, 1994.

15. "Woundhealingsocietyfoundation.org," 13 2 2017. Online. Available: www.woundhealingsoci-etyfoundation.org/About.aspx.
16. P. D. Dale, P. K. Maini and J. A. Sherratt, "Mathematical modeling of corneal epithelial wound healing," *Mathematical Biosciences*, vol. 124, no. 2, pp. 127–147, 1994.
17. J. E. Grey, "Venous and arterial leg ulcers," *BMJ*, vol. 332, no. 7537, pp. 347–350, 2006.
18. N. D. Evans, R. O. Oreffo, E. Healy, P. J. Thurner and Y. H. Man, "Epithelial mechanobiology, skin wound healing, and the stem cell niche," *Journal of the Mechanical Behavior of Biomedical Materials*, vol. 28, pp. 397–409, 2013.
19. B. Reid and M. Zhao, "The electrical response to injury: molecular mechanisms and wound healing," *Advances in Wound Care*, vol. 3, no. 2, pp. 184–201, 2014.
20. B. Song, M. Zhao, J. V. Forrester and C. D. McCaig, "Electrical cues regulate the orientation and frequency of cell division and the rate of wound healing in vivo," *Proceedings of the National Academy of Sciences*, vol. 99, no. 1, pp. 13577–13582, 2002.
21. C. D. McCaig, "Controlling cell behavior electrically: current views and future potential," *Physiological Reviews*, vol. 85, no. 3, pp. 943–978, July 2005.
22. G. Thakral, J. LaFontaine, B. Najafi, T. K. Talal, P. Kim and L. A. Lavery, "Electrical stimulation to accelerate wound healing," *Diabetic Foot & Ankle*, vol. 4, no. 1, p. 22081, 2013.
23. J. I. Hoare, A. M. Rajnicek, C. D. McCaig, R. N. Barker and H. M. Wilson, "Electric fields are novel determinants of human macrophage functions," *Journal of Leukocyte Biology*, vol. 99, no. 6, pp. 1141–1151, 2016.
24. A. Guo, B. Song, B. Reid, Y. Gu, J. V. Forrester, C. A. Jahoda and M. Zhao, "Effects of physiological electric fields on migration of human dermal fibroblasts," *Journal of Investigative Dermatology*, vol. 130, no. 9, pp. 2320–2327, 2010.
25. A. Sebastian, F. Syed, D. A. McGrouther, J. Colthurst, R. Paus and A. Bayat, "A novel in vitro assay for electrophysiological research on human skin fibroblasts: degenerate electrical waves downregulate collagen I expression in keloid fibroblasts," *Experimental Dermatology*, vol. 20, no. 1, pp. 64–68, 2011.
26. M. Rouabhia, H. J. Park and Z. Zhang, "Electrically activated primary human fibroblasts improve in vitro and in vivo skin regeneration," *Journal of Cellular Physiology*, vol. 231, no. 8, pp. 1814–1821, 2016.
27. M. Rouabhia, H. Park, S. Meng, H. Derbali and Z. Zhang, "Electrical stimulation promotes wound healing by enhancing dermal fibroblast activity and promoting myofibroblast trans-differentiation," *PLoS One*, vol. 8, no. 8, 2013.
28. Y. Wang, M. Rouabhia and Z. Zhang, "Pulsed electrical stimulation benefits wound healing by activating skin fibroblasts through the TGFβ1/ERK/NF-κB axis," *Biochimica et Biophysica Acta (BBA)-General Subjects*, vol. 1860, no. 7, pp. 1551–1559, 2016.
29. D. J. Cohen, W. J. Nelson and M. M. Maharbiz, "Galvanotactic control of collective cell migration in epithelial monolayers," *Nature Materials*, vol. 13, no. 4, pp. 409–417, 2014.
30. L. Li, W. Gu, J. Du, B. Reid, X. Deng, Z. Liu, Z. Zong, H. Wang, B. Yao and C. Yang, "Electric fields guide migration of epidermal stem cells and promote skin wound healing," *Wound Repair and Regeneration*, vol. 20, no. 6, pp. 840–851, 2012.
31. J. Gao, V. K. Raghunathan, B. Reid, D. Wei, R. C. Diaz, P. Russell, C. J. Murphy and M. Zhao, "Biomimetic stochastic topography and electric fields synergistically enhance directional migration of corneal epithelial cells in a MMP-3-dependent manner," *Acta Biomaterialia*, vol. 12, pp. 102–112, 2015.
32. H. Bai, C. D. McCaig, J. V. Forrester and M. Zhao, "DC electric fields induce distinct preangio-genic responses in microvascular and macrovascular cells," *Arteriosclerosis, Thrombosis, and Vascular Biology*, vol. 24, no. 7, pp. 1234–1239, 2004.
33. H. Bai, J. V. Forrester and M. Zhao, "DC electric stimulation upregulates angiogenic factors in endothelial cells through activation of VEGF receptors," *Cytokine*, vol. 55, no. 1, pp. 110–115, 2011.
34. R. C. Gomes, H. E. Brandino, A. de Sousa, N. Teixeira, M. F. Santos, R. Martinez and R. R. de Jesus Guirro, "Polarized currents inhibit in vitro growth of bacteria colonizing cutaneous ulcers," *Wound Repair and Regeneration*, vol. 23, no. 3, pp. 403–411, 2015.

35. M. R. Asadi and G. Torkaman, "Bacterial inhibition by electrical stimulation," *Advances in Wound Care*, vol. 3, no. 2, pp. 91–97, 2014.

36. L. C. Kloth, "Electrical stimulation technologies for wound healing," *Advances in Wound Care*, vol. 3, no. 2, pp. 81–90, 2014.

37. W. R. Gault and P. Gatens Jr, "Use of low intensity direct current in management of ischemic skin ulcers," *Physical Therapy*, vol. 56, no. 3, pp. 265–269, 1976.

38. C.-C. Chen and M. I. Johnson, "A comparison of transcutaneous electrical nerve stimulation (TENS) at 3 and 80 pulses per second on cold-pressor pain in healthy human participants," *Clinical Physiology and Functional Imaging*, vol. 30, no. 4, pp. 260–268, 2010.

39. E. Bosi, G. Bax, L. Scionti, V. Spallone, S. Tesfaye, P. Valensi, D. Ziegler, F. E. T. S. Group and others, "Frequency-modulated electromagnetic neural stimulation (FREMS) as a treatment for symptomatic diabetic neuropathy: results from a double-blind, randomised, multicentre, long-term, placebo-controlled clinical trial," *Diabetologia*, vol. 56, no. 3, pp. 467–475, 2013.

40. J. Colthurst and P. Giddings, "A retrospective case note review of the Fenzian electrostimulation system: a novel non-invasive, non-pharmacological treatment," *The Pain Clinic*, vol. 19, no. 1, pp. 7–14, 2007.

41. S. Hampton and L. King, "Healing an intractable wound using bio-electrical stimulation therapy," *British Journal of Nursing*, vol. 14, no. 15, 2005.

42. G. Torkaman, "Electrical stimulation of wound healing: a review of animal experimental evidence," *Advances in Wound Care*, vol. 3, no. 2, pp. 202–218, 2014.

43. G. Talebi, G. Torkaman, M. Firoozabadi and S. Shariat, "Effect of anodal and cathodal microamperage direct current electrical stimulation on injury potential and wound size in guinea pigs," *Journal of Rehabilitation Research and Development*, vol. 45, no. 1, p. 153, 2008.

44. R. Latta, C. Clausen and L. C. Moore, "General method for the derivation and numerical solution of epithelial transport models," *Journal of Membrane Biology*, 82, pp. 67–82, 1984.

45. G. J. Garcia, R. C. Boucher and T. C. Elston, "Biophysical model of ion transport across human respiratory epithelia allows quantification of ion permeabilities," *Biophysical Journal*, vol. 104, no. 3, pp. 716–726, 2013.

46. M. H. Levin, J. K. Kim, J. Hu and A. Verkman, "Potential difference measurements of ocular surface Na^+ absorption analyzed using an electrokinetic model," *Investigative Ophthalmology & Visual Science*, vol. 47, no. 1, pp. 306–316, 2006.

47. H. Lodish, A. Berk, A. Amon, A. Bretscher, C. Kaiser and M. Kriefer, *Molecular Cell Biology*, 7 ed., New York: W.H. Freeman, 2013.

48. J. A. Novotny and E. Jakobsson, "Computational studies of ion-water flux coupling in the airway epithelium. I. Construction of model," *American Journal of Physiology-Cell Physiology*, vol. 270, no. 6, pp. C1751–C1763, 1996.

49. A. Verkman and R. J. Alpern, "Kinetic transport model for cellular regulation of pH and solute concentration in the renal proximal tubule," *Biophysical Journal*, vol. 51, no. 4, pp. 533–546, 1987.

50. T. Hartmann and A. Verkman, "Model of ion transport regulation in chloride-secreting airway epithelial cells. Integrated description of electrical, chemical, and fluorescence measurements," *Biophysical Journal*, vol. 58, no. 2, pp. 391–401, 1990.

51. M. Duszyk and A. S. French, "An analytical model of ionic movements in airway epithelial cells," *Journal of Theoretical Biology*, vol. 151, no. 2, pp. 231–247, 1991.

52. J.-D. Horisberger, "ENaC-CFTR interactions: the role of electrical coupling of ion fluxes explored in an epithelial cell model," *European Journal of Physiology*, vol. 445, no. 4, pp. 522–528, 2003.

53. I. H. Quraishi and R. M. Raphael, "Computational model of vectorial potassium transport by cochlear marginal cells and vestibular dark cells," *American Journal of Physiology-Cell Physiology*, vol. 292, no. 1, pp. C591–C602, 2007.

54. H. Zhu and A. Chauhan, "Tear dynamics model," *Current Eye Research*, vol. 32, no. 3, pp. 177–197, 2007.

55. C. V. Falkenberg and E. Jakobsson, "A biophysical model for integration of electrical, osmotic, and pH regulation in the human bronchial epithelium," *Biophysical Journal*, vol. 98, no. 8, pp. 1476–1485, 2010.

56. D. L. O'Donoghue, V. Dua, G. W. Moss and P. Vergani, "Increased apical Na$^+$ permeability in cystic fibrosis is supported by a quantitative model of epithelial ion transport," *The Journal of Physiology*, vol. 591, no. 15, pp. 3681–3692, 2013.

57. V. Lew, H. Ferreira and T. Moura, "The behaviour of transporting epithelial cells. I. Computer analysis of a basic model," *Proceedings of the Royal Society of London B: Biological Sciences*, vol. 206, no. 1162, pp. 53–83, 1979.

58. M. Friedman, "Mathematical modeling of transport in structured tissues: corneal epithelium," *American Journal of Physiology-Renal Physiology*, vol. 234, no. 3, pp. F215–F224, 1978.

59. S. C. Chapra and R. P. Canale, *Numerical Methods for Engineers*, vol. 2, New York: McGraw-Hill, 1988.

60. L. Euler, *Institutiones Calculi Differentialis*, Teubner, 1755.

61. I. Newton, *De analysi per aequationes numero terminorum infinitas*, 1711.

62. R. Robinson and R. Stokes, "Electrolyte solutions," *Butterworths Scientific Publications*, 1959.

63. N. J. Willumsen and R. C. Boucher, "Shunt resistance and ion permeabilities in normal and cystic fibrosis airway epithelia," *American Journal of Physiology-Cell Physiology*, vol. 256, no. 5, pp. C1054–C1063, 1989.

64. G. E. Lindenmayer, A. Schwartz and H. K. Thompson, "A kinetic description for sodium and potassium effects on (Na^{++} K$^+$)-adenosine triphosphatase: a model for a two-nonequivalent site potassium activation and an analysis of multiequivalent site models for sodium activation," *The Journal of Physiology*, vol. 236, no. 1, pp. 1–28, 1974.

65. H. Matsui, C. W. Davis, R. Tarran and R. C. Boucher, "Osmotic water permeabilities of cultured, well-differentiated normal and cystic fibrosis airway epithelia," *Journal of Clinical Investigation*, vol. 105, no. 10, p. 1419, 2000.

66. A. M. Hassan and M. El-Shenawee, "Biopotential signals of breast cancer versus tumor types and proliferation stages," *Physical Review E*, vol. 85, p. 021913, 2012.

67. A. M. Hassan and M. El-Shenawee, "Diffusion–drift modeling of a growing breast," *IEEE Transactions on Biomedical Engineering*, vol. 56, no. 10, pp. 2370–2379, 2009.

68. A. M. Hassan and M. El-Shenawee, "Modeling biopotential signals and current densities of multiple breast cancerous cells," *IEEE Transactions on Biomedical Engineering*, vol. 57, no. 9, pp. 2099–2106, 2010.

69. A. M. Hassan, B. Reid, F. Ferreira and M. Zhao, "Drift-diffusion modeling of the electric signals generated by healing wounds," in *Proceedings of the IEEE International Symposium on Antennas and Propagation and USNC/URSI National Radio Science Meeting*, Fajardo, Puerto Rico, 2016.

70. J. Van Egeraat and J. Wikswo, "A model for axonal propagation incorporating both radial and axial ionic transport," *Biophysical Journal*, vol. 64, no. 4, pp. 1287–1298, 1993.

71. A. Pietak and M. Levin, "Exploring instructive physiological signaling with the bioelectric tissue simulation engine," *Frontiers in Bioengineering and Biotechnology*, vol. 4, p. 55, 2016.

72. C. J. Crasto, S. H. Koslow, J. M. Bower and D. Beeman, "Constructing realistic neural simulations with GENESIS," In C. J. Crasto, (Ed). *Neuroinformatics*, Totowa NY: Humana Press. pp. 103–125, 2007.

73. J. Keener and J. Sneyd, *Mathematical Physiology: I: Cellular Physiology*, New York: Springer Science & Business Media, 2010.

12

Electrical Shock Trauma

Colin McFaul
University of Chicago

Mei Li
Shanghai Power Hospital

Ze Liang
Peking Union Medical College

Raphael C. Lee
Chicago Electrical Trauma Research Institute, University of Chicago

CONTENTS

12.1 Introduction

The industrialization of electrical power has been one of the most impactful engineering feats in the history of humanity. As electric power penetrates further into society, it poses greater risk to human society in terms of safety. Many citizens have experienced electric shock at least once in their lifetime. The pain and fear generated from encounters with electricity usually prevents us from further tampering with such a dangerous force. However, no matter how careful, accidents can and do occur, especially among electrical workers who handle commercial electrical power lines every day. The purpose of this chapter is to provide a basic overview of the harmful effects of electrical force from both the engineering and medical perspectives.

The incidence of clinical manifestations following electrical shock injury is well documented. Often survivors never seek attention after less severe electrical shocks, rather they manage the injuries themselves. Furthermore, there is considerable variation in how electrical injury and safety is managed across various countries. In developing countries the expense of imposing safety practices is often not the top priority, resulting in high rates of injury. A study of major burn injuries in rural southern Turkey by Nursal et al. (2003) during a 1-year (2000–2001) period indicated that 21% of burn patients were victims of electrical injury. In highly industrialized nations, major electrical injury rates are on the decline. In the United States, electrocution remains the fifth leading cause of fatal occupational injury with an estimated economic impact of more than 1 billion dollars annually (Bureau of Labor Statistics 2017). The rates of injury are highest among electrical workers, mostly caused by "live" electrical equipment, such as wiring, light fixtures, and overhead power lines (McCann et al. 2003). More than 90% of these injuries occur in men, mostly between the ages of 20 and 34, with 4–8 years of experience on the job (Gourbière, Cabanes, and Lambrozo 1992). Another study found that the average age of victims was 37.5 years and the average experience was 11.3 years. In yet another study of the incidence in a 9-year period 96% of victims were male, and the mean age was 32.7 years (Hunt 1992). For survivors, the injury pattern is very complex, with a high disability rate due to accompanying neuromuscular and neuropsychological consequences.

Away from the workplace, most electrical injuries are due to either indoor household low-voltage (<1,000 V) electrical contact or outdoor lightning strikes (National Safety Council 2017). An epidemiological study conducted in India reveals that 60% of high-voltage (>1,000 V and high-current capacity) electric injuries were due to exposed electric wires on farm or agricultural land. While low-voltage electric shocks happened mainly at home (47%) and at professional utility places (29%) (McCann et al. 2003). In the United States, domestic household 60 Hz electrical shocks are common and may result in minor peripheral neurological symptoms or skin surface burns. More complex injuries may result depending on the current path, particularly following oral contact with household appliance cord disclosures or outlets by small children (National Safety Council 2017). Compared to a high-voltage shock that is usually mediated by an arc, low-voltage shocks are more likely to produce a prolonged, "no-let-go" contact with the power source. This "no-let-go" phenomenon is caused by an involuntary, current-induced, muscle spasm (Dalziel and Lee 1969). For 60 Hz electrical current, the "no-let-go" threshold for axial current passage through the forearm is 16 mA for males and 11 mA for females (Dalziel and Lee 1969; Dalziel, Ogden, and Abbott 1943).

There are roughly 30 human deaths annually in the United States due to lightning related electrical shocks and approximately ten times that number of injuries (Holle 2015; National Weather Service 2017). The range of lightning injury extent is quite broad, depending upon the magnitude of exposure and the condition of the victim. Usually lightning hits result in surface burns, central neurological damage similar to blunt head trauma, peripheral neurologic injury, and cardiac damage (Whitcomb, Martinez, and Daberkow 2002). Radiofrequency and microwave injuries result from industry related contacts and are less common than lightning injuries. Nonetheless, they represent an important medical problem to understand. At higher frequencies, when the wavelength is short enough to couple at the atomic level, the fields can be ionizing as well as possibly causing molecular heating. Electrical trauma may produce such complex patterns of injury because of variations in the source of the electricity, differences in tissue-current interactions by electrical frequency, the variation in current density along its pathway through the body, and variations in body size, body position, and use of protective gear. No two cases are the same.

12.2 Electrical Transport within Tissues

The fundamental bioengineering perspective is that the human body is considered to be a compartmentalized (or lumped element) conducting dielectric. It consists of about 60% water by weight: 33% intracellular and 27% extracellular (Duling 1983). Body fluid in both the intracellular and extracellular compartments is highly electrolytic, and these two compartments are separated by a relatively impermeable, highly resistive plasma membrane. Current within the body is carried by mobile ions in the body fluid. The concentration of mobile ions results in a conductivity of approximately 1.4 S m^{-1} in physiological saline. While electrons are the charge carriers in metallic conductors or electrical arcs, in the human body the charge carriers are ions. The conversion from one to the other occurs at the skin surface through electrochemical reactions (Geddes and Baker 1967).

At low frequencies (i.e., below radio frequencies), the electric current passing across the body distributes such that the electric field strength is nearly uniform throughout any plane perpendicular to the current path (Daniel et al. 1988; Lee and Kolodney 1987; Sances et al. 1981). As a consequence, the current density distribution depends on the relative electrical conductivity of various tissues and the frequency of the current. Experimental data support this basic concept. Sances et al. (1981) measured the current distribution in the hind limb of anesthetized hogs. They found that major arteries and nerves experienced the largest current density because of their higher conductivity. It was also observed that skeletal muscles carried the majority of the current due to their predominant volumetric proportions.

Anatomically, upper limbs are most involved in electric shocks, especially the right upper limb, as would be expected from dominant hand interactions with electrical sources (Sokhal et al. 2017). Cela et al. (2011) modeled this using a multiresolution admittance method. This model was applied to predict the damage in skeletal muscle caused by cell lysis and to simulate the injury pattern. The simulation found that current density increases towards the distal part of the arm as the cross sectional area decreases. The wrist has particularly high current density and damage due to the constriction and the high fraction of less conductive bone. The overall impedance of this arm model is 599 Ω, which is consistent with the estimated resistance of the human body (Cela, Lee, and Lazzi 2011). Computational models of human high-voltage electrical shock suggest that the induced tissue electric field strength in the extremities is high enough to electroporate skeletal muscle and peripheral nerve cell membranes (Diller 1994; Lee 1997; Reilly 1994; Tropea and Lee 1992) and to possibly cause electroconformational denaturation of membrane proteins.

Within tissues, low-frequency current distribution is determined by the density, shape, and size of cells. Cellular membranes are insulating ion transport barriers that shield the cytoplasmic fluid from electrical current. The higher the cell density in tissues, the lower the interstitial area available for ionic current which makes tissues less conductive. As cell size increases, the membrane has less impact on a cell's electrical properties, because the volume fraction of the cell occupied by the membrane is inversely proportional to the total cell size (Gaylor, Prakah-Asante, and Lee 1988). Similarly, the conductivity of skeletal muscle parallel to the long axis of the muscle cells is greater than that perpendicular to this axis. Solid volume fraction of the extracellular matrix can also be important in certain tissues and anatomic locations. For example, the resistivity of cortical bone and epidermis is higher than other tissues because their free water content is lower, as evidenced in the recent work by Kalkan et al. (2004).

At higher frequencies, in the RF and microwave ranges, the current distribution is dependent on different parameters. The cell membrane is no longer an effective barrier to

TABLE 12.1

Frequency – Wavelength Regimes with General Applications and Harmful Effects

Field Frequency (cycles/s)	Energy Coupling Mechanism	Tissue Damage
D.C. to 10^3	Ionic Currents	Joule Heating
	Forces on Cell Structures	Membrane Poration
10^3 to 10^7	Ionic Currents	Joule Heating
	Field Energy Absorption by cells	Cell spinning
10^7 to 10^9	Field Energy Absorption by proteins	Macromolecular Heating
10^9 to 10^{11}	Field energy absorption by water	Microwave Heating of water
10^{11} to 10^{15}	Field Energy Absorption by atomic bonds	Photo-optical protein damage

current passage, and capacitive coupling of power across the membrane readily permits current passage into the cytoplasm. Frequency-dependent factors like energy absorption and skin-depth effects govern the field distribution in tissues. At the highest frequency ranges, including light and shorter wavelengths, other effects such as scattering and quantum absorption effects become important in governing field distribution in tissues. Table 12.1 provides a categorization of frequency regimes, with the corresponding wavelength spectrum, their common applications, and their effects on tissues as a result of electrical injury. Mechanisms of biological effects are different in each regime. A discussion of injury mechanisms must also be separated according to the frequency regime.

12.3 Physicochemistry of Tissue Injury

12.3.1 Low-Frequency Electric Shocks

The pathophysiology of tissue electrical injury is complex, involving thermal, electroporation, and electrochemical interactions (Bhatt, Gaylor, and Lee 1990; Block et al. 1995; Kalkan et al. 2004; Lee and Astumian 1996) and blunt mechanical trauma secondary to thermoacoustic blast from high-energy arc (Capelli-Schellpfeffer et al. 1998). The various modes of trauma lead to complex patterns of injury, which remain incompletely described.

The understanding of electric injuries has deepened from simple burns by Joule heating to complicated models of cell damages. These new concepts are helping physicians with better management of electrical injury patients (Koumbourlis 2002). In the most general terms, tissue damage exists when proteins and other biomolecules, cellular organelle membranes or water content is altered. Among all the components of the cells and tissues, which can be damaged by an electrical shock, it is the thin cell membrane, which has the greatest vulnerability. Thus, the cell membrane appears to be most important determinate of tissue injury accumulation.

The most important function of the cell membrane is to provide a diffusion barrier against free ion diffusion (Parsegian 1969). Because most metabolic energy of mammalian cells is used in maintaining transmembrane ionic concentration differences (Mandel 1987), the importance of the structural integrity of the lipid bilayer is apparent. The conductance of electropermeabilized membranes may increase by several orders of magnitude. ATP production and in turn, ATP-fueled protein ionic pumps, cannot keep pace, leading to metabolic energy exhaustion. Cell necrosis results if the membrane is not sealed. Thus, in discussing tissue injury resulting from electrical shock, the principal focus is directed at kinetics of cell membrane injury and the reversibility of that process. A simulation study of membranes by Tarek (Tarek 2005) explains the electroporation phenomena in bilayers.

12.3.1.1 Direct Electric Force Mediated Injury

Cells within an applied DC or low-frequency electric field will experience electric forces which will act most forcefully across and along the surface of the cell membrane. The forces acting across the membrane can alter membrane protein conformation and disrupt the structural integrity of the lipid bilayer. The magnitude of the forces acting across the membrane is related to the induced transmembrane potential V_m. V_m depends on a variety of factors, such as the intracellular and extracellular medium conductivity, cell shape and size, the external electric field strength E as well as how the electric field vector orients with respect to the point of interest on the cell membrane (Gaylor, Prakah-Asante, and Lee 1988; Kalkan et al. 2004; Lee 1997).

Given that most cells are either somewhat spheroidal or cylindrical in shape, the relationship between the externally applied electric field and the induced transmembrane potential can be simplified to either of two simple forms. Under physiologic tissue conditions, the peak magnitude of induced transmembrane potential $V_m\left(V^p_m\right)$ at the electrode-facing poles of spherical cells can be expressed as

$$V^p_m = 1.5\, R_{cell} \cdot \cos\cdot(\phi)\cdot\left(1+\left(f/f_s\right)^2\right)^{-1/2} \cdot E_{peak}, \qquad (12.1)$$

where R_{cell} is the radius of the cell, E_{peak} is the peak field strength in the tissue surrounding the cell, ϕ is the angle off axis from the field direction, f_s is the sub-β-dispersion frequency limit below which the cell charging time is short compared to rate of field change, and f is the field frequency (Gaylor, Prakah-Asante, and Lee 1988). For cylindrically shaped cells, such as skeletal muscle and nerve cells, aligned in the direction of the field (herein assigned the z coordinate), the induced transmembrane potential takes a different form. Under these circumstances an electrical space constant parameter becomes useful in describing the electrical properties of the cell. The induced transmembrane potential can be expressed as a function of z:

$$V^p_m(z) \approx A\cdot\lambda_m \sinh\left(z/\lambda_m\right)\left(1+\left(f/f_s\right)^2\right)^{-1/2}\cdot E_{peak} \qquad (12.2)$$

where λ_m is the electrical space constant of the cell, A is a variable that depends on cell length, and the position $z = 0$ corresponds to the mid-point of the cell (Ho and Mittal 1996). The bottom of Figure 12.1 illustrates schematically the spatial variation of $V^p_m(z)$ on the cell size for both of these cases. Of course, physically larger cells like skeletal muscle and peripheral nerve oriented in the direction of the electrical field would experience an induced transmembrane potential of greater magnitude than smaller cells.

Equations 12.1 and 12.2 are valid as long as the electrical properties of the cell membrane remain constant. The characteristic transmembrane potential of mammalian cells has a magnitude of less than 140 mV (Cevc 1990). When an extracellular imposed electric field results in an induced transmembrane potential difference magnitude of greater than 200–300 mV across a mammalian cell membrane, molecular alterations occur that can lead to membrane disruption with subsequent loss of membrane transport barrier function (Gaylor, Prakah-Asante, and Lee 1988). Gaylor et al. also showed that crowding of cells

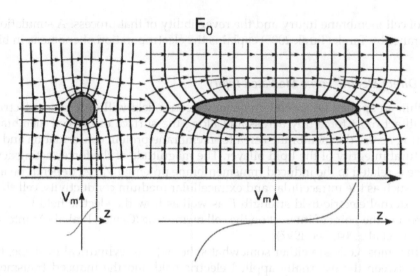

FIGURE 12.1
Top: Dependence of the induced transmembrane potential difference on cell size and position when cells are exposed to the same electric field. Electrical current lines are the same as electric field lines (shown as stream lines with arrows). Constant voltage lines are shown in darker color without arrows. Bottom: The transmembrane potential difference as a function of position along the direction of the applied electric field. The longer cell has a much larger transmembrane potential at its ends than the shorter cell.

increases the induced transmembrane potential by preventing the electric field lines from diverting around a given cell. One effect of this is that cells in the interior of a muscle are more susceptible to direct damage from an applied electric field than are cells that are adjacent to more conductive tissue.

The principal mechanisms of cell membrane molecular alteration (i.e., membrane damage) mediated by electrical forces are electroporation of the lipid bilayer and electro-conformational denaturation of the membrane proteins. Electro-conformational damage to membrane proteins has been well documented for voltage-gated membrane protein channels (Chen and Lee 1994; Lee et al. 1995). The processes occur quickly, on the order of milliseconds or less, after strong fields are applied.

Electroporation is the biophysical process of cell membrane disruption resulting from an induced membrane electrical field of such magnitude that reordering of lipids in the lipid bilayer takes place (Chen and Lee 1994; Lee et al. 1995; Weaver and Chizmadzhev 1996). Investigation of electroporation of many cells within a tissue was initially driven by the need for a better understanding of the pathophysiology of electrical injury (Glaser et al. 1988; Lee et al. 1988; Neu and Krassowska 1999). In the early 1990s, it was studied in connection with cardiac defibrillation shocks (Tung 1992; Tung et al. 1994). More recently, tissue electroporation has begun to be envisioned as a potential therapeutic tool in the medical field. It has found useful applications at both the single and multicellular level in (1) enhanced cancer tumor chemotherapy (electrochemotherapy, Heller et al. 1998; Mir et al. 1998); (2) localized gene therapy (Aihara and Miyazaki 1998; Mir et al. 1999); (3) transdermal drug delivery and body fluid sampling (Pliquett, Langer, and Weaver 1995; Prausnitz et al. 1996; Teissié et al. 1999); (4) introduction of foreign DNA into cells; (5) introduction of enzymes, antibodies, viruses, and other agents or particles for intracellular assays; (6) cell fusion; (7) inserting or embedding macromolecules into the cell membrane; (8) sampling microenvironments across membranes (Woods, Gandhi, and Ewing 2005);

(9) gene delivery in human embryonic stem cells (Kim et al. 2005); and (10) gene transfer in whole embryos (Pierreux et al. 2005) and gene repair in mammalian cells (Hu et al. 2005). Recent reviews and books published have extensively treated this subject (Chang et al. 2012; Ho and Mittal 1996; Jordan, Neumann, and Sowers 2013; Lynch and Davey 2012; Neumann, Kakorin, and Tœnsing 1999; Teissié et al. 1999; Weaver 1993; Weaver and Chizmadzhev 1996). Electroporation is further discussed in Chapter 7.

The process of cell membrane electroporation can be simulated as a chemical reaction that involves the rearrangement of phospholipids in the bilayer portion of the cell membrane. Bier et al. (2004) constructed a thermodynamic model of this process. It is driven by energy differences of the minimum energy state in pore formation and the bilayer state equaling the line tension minus the Kelvin Polarization stresses within the defect. This leads to an estimate of pore radius of 0.36 nm, consistent with previous reports (Bier et al. 2004).

Whether cells survive electroporation depends on whether the defects are transient or stable. Stability of defects is governed by the magnitude of the imposed transmembrane potential, the duration for which it is imposed, membrane composition and the membrane temperature. The time required to electroporate a cell is also dependent on these same variables and typically ranges from tens of microseconds to milliseconds. After application of a brief electroporating field pulse, the transiently electroporated membrane will spontaneously seal. Sealing follows removal of water from the membrane defects. Sealing kinetics are often orders of magnitude slower than the field relaxation because the forces driving the molecular sealing events are not as strong as those caused by the electroporating electric field. Sealing of electropores requires reordering of membrane lipids and removal of water molecules from the pore, both time- and energy-consuming processes (Bier et al. 1999; Gabriel and Teissié 1997; Gabriel and Teissié 1998).

The threshold transmembrane potential for induction of membrane electroporation is remarkably similar across cell types. The threshold V_m for electroporation has been found to be in the range 300–350 mV (Bier et al. 1999; Gabriel and Teissié 1997; Gabriel and Teissié 1998; Gowrishankar, Chen, and Lee 1998). Several authors have developed models to explain the experimentally observed values of V_m required for electroporation and associated transmembrane aqueous dynamics (Chizmadzhev, Arakelyan, and Pastuhenko 1979; Glaser et al. 1988). Using empirical data as parameters in an asymptotic approximation (39), the threshold V_m is predicted to be approximately 250 mV, consistent with reported experimental data.

Generally, for most media-suspended, isolated cells with a typical diameter of 10–20 μm, the DC field strength threshold for electroporation is in the range of 1 kV cm^{-1}. By comparison, the fields required to alter large cells are much less. Due to their relatively long length, skeletal muscle cells, up to 8 cm long in large animals, and nerve cells, up to 2 m long, have much lower electroporation thresholds. Therefore, muscle and nerve cell membranes are likely to be damaged with electrical fields as small as 60 V cm^{-1}.

The distribution of electropore formation in a cell placed in an applied field was addressed by DeBruin and Krassowska (1999a,b). Expanding from previous theoretical models and including the fact that the membrane charging time of about 1 μs is very short compared to a 1 ms field duration, they concluded that supraphysiological V_m at the pole caps is large enough to create pores, and thereby effectively to prevent a further increase in V_m in these areas. This confirms early experimental findings which show a saturation of V_m that is independent of the field strength for high-voltage shocks (Hibino et al. 1991; Kinosita et al. 1992; Knisley and Grant 1995). After the effect of ionic concentrations is included, DeBruin and Krassowska's model is able to confirm asymmetries in V_m observed in respect to the hyperpolarized (anode-facing) and hypopolarized (cathode-facing) pole of a cell (Gabriel and

Teissié 1997; Gabriel and Teissié 1998; Hibino, Itoh, and Kinosita 1993). Although the pore sealing time in the range of seconds predicted by the model is in agreement with some published experimental results (Neumann et al. 1992), others have found longer sealing times in the range of several minutes (Bier et al. 1999; Gabriel and Teissié 1997; Rols and Teissié 1990). This might be explained by the fact that (1) this model is based on pure lipid bilayers instead of cell membranes embedded with proteins, and (2) it only considers primary pores formed by V_m during the shock and not the secondary pores formed after the external field pulse ends, which provide transport routes for macromolecules.

Bhatt et al. (1990) measured electroporation damage accumulation using isolated, cooled *in vitro* rat *biceps femoris* muscles. After the initial impedance measurement, an electric field pulse was delivered to the muscle creating tissue field pulse amplitudes ranging between 30 and 120 V cm^{-1}, in the range of typical forearm field strengths in high-voltage electrical shock. The duration of the DC pulses ranged from 0.5 to 10 ms. These short pulses reduce Joule heating to insignificant levels. Field pulses were separated by 10 s to allow thermal relaxation. The drop in the low-frequency electrical impedance in the muscle tissue following the application of short-duration DC pulses indicated skeletal muscle membrane damage. A decrease in muscle impedance magnitude occurs following DC electric field pulses that exceed 60 V cm^{-1} magnitude and 1 ms duration. These results indicate that the field strength, pulse duration, and number of pulses are all factors that determine the extent of electroporation damage.

Based on these results, Block et al. (1995) electrically shocked fully anesthetized female Sprague-Dawley rats through cuff-type electrodes wrapped around the base of the tail and one ankle using a current-regulated DC power supply. The objective was to determine whether electroporation of skeletal muscle tissue *in situ* could lead to substantial necrosis. The study involved histopathological analysis and diagnostic imaging of an anesthetized animal hind limb. A series of 4 ms DC-current pulses, each separated by 10 s to allow complete thermal relaxation back to baseline temperature before the next field pulse, was applied. The electric field strength produced in the thigh muscle was estimated to range from 37 to 150 V cm^{-1}, corresponding to applied currents ranging from 0.5 to 2 A. These tissue fields were suggested to be on the same level as that experienced by many victims of high-voltage electrical shock. Muscle biopsies were obtained from the injured as well as the collateral control legs six hours post shock, and subjected to histopathological analysis. Sections of electrically shocked muscle revealed extensive vacuolization and hypercontraction-induced degeneration band patterns, which were not found in un-shocked contralateral controls (Figure 2 of Block et al. 1995)). The fraction of hypercontracted muscle cells increased with the number of applied pulses. These results are consistent with the investigators' hypothesis that non-thermal electrical effects alone can induce cellular necrosis. The pathologic appearance of the shocked muscle was similar to that seen in malignant hyperthermia, indicating that electroporation may lead to Ca^{2+}-influx into the sarcoplasm. A similar muscle injury pattern has been described in a human electrical injury victim published by deBono (1999) in a clinical case report. These results suggested that direct electrical injury of skeletal muscle *in situ* can lead to the commonly seen pattern of injury in electrical shock victims even in the absence of pathologically significant Joule heating.

12.3.1.2 Thermal "Burn" Injury

Passage of electrical current through electrically conducting media leads to Joule heating that can lead to severe burn injury in electrical shock victims. Burn injury is used here to specifically refer to tissue injury by damaging supraphysiological temperatures. Burn effects are related to lysis of cell membranes and protein denaturation, often followed by recognizable changes in the optical properties of tissue. There are two different potential outcomes for the denatured protein, which depend on the initial molecular structure and configuration. The first occurs when the native folded conformational state of the protein, held by intramolecular bonds, is different from the most favored conformation without intramolecular bonds (the thermodynamically lowest energy level). When this protein is heated, the intramolecular bonds are broken and it denatures to one of several preferred lower energy states from which it will not spontaneously return to the native conformation. Conceivably, if the primary structure of the protein is undamaged it may be plausible to reconfigure the protein using chaperone-assisted mechanisms similar to those which establish its initial folding after biosynthesis. The second possibility occurs when the native folded state of the protein is the same as the most energetically preferred conformation in the absence of intramolecular crosslinks. In this case, the protein is able to spontaneously refold to its native state.

The speed of the transition from natural to denatured states is governed by the Arrhenius rate equation which states that when the kinetic energy of the molecule exceeds a threshold magnitude E^i_a (for activation energy), the transition to the ith state will occur (in this case from natural to denatured state). For a large number of molecules at temperature T, the fraction Γ with a kinetic energy above E_a is governed by the Maxwell-Boltzmann relation (Eyring, Lin, and Lin 1980),

$$\Gamma^i = \exp\left(-E^i_a/k_B T\right) \tag{12.3}$$

where k_B is Boltzmann's constant. Because the strength of bonds retaining the folding conformation of macromolecules is dependent on the nature of the chemical bond, the value of E^i_a is dependent on molecular structure. Despite this complexity, the net rate of denaturation of cellular structures containing many different proteins is also often describable in terms of Equation 12.3. For example, the accuracy of this equation in describing thermal damage to cell membranes has been reported to be reasonable (Cravalho et al. 1992; Moussa et al. 1977; Rocchio 1989). Even the thermal injury to intact tissues like human skin is reasonably described by the simple Equation 12.3. It has been known for more than 50 years that the rate at which damage accumulates in heated skin can be estimated by convolving Equation 12.3 with the temperature history. The resulting expression is called the "heat damage" equation (Henriques Jr 1947).

$$d\Omega/dt = A \cdot \Gamma \tag{12.4}$$

where Ω is a parameter reflective of the extent of damage and A is a frequency factor that describes how often a configuration from which reaction is energetically possible occurs, which is also dependent on molecular structure. The shape of the temperature-time curve predicted by Equation 12.4 is the same as the human skin temperature vs. time scald burn curve measured by Henriques and Moritz (Moritz and Henriques Jr 1947). This temperature–time curve shape has also been obtained for heat damage to isolated cells (Cravalho et al. 1992).

Because the lipid bilayer structure is supported only by entropic energy gradients, the lipid bilayer is the most vulnerable cell structure to thermal damage (Gershfeld and Murayama 1988). Even at temperatures of only 6°C above normal (i.e., 43°C) the structural integrity of the lipid bilayer is lost (Moussa, Tell, and Cravalho 1979). In effect, the warmed lipid bilayer goes into solution, rendering the membrane freely permeable to small ions. At slightly higher temperatures, published reports indicate that the contractile mechanism of muscle cells is destroyed immediately following exposure to 45°C and above (Gaylor 1989). Experiments on fibroblasts demonstrated that heat-induced membrane permeabilization also begins to appear above 45°C (Merchant et al. 1998).

Bischof et al. (1995) investigated the effect of supraphysiological temperatures on isolated rat muscle cells using a thermally controlled microperfusion stage. Cells were loaded with the membrane permeable fluorescent dye precursor calcein-AM. After entering the cell, the precursor is converted by nonspecific esterases into the membrane impermeable fluorescent calcein. Using quantitative fluorescent microscopy, these authors measured time-resolved dye leakage from the muscle cells at several supraphysiological temperatures. In addition, using Equations 12.3 and 12.4, the authors determined the activation energy necessary to thermally induce membrane permeabilization in the isolated muscle cells to be 32.9 kcal mol^{-1} (Bischof et al. 1995). Reported activation energy values for thermal damage in other cell types are in the range from 30 to 140 kcal mol^{-1} (Cravalho et al. 1992).

During high-energy electrical shock, both thermal and direct electrical injury processes evolve with time. Both correlate with the square of the tissue electric field strength but, because of tissue material properties, often have different anatomical tissue injury distributions. Figure 12.2 illustrates the difference between electroporation damage and thermal damage. Panel A shows the development of electrical lysis of cells in the muscle caused by a model shock (Cela, Lee, and Lazzi 2011). In this case, a 0.5 s, 4.5 kV alternating current shock was applied between the palm and the shoulder, modeling a worst-case scenario 10 kV shock between the hands. Panel B shows the thermal injury function Ω resulting from a similar 1 s model shock. Joule heating is highest in the regions of the highest current density. These are the regions where the current is constrained to a smaller cross section area. The most notable such regions are the wrist and the point of electrical contact (the palm in this case). Figure 12.2 shows the difference between electroporation and thermal

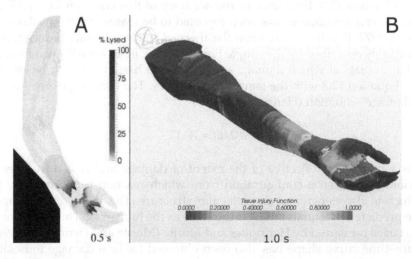

FIGURE 12.2

Typical electric injury pattern of an electrical shock in a human arm. (A) Injury due to electrical lysis of muscle cells after a 0.5 s shock. Reprinted from Cela, Lee, and Lazzi (2011) with permission (© 2011 IEEE). (B) Thermal injury function Ω due to joule heating after a 1 s shock. Thermal damage is highest at the point of electrical in the palm and the wrist (red), due to lower cross sections increasing the local current density. Note that the two damage scales are not directly comparable.

damage: regions that show no thermal damage can show electroporation damage, and regions that show significant thermal damage can show little to no electroporation injury. It is important to point out that a thermal injury function value $\Omega = 1$ in a given region does not correspond to thermal injury of all cells in that region. Ω can take on any positive value. Specifically, $\Omega = 1$ corresponds to approximately 63% of cells being thermally damaged.

12.3.1.3 Electro-Conformational Denaturation of Transmembrane Proteins

Imposed supraphysiological transmembrane potential differences can produce electroconformational changes of membrane proteins, ion channels, and ion pumps. Approximately 30% of cell membrane consists of proteins, some of them embedded into the bilayer, others spanning across the entire membrane. Many of them carry electric charges from amino acids with acidic or basic side groups that can be acted on directly by an intense V_m (charge separation or charge induction through dissociation). In addition, each amino acid has an electrical dipole moment of about 3.5 D (1 Debye = 3.336×10^{-30} C m) giving the proteins an overall dipole moment that, in the case of an α-helical protein structure, can reach 120 D (Tsong and Astumian 1987). In a strong external electric field, those molecules will orient themselves and thereby change their conformation to increase the effective dipole moment in the direction of that field.

If the field strength becomes sufficiently intense, those field-induced changes can cause irreversible damage to membrane proteins. In particular, ion channels and pumps with their selective voltage-gated charge transport mechanisms (e.g., Ca^{2+}-specific channel) are highly sensitive to differences in V_m. Chen et al. investigated the effects of large magnitude V_m pulses on voltage-gated Na^+ and K^+ channel behavior in frog skeletal muscle membrane using a modified double vaseline-gap voltage clamp. They found in both channel types, but more drastically in K^+ channels, reductions of channel conductance and ionic selectivity by the imposed V_m (Chen and Lee 1994). Further, these authors were able to demonstrate that these changes are not caused by the field-induced channel currents (Joule heating damage) but rather by the magnitude and polarity of the imposed V_m (Chen et al. 1998). In the most recent work, Clausen et al. (Clausen and Gissel 2005) studied the effects of shock and electroporation on the acute loss of force in skeletal muscles and the role of the Na^+ and K^+ pumps in the force recovery after electroporation. Ionic pumps alone are sufficient to compensate a simple mechanical leakage. They report that electroporation induces reversible depolarization, partial rundown of Na^+, K^+ gradients, cell membrane leakage, and loss of force. The consequences of this effect may underlie the transient nerve and muscle paralysis in electrical injury victims.

12.3.2 Radiofrequency (RF) and Microwave Burns

Every year, a few cases of RF (radio frequency) or microwave field injuries require medical attention in the United States. The victims are usually industrial workers. Above the low-frequency regime (>10 kHz), tissue response strongly depends upon the field frequency. In the 10–100 MHz RF range, two types of tissue heating occur, Joule and dielectric heating, with Joule heating outweighing dielectric heating. Small molecules like water, when not bound, are able to follow the field up to the gigahertz range (Chou 1995). However, at microwave frequencies (100 MHz to 100 GHz), dielectric heating is more significant than Joule heating because both bound and free water is excited by microwave radiation. Molecular dipoles of macromolecules have lower natural frequencies, so that their most efficient induction frequency is in the radiofrequency range.

Exposure to ambient microwave fields is known to cause burn trauma. Microwave burns have different clinical manifestations than low-frequency electrical shocks (Alexander, Surrell, and Cohle 1987; Nicholson, Grotting, and Dimick 1987; Rhoon et al. 1992; Sneed et al. 1992). At low frequency, the epidermis is a highly resistive barrier, whereas in the microwave regime, electrical power readily passes the epidermis in the form of capacitive coupling with very little energy dissipation. Consequently, the epidermis may not be burned unless it is very moist. The microwave field penetration into tissue has a characteristic depth in the range of 1 cm, resulting in direct heating of subepidermal tissue water. The rate of tissue heating is dependent not only on the amplitude of tissue electric field but also on the density of dipoles. For example, microwave heating is much slower in fatty tissues (Alexander, Surrell, and Cohle 1987; Surrell et al. 1987).

12.3.3 Lightning Injury

Lightning arcs result from dielectric breakdown in air caused by buildup of free electrical charges on the surface of clouds. The current through an arc can be enormous, but the duration is quite brief (1–10 ms). The primary current is confined to the surface of conducting objects connected by the arc. Peak lightning current ranges between 30,000 and 50,000 A, which is able to generate temperatures near 30,000 K. This abrupt heating generates a high-pressure thermoacoustic blast wave known as thunder.

An individual directly struck by lightning will experience current for a brief period of time. Initially, the surface of the body is charged by the high electric field in the air. This can cause breakdown of the epidermis, and several hundred amperes to flow through the body for a 1–10 µs period, which is long enough to induce electroporation. Following this, a much smaller current persists for several milliseconds, in which time the body is discharging into the ground. The duration of current flow is relatively short, so there is no substantial heating except a breakdown of the epidermis. However, disruption of cell membrane can wreak havoc on nerve and muscle tissues.

When lightning reaches the ground, it spreads out radially from the contact point. A substantial shock current can be experienced by a person walking nearby, if their feet are widely separated. For example, with an average lightning current of 20,000 A, a step length of 50 cm, and an individual located 10 m away from strike point, the voltage drops between the legs can reach 1500 V. This can induce a 2–3 A current flow through the body between the legs for a 10 µs period.

12.4 Common Clinical Syndromes Following Electrical Injury

Clinical manifestations of electrical shock depend on the magnitude, frequency, and duration of the imposed fields within the tissues that exist in the current path through the body. It is no surprise that workers coming in contact with high energy industrial electrical power sources experience rapid Joule heating of tissues throughout the current path. Total thermal destruction of tissues throughout the current path can result. Because of the high heat capacity of water, thermal injury dynamics accrue on a time frame of seconds in most cases. With more rapid kinetics, electroporation of tissues, especially skeletal muscle and peripheral nerve can occur.

Brief accidental electrical shocks involving several hundred volts are common among electricians and others working with electrical power. This may not result in a large thermal burn but will result in neuromuscular dysfunction and pain. Electroporation is the most likely pathophysiologic process linking the neuromuscular dysfunction to the electrical shock. Acute symptoms most often resolve in a few days. However, many of these shock victims will develop late generalized musculoskeletal pain, loss of balance control, and neuropsychological symptoms. Although the precise mechanisms linking a local brief electrical shock to generalized peripheral and central neurological problems remains under investigation, it is clear that these sequelae are common (Aase et al. 2014; Kelley et al. 1999; Pliskin et al. 1999; Ramati et al. 2009).

The most common anatomical contact point with of electrical current is to the arm and hand. Regarding the pattern of thermal injury, Joule heating is mostly concentrated at the wrist because of the small cross-sectional area and the lower conductivity of skin and bone. The second skin burn wound is usually at the flexor aspect of the elbow, and the third at the armpit. As the energy decreases along the arm, so does the damage. The skin burn wound varies depending on the condition of the victim when the incident happens. Where the skin is burned along the current path, the deeper tissues are as well. Patients can suffer from long-term rarefaction of bone and protracted residual wounds for months to years after recovery.

Electrical injury causes damage to the peripheral nerves and spinal cord, which can lead to cognitive and emotional changes. Patients exhibit lower attention, verbal memory, learning ability, and executive function, while experiencing higher incidents of depression and poor anger control. Research shows the relationship with changes in both cerebra and cognitive circuits, for example, including hypermetabolism in the cerebellum-limbic system.

12.5 Diagnostic Imaging of Electrical Injury

Because most of the damage caused by electrical shock occurs beneath the skin, it is important to discuss how to achieve tissue injury detection and localization. There are two basic cellular abnormalities in electrical injury: altered protein structure and disrupted cell membranes. In addition, there can be blood coagulation, tissue edema, elevated tissue pressures, and other abnormalities that affect molecular transport. From the clinical perspective, it is important to recognize areas of damaged cells and interrupted blood flow.

Magnetic resonance imaging (MRI) methods are particularly well suited for detection of changes in protein folding, disruption of cell membranes and tissue edema. Most useful are MRI methods based upon measurement of water proton behavior. Since water behavior will change in the presence of denatured proteins, and osmotic swelling will follow disruption of cell membranes, the typical MRI equipment in hospitals can measure these changes associated with electrical injury.

Technetium[99m]-PYP (pyrophosphate) is widely used as a radiolabel tracer for various forms of soft tissue injury including electrical trauma because it is believed to follow the calcium movement in cellular function (Shen and Jennings 1972). Increased tracer accumulation in muscle tissue indicates loss of cell membrane integrity, tissue edema and is predictive of tissue injury. The in vivo rat hind limb electrical injury model described by Block et al. (1995) monitored the uptake of Tc^{99m}-PYP in the electrically shocked tissue as a function of the magnitude of DC current. Either 0.5, 1.0 or 1.85 A of direct current was applied to the rat's hind limb, and compared to intravenous saline infusions as the sham-treatment. Their results indicated that Tc^{99m}-PYP does accumulate in electroporated tissue and the level of the tracer accumulation is positively correlated to the tissue field pulses applied. This indicates that quantitative imaging of Tc^{99m}-PYP uptake may be developed further as an indicator of the extent of electroporation or other membrane injury.

A recent report by Park et al. (2017) measured cerebral blood volume (CBV) of electrical injury patients. In that study, electric injury patients exhibiting cognitive dysfunction were imaged to measure CBV. It was found that greater CBV correlated with various clinical measures of cognitive function. Because CBV can be measured with gadolinium contrast enhanced MRI, this may allow more quantitative means of diagnosing electrical injury and the concomitant cognitive impairment, as well as leading to more effective treatment.

12.6 Summary and Conclusions

Given the importance of electrical power to human culture, the problem of electrical injury is one that will continue to exist for the foreseeable future. Electrical injury has been poorly understood and less than optimally managed in the past. Better understanding of injury mechanisms, anatomical patterns of injury, and therapy are required. A prompt, accurate clinical diagnosis of electrical injury is one of the most difficult tasks in the medical field (Hunt 1992) because it usually calls upon an understanding of the complex interactions between the electric current and human tissue. Specifically, an accurate and complete diagnosis is complicated by:

1. The exact tissue damage mechanism and damage level depends on several deterministic parameters including the characteristics of the power source (DC or AC current, voltage, frequency, etc.), path, and duration of the closed circuit, area and impedance of the skin contract points. Clinical injury assessment and management priority setting requires four-dimensional assessment in order to arrive at a correct diagnosis.

2. Electrical damage to the tissues is not easily detectable by visual inspection or physical examination. Often neuromuscular and neuropsychological sequelae will not manifest themselves for months after healing. Furthermore, tissue injured by direct electrical force mediated processes may initially appear viable, only to become visibly necrotic at a later point (in a number of days) (Artz 1967; Baxter 1970; Hammond and Ward 1994).

Rehabilitation and reconstruction needs in the electrically injured are usually not obvious at the initial evaluation. The reintegration of the individual into their pre-injury living situation often becomes a real challenge. Aside from physically obvious impairments (loss of limb, etc.) it is not uncommon for an electrician to develop a phobia towards electricity after being injured. The more in-depth understanding of the underlying mechanism of injury will lead to a more specific treatment regime that may prevent some of the late sequelae of electrical injury.

Acknowledgments

Parts of the research presented were funded by grants from the Electric Power Research Institute (RP WO-2914 and RP WO-9038), the National Institutes of Health (NIGMS 5-R01 GM53113), and Commonwealth Edison. The authors thank Zhou-xian Pan for assistance in editing this chapter.

References

Aase, Darrin M., Joseph W. Fink, Raphael C. Lee, Kathleen M. Kelley, and Neil H. Pliskin. 2014. "Mood and Cognition after Electrical Injury: A Follow-up Study." *Archives of Clinical Neuropsychology: The Official Journal of the National Academy of Neuropsychologists* 29 (2): 125–130. doi:10.1093/arclin/act117.

Aihara, Hiroyuki, and Jun-ichi Miyazaki. 1998. "Gene Transfer into Muscle by Electroporation in Vivo." *Nature Biotechnology* 16 (9): 867–870.

Alexander, Randell C., James A. Surrell, and Stephen D. Cohle. 1987. "Microwave Oven Burns to Children: An Unusual Manifestation of Child Abuse." *Pediatrics* 79 (2): 255–260.

Artz, Curtis P. 1967. "Electrical Injury Simulates Crush Injury." *Surgery, Gynecology & Obstetrics* 125 (6): 1316.

Baxter, Charles R. 1970. "Present Concepts in the Management of Major Electrical Injury." *Surgical Clinics of North America* 50 (6): 1401–1418.

Bhatt, Deepak L., Diane C. Gaylor, and Raphael Lee. 1990. "Rhabdomyolysis Due to Pulsed Electric Fields." *Plastic and Reconstructive Surgery* 86 (1): 1–11.

Bier, Martin, Stephanie M. Hammer, Daniel J. Canaday, and Raphael Lee. 1999. "Kinetics of Sealing for Transient Electropores in Isolated Mammalian Skeletal Muscle Cells." *Bioelectromagnetics* 20 (3): 194–201. doi:10.1002/(SICI)1521-186X(1999)20:3<194::AID-BEM6>3.0.CO;2-0.

Bier, Martin, Thiruvallur R. Gowrishankar, Wei Chen, and Raphael Lee. 2004. "Electroporation of a Lipid Bilayer as a Chemical Reaction." *Bioelectromagnetics* 25 (8): 634–637.

Bischof, John C., Joseph Padanilam, W. H. Holmes, Robert M. Ezzell, Raphael Lee, Ronald G. Tompkins, Martin L. Yarmush, and Mehmet Toner. 1995. "Dynamics of Cell Membrane Permeability Changes at Supraphysiological Temperatures." *Biophysical Journal* 68 (6): 2608–2614. doi:10.1016/S0006-3495(95)80445-5.

Block, Thomas, John Aarsvold, Kenneth L. Matthews II, Robert A. Mintzer, L. Philip River, M. Capelli-Schellpfeffer, Robert L. Wollmann, Satish Tripathi, Chin-Tu Chen, and Raphael Lee. 1995. "The 1995 Lindberg Award: Nonthermally Mediated Muscle Injury and Necrosis in Electrical Trauma." *Journal of Burn Care & Research* 16 (6): 21A–31A.

Bureau of Labor Statistics. 2017. "Industry Injury and Illness Data." *Injuries, Illnesses, and Fatalities.* Accessed July 14. www.bls.gov/iif/oshsum.htm.

Capelli-Schellpfeffer, Mary, Raphael Lee, Mehmet Toner, and Kenneth R. Diller. 1998. "Correlation between Electrical Accident Parameters and Injury." *IEEE Industry Applications Magazine* 4 (2): 25–31,41. doi:10.1109/2943.655657.

Cela, Carlos J., Raphael Lee, and Gianluca Lazzi. 2011. "Modeling Cellular Lysis in Skeletal Muscle due to Electric Shock." *IEEE Transactions on Biomedical Engineering* 58 (5): 1286–1293.

Cevc, Gregor. 1990. "Membrane Electrostatics." *Biochimica et Biophysica Acta (BBA)-Reviews on Biomembranes* 1031 (3): 311–382.

Chang, Donald C., Bruce M. Chassy, James Saunders, and Arthur E. Sowers. 2012. *Guide to Electroporation and Electrofusion.* San Diego: Academic Press. (1992).

Chen, Wei, and Raphael Lee. 1994. "Altered Ion Channel Conductance and Ionic Selectivity Induced by Large Imposed Membrane Potential Pulse." *Biophysical Journal* 67 (2): 603–612. doi:10.1016/S0006-3495(94)80520-X.

Chen, Yu Han, Yan Chen, and Dean Astumian. 1998. "Electric Field-Induced Functional Reductions in the K+ Channels Mainly Resulted from Supramembrane Potential-Mediated Electroconformational Changes." *Biophysical Journal* 75 (1): 196–206. doi:10.1016/S0006-3495(98)77506-X.

Chizmadzhev, Yuri A., Valeri B. Arakelyan, and Vassili F. Pastushenko. 1979. "Electric Breakdown of Bilayer Lipid Membranes." *Journal of Electroanalytical Chemistry and Interfacial Electrochemistry* 104 (January): 63–70. doi:10.1016/S0022-0728(79)81008-6.

Chou, C. K. 1995. "Radio Frequency Hyperthermia in Cancer Therapy." In *Biologic Effects of Nonionizing Electromagnetic Fields,* edited by J Bronzino, 1424–1428. Boca Raton, FL: CRC Press.

Clausen, Torbin, and Hanne Gissel. 2005. "Role of Na+, K+ Pumps in Restoring Contractility Following Loss of Cell Membrane Integrity in Rat Skeletal Muscle." *Acta Physiologica Scandinavica* 183 (3): 263–271. doi:10.1111/j.1365-201X.2004.01394.x.

Cravalho, Ernest, Mehmet Toner, Diane Gaylor, and Raphael Lee. 1992. *Response of Cells to Supraphysiological Temperatures: Experimental Measurements and Kinetic Models.* Cambridge, NY: Cambridge University Press.

Dalziel, Charles F., and W. Ralph Lee. 1969. "Lethal Electric Currents." *IEEE Spectrum* 6 (2): 44–50. doi:10.1109/MSPEC.1969.5213962.

Dalziel, Charles F., Eric Ogden, and Curtis E. Abbott. 1943. "Effect of Frequency on Let-Go Currents." *Electrical Engineering* 62 (12): 745–749. doi:10.1109/EE.1943.6436039.

Daniel, Rollin K., Paul A. Ballard, Paul Heroux, Ronald G. Zelt, and Courtney R. Howard. 1988. "High-Voltage Electrical Injury: Acute Pathophysiology." *The Journal of Hand Surgery* 13 (1): 44–49. doi:10.1016/0363-5023(88)90198-0.

DeBono, Raymond. 1999. "A Histological Analysis of a High Voltage Electric Current Injury to an Upper Limb." *Burns* 25 (6): 541–547. doi:10.1016/S0305-4179(99)00029-7.

DeBruin, Katherine A., and Wanda Krassowska. 1999a. "Modeling Electroporation in a Single Cell. I. Effects of Field Strength and Rest Potential." *Biophysical Journal* 77 (3): 1213–1224. doi:10.1016/S0006-3495(99)76973-0.

DeBruin, Katherine A., and Wanda Krassowska. 1999b. "Modeling Electroporation in a Single Cell. II. Effects of Ionic Concentrations." *Biophysical Journal* 77 (3): 1225–1233. doi:10.1016/S0006-3495(99)76974-2.

Diller, Kenneth R. 1994. "The Mechanisms and Kinetics of Heat Injury Accumulation." *Annals of the New York Academy of Sciences* 720 (1): 38–55. doi:10.1111/j.1749-6632.1994.tb30433.x.

Duling, Brian R. 1983. "The Kidney." In *Physiology,* 824. St. Louis, MO: The C. V. Mosby Company.

Eyring, Henry J., Sheng H. Lin, and S. M. Lin. 1980. *Basic Chemical Kinetics.* New York: John Wiley & Sons Inc.

Gabriel, Bruno, and Justin Teissié. 1997. "Direct Observation in the Millisecond Time Range of Fluorescent Molecule Asymmetrical Interaction with the Electropermeabilized Cell Membrane." *Biophysical Journal* 73 (5): 2630–2637. doi:10.1016/S0006-3495(97)78292-4.

Gabriel, Bruno, and Justin Teissié. 1998. "Mammalian Cell Electropermeabilization as Revealed by Millisecond Imaging of Fluorescence Changes of Ethidium Bromide in Interaction with the membrane 1 Presented at the 14th BES Symposium in Vingstedcentret (Denmark), 1998.1." *Bioelectrochemistry and Bioenergetics* 47 (1): 113–118. doi:10.1016/S0302-4598(98)00174-3.

Gaylor, Diane. 1989. "Role of Electromechanical Instabilities in Electroporation of Cell Membranes." *PhD Thesis.* MIT, Cambridge.

Gaylor, Diane, Kwaku Prakah-Asante, and Raphael Lee. 1988. "Significance of Cell Size and Tissue Structure in Electrical Trauma." *Journal of Theoretical Biology* 133 (2): 223–237. doi:10.1016/S0022-5193(88)80007-9.

Geddes, Leslie A., and Lee E. Baker. 1967. "The Specific Resistance of Biological Material—A Compendium of Data for the Biomedical Engineer and Physiologist." *Medical and Biological Engineering* 5 (3): 271–293.

Gershfeld, Norman L., and Makio Murayama. 1988. "Thermal Instability of Red Blood Cell Membrane Bilayers: Temperature Dependence of Hemolysis." *The Journal of Membrane Biology* 101 (1): 67–72. doi:10.1007/BF01872821.

Glaser, Ralf W., Sergei L. Leikin, Leonid V. Chernomordik, Vasili F. Pastushenko, and Artjom I. Sokirko. 1988. "Reversible Electrical Breakdown of Lipid Bilayers: Formation and Evolution of Pores." *Biochimica et Biophysica Acta (BBA) - Biomembranes* 940 (2): 275–287. doi:10.1016/0005-2736(88)90202-7.

Gourbière, Elisabeth, Jean Cabanes, and Jacques Lambrozo. 1992. "Work—Related Electrical Burns among Workers of Electricite de France: A Review of 938 Cases during the Ten-Year Period 1980 to 1989." In *1992 14th Annual International Conference of the IEEE Engineering in Medicine and Biology Society*, 7: 2821–2823 doi:10.1109/IEMBS.1992.5761709.

Gowrishankar, Thiruvallur R., Wei Chen, and Raphael Lee. 1998. "Non-Linear Microscale Alterations in Membrane Transport by Electropermeabilizationa." *Annals of the New York Academy of Sciences* 858 (1): 205–216. doi:10.1111/j.1749-6632.1998.tb10154.x.

Hammond, Jeffrey, and C. Gillon Ward. 1994. "The Use of Technetium-99 Pyrophosphate Scanning in Management of High Voltage Electrical Injuries." *The American Surgeon* 60 (11): 886–888.

Heller, Richard, Mark J. Jaroszeski, Douglas S. Reintgen, Chris A. Puleo, Ronald C. DeConti, Richard A. Gilbert, and Lewis F. Glass. 1998. "Treatment of Cutaneous and Subcutaneous Tumors with Electrochemotherapy Using Intralesional Bleomycin." *Cancer* 83 (1): 148–157. doi:10.1002/(SICI)1097-0142(19980701)83:1<148::AID-CNCR20>3.0.CO;2-W.

Henriques Jr, F. C. 1947. "Studies of Thermal Injury; the Predictability and the Significance of Thermally Induced Rate Processes Leading to Irreversible Epidermal Injury." *Archives of Pathology, Chicago* 43 (5): 489–502.

Hibino, Masahiro, Masaya Shigemori, Hiroyasu Itoh, K. Nagayama, and Kazuhiko Kinosita. 1991. "Membrane Conductance of an Electroporated Cell Analyzed by Submicrosecond Imaging of Transmembrane Potential." *Biophysical Journal* 59 (1): 209–220. doi:10.1016/S0006-3495(91)82212-3.

Hibino, M., H. Itoh, and K. Kinosita. 1993. "Time Courses of Cell Electroporation as Revealed by Submicrosecond Imaging of Transmembrane Potential." *Biophysical Journal* 64 (6): 1789–1800. doi:10.1016/S0006-3495(93)81550-9.

Ho, S. Y., and Gauri S. Mittal. 1996. "Electroporation of Cell Membranes: A Review." *Critical Reviews in Biotechnology* 16 (4): 349–362. doi:10.3109/07388559609147426.

Holle, Ronald L. 2015. "A Summary of Recent National-Scale Lightning Fatality Studies." *Weather, Climate, and Society* 8 (1): 35–42. doi:10.1175/WCAS-D-15-0032.1.

Hu, Yiling, Hetal Parekh-Olmedo, Miya Drury, Michael Skogen, and Eric B. Kmiec. 2005. "Reaction Parameters of Targeted Gene Repair in Mammalian Cells." *Molecular Biotechnology* 29 (3): 197–210. doi:10.1385/MB:29:3:197.

Hunt, John L. 1992. "Soft Tissue Patterns in Acute Electric Burns." In *Electrical Trauma: The Pathophysiology, Manifestations, and Clinical Management*, 83–104. Cambridge, NY: Cambridge University Press.

Jordan, Carol A., Eberhard Neumann, and Arthur E. Sowers. 2013. *Response of Cells to Supra-physiological Temperatures: Experimental Measurements and Kinetic Models*. New York: Springer Science & Business Media.

Kalkan, Tunaya, Mustafa Demir, A. S. M. Sabbir Ahmed, Sukru Yazar, S. Dervisoglu, H. B. Uner, and Oguz Çetinkale. 2004. "A Dynamic Study of the Thermal Components in Electrical Injury Mechanism for Better Understanding and Management of Electric Trauma: An Animal Model." *Burns* 30 (4): 334–340. doi:10.1016/j.burns.2003.11.009.

Kelley, Kathleen M., Tatiana A. Tkachenko, Neil H. Pliskin, Joseph W. Fink, and Raphael Lee. 1999. "Life after Electrical Injury: Risk Factors for Psychiatric Sequelae." *Annals of the New York Academy of Sciences* 888 (1): 356–363.

Kim, Jae-hwan, Hyun-jin Do, Seong-jun Choi, Hyun-jung Cho, Kyu-hung Park, Heung-Mo Yang, Sang-Hwa Lee, et al., 2005. "Efficient Gene Delivery in Differentiated Human Embryonic Stem Cells - ProQuest." *Experimental & Molecular Medicine* 37 (1): 36–44.

Kinosita, K., Masahiro Hibino, Hiroyasu Itoh, Masaya Shigemori, Ken 'ichi Hirano, Yutaka Kirino, and Tsuyoshi Hayakawa. 1992. "Events of Membrane Electroporation Visualized on a Time Scale from Microsecond to Seconds." In Chang, Donald C., Bruce M Chassy, James A. Saunders and Arthur E. Sowers, In *Guide to Electroporation and Electrofusion*, edited by Chang, Donald C., Bruce M. Chassy, James A. Saunders, and Arthur E. Sowers, 29–46. San Diego, CA: Academic Press.

Knisley, Stephen B., and Augustus O. Grant. 1995. "Asymmetrical Electrically Induced Injury of Rabbit Ventricular Myocytes." *Journal of Molecular and Cellular Cardiology* 27 (5): 1111–1122.

Koumbourlis, Anastassios C. 2002. "Electrical Injuries." *Critical Care Medicine* 30 (11 Suppl): S424–430.

Lee, Raphael. 1997. "Injury by Electrical Forces: Pathophysiology, Manifestations, and Therapy." *Current Problems in Surgery* 34 (9): 677, 679–764.

Lee, Raphael, and Michael S. Kolodney. 1987. "Electrical Injury Mechanisms: Dynamics of the Thermal Response." *Plastic and Reconstructive Surgery* 80 (5): 663–671.

Lee, Raphael, and R. Dean Astumian. 1996. "The Physicochemical Basis for Thermal and Non-Thermal 'burn' Injuries." *Burns* 22 (7): 509–519. doi:10.1016/0305-4179(96)00051-4.

Lee, Raphael, Diane C. Gaylor, Deepak Bhatt, and David A. Israel. 1988. "Role of Cell Membrane Rupture in the Pathogenesis of Electrical Trauma." *Journal of Surgical Research* 44 (6): 709–719.

Lee, Raphael, John N. Aarsvold, Wei Chen, R. Dean Astumian, Mary Capelli-Schellpfeffer, Kathleen M. Kelley, and Neil H. Pliskin. 1995. "Biophysical Mechanisms of Cell Membrane Damage in Electrical Shock." In *Seminars in Neurology*, 15, 367–374. New York: Thieme Medical Publishers, Inc.

Lynch, Paul, and Michael Raymond Davey. 2012. *Electrical Manipulation of Cells*. Springer Science & Business Media.

Mandel, Lazaro J. 1987. "Bioenergetics of Membrane Transport Processes." *Membrane Physiology*, 295–310. doi:10.1007/978-1-4613-1943-6_18.

McCann, Michael, Katherine L. Hunting, Judith Murawski, Risana Chowdhury, and Laura Welch. 2003. "Causes of Electrical Deaths and Injuries among Construction Workers." *American Journal of Industrial Medicine* 43 (4): 398–406. doi:10.1002/ajim.10198.

Merchant, Fatima A., W. H. Holmes, Mary Capelli-Schellpfeffer, Raphael C. Lee, and Mehmet Toner. 1998. "Poloxamer 188 Enhances Functional Recovery of Lethally Heat-Shocked Fibroblasts." *Journal of Surgical Research* 74 (2): 131–140. doi:10.1006/jsre.1997.5252.

Mir, Lluis, L. Frank Glass, Gregor Sersa, Justin Teissie, C. Domenge, Damijan Miklavcic, Mark J. Jaroszeski, et al., 1998. "Effective Treatment of Cutaneous and Subcutaneous Malignant Tumours by Electrochemotherapy." *British Journal of Cancer* 77 (12): 2336–2342.

Mir, Lluis, Michel F. Bureau, Julie Gehl, Ravi Rangara, Didier Rouy, Jean-Michel Caillaud, Pia Delaere, Didier Branellec, Bertrand Schwartz, and Daniel Scherman. 1999. "High-Efficiency Gene Transfer into Skeletal Muscle Mediated by Electric Pulses." *Proceedings of the National Academy of Sciences* 96 (8): 4262–4267. doi:10.1073/pnas.96.8.4262.

Moritz, Alan Re, and F. C. Henriques Jr. 1947. "Studies of Thermal Injury: II. The Relative Importance of Time and Surface Temperature in the Causation of Cutaneous Burns." *The American Journal of Pathology* 23 (5): 695.

Moussa, N. Albert, J. J. McGrath, Ernest G. Cravalho, and Panayiotis J. Asimacopoulos. 1977. "Kinetics of Thermal Injury in Cells." *Journal of Biomechanical Engineering* 99 (3): 155–159. doi:10.1115/1.3426283.

Moussa, N. Albert, E. N. Tell, and Ernest G. Cravalho. 1979. "Time Progression of Hemolysis of Erythrocyte Populations Exposed to Supraphysiological Temperatures." *Journal of Biomechanical Engineering* 101 (3): 213–217.

National Safety Council. 2017. "Research and Statistical Services." *NSC Research & Statistical Services*. Accessed July 24. www.nsc.org/Measure/Pages/safety-management-research-statistical-services.aspx.

National Weather Service. 2017. "NWS Lightning Fatalities." Accessed July 27. www.lightningsafety.noaa.gov/fatalities.shtml.

Neu, John C., and Wanda Krassowska. 1999. "Asymptotic Model of Electroporation." *Physical Review E* 59: 3471.

Neumann, Eberhard, Andreas Sprafke, Elvira Boldt, and Hendrik Wolf. 1992. "Biophysical Considerations of Membrane Electroporation." In *Guide to Electroporation and Electrofusion*, edited by DC Chang, BM Chassy, J Saunders, and AE Sowers, 77–90. San Diego, CA: Academic Press.

Neumann, Eberhard, Sergej Kakorin, and Katja Tœnsing. 1999. "Fundamentals of Electroporative Delivery of Drugs and Genes." *Bioelectrochemistry and Bioenergetics* 48 (1): 3–16. doi:10.1016/S0302-4598(99)00008-2.

Nicholson, C. Phifer, James C. Grotting, and Alan R. Dimick. 1987. "Acute Microwave Injury to the Hand." *The Journal of Hand Surgery* 12 (3): 446–449. doi:10.1016/S0363-5023(87)80021-7.

Nursal, Tarik Z., Sedat Yildirim, Akin Tarim, K. Caliskan, Ali Ezer, and Turgut Noyan. 2003. "Burns in Southern Turkey: Electrical Burns Remain a Major Problem." *Journal of Burn Care & Research* 24 (5): 309–314.

Park, Chang-hyun, Cheong Hoon Seo, Myung Hun Jung, So Young Joo, Soyeon Jang, Ho Young Lee, and Suk Hoon Ohn. 2017. "Investigation of Cognitive Circuits Using Steady-State Cerebral Blood Volume and Diffusion Tensor Imaging in Patients with Mild Cognitive Impairment Following Electrical Injury." *Neuroradiology*, July, 1–7. doi:10.1007/s00234-017-1876-1.

Parsegian, Adrian. 1969. "Energy of an Ion Crossing a Low Dielectric Membrane: Solutions to Four Relevant Electrostatic Problems." *Nature* 221 (5183): 844–846.

Pierreux, Christophe, Aurelie Poll, Patrick Jacquemin, Frederic Lemaigre, and Guy Rousseau. 2005. "Gene Transfer into Mouse Prepancreatic Endoderm by Whole Embryo Electroporation." *Journal of the Pancreas* 6 (2): 128–135.

Pliquett, Uwe, Robert Langer, and James C. Weaver. 1995. "Changes in the Passive Electrical Properties of Human Stratum Corneum due to Electroporation." *Biochimica et Biophysica Acta (BBA) - Biomembranes* 1239 (2): 111–121. doi:10.1016/0005-2736(95)00139-T.

Pliskin, Neil H., Joseph Fink, Aaron Malina, Sharon Moran, Kathleen M. Kelley, Mary Capelli-Schellpfeffer, and Raphael Lee. 1999. "The Neuropsychological Effects of Electrical Injury: New Insights." *Annals of the New York Academy of Sciences* 888 (1): 140–149.

Prausnitz, Mark R., Caroline S. Lee, Cindy H. Liu, Judy C. Pang, Tej-Preet Singh, Robert Langer, and James C. Weaver. 1996. "Transdermal Transport Efficiency during Skin Electroporation and Iontophoresis." *Journal of Controlled Release* 38 (2): 205–217. doi:10.1016/0168-3659(95)00121-2.

Ramati, Alona, Neil H. Pliskin, Sarah Keedy, Roland J. Erwin, Joseph W. Fink, Elena N. Bodnar, Raphael C. Lee, Mary Ann Cooper, Kathleen Kelley, and John A. Sweeney. 2009. "Alteration in Functional Brain Systems after Electrical Injury." *Journal of Neurotrauma* 26 (10): 1815–1822. doi:10.1089/neu.2008.0867.

Reilly, J. Patrick. 1994. "Scales of Reaction to Electric Shock." *Annals of the New York Academy of Sciences* 720 (1): 21–37. doi:10.1111/j.1749-6632.1994.tb30432.x.

Rhoon, Gerard C. Van, Jacoba van der Zee, Maria Pia Broekmeyer-Reurink, Andries G. Visser, and Huibert S. Reinhold. 1992. "Radiofrequency Capacitive Heating of Deep-Seated Tumours Using Pre-Cooling of the Subcutaneous Tissues: Results on Thermometry in Dutch Patients." *International Journal of Hyperthermia* 8 (6): 843–854. doi:10.3109/02656739209005031.

Rocchio, Catherine Mary. 1989. "The Kinetics of Thermal Damage to an Isolated Skeletal Muscle Cell." Massachusetts Institute of Technology, Department of Electrical Engineering and Computer Science.

Rols, Marie-Pierre, and Justin Teissié. 1990. "Electropermeabilization of Mammalian Cells. Quantitative Analysis of the Phenomenon." *Biophysical Journal* 58 (5): 1089–1098. doi:10.1016/S0006-3495(90)82451-6.

Sances, Anthony, Joel Myklebust, Sanford Larson, Joseph Darin, Thomas Swiontek, Thomas Prieto, Michael Chilbert, and Joseph Cusick. 1981. "Experimental Electrical Injury Studies. " *Journal of Trauma-Injury Infection & Critical Care* 21 (9): 589–597.

Shen, Anthony C., and Robert B. Jennings. 1972. "Kinetics of Calcium Accumulation in Acute Myocardial Ischemic Injury." *The American Journal of Pathology* 67 (3): 441–452.

Sneed, Penny K., Philip H. Gutin, Paul R. Stauffer, Theodore L. Phillips, Michael D. Prados, Stuart Suen, Sharon A. Lamb, and Brigid Ham. 1992. "Thermoradiotherapy of Recurrent Malignant Brain Tumors." *International Journal of Radiation Oncology Biology Physics* 23 (4): 853–861.

Sokhal, Ashok Kumar, Krishna Govind Lodha, Manoj Kumari, Rajkumar Paliwal, and Sitaram Gothwal. 2017. "Clinical Spectrum of Electrical Burns – A Prospective Study from the Developing World." *Burns* 43 (1): 182–189. doi:10.1016/j.burns.2016.07.019.

Surrell, James A., Randell C. Alexander, Stephen D. Cohle, F. R. Lovell Jr, and R. A. Wehrenberg. 1987. "Effects of Microwave Radiation on Living Tissues." *Journal of Trauma and Acute Care Surgery* 27 (8): 935–939.

Tarek, Mounir. 2005. "Membrane Electroporation: A Molecular Dynamics Simulation." *Biophysical Journal* 88 (6): 4045–4053. doi:10.1529/biophysj.104.050617.

Teissié, Justin, Natalie Eynard, Bruno Gabriel, and Marie-Pierre Rols. 1999. "Electropermeabilization of Cell Membranes." *Advanced Drug Delivery Reviews*, 35 (1): 3–19. Enhanced Drug Delivery Using High-Voltage Pulses, doi:10.1016/S0169-409X(98)00060-X.

Tropea, B. I., and R. C. Lee. 1992. "Thermal Injury Kinetics in Electrical Trauma." *Journal of Biomechanical Engineering* 114 (2): 241–250.

Tsong, Tian Yow, and R. Dean Astumian. 1987. "Electroconformational Coupling and Membrane Protein Function." *Progress in Biophysics and Molecular Biology* 50 (1): 1–45. doi:10.1016/0079-6107(87)90002-2.

Tung, Leslie. 1992. "Electrical Injury to Heart Muscle Cells." In *Electrical Trauma: The Pathophysiology, Manifestations, and Clinical Management*. edited by R. C. Lee, E.G. Cravalho, and J. R. Burke, 361–400. New York: Cambridge University Press.

Tung, Leslie, Oscar Tovar, Michel Neunlist, Sandeep K. Jain, and Rory J. O'neill. 1994. "Effects of Strong Electrical Shock on Cardiac Muscle Tissuea." *Annals of the New York Academy of Sciences* 720 (1): 160–175. doi:10.1111/j.1749-6632.1994.tb30444.x.

Weaver, James C. 1993. "Electroporation: A General Phenomenon for Manipulating Cells and Tissues." *Journal of Cellular Biochemistry* 51 (4): 426–435. doi:10.1002/jcb.2400510407.

Weaver, James C., and Yu. A. Chizmadzhev. 1996. "Theory of Electroporation: A Review." *Bioelectrochemistry and Bioenergetics* 41 (2): 135–160. doi:10.1016/S0302-4598(96)05062-3.

Whitcomb, Darren, Jorge A. Martinez, and Dayton Daberkow. 2002. "Lightning Injuries." *Southern Medical Journal* 95 (11): 1331–1335.

Woods, Lori A., Parul U. Gandhi, and Andrew G. Ewing. 2005. "Electrically Assisted Sampling across Membranes with Electrophoresis in Nanometer Inner Diameter Capillaries." *Analytical Chemistry* 77 (6): 1819–1823. doi:10.1021/ac048589y.

13

Epidemiologic Studies of Extremely Low Frequency Electromagnetic Field

Leeka Kheifets and Andrew S. Park
University of California-Los Angeles

John Swanson
National Grid

Ximena Vergara
Electric Power Research Institute
University of California-Los Angeles

CONTENTS

13.1 Introduction

Given the ubiquitous nature of extremely low frequency (ELF) electromagnetic fields (EMF), there is concern regarding their potential to adversely affect human health. Numerous health effects have been studied in relation to EMF exposure: cancer, reproductive disorders, as well as neurodegenerative and cardiovascular diseases. Cancer, especially childhood leukemia, has received the most attention.

A number of reviews on the potential of EMF to cause damage to health have been conducted.[1-5] The general consensus is that any evidence for effects below 100 μT comes primarily from epidemiologic evidence, rather than from laboratory or animal studies.

EMFs are imperceptible, ubiquitous, have multiple sources, and can vary greatly over time and short distances.[6] In the absence of a biological mechanism that would focus attention on one particular metric of exposure, and with developments in technology, exposure assessment of EMF has varied over the years. Exposure assessment methods used in epidemiologic studies improved markedly through the 1980s and 1990s. Most of the epidemiologic studies discussed below use the time-weighted average (TWA) measurement to characterize exposure. Furthermore, with technological advances in assessing exposures and increased study sample size, higher exposures, i.e., >0.4 μT, have been explored. Although epidemiologic evidence is not conclusive, it is generally agreed that the possibility of a causal association between EMF and adverse health outcomes cannot be excluded and that epidemiologic studies of childhood leukemia provide the strongest evidence of an association.

Epidemiologic evidence is a major contributor to the understanding of the potential effects of EMF on health. The International Agency for Research on Cancer (IARC) classified EMF as a "possibly carcinogenic to humans," or a Group 2B carcinogen[1]; this classification, confirmed by World Health Organization (WHO),[5] was based on consistent epidemiological evidence of an association between exposure to these fields and childhood leukemia, and laboratory studies in animals and cells, which were not supportive of EMF causing cancer. Although the body of evidence is always considered as a whole, using the weight of evidence approach that incorporates different lines of scientific enquiry, the epidemiologic evidence is viewed as most relevant to human health, and thus is given the greatest weight.

Epidemiologic data are routinely and critically assessed to shed light on the potential of EMF to cause harm to health. In this chapter, we review a large body of available epidemiologic evidence for a variety of diseases. Depending on the number of available studies, we often focus on the key studies as summary or discussion of all studies is not feasible. When the number of studies is very large (for example, as with occupational studies and cancer), we largely rely on the pooled or meta-analysis. In addition to an up-to-date review of the epidemiologic evidence, we discuss exposure assessment and other methodologic concepts and concerns that affect the interpretation of the evidence.

13.2 Methodology of Epidemiologic Studies of EMF

13.2.1 Exposure Assessment

13.2.1.1 Exposure Assessment in Residential Studies

13.2.1.1.1 Wire Codes

The underpinning of wire codes as a surrogate for EMF exposure is that, across an entire living space, the outdoor electric line and the associated grounding system are the dominant source of long-term magnetic field exposure, and the characteristics of those lines provide an indication of the likely magnetic field exposure level. Further, unless the lines were modified over time or homes were demolished, they also provide an estimate of past exposure.

In the first study by Wertheimer and Leeper[7] published in 1979, each subject's exposure was categorized on the basis of (a) the type of electric utility wiring adjacent to the residence, i.e., transmission lines and primary and secondary distribution lines of various types, and (b) the distance from that wiring to the residence. This categorical exposure is referred to as the "wire code." (See Table 13.1 for a list of the epidemiologic studies using wire codes and other exposure surrogates.) Wertheimer and Leeper[7]

TABLE 13.1

Epidemiologic Studies of the Association between EMF and Childhood Leukemia

Reference	Study Population	Study Design Cases/Controls	Exposure	High Category RR (95% CI)
Residential Studies				
Wertheimer and Leeper[7]	Cases: deaths, <19 years old (y.o.). Birth certificate controls, Colorado	Case-control 155/155	Wire code	HCC 3.0 (1.8–5.0)
Fulton et al.[11]	Cases: <20 y.o. Controls: birth certificates. Rhode Island	Case-control 119/240	Wire code	No association
Tomenius[12]	Cases: <19 y.o. Birth certificate controls, Sweden	Case-control 243/212	Measured fields (spot front door)	≥0.3 µT 0.3 (NR)
Savitz et al.[9]	Cases: <15 y.o. Controls: random digit dialing (RDD). Denver, Colorado	Case-control WC—97/259 MF—36/207	Wire code Measured fields (spot, child's bedroom)	HCC 2.7 (0.9–8.0) ≥0.25 µT 1.9 (0.7–5.6)
Myers et al.[13]	Cases: <15 y.o. Controls: birth register. Yorkshire, England	Case-control 243/212 (all cancers)	Distance Calculated fields	<25 m 1.1 (0.5–2.6) ≥0.1 µT 0.4 (0.0–4.1)
London et al.[14]	Cases: <10 y.o. Controls: friends & RDD. Los Angeles, California	Case-control WC—211/205 MF—162/143	Wire code Measured (24-h bedroom)	VHCC 2.1 (1.1–4.3) ≥0.27 µT 1.5 (0.7–3.3)

(Continued)

TABLE 13.1 (*Continued*)

Epidemiologic Studies of the Association between EMF and Childhood Leukemia

Reference	Study Population	Study Design Cases/Controls	Exposure	High Category RR (95% CI)
Feychting and Ahlbom[15]	Residents within 300 m of power line. Cases: <15 y.o. Controls: random from cohort. Sweden	Nested Case-control 38/554	Distance Calculated fields	≤50 m 2.9 (1.0–7.3) ≥0.3 μT 3.8 (1.4–9.3)
Verkasalo et al.[16]	Residents within 500 m of power line. <17 y.o, 1974–1990. Finland	Cohort 35 cases	Calculated fields	≥0.2 μT 1.6 (0.3–4.5)
Coghill et al.[17]	Cases from advertising and various referrals Controls identified by parents of cases	Case-control 56/56	Measured fields (24-h in home)	≥0.4 μT NR[a]
Tynes and Haldorsen[18]	Wards with high-voltage power lines. <15 y.o. Controls: random from cohort. Norway	Nested Case-control 139/546	Distance Calculated fields	≤50 m 0.6 (0.3–1.3) ≥0.14 μT 0.3 (0.0–2.1)
Fajardo-Gutierrez et al.[19]	Cases and controls hospital based, Mexico	Case-control 81/77	Wire code	VHCC 2.6 (1.3–5.4)
Petridou et al.[20]	<14 y.o. 1993–1994; Hospital controls. Greece	Case-control 117/202	Wire code	VHCC 1.6 (0.3–9.4)
Linet et al.[21]	Cases (ALL): <15 y.o. Controls: RDD. U.S.	Case-control WC—402/402 MF—162/143	Wire code Measured fields (time weighted average [TWA])	VHCC 0.9 (0.5–1.6) ≥0.2 μT 1.5 (0.9–2.6)
Michaelis et al.[22]	Cases: <15 y.o. Controls: govt. office residents' registry. Germany	Case-control 176/414	Measured fields (24-h bedroom)	≥0.2 μT 2.3 (0.8–6.7)
Dockerty et al.[23]	Cases: <15 y.o. Controls: birth certificate. New Zealand	Case-control 115/117	Measured fields (24-h bedroom)	≥0.2 μT 15.5 (1.1–224)
Lin et al.[24] and Li et al.[25]	Three districts with many high-voltage transmission lines (HVTL) Taiwan	SIR 28 cases	Distance	<100 m 2.7 (1.1–5.6)
McBride et al.[26]	Cases: <15 y.o. Controls: health insurance records. Canada	Case-control WC—303/309 Personal—293/339 MF—272/304	Wire code Measured fields (48-h personal) Measured fields (24-h bedroom)	VHCC 0.8 (0.4–1.6) ≥0.2 μT 1.1 (0.7–1.6) ≥0.2 μT 1.3 (0.7–2.3)
Green et al.[27,28]	Cases: <15 y.o. Controls: telephone marketing lists. Canada	Case-control WC—79/125 Personal—88/133 MF—21/46	Wire code Measured fields (spot) Measured fields (48-h personal)	VHCC 0.8 (0.2–2.9) ≥0.13 μT 1.1 (0.3–4.1) ≥0.14 μT 4.5 (1.3–15.9)
UKCCS[29,30]	Cases: <15 y.o. Controls: health services. United Kingdom	Case-control 1,094/1,096	Distance Measured fields[b]	0–49 m 0.8 (0.4–1.4) ≥0.4 μT 1.7 (0.4–7.1)

(Continued)

TABLE 13.1 (*Continued*)

Epidemiologic Studies of the Association between EMF and Childhood Leukemia

Reference	Study Population	Study Design Cases/Controls	Exposure	High Category RR (95% CI)
Bianchi et al.[31]	Cases: <15 y.o. Controls in Varese province, Italy	Case-control 101/412	Calculated fields	≥0.1 µT 4.5 (0.9–23.2)
Schuz et al.[32]	Cases: <15 y.o. Childhood Cancer Registry. Controls: population registration files. West Germany	Case-control 514/1,301	Measured fields (24-h residential)	≥0.4 µT 5.9 (0.8–44.1)
Mizoue et al.[33]	City in Japan	IRR 3 cases	50% + of the area fell within 300 m	0–300 m 2.2 (0.5–9.0)
Perez et al.[34]	Cases: <15 y.o. 1996–2000 Cuba Methods unclear	Case-control Numbers NR	Spot measurements	≥0.5 µT 6.72 (NR)
Kabuto et al.[35]	Cases: <15 y.o. from five major Childhood Cancer study groups; Controls: population registry. Japan	Case-control 312/603	Distance 1-week bedroom measurements	0–50 m 3.1 (1.3–7.1) ≥0.4 µT 2.8 (0.8–9.6)
Mejia-Arangure et al.[36]	Cases: <16 y.o. cancer institutions in Mexico City; Controls: institutions with disabilities	Case-control (Only Down syndrome) 42/124	Spot measurements	>0.6 µT 3.7 (1.1–13.1)
Feizi et al.[37]	Cases: <15 (ALL) Children's Hospital; Controls: hospital Controls. Iran	Case-control 60/59	Calculated fields	≥0.45 µT 3.6 (1.1–12.4)
Yang et al.[38]	Cases: <15 y.o. at the Children's Medical Center in Shanghai, China	Case-only XRCC1 Ex9þ16A gene and MF 123 Cases	Transformers or power lines within 50 m	Interaction with 0–50 m 4.4 (1.4–13.5)
Malagoli et al.[39]	Cases: <14 y.o. in nation-wide registry in Italy; Controls: Municipal databases	Case-control 28/131	Calculated fields	≥0.4 µT 2.1 (0.2–26.2)
Sohrabi et al.[40]	Cases: 0–18 y.o. (ALL) Hospital Cases and Controls. Iran	Case-control 300/300	Distance	<600 m 2.6 (1.7–3.9)
Does et al.[41]	Cases: <15 y.o. Hospital ascertainment Controls: birth certificate. Northern California	Case-control 245/269	Wire code 30-min indoor	HCC 1.2 (0.9–1.6) >0.3 µT 0.6 (0.1–2.4)
Wunsch-Filho et al.[42]	Cases: Eight hospitals; State of São Paulo birth registry, Brazil	Case-control 162/565	Distance 24-h bedroom	0–50 m 3.6 (0.4–31.4) ≥0.3 µT 1.1 (0.3–3.6)
Jirik et al.[43]	Hospital based, matched on village/town, Czech Republic	Case-control 82/81	Measured details unavailable	≥0.4 µT 0.9 (0.4 2.2)
Sermage-Faure et al.[44]	Cases: <15 y.o. Registry Controls: tax database. France	Case-control 2,779/30,000	Distance	0–49 m 1.7 (0.9–3.6)

(Continued)

TABLE 13.1 (*Continued*)

Epidemiologic Studies of the Association between EMF and Childhood Leukemia

Reference	Study Population	Study Design Cases/Controls	Exposure	High Category RR (95% CI)
Abdul Rahman et al.[45] and Ba Hakim et al.[46]	Cases: <15 y.o. from two hospitals, Non-cancer hospital controls. Malaysia	Case-control 108/118	Distance[c] Spot front door ≥0.3 µT	<200 m 0.9 (0.4–2.2) 0.8 (0.3–2.0)
Pedersen et al.[47,48]	Cases: <15 y.o. Controls: Central Population Registry. Denmark 1968–2003	Case-control 1,536/3,072	Distance Calculated fields[d] ≥0.4 µT	0–199 m NR 1.7 (0.5–5.5)
Bunch et al.[49,50]	Cases: <15 y.o. in the Registry of Childhood Tumours Controls: birth registers. United Kingdom	Case-control 9,645/9,647 9,653/9,653	Distance Calculated fields[e] ≥0.4 µT	0–49 m 0.8 (0.4–1.4) 0.5 (0.2–1.6)
Salvan et al.[51]	0–10 y.o. 1998–2001, Italy Population controls	Case-control 745/1,475	24–48-h bedroom >0.2 µT	0.9 (0.5–1.7)
Crespi[52] and Kheifets[53]	Cases <16 y.o. born in and diagnosed in California birth controls	Case-control 5,788/5,788	Distance Calculated fields ≥0.4 µT	0–50 m 1.4 (0.7–2.7) 1.5 (0.7–3.2)
Pooled Analyses				
Greenland et al.[54]	12 studies of measured or calculated fields	Pooled analyses 2,656/7,084	Magnetic fields ≥0.3 µT	1.7 (1.2–2.3)
Ahlbom et al.[55]	9 studies of measured or calculated fields	Pooled analyses 3,203/10,338	Magnetic fields ≥0.4 µT	2.0 (1.3–3.1)
Kheifets et al.[56]	14 studies published since 2000	Pooled analyses 10,865/12,853	Distance Magnetic fields ≥0.3 µT	0–50 m 1.6 (1.0, 2.5) 1.4 (0.9–2.4)

HCC, high current configuration; NR, not reported; OHCC, ordinary high current configuration; OLCC, ordinary low current configuration; VHCC, very high current configuration; VLCC, very low current configuration.

[a] Reported for electric fields only.

[b] Phase I: 90 min in family room + spot measurement in bedroom; Phase II: 48-h bedroom and spot measurement in school only for highest 10% in Phase I.

[c] Abdul Rahman et al. (2004) originally reported OR 2.3 (1.2–4.5) for distance <200 m.

[d] Olsen et al.[57] originally reported OR of around 6.0 for calculated fields before latest update.

[e] Draper et al.[67] and Kroll et al.[113] originally reported OR of around 2.0 for distance and magnetic fields before latest update.

initially used a dichotomous exposure classification wherein subjects were classified as living in either high- or low-current configuration (HCC or LCC) homes. Later, they introduced a finer degree of resolution into their wire code classification system, partly by using the size of conductors as a surrogate for likely electrical current load, to produce a four-category scheme: very low current configuration (VLCC), ordinary low current configuration (OLCC), ordinary high current configuration (OHCC), and very high current configuration (VHCC).[8] Subsequent studies added a fifth category (underground) and refined the categories to improve the fit to magnetic fields (Savitz et al.[9] and Kaune and Savitz[10]).

Wire coding does not require resident participation, thus, exposure assessment without intrusion is possible for cancer cases and controls (cancer-free comparison subjects) with verified addresses, and study size was therefore maximized and participation bias minimized. The necessary data can be gathered quite efficiently and has even, in some cases, been automated.[58] However, as an estimate of magnetic field, wire codes introduce considerable misclassification[59] and, as more direct measurement or calculation methods have been developed, their use in epidemiologic studies has largely been superseded.

13.2.1.1.2 Spot Measurements

Before data logging instruments were available, measurements could only be "spot measurements," i.e., of the magnetic field at one location and one moment in time. A single-axis meter could be used to measure the field in a specified direction, e.g., vertical, or in three orthogonal directions, allowing the resultant total field to be calculated, or, when they became available, three-axis meters could be used to measure the total field directly. If access to the home was not possible, spot measurements could be performed at the front door. If access was possible, locations of the measurements would be specified so as to make the measurement as representative as possible of the field experienced by a subject in that home: typically the bed, and/or the middle of one or more rooms, and/or the room corners.

To overcome the limitations of the measurement being at only one instant in time, various strategies have been adopted, including adjusting the measurement using information on electrical loads or on seasonal variations. Measurements are sometimes specified under "low-power" or "high-power" conditions, with domestic appliances turned off or on to simulate the variation in field as power use in the home varies.

If measurements are to be performed at all, spot measurements are the least resource-intensive way of performing them, and, in the early years of EMF research, were all that the technology allowed. However, the uncertainties caused by measuring at only one instant of time (particularly as there is a strong diurnal variation not captured by spot measurements) mean that spot measurements are now considered inferior to long-term measurements.

13.2.1.1.3 Long-Term Measurements

The development of logging instruments allowed measurements to be made over extended periods of time, with the subsequent summary being typically either the arithmetic or geometric mean. Measurement times of 24h up to 1week have been used, allowing an average over the diurnal variation of fields. Long-term measurements are more expensive, yet still do not allow for annual variations or trends over longer periods of time or for any changes in relevant features of the surrounding wiring.

These measurements are vulnerable to changes in the location of a local source of high magnetic field, e.g., when a domestic appliance is close to the meter. To reduce the impact of any such "outlier," studies have attempted to place the meter away from appliances and some analyzed the measurements using the geometric rather than the arithmetic mean. Despite these limitations, when pooled analyses have defined inclusion criteria on quality grounds, a criterion for measurement studies has often been a minimum of 24h measurements, as a mark of a higher-quality EMF exposure surrogate.

13.2.1.1.4 Personal-Exposure Measurements

Few studies employed the use of personal EMF meters to measure exposure. Personal-exposure measurements would be the gold standard for many exposures, and evidence suggests strong correlation between household exposure and personal-measurements[10,29]; thus, use of personal measurements might be appropriate in the prospective studies of EMF. However, in case-control studies personal measurements might be biased as disease status might alter behavior patterns and thereby differentially affect personal exposure measurements. Personal measurements are even more problematic in case-control studies of children as exposure at young age is highly age-dependent, and measurements made in the few years after the etiologically relevant time period may differ from those made in the time period of interest.

13.2.1.1.5 Distance and Calculated Field

Several studies have used distance from residence to overhead (or more rarely, underground) transmission lines as an exposure surrogate, sometimes complemented by calculated fields which seek to capture historical exposure levels. Calculated fields are based on distance, power-line load data, and other information for power lines specific to the time period of interest. In studies based on distance or calculated fields, subject participation is not required, thus minimizing selection and participation bias, and such studies can efficiently include large number of subjects.

Calculated fields reconstruct exposure from a particular power line with reasonable accuracy. In a home close to a high-voltage power line the dominant source of exposure will likely be that power line, so calculated fields assess the EMF exposure in these scenarios well. However, they fail to identify high exposures from other sources leading to some homes being incorrectly classified as low exposure. This slightly reduces the power of a study as such bias will be non-differential between cases and controls.

13.2.1.1.6 Electric Fields

Exposure assessment for electric fields is particularly difficult. Power lines may carry no current at all and thus produce no magnetic fields, but they still may be energized and produce similar electric field as when fully loaded. Similarly, in the home, an electrical appliance may be off and produce no magnetic field, but if remaining plugged into a power outlet produce electric fields. Electric fields are affected by conducting objects including the ground, most building materials, and human beings, in ways in which magnetic fields are not, such as attenuating the field, perturbing it and creating local areas of high electric fields. Calculation of electric fields in the presence of trees or buildings is difficult, thus it is better to measure the electric field than to rely on calculations. Appliances can result in high electric-field exposures, though these fields diminish with distance to the levels present from other sources after about a meter away.

13.2.1.2 Exposure Assessment in Occupational Studies

The starting point for almost all assessments of occupational exposure to EMF in epidemiological studies is the job, using some form of job-exposure matrix (JEM). The JEM may be constructed based on measurements on samples of workers or on expert judgment.

"Job" is not, however, always a good predictor of exposure, either because a given "job" encompasses activities with different exposures (contrast "electricians" who perform maintenance of live circuits with those who construct new-build and work on unenergized equipment), or because exposure is determined by work location rather than job (e.g., managers and clerical workers, not jobs attributed with high exposures, may work in power stations and experience high fields). Thus, individual exposures will differ from JEM measurements due to differences in job conditions and work practices. This is even more problematic for JEMs that cover multiple industries, as jobs may be defined differently by various industries. Assigning subjects an exposure determined by the JEM ignores several uncertainties, such as biases due to uncontrolled confounding.[60]

Kelsh, Kheifets, and Smith[61], analyzing a large occupational database from the electricity industry, found that the variance components of the nested factors of utility, worker, and day together comprised about 68% of the variability (15.7%, 24.7%, and 27.6%, respectively), whereas work environment was associated with about 24% of the variability. Occupation contributed only 5% of the total variability. Bowman, Touchstone, and Yost,[62] analyzing a different database, found that the U.S. Bureau of Occupational Classification occupation accounted for 30% of the MF variance, but they were not including within-worker variability in the total variance.

To improve the exposure estimates, additional information or dimensions can be added to augment "job", particularly for industry-specific JEMs. For a power-station worker study, Renew, Cook, and Ball[63] used specific power-station layout information and load data from relevant years to expand the JEM into a three-dimensional Job-Site-Year Exposure Matrix. Coble et al.[64] incorporated information from interviews about tasks, sources, and distances. More recently, methods have been developed to combine measurement data with expert judgment and to quantify exposure uncertainty.[65]

Even cruder approaches, such as relying on a simple job or population-based JEM, to classify occupational exposures have been used in studies of parental exposures and cancers in their offspring.

13.2.2 Key Aspects of Study Design

13.2.2.1 Case Ascertainment: Source and Type of Outcome Information

Many residential studies, particularly of cancer, ascertain cases from a disease registry. These are often reasonably complete, though it is in the nature of such registers and of all medical records that any people with a disease who do not engage with the health system to the extent necessary to appear on the relevant register will be atypical of the population in other ways as well.

With registries based on incidence of a disease, incomplete ascertainment is possible if a subset of cases of the disease are misdiagnosed or masked by other symptoms and not recorded. When case ascertainment is based on prevalence, biases may be introduced for diseases of long duration such meningiomas (type of brain tumors) or Alzheimer's disease. When case ascertainment is based on death certificates, the problem is more serious as commonly the immediate cause of death does not necessarily reflect health conditions present before death, and recording of other conditions (contributing causes) is variable. The validity of cause of death on the death certificate is very problematic for some diseases (such as Alzheimer's or subsets of cardiovascular disease) and reasonably good for others (such as amyotrophic lateral sclerosis (ALS) that is distinct and rapidly fatal).

Ascertainment of cases from hospital records may also be reasonably complete, but are not necessarily linked to a well-defined source population. Hospital or clinic-based studies may be selective and influenced by factors such as wealth or education. Bias may be compounded if subjects move to attend specialist facilities.[42]

Ascertainment of cases by self-reporting or word-of-mouth referral is highly likely to be selective.[17] While not necessarily creating a bias itself (if, for example, the controls in a case-control study are still carefully enough matched to the cases), such studies should be critically examined.

No single source of case ascertainment is likely to be 100% complete. For some cancers, cancer registries may be nearly complete and sufficient. For some other diseases, any individual source is incomplete, and combining multiple sources improves ascertainment.

13.2.2.2 Control Selection

In a case-control study, a source population must be defined that represents a study population from which cases arose. Controls are randomly selected from the source population, typically matched to cases only on characteristics not under study and not related to exposure. In practice, defining a source population is particularly difficult, and resulting biases from control selection or control participation are known or surmised to be present in many studies.

Where comprehensive population registers exist, selection of controls is likely to be free from selection bias (see below for participation bias). Likewise, if the study is concerned with exposure perinatally, birth registers are likely to be reasonably complete in most developed countries, and hence unbiased.

If such registers are not available, alternatives have been used such as insurance lists or enrollment in health-care organizations. These alternatives for control selection introduce obvious scope for bias, as more participation comes from higher socioeconomic status (SES) groups. Likewise, past methods of recruitment using random telephone digit dialing are also prone to SES biases.

Controls selected from hospital admissions for diseases or from cancer registries other than the one under investigation have strengths, such as similarity in participation rates and SES status to cases, but are still prone to bias as different diseases might have different referral patterns or catchment area and different socioeconomic profiles. These methods also depend on the assumption that the exposure in question, in this case EMF, affects only the disease being investigated and not for other diseases from which controls are chosen.

Finally, neighborhood, friend, or relative controls, while having obvious advantages, might lead to inadvertent overmatching on exposure.

13.2.2.3 Residential Studies

As most of diseases of interest are relatively rare and past exposures are not readily identifiable, most residential studies are of case-control design. In studies with calculated or modeled exposure subject participation is not necessary, so control selection is the primary bias under operation. In studies with measurements made inside the home subject participation is required and introduces bias by variable willingness to participate. Even among cases, participation rates in such studies are not 100%, but controls have less incentive to participate and do so at much lower rates than cases, on the order of 50% for interview studies and even lower for measurement studies.[66] These participation rates are very likely to introduce potential bias: better-educated control families are more likely to participate, for example.

Different studies of childhood cancer assess exposure at various time points or periods: (1) at the residence at the time of diagnosis, (2) a specified short interval before diagnosis, (3) at birth, or (4) cumulatively, for all homes occupied during a child's life up to diagnosis. Similar choices are made for other diseases, and ideally these windows of exposure should be informed by etiological hypotheses. However, in reality, they may be determined by practical issues to do with accessibility to information and resources. In measurement studies, for example, there is a strong incentive to assess the subject's current home as identification and access are easier. Conversely, the need to use birth registers for control selection has limited several studies' focus to perinatal exposure.[52,67]

It is thought that residential exposure is a better exposure proxy for children than for adults, both because children spend more time at home and because they do not encounter occupational exposures which are presumably higher.[68]

13.2.2.4 Occupational Studies

Occupational studies are often either retrospective cohort studies or case-control studies nested within a cohort. In such studies, which are commonly record-based, issues of control selection and participation and thus the biases introduced are usually reduced.

However, the health experience of a whole cohort, particularly a cohort of working or formerly working people, is likely to be different from the population as a whole which includes persons unable to perform work. A bias may manifest usually described as the "healthy worker effect," meaning that relative comparisons within a given cohort are usually more informative than the absolute experience of that cohort as compared to the general population.

Other types of occupational studies, known as proportionate mortality studies, are based on death certificates alone, and thus have many limitations. In such studies, the population at risk is unknown. Thus, an apparent increase in the proportion of deaths from one disease among exposed workers may be due to a decrease in the proportions of deaths from other causes in the comparison group. In addition, the validity of the study results depends upon the accuracy of the occupational information reported on death certificates and the extent to which job titles alone reflect exposure to magnetic fields. Such studies are considered to be of a preliminary nature.

13.2.2.5 Common Biases

In any epidemiologic study, the method used for ascertaining subjects can have a bearing on the results. Incomplete ascertainment will reduce the power of the study, but will not in itself introduce a bias. Bias occurs if, in a retrospective cohort study, selection or choice of the exposed or unexposed subjects is somehow related to the outcome of interest or if the follow-up differs by exposure and outcome. In a case-control study, a bias can occur if the cases and/or controls that are included have different characteristics from the source population.

Strictly speaking, a bias in the result is introduced only if these differences in observed subjects' characteristics are related to exposure, so that the exposure of the included subjects is systematically higher or lower than it should be. In practice, however, residential exposure to magnetic fields are known to relate to different population characteristics, all broadly related to SES. High-magnetic-field homes tend to be older, of smaller dimensions, in areas densely populated, on busier roads, occupied by families with lower education, lower socioeconomic status and younger children; low-magnetic-field homes tend to be larger with wider footprints and located in areas of higher socioeconomic status. In addition, higher fields (or wire-code classifications) have been reported in homes located in urban and suburban areas versus rural (United States, also seen weakly in United Kingdom), flats and apartments vs. single-family homes, and terraced vs. detached houses (United States and United Kingdom), in homes on or near busier roads (United States, United Kingdom), in homes with conducting water pipes rather than with local grounding systems (United States) and with shorter occupancy (United States). Given these wide-reaching plausible linkages, bias in subject ascertainment is likely, and certainly any bias related to SES factors can impact study findings.

Residential mobility is also a key factor in understanding the biases operating in a study.[53] It may introduce a bias if, directly or indirectly, it acts as a selection factor (e.g., if only more mobile subjects enter the catchment area, or conversely, if exposure in relevant homes depends on access and consent from a subject living in the home), and in the case of childhood leukemia, residential mobility may also be a risk factor or associated with risk factors, and thus act as a confounder.

There is evidence that these various biases impact the outcome of many EMF studies.[66] In principle, confounding may be addressed in the analysis by adjusting for factors such as SES. In practice, it is difficult to achieve confidence that the risk of bias, once introduced, has been completely removed. Rarely do epidemiologic studies account for all biases, instead bias analysis may be carried out to understand magnitude and direction of changes in risk estimates.[69]

13.3 Leukemia

13.3.1 Background

Leukemias are cancers of the blood and bone marrow. The classification of leukemias is conventionally based on the cell types of origin (lymphocytes, myelocytes, monocytes) and on the rate at which the disease progresses (acute and chronic).

The age distribution of leukemias is bimodal, with a first peak occurring at age 4 years, a decline at ages 15–29 years, and then a slow rise throughout the rest of life. Leukemia is the most common childhood malignancy, constituting more than half of all childhood cancers. Acute lymphocytic leukemias (ALLs) account for 75% of all cases of childhood leukemia; the most common types in adults are acute myeloid (AML) and chronic lymphocytic (CLL) leukemias.

The age-standardized rate of leukemia for children younger than 15 years has been estimated to be 3.5 per 100,000 per year for females and 4.2 per 100,000 per year for males in the developed world and 2.2 per 100,000 per year for females and 2.9 per 100,000 per year for males in the developing world.[70] For adults, rates for each type of leukemia have changed very little over the past 20 years. For children, however, incidence rates have risen slightly; similar or more pronounced increases have occurred for other childhood cancers.[71] Some of these increases might be attributable to improved diagnosis.

Environmental, occupational, and genetic factors have been associated with one or more types of leukemia. Increased risks have been associated with radiation exposure (all types of leukemia except CLL), cigarette smoking (parental smoking for childhood leukemia), and exposure to the human T cell leukemia virus type one (HTLV-1) (associated with adult T-cell leukemia and lymphoma). Occupational exposures associated with increased risk are benzene (AML), the manufacturing processes of styrene & butadiene production (lymphoid leukemia) and petroleum refining (AML & to a lesser extent CLL). Genetic risk factors include the chromosomal and congenital abnormalities of Fanconi's anemia, along with Down's, Bloom's, Kleinfelter's, and trisomy G syndromes.[72]

In general, the relationship between SES and childhood leukemia is weak and inconsistent.[73] The causes of leukemia, especially childhood leukemia, are not well understood. In addition, the presently known or suspected risk factors are likely to account for only a small proportion of all cases.[74]

13.3.2 Childhood Leukemia

13.3.2.1 Residential Exposure to Magnetic Fields

13.3.2.1.1 Wire Codes

In the first study by Wertheimer and Leeper[7] in 1979, each subject's exposure was categorized using wire codes. Based on cases occurring between 1950 and 1973, they reported that childhood leukemia mortality was associated with residence in HCC homes. However, methodological problems, such as non-blind exposure assessment, reliance on death certificates, unconventional analysis and the lack of evaluation of confounding, rendered this study difficult, if not impossible, to interpret. It did, nevertheless, generate a hypothesis that has been followed up by multiple other studies (Table 13.1).

A childhood cancer investigation by Savitz et al.[9] conducted in the same geographical area, was designed to replicate the Wertheimer and Leeper[7] study and to improve upon it through comprehensive ascertainment of incident cases, assessment of potential confounders, and "blind" exposure assessment. In addition to wire coding, they included point-in-time or "spot" magnetic field measurements in all available residences. In general, higher magnetic fields were registered in the OHCC and especially VHCC residences, but the wire code/magnetic field correlation was weak. Savitz et al.[9] reported positive associations of wire code with childhood leukemia. The risk for spot measurements was lower and less precise, partially owing to the reduced number of homes available for measurement. The results for the wire code and leukemia investigations were basically consistent with those of Wertheimer and Leeper,[7] with the additional evidence that wire code may serve as a weak indicator of contemporary measured magnetic fields.

London et al.[14] conducted an incidence study of childhood leukemia similar in its basic design to the study by Savitz et al.[9] but with 24 h bedroom measurements added to the exposure assessment. Similar results emerged: (1) residential magnetic field strength correlated weakly with wire code and was not associated with childhood leukemia (albeit using a low cut-point), and (2) a trend of increased leukemia risk across wire code, with elevated leukemia risk among the VHCC sample relative to the referent. As compared to wire code configuration, lower risks for measurements were interpreted as an indication that the association might not be with magnetic fields, but with something else associated with wire codes, despite wire codes having been developed as a measure of magnetic fields (known as the wire code paradox). Subsequently, several studies included wire codes, but their focus was on residential measurements and use of higher magnetic field cutpoints.[21,26,27] As a result, the wire code paradox seems to be resolved, as they reported stronger risks for measured fields than for wire codes.

13.3.2.1.2 Household and Personal Exposures

The majority of epidemiologic studies on EMF and childhood leukemia use residential EMF exposure measurements: either spot measurements[9,12,27] or area (mostly bedroom) magnetic field measurements of 24 h and longer.[17,21,22,26,27,29,55,75–77] The largest studies yet conducted incorporating household and personal EMF measurements were in the late 1990s and early 2000s, in the United States, Canada, United Kingdom, and Germany. These studies all used 24 or 48 h logging of fields, in some cases supplemented by spot measurements at different locations in the home and measurements at schools, and all sought information on possible confounding factors. In some studies, bias in control selection or through differential participation rates of cases and controls is present,[66] but broadly speaking, these studies enhanced the level of quality that has not subsequently improved. Although most of these studies observed elevated odds ratios (ORs) for higher fields,

95% confidence intervals (95% CIs) around many of these effect estimates are wide due to small numbers of highly exposed subjects. Given the rarity of both the disease and high exposure, securing enough highly exposed cases needed for statistically stable estimates is quite difficult, nevertheless, as time went on higher and higher cutpoints were used.

Only two studies employed the use of personal EMF meters to measure exposure, with conflicting results.[26,28]

13.3.2.1.3 Exposure Based on Distance and Calculated fields

Both Feychting and Ahlbom[15] and Tynes and Haldorsen[18] used a nested case-control study approach to identify leukemia cases within defined cohorts during specific time periods and calculated field measurements. The risk of childhood leukemia was elevated for children exposed to 0.3 µT or greater in Feychting and Ahlbom[15]; however, there was no elevated risk of leukemia among those exposed to 0.14 µT and greater in Tynes and Haldorsen.[18] No analysis for higher cutpoints was presented. A study from Finland[16] using similar design showed a non-significant elevated risk of childhood leukemia among those with 0.2 µT and greater exposure.

A study in the United Kingdom that found an association between childhood leukemia and the distance between home address at birth and the nearest high-voltage overhead line[67] renewed the interest in distance to transmission lines. However, the apparent risk was found to extend out to some 600 m, a distance greater than would be expected if magnetic fields from the high-voltage lines were a causal agent since the fields, which typically fall inversely with distance, are very small beyond 100 m. This study was extended to cover more recent time periods and lower line voltages. The updated study found higher risks in the earlier decades declining in the latest decades, with no overall elevated risks. In France and California, two large studies found that living less than 50 m from a 200 + kV lines may be associated with a small and imprecise risk of childhood leukemia.[44,52] No increase in risk was observed farther from those lines, and no increase in childhood leukemia risk was detected within 50 m of the lower-voltage lines.

13.3.2.2 Electric Appliance Exposure

Studies that have evaluated risks of childhood leukemia[14,23,78,79] associated with use of electric appliances are based on interviews of subjects' mothers to assess exposure information. Positive findings were observed in only a couple of these studies. In one study, an elevated risk of leukemia, but no exposure–response, was noted among children watching black-and-white television[14]; in another study, a rise in leukemia with an increasing number of hours children watched television, regardless of the child's distance from the television set was observed.[78] Risks were increased for postnatal exposure to a few other appliances in one study,[78] with no exposure-response relationship. Postnatal use of electric blankets[23,78,79] and hair dryers[14,78] were linked with modestly elevated risks in more than one study, but there was no evidence of exposure–response relationships. Overall, the small number of studies, evaluation of one appliance at a time, recall of use by parents leading to a very large exposure misclassification, and the absence of good measurement data within the studies preclude straightforward interpretation of results.

13.3.2.3 Residential Exposure to Electric Fields

Eight epidemiological studies investigated whether there are associations for childhood leukemia with residential electric fields. Unlike studies of residential magnetic-field exposure and childhood leukemia, epidemiological studies of residential electric fields have been predominately negative (see Kheifets et al.[80] for a detailed review).

13.3.2.4 Parental Exposure

Of the studies that have examined parental occupation and childhood cancer,[79] none have found any association with parental exposure to EMF and childhood leukemia. London et al.[14] reported an association between a mother's exposure during pregnancy to non-ionizing radiation and risk of childhood leukemia. However, the exposure question did not focus on EMF and is likely to reflect exposures to higher than power frequencies. Recent meta-analysis[81] also reports that neither paternal nor maternal EMF exposure is associated with childhood leukemia.

Two studies[9,78] observed small increases in the risk of childhood leukemia with the prenatal use of electric blankets, one study finding an exposure–response trend. In general, based on these studies, there is little evidence of elevated risk of leukemia in offspring associated with mothers' prenatal use of other types of electric appliances.

13.3.2.5 Survival Analyses

Hypothesizing that EMF may promote growth of leukemia cells, investigators have studied the relationship between magnetic fields and length of remission and overall survival of children diagnosed with childhood leukemia. A hypothesis generating cohort study in the United States of children with ALL[82] and subsequently another study in Germany following cases from a previous case-control study on EMF and risk of ALL showed poorer survival from ALL for EMF exposures $\geq 0.3\,\mu T$ (or $\geq 0.2\,\mu T$[83]), but based on small numbers. These two studies were part of a subsequent pooled analysis of case-control studies, which also included studies from Denmark, Japan, United Kingdom, and United States, where cases were followed up 10 years for relapse, second neoplasm and survival.[84] There was little indication of an effect of EMF on event-free survival or overall survival of ALL or for different subtypes of ALL.

13.3.2.6 Pooled Analyses

The accumulated epidemiologic literature on EMF and childhood leukemia now comprises multiple studies, generally, when taken individually, statistically imprecise and with variable findings. Interpreting the cumulative result of the individual studies is problematic. Combining results in a 'pooled analysis' overcomes some of these difficulties and offers the most powerful approach to provide a cohesive assessment of the epidemiologic data of EMF and childhood leukemia. Pooled analysis, considered the gold standard for synthesizing results from multiple studies, allows for comparison across different metrics and studies, is free of artifacts introduced by analytic differences or selective reporting by original authors, and for derivation of statistically more stable results.[82] Pooled analyses use raw data from the component studies, and thus can apply identical epidemiologic assumptions, such as categorization, metrics, etc., and statistical procedures to all included studies. The choices of cutpoints, reference groups, metrics, etc. in a pooled analysis may differ from the choices made in the original studies resulting in changes to the study-specific effect estimates. Despite strengths, results from pooled analyses are prone to the same biases operating in the original studies.

A sequence of three key pooled analyses represents the most powerful attempt to provide a cohesive assessment of EMF and childhood leukemia epidemiologic data.[54–56] These analyses come to similar conclusions.

In the pooled analysis by Greenland et al.[54] 12 studies using measured or calculated fields were identified; the study included a total of 2,656 cases and 7,084 controls. For this analysis, the metric of choice was the time-weighted average. The estimated OR for childhood leukemia was 1.68 (95% CI: 1.23–2.31) for exposures greater than 0.3 μT as compared to exposures less than 0.1 μT, controlling for age, sex, and study.

Using more stringent inclusion criteria, Ahlbom et al.[55] included nine studies using measured and calculated fields, which overlapped with previous pooling. There were a total of 3,203 cases and 10,338 controls in the pooled sample. Using the geometric mean as the metric of choice, the estimated OR for childhood leukemia was 2.00 (95% CI: 1.27–3.13) for exposures greater than or equal to 0.4 μT as compared to exposures less than 0.1 μT, controlling for age, sex, SES (in measurement studies only), and East/West (in German study only).

More recently, Kheifets et al. identified 14 studies published since the two previous 2000 pooled analyses, of which seven met their inclusion criteria.[56] A total of 10,865 cases and 12,853 controls were included in the pooled analysis which focused on 24 h magnetic field measurements or calculated fields in residences. The OR for exposure above 0.3 μT compared to <0.1 μT was 1.44 (95% CI: 0.88–2.36). Without the most influential study, from Brazil,[42] which is suspected to be particularly prone to bias, the ORs increased and became similar to previous pooled analysis. All three analyses, while focusing on overlapping but distinct set of studies, come to similar conclusions. A fourth childhood leukemia pooled analysis was designed principally to specifically test the hypothesis that the childhood leukemia association is stronger for night-time exposure than for total exposure.[85] The findings did not support a stronger association for the night-time exposure, but agreed with an overall findings of other pooled analyses.

The pooled analyses are often presented as finding an elevated risk for exposures above a specified threshold (0.3 or 0.4 μT), implying a step-function exposure–response relationship, and for example, attributable fractions are often calculated on this basis.[69,86] The fact that the risk for >0.4 μT is greater than for 0.3 μT, and that there are elevated risks reported for lower exposure categories, albeit small and imprecise, is compatible with a progressive exposure–response relationship, but the data are insufficient to draw any deductions about exposure-response with certainty.[87]

13.3.3 Adult Leukemia

13.3.3.1 Residential Exposure

The first study of residential exposures and adult cancer was also conducted by Wertheimer and Leeper.[8] The focus was on total cancers, and leukemia did not contribute to the elevated risk found for all cancers combined.

Several other studies have attempted to examine the risk of adult leukemia in populations residing near power lines.[88–91] These studies are based on small numbers and very crude exposure assessment methods. The overall results are negative with a few hints of a small non-significant elevation of risk in some studies.

Since then, other studies on residential EMF exposure and adult leukemia have shed more light on the plausible relationship (Table 13.2) adding spot measurements and calculated fields to the exposure assessment mix.[91–99] A small increased risk for all leukemia was observed in some of these studies. Of note is a reanalysis of the Swedish study[100] that

TABLE 13.2

Epidemiologic Studies of Residential Exposure and Meta-Analysis of Occupational Exposure to Magnetic Fields and Adult Leukemia

Reference	Study Population	Study Design Cases/Controls	Exposure	High Category RR (95% CI)
Residential Studies				
Severson et al.[93]	ANLL aged 20–79 (y.o.); registry RDD controls. United States	Case-control 114/133	Spot measurements	≥0.2 µT 1.0 (0.3–3.2)
Youngson et al.[91]	≥15 y.o., 1979–1985. North West and Yorkshire, United Kingdom	Case-control 3,144/3,144	Distance Calculated fields	0–50 m 1.3 (0.99–1.7) ≥0.3 µT 1.9 (0.8–4.4)
Feychting and Ahlbom[92]	≥16 y.o. Residents within 300 m of power line. Controls: random from cohort. Sweden	Case-control 325/1,091	Distance Historically calculated fields	0–50 m 1.2 (0.7–2.0) ≥0.2 µT 1.0 (0.7–1.7)
Verkasalo et al.[94]	≥20 y.o. Residents within 500 m of line. Finland	Case-Cohort 196 cases	Cumulative Calculated fields	≥0.3 µT 0.5 (0.2–1.7)
Li et al.[95]	Cancer registry (1987–1992). Controls: Other cancers except brain, breast and several others. Taiwan	Case-control 870/889	Calculated exposure in year of diagnosis	0–50 m 2.0 (1.4–2.9) >0.2 µT 1.4 (1.0–1.9)
Lowenthal et al.[96]	Subjects from 1972 to 1980. Tasmania	Case-control 854/854	Distance	0–50 m 2.1 (0.9–4.9)
Fazzo et al.[99]	Population of a district built under a 60 kV; Italy	Cohort N = 142	Distance	0–28 m 0 cases
Marcilio et al.[97]	Death certificates. Controls random from other causes deaths, except those associated with MF Brazil	Case-control 1,857/4,706	Distance Calculated Fields	0–50 m 1.5 (0.99–2.2) >0.3 µT 1.6 (0.9–2.9)
Elliott et al.[98]	15–74 y.o.; Controls Other cancers: except brain, breast, melanoma, and several others. United Kingdom	Case-control 7,823/23,469	Distance Calculated Fields in year of diagnosis	0–50 m 1.1 (0.8–1.5) >1 µT 1.0 (0.6–1.9)
Meta-Analysis and Pooled Analyses of Occupational Studies				
Kheifets et al.[101]	Studies of utility workers	Pooled analysis of six cohorts	Detailed Measurement data	per 10 µT-years 1.1 (0.98–1.2)
Kheifets et al.[102]	Occupational studies published between 1981 and 2007	Meta-analysis of 56 studies	Study-specific	1.16 (1.1–1.2)

added occupational exposure (based on JEM for occupation held in the year preceding the reference date), which reported a high risk of 3.7 (95% CI: 1.5–9.4) when both residential and occupational exposures were ≥0.2 µT (not shown).

13.3.3.2 Electric Appliance Exposure

In a case-control study of adult AML and CML in Los Angeles County that used cases and matched neighborhood controls,[103] use of electric blankets was not related to leukemia risk. Lovely et al.[104] examined adult leukemia risk and personal appliance use based on the study of Severson et al.[93] mentioned above. Most noteworthy in this analysis was a small elevation in risk for ever/never use of electric razors (Relative Risk (RR) = 1.3, 95% CI: 0.8–2.2), and a larger increase in risk with increased duration of daily use of electric razors (RR = 2.4, 95% CI: 1.1–5.5 for the highest relative to the lowest category). However, the finding was due to bias introduced by proxy-reported information, in actuality there was no association between leukemia risk and either use vs. no use or duration of use of electric razors.[105]

13.3.3.3 Occupational Studies

Studies on occupational exposure to EMF and adult leukemia have mostly linked job titles with cancer incidence or mortality. In a meta-analysis of 39 papers by Kheifets et al.[106] there was a small increased risk of leukemia associated with work in electric occupations. However, jobs thought to have higher magnetic field exposure (welders, electricians, linemen, and power plant operators) did not have higher risks than electric workers who generally have lower exposures (installers, engineers, and television or radio repairmen). Twenty-one studies published since this meta-analysis were included in an update by Kheifets.[102] Pooled risk estimates were lower than in past meta-analyses, and leukemia subtypes showed no consistent pattern when past and present meta-analyses were compared. When combined with studies in the original meta-analysis there was no clear pattern of EMF exposure and risk. Overall, results (Table 13.2) do not support a hypothesis that magnetic field exposures are responsible for the observed small excess risk (RR = 1.2, 95% CI: 1.1–1.2). Findings were not sensitive to assumptions, influential studies, weighting schemes, publication bias, study characteristics, or funding source.

13.3.4 Summary Leukemia

There is enough consistency in the results from the large body of research on childhood leukemia, which, while of variable quality, includes sufficient high-quality studies to reach a general agreement that exposures above 0.3–0.4 μT are associated with an elevated risk of childhood leukemia as compared to exposures less than 0.1 μT; this relative risk has been estimated to be less than 2, based on pooled analyses. This is unlikely to be due to chance but may be at least partly due to bias. A convincing explanation for this association is lacking. For other exposure measures and for adult leukemia the evidence is considerably weaker.

13.4 Brain Cancer

13.4.1 Background

Of all nervous system cancers, 90% occur in or around the brain. Several cancers of the brain and nervous system ("brain cancer") are rapidly fatal but fairly rare, with an incidence rate of 6 per 100,000 people per year in the United States.[107] Glioblastoma and astrocytoma are two subtypes of brain cancer that have been examined in relation to EMF exposure. Brain cancers are more common among males than females. Malignant neoplasms of the brain and other parts of the nervous system are the second most common form of cancer in children aged 0–19 years, representing more than one-fifth of all childhood malignancies.

There are few clearly recognized risk factors for childhood and adult brain cancer. Established risk factors for childhood brain tumors are limited to ionizing radiation exposure and certain cancer syndromes. Advanced parental age, birth defects, markers of fetal growth, CT scans, maternal diet (particularly N-nitrosamides), and residential pesticide exposure are suggested by larger studies and meta-analyses.[108] For adults, in addition to ionizing radiation, occupational exposures linked to brain cancer risk in some studies are organic solvents and pesticides. Excess risks have been found among farmers and painters, but the specific agents responsible for these risks remain unidentified. Brain cancers have also been linked to exposure to N-nitroso compounds and halomethanes. People with a family history of cancer, certain genetic diseases, or head injury may have an elevated risk of brain tumors. Tobacco and alcohol use has not been linked to brain cancer risk. Thus, the causes of both childhood and adult brain cancers are not well understood. Presently known or suspected factors appear to account for only a small proportion of all cases.

13.4.2 Childhood Brain Cancer

13.4.2.1 Residential Exposure

Several of the previously described childhood cancer studies examined brain cancer in addition to leukemia and other childhood tumors, though few focused on childhood brain cancer specifically (Table 13.3).

13.4.2.1.1 Wire Codes

Two studies based in Denver, Colorado[7,9] found an association between wire codes and brain tumors. In the largest study of childhood brain tumors and wire codes, Preston-Martin et al.[111] found that brain cancer risk was not related to measured fields or "high" (HCC or VHCC) wire codes. A companion study[115] also found no association between "high" wire code and occurrence of brain tumors.

13.4.2.1.2 Household Exposures

Far fewer studies of childhood brain tumors have measured magnetic fields: two used spot measurements[9,12] and three used long-term measurements.[29,112,114] Although some of these studies observed elevated ORs for higher fields, for all but one, confidence intervals around these estimates of effect include the null value, due to even smaller numbers of highly exposed subjects than for childhood leukemia. The one finding of statistical significance was based on three cases and one control. Overall, evidence appears to be weaker than that for leukemia, despite the fact that, in studies examining both outcomes, the same biases apply.

No studies employed the use of personal EMF meters to measure exposure in childhood brain tumor studies.

13.4.2.1.3 Exposure Based on Distance and Calculated Fields

Most of the distance/calculated field studies also included childhood brain tumors. Similar to household exposures, results are weaker than for leukemia, for example, in the study by Feychting and Ahlbom,[15] none of the exposure metrics were significantly associated with brain cancer. One possible exception is Finland,[16] but three of the tumors were diagnosed in one 18-year-old boy who had neurofibromatosis type 2. In addition, the Draper et al.[67] study reported raised risks for leukemia but not brain tumors for earlier time periods.

TABLE 13.3

Epidemiologic Studies of the Association between EMF and Childhood Brain Tumors

Reference	Study Population	Study Design Cases/Controls	Exposure	High Category RR (95% CI)
Residential Studies				
Wertheimer and Leeper[7]	Cases: deaths <19 (y.o). Controls: BC. Colorado	Case-control 66/66	Wire code	HCC 2.4 (1.0–5.4)
Tomenius[12]	Cases: <19 y.o. Controls: BC. Stockholm, Sweden	Case-control 294/253	Measured field (front door)	≥0.3 µT 3.7 (–)
Savitz et al.[9]	Cases: <15 y.o. Controls: random digit dialing (RDD). Denver, Colorado	Case-control WC—59/259 MF—25/207	Wire Code Measured fields (Spot bedroom)	HCC 1.9 (0.5–8.0) ≥0.25 µT 1.0 (0.2–4.8)
Myers[13]	Solid tumors 0–15 y.o. from 1970 to 1979. United Kingdom	Case-control 194/311	Calculated fields	≥0.3 µT 3.1 (0.3–31.8)
Feychting and Ahlbom[15]	Residents within 300 m of power line. Cases: <15 y.o. Controls: random from cohort. Sweden	Nested Case-control 33/549	Distance Historically calculated fields	≤50 m 0.5 (0.0–2.8) ≥0.3 µT 1.0 (0.2–3.9)
Verkasalo et al.[16]	<17 y.o., Residents within 500 m of power lines. Finland	Cohort N = 39 cases	Historically calculated fields	≥0.2 µT 2.3 (0.8–5.4)
Lin[109]	Hospital-based Taiwan[a]	Case-control 216/422	Distance	0–50 m 1.1 (0.5–2.4)
Preston-Martin et al.[110]	Cases: <20 y.o.; Controls: RDD. Los Angeles, California	Case-control 833/1,666	Wire code Measured fields	VHCC (0.6–2.2) ≥0.3 µT 1.7 (0.6–5.0)
Gurney et al.[111]	Cases: <20 y.o.; Controls: random digit dialling. United States	Case-control 120/240	Wire code	VHCC 0.5 (0.2–1.6)
Tynes and Haldorsen[18]	<15 years Residents in ward with high-voltage power lines. Controls: random from cohort. Norway	Nested Case-control 144/599	Distance Historically calculated fields	≤50 m 0.8 (0.4–1.6) ≥0.14 µT 0.7 (0.2–2.1)
UKCCS[29]	Cases: <15 y.o. Controls: health services. United Kingdom	Case-control 390/393	Measured fields[b]	≥0.4 µT 0 cases/2 cont
Schuz et al.[112]	Cases: <15 y.o. Registry Controls: population registration. Germany	Case-control 64/414	Measured fields (24-h residential)	≥0.2 µT 1.7 (0.3–8.8)
Draper[67] and Kroll et al.[113]	Cases: <15 y.o. Registry of Childhood Tumours Controls: birth registers. United Kingdom	Case-control	Distance Calculated fields	<200 m (0.7–1.3) ≥0.4 µT 0.6 (0.2–2.1)
Saito et al.[114]	Cases: <15 y.o. from CC groups; Controls: population registry. Japan	Case-control 55/99	1-week bedroom measurements	≥0.4 µT 10.9 (1.1–113)
Olsen et al.[57] and Pedersen et al.[47,48]	Cases: <15 y.o. 1968–2003; Controls: population registry. Denmark	Case-control 1,324/3,972	Calculated fields	≥0.4 µT 1.3 (0.4–4.3)
Crespi[52] and Kheifets[53]	Cases <16 y.o. registry; birth controls. California	Case-control 3,308/3,308	Distance	0–50 m 1.2 (0.4–3.4)
Pooled Analyses				
Kheifets et al.[56]	Based on ten studies from 1979 to 2010	Pooled 8,372/11,494	Measured and Calculated fields	≥0.4 µT 1.1 (0.6–2.1)

[a] Abstract only.

[b] Phase I: 90 min in family room + spot measurement in bedroom; Phase II: 48-h bedroom and spot measurement in school only for highest 10% in Phase I.

13.4.2.2 Electric Appliance Exposure

Four studies examined brain tumor occurrence and use of appliances by children or their mother during pregnancy.[110,111,116,117] No consistent or remarkable associations were reported in any of the studies. Positive associations with certain appliances found in individual studies were generally not replicated in other studies.

13.4.2.3 Parental Exposure

Six case-control studies have examined the occurrence of childhood brain cancer or neuroblastoma among the children and paternal occupation, including work that presumably exposed them to EMF.[118–126] As in most occupational studies, exposure assessment was based on job titles, a method that may not be very precise and particularly problematic when a broad set of occupations from many industries is considered. Elevated relative risks (above 2.0) reported in the first two studies were not confirmed in later studies. The predominance of positive findings in earlier reports could be due to selective reporting, as many occupations were examined. A recent review by a Brain Tumor Epidemiology Consortium[108] referenced earlier, concluded that parental occupational ELF exposure in different exposure time windows are inconsistent.

Some additional information regarding parental occupations and childhood brain tumor is provided by reanalyses of the childhood brain cancer studies.[110,118,125–128] These studies further support the absence of an association.

13.4.2.4 Pooled Analyses

Only one pooled analysis, of measured or calculated fields and brain tumors, was conducted. Kheifets et al. identified 16 studies published in 1979–2010, of which 10 met their inclusion criteria.[129] A total of 10,865 cases and 12,853 controls were included in the pooled analysis, which focused on 24 h magnetic field measurements or calculated fields in residences. The OR for exposure above $0.4\,\mu T$ compared to $<0.1\,\mu T$ was 1.14 (95% CI: 0.61–2.13), controlling for age and gender, thus providing little evidence for an association between ELF exposure and childhood brain tumors. Other analyses employing alternate cutpoints, further adjustment for confounders, exclusion of particular studies, stratification by type of measurement or type of residence, and a nonparametric estimate of the exposure–response relation also did not reveal evidence of increased childhood brain tumor risk associated with ELF exposure.

13.4.3 Adult Brain Cancer

13.4.3.1 Residential Exposure

Few studies have examined the potential association between brain cancer and residential exposure in adults, and none have looked at appliance use. Cancer of the brain or nervous system by subtype was examined in several studies of adult cancers, first by wire codes or distance (data not shown)[97,98,130] and later with measurements or calculated fields[92,95,97,98,131–133] with predominantly null results (see Table 13.4). Most notable is a study by Feychting and Ahlbom[92] which showed no evidence of an association between residential EMF exposure and adult brain cancer, regardless of the method of estimating exposure. Results from a large adult glioma study[132] and residential EMF exposure

TABLE 13.4

Epidemiologic Studies of Residential Exposure and Meta-Analysis of Occupational Exposure to Magnetic Fields and Adult Brain Tumors

Reference	Study Population	Study Design Cases/Controls	Exposure	High Category RR (95% CI)
Residential Studies				
Feychting and Ahlbom[92]	Residents within 300 m of power line. Cases: ≥16 y.o. Controls: random from cohort. Sweden	Case-control 325/1,091	Distance Calculated fields	0–50 m 1.0 (0.6–1.8) ≥0.2 µT 0.7 (0.4–1.3)
Verkasalo et al.[131]	Residents within 500 m of power line. ≥20 y.o., Finland	Cohort Cases 301	Cumulative Calculated fields	≥2.0 µT–years 0.9 (0.3–1.9)
Li et al.[95]	Taiwan cancer registry (1987–1992). Controls: Other cancers excluding brain, breast and several others.	Case-control 577/552	Calculated exposure in year of diagnosis	0–50 m 1.3 (0.8–2.1) >0.2 µT 1.1 (0.8–1.6)
Wrensch et al.[132]	Cases: Northern California Cancer Center Controls RDD, United States	Case-control 492/462	Spot Measurements	>0.3 µT 1.7 (0.8–3.6)
Klaeboe et al.[133]	>16 y.o. Power line corridor. Controls: random from cohort. Norway	Nested CC 454/908	Calculated fields	≥0.2 µT 1.3 (0.7–2.3)
Marcilio et al.[97]	Death certificates. Controls random from other causes deaths, except those associated with MF. Brazil	Case-control 2,357/4,706	Distance Calculated fields	0–50 m 1.1 (0.7–1.6) >0.3 µT 1.2 (0.6–2.1)
Baldi et al.[130]	Population-based study from 1999 to 2001. Gironde, France	Case-control 221/642	Proximity to power lines	0–100 m 1.5 (0.7–3.1)
Elliott et al.[98]	15–74 y.o.; Controls Other cancers: except brain, breast, melanoma, and several others. United Kingdom	Case-control 6,781/20,343	Distance Calculated fields diagnosis year	0–50 m 1.2 (0.9–1.7) >1 µT 1.0 (0.5–2.2)
Meta-Analysis and Pooled Analyses of Occupational Studies				
Kheifets et al.[101]	Studies of utility workers	Pooled of six cohorts	Detailed Measurement data	per 10 µT-years 1.1 (0.98–1.3)
Kheifets et al.[102]	Occupational studies published 1983–2007	Meta of 47 studies	Study-specific	1.14 (1.1–1.2)

assessed through spot measurements, wire codes, and distance from electrical facilities did not support an association. For residences with measurements above 0.3 µT, there was a suggestion of increased risk; however, the number of cases and controls in this category was small. Other studies are even more problematic as some use other cancers[98,134] or other deaths as controls.[97]

In Feychting et al.[100] residential and occupational exposures were combined by incorporating estimates of occupational magnetic field exposure into Feychting and Ahlbom's earlier residential study[92]; unlike results for leukemia, it found no association between exposure and central nervous system tumors in adults exposed to higher levels of magnetic fields both at home and at work. Although the study has limitations, particularly that the occupational magnetic field measurements were from a different study whose applicability is questionable, the study advanced the EMF exposure assessment with its efforts to incorporate both residential and occupational exposures.[135] A subsequent study from Norway that also combined occupational exposures also did not find an association (OR = 1.0, 95% CI: 0.4–27) for combined exposure.[133]

13.4.3.2 Occupational Studies

Many epidemiologic studies have examined the possible association between occupational EMF exposure and brain cancer. In 1995, Kheifets et al.[136] conducted a review of 52 occupational studies; of these, 29 represented original research published meeting inclusion criteria for the meta-analysis. These studies examined populations in 12 different countries, although most were conducted in the United States and Scandinavia. While most studies presented a small elevation in risk, there was considerable heterogeneity in the results. An inverse-variance weighted pooling of all the data resulted in a small but significant overall increase in risk among individuals employed in the broadly defined group of electrical occupations. Relative risk was higher for some specific jobs and for gliomas. The meta-analysis findings were not affected by inclusion of unpublished data, influence of individual studies, weighting schemes, or model specification. Kheifets[137] also reviewed the studies published since the 1995 meta-analysis[100,138–149] and concluded that these studies mainly showed no risk.

Although positive associations have been reported in some studies with employment in "electrical occupations," these studies have often had methodological limitations, such as reliance on a single job title for exposure assessment particularly in earlier studies. More rigorous studies on workers in the electricity supply industries with a specific focus on occupations with high potential for EMF exposure[150–152] have had fewer of these limitations. In a comparative analysis by Kheifets et al.[101] conclusions based on these more rigorous studies were compatible with a weak association between magnetic fields and brain cancer; based on a combined analysis of data, the relative risk per 10 µT-years of exposure was 1.12 (95% CI: 0.98–1.28). However, results were also compatible with chance fluctuation. A new understanding emerged from this pooled analysis: what previously appeared to be important differences in results across studies are small and not from methodologic differences.

Twenty occupational brain cancer studies published since the 1995 meta-analysis were included in an update.[102] Pooled risk estimates were lower than in past meta-analyses for both all brain cancers and gliomas. When added to the studies in the original meta-analysis there was no clear pattern of EMF exposure and risk. Overall, results (Table 13.4) do not support a hypothesis that magnetic field exposures are responsible for the observed small excess risk (RR = 1.14, 95% CI: 1.1–1.2). Findings were not sensitive to assumptions, influential studies, weighting schemes, publication bias, study characteristics, or funding source.

Since the last update to the meta-analysis several new studies have been published (e.g., Baldi and Turner[153]). The INTEROCC study which was a multicenter case-control study, using a subset of seven country-specific, occupational data collected as part of the INTERPHONE study, reported excess glioma risk only among workers with more recent exposure (1–4 years).

13.4.4 Summary Brain Cancer

Brain-cancer studies have shown inconsistent results. Based on the pattern of results when considering all epidemiologic studies of childhood brain tumors and residential magnetic fields, particularly looking at studies that included both leukemia and brain cancer, results for brain tumors are generally less consistent and indicate smaller and less precise risks than for leukemia. However, there are more studies for childhood leukemia compared to childhood brain tumors, and leukemia studies tend to be larger and capture more exposed subjects as confirmed by comparison of pooled analysis of childhood leukemia and brain cancer studies. For adult brain tumor studies, both occupational and residential, the evidence is weaker still.

13.5 Breast Cancer

13.5.1 Background

Breast cancer is the most commonly occurring malignancy in women in the United States and the second most worldwide.[154] A considerable body of epidemiologic research has identified numerous factors that affect the risk of developing breast cancer in females. The disease occurs most frequently among women who are white, higher social class, without children or with few children (low parity), and who had their first child at a late age. Other risk factors include early age of menarche (menses), late age of menopause, obesity for postmenopausal women, proliferative fibrocystic disease, and a first degree relative with breast cancer, especially if that cancer was diagnosed at a young age. Considerably less is known about male breast cancer but indications are that genetic and environmental factors including obesity, familial history and endocrine factors play a causative role. Occupational studies indicate elevated rates of breast cancer among men in jobs such as newspaper printing, soap and perfume manufacturing, and health care.

Breast cancer incidence rates are highest in North America and northern Europe and lowest in Asia and Africa. Until recently, the search to possibly explain this pattern had focused on the societal differences in dietary and female reproductive patterns in societies with different degrees of industrialization. However, the role of diet in the etiology of breast cancer remains uncertain and reproductive risk factors apparently account for only a fraction of the excess disease reported in modernized societies.[137]

Factors proposed to contribute to the greater occurrence of breast cancer in industrialized compared to non-industrialized societies are the use of electric power and higher exposures to light at night or to magnetic fields. Stevens[155] hypothesized that EMF and light at night can affect breast cancer through suppression of melatonin, an important regulating hormone of circadian rhythm. Epidemiologic investigations addressing the potential link between breast cancer and exposure to magnetic fields include occupational studies and residential studies that examine breast cancer risk in relation to proximity to electric installations and the use of electric blankets.

13.5.2 Female Breast Cancer

13.5.2.1 Residential Exposure

Several studies of residential exposure and other adult cancers examined risk of breast cancer in populations residing near power lines. One of these studies found an association between premenopausal but not postmenopausal breast cancer and wiring configuration.[8] Two other studies[89,90] did not detect any associations and one found a non-significant risk for subjects within 152 m of transmission line or substation[156] (data not shown). Several

TABLE 13.5

Epidemiologic Studies of Residential and Occupational Exposure to Magnetic Fields and Breast Cancer

Reference	Study Population	Study Design Cases/ Controls	Exposure	High Category RR (95% CI) Female	High Category RR (95% CI) Male
Residential Studies					
Feychting et al.[157]	Residents within 300 m of power line. ≥16 years old (y.o.). Controls: random from cohort. Sweden	Case-control F: 699/699 M: 9/72	Historically calculated fields	0–50 m 0.8 (0.5–1.3) ≥0.2 µT 1.0 (0.7–1.5)	0–50 m 1.4 (0.1–15.0) ≥0.2 µT 2.1 (0.3–14.1)
Verkasalo et al.[131]	Residents within 500 m of power line. ≥20 y.o., Finland	Cohort 1,229	Cumulative Calculated	≥2.0 µT–years 0.8 (0.5–1.1)	—
Li et al.[95]	Cancer registry (1987–1992). Controls: other cancers excluding brain, breast and several others. Taiwan	Case-control 1,980/1,880	Calculated exposure in year of diagnosis	0–50 m 1.0 (0.8–1.3) >0.2 µT 1.1 (0.9–1.3)	—
Davis et al.[159]	Population-based study, 20–74 RDD controls in Washington State	Case-control 744/711	2 day bedroom nighttime	VHCC 0.8 (0.5–1.3) ≥0.073 µT 0.9 (0.7–1.4)	—
London et al.[160]	Cohort of residents in Los Angeles County, 45–74 y.o.	Nested case-control 347/286	1 week bedroom night time	VHCC 0.8 (0.5–1.2) ≥0.4 µT 1.2 (0.5–3.0)	—
Schoenfeld et al.[161]	Same home 15 years; 20–74; RDD controls. United States	Case-control 576/585	24-h night time	≥0.14 µT 0.99 (0.9–1.4)	
Kliukiene et al.[158]	≥16 y.o. Cohort near power lines. Norway	Nested CC 1,830/3,658	Calculated fields	≥0.2 µT 1.4 (1.0–1.8)	
Elliott et al.[98]	15–74 y.o.; Controls Other cancers: except brain, breast, melanoma, and several others. United Kingdom	Case-control 29,202/29,202 (50% sample)	Distance Calculated fields in year of diagnosis	0–50 m 1.1 (0.9–1.2) >1 µT 1.1 (0.8–1.5)	—
Meta-Analysis of Occupational Studies					
Chen et al.[162]	Occupational studies 1990–2010[a]	23 studies (7 occupational)	Study-specific	1.1 (1.0–1.2)	
Sun et al.[163]	Occupational studies 1991–2005[a]	18 studies (16 occupational)	Study-specific	—	1.3 (1.2–1.5)

[a] Included residential studies—only occupational result presented here.

large breast cancer studies added measurements or used calculated fields (Table 13.5). No risk has been identified in any of the calculated field studies.[95,98,131,157,158]

Importantly, three large and well-conducted breast cancer residential studies which incorporated measurements into their design found no association with exposure to magnetic fields.[159–161] It should be noted however, that higher cutpoints have not been evaluated.

While some studies found elevated risk in premenopausal and/or estrogen receptor positive (ER+) breast cancer (e.g. Feychting[157]), others did not.[158–160] Studies that combined residential and occupational exposure did not find substantial changes in risk when both exposures were considered.[146,164]

13.5.2.2 Electric Blankets

Two early case-control studies[165,166] did not support the hypothesis that the use of electric blankets increases the risk of postmenopausal or premenopausal breast cancer. Vena et al.[165] combined these two studies and found elevated risk among women who reported some use of blankets throughout the night (RR = 1.5, 95% CI: 1.1–1.9) in the previous 10 years; however, the risk was not the highest among the highest exposure group, that is, those who reported daily use of the blankets in season and continuously throughout the night for 10 years (RR = 1.2, 95% CI: 0.8–1.9). Subsequent studies have been inconsistent and meta-analysis of eight studies did not find a risk (OR = 1.0, 95% CI: 0.95–1.1).[162]

13.5.2.3 Occupational Studies

Few occupational studies of electrical workers included sufficient numbers of females to address the potential association of occupational EMF exposure and development of breast cancer. Albeit based on small numbers, four studies found no elevation in risk of breast cancer among females working in occupations with potential exposure to EMF as compared to low exposure occupations.[167–170]

One large study[171] used computerized mortality files from the National Center for Health Statistics for the years 1985–1989. Death certificates included the occupation and industry in which the decedent usually worked, coded according to the 1980 U.S. Census. Excluded were women whose occupation was listed as "homemaker" and those whose death certificate provided no occupational data; these two groups made up more than half of the database. Seven electrical occupations used in previous studies were included, along with seven other occupations, such as computer programmers and telephone operators, presumed to have a large number of female workers and some potential for above-background EMF exposure. All other occupations were considered unexposed. Among 27,882 breast cancer cases and 110,949 controls, 68 cases and 199 controls had been employed in traditional electrical occupations. The relative risk for breast cancer among those employed in electrical occupations was 1.4 (95% CI: 1.0–1.8). In a more detailed analysis, the association was the strongest for the managerial/professional class, and for those 45–54 years of age. The relative risks for the other occupations with potential exposure were around 1.0 or lower. In a separate analysis of the same data, but with a different approach to exposure grouping, Cantor et al.[172] did not find an association of female breast cancer and potential workplace exposure to EMF.

Aside from being a death certificate study, the authors could not adjust for many risk factors known to be associated with breast cancer, including reproductive and family histories. Working in male-dominated jobs may have favored nulliparity, delayed childbearing, or other characteristics related to risk of breast cancer. The authors attempted to control for some of these characteristics by adjusting for social class. However, it is not clear how effectively social class was determined, and at best it can serve only as a partial control for known risk factors of breast cancer.

Although some earlier registry-based studies provided some support for a possible association between EMF exposure and female breast cancer,[173] the most recent very large study, which incorporated exposure measurements in female workers, did not find an association.[164] Similarly, a meta-analysis did not find an association between occupational studies in females and risk of breast cancer.[162]

13.5.3 Male Breast Cancer

13.5.3.1 Residential Exposure

Male breast cancer accounts for ~1% of all breast cancer cases; thus, most studies have included only female breast cancer. The only residential study that included male breast cancer (Feychting et al. 1998[157]) reported an elevation in risk, but the results were not significant and were based on only two exposed/nine total cases of male breast cancer (OR = 2.1, 95% CI: 0.3–14.1).

13.5.3.2 Occupational Studies

As described earlier, many studies have examined cancer in electrical occupations. As part of that examination, many considered breast cancer as one of the outcomes. Male breast cancer is rare and most of the studies are not based on sufficiently large populations, so estimates of risk for male breast cancer often are not included in tables of results unless an excess risk has been observed.[169,170,174–178] This makes it difficult to evaluate the potential for the excess risk of male breast cancer. Nevertheless, several reports[167,179–182] are suggestive of a positive association, while negative results were reported by Loomis[134] and Camarano.[183] The large studies of electrical workers[150–152,184] did not identify any excess of male breast cancer.

Recently, the largest case-control study[185] of male breast cancer (115 cases) and occupational exposure to magnetic fields reported an elevated risk in the highest category (OR = 1.9, 95% CI: 0.8, 4.5) for exposure ≥0.6 μT, but no risk in the intermediate category 0.3 to <0.6 μT.

A meta-analysis reports small risk[163] (OR = 1.3, 95% CI: 1.2–1.5) based on job titles in 16 occupational studies, but more rigorous analysis is warranted.

13.5.4 Summary Breast Cancer

For male and female breast cancer, the research began with a biological hypothesis that magnetic fields could affect melatonin production, which was initially supported by early studies. More rigorous epidemiologic studies that followed showed no effect. Thus, it appears that EMF fields are not involved in the development of breast cancer.[5]

13.6 Lung Cancer

Of the many studies[151,152,169,174,176–178,183,184,186] that have examined the possible association between electrical occupations or extremely low-frequency magnetic field exposure and lung cancer, only two[170,175] report some elevation in risk.

Armstrong et al.[138] reported an association between lung cancer and cumulative high frequency electromagnetic transients, or pulsed electromagnetic fields (PEMFs). In this study of EMF exposure and lung cancer, some residual confounding from smoking may possibly remain, because (a) smoking is a strong risk factor for lung cancer, and (b) the length of employment is likely to be strongly correlated with both cumulative PEMF exposure and the amount and length of smoking, rather than just current smoking status.

In summary, presently available evidence does not suggest an association between EMF exposure and lung cancer. The study of lung cancer and PEMFs may be relevant to exposure from cell phones and thus might need replication.

13.7 Other Cancers

Sporadic reports of elevated risks for other cancers have appeared in the literature, most notably for malignant melanoma,[187] but none have been sufficiently suggestive to warrant presentation here, particularly as the recent UK study did not identify risk for malignant melanoma.[98] Finally, cancers of the prostate and pituitary gland could be of interest because of their roles in the production of hormones. Patterns of risk for these cancers in relation to jobs with exposure to magnetic fields remain largely unexplored.

13.8 Cardiovascular Disease

Concerns about cardiovascular changes resulting from EMF exposure originated from descriptions in the 1960s and early 1970s of the symptoms among Russian high-voltage switchyard operators and workers.[188] Although these reports remain unconfirmed,[189] investigations into cardiovascular disease continues and focused on direct cardiac effects of EMF exposure, mostly related to heart rate variability and subsequent acute cardiovascular events.

Sastre et al.[190] hypothesized an association between exposure to EMF and acute cardiovascular disease. This hypothesis was based on two independent lines of evidence. The first was experimental data in which intermittent 60 Hz magnetic fields were found to reduce the normal heart rate variability.[190] The second came from several prospective cohort studies which indicated that reductions in some components of the variation in heart rate increase the risk for (1) heart disease,[191–193] (2) overall mortality rate in survivors of myocardial infarction,[194–196] and (3) risk for sudden cardiovascular death.[197] Thus, Savitz et al.[198] postulated that occupational EMF exposure would increase the risk for cardiac arrhythmia-related conditions and acute myocardial infarction, but not for chronic cardiovascular disease. As postulated, they observed an increased risk of acute myocardial infarction (AMI) AMI and arrhythmia related death with high EMF exposure, but not for chronic cardiovascular disease (Table 13.6).

Other studies were unable to replicate their findings.[99,200,201,203,204,206,208–211] Similarly, using morbidity as the outcome measure Johansen et al.[205] and Ahlbom et al.[207] did not observe any association. The Ahlbom et al. study is particularly informative, as it focused on high validity of the AMI diagnoses, elicited high participation rates in this population

TABLE 13.6

Epidemiologic Studies of Cardiovascular Disease in Relation to EMF

Reference	Study Population	Study Design	Exposure	RR (95% CI) High Category AMI	RR (95% CI) High Category CHD
Residential Studies					
Perry et al.[199]	AMI discharge from hospital; neighborhood controls	Case-control 596/596 Incidence	Measurements at front door	Mean difference zero	
Fazzo et al.[99]	Population of a district built under a 60 kV line 1954 and 2003. Italy	Cohort N = 142 Incidence	Residence within 28 m of the line		SMR 2.8 (1.3–6.3)
Occupational Studies					
Baris et al.[200]	Workers employed in electrical company between 1970 and 1988. Quebec	Cohort N = 21,744 Mortality	Job exposure matrix		RR 0.9 (0.7–1.1)
Johansen et al.[201]	Male utility workers, employed between 1990 and 1993, followed 1974–1993	Cohort N = 21,236 Mortality	JEM based on measurements	SMR 1.0 (O = 160)	
Savitz et al.[198] and van Wijngaarden et al.[202]	Male utility workers, employed between 1950 and 1986, followed to 1988	Cohort N = 138,903 Mortality	Duration of work in jobs with elevated EMF	RR 1.6 (1.5–1.8)	RR 1.0 (0.9–1.8)
Kelsh and Sahl[145] and Sahl et al.[203]	Utility workers, employed between 1960 and 1991, followed to 1992	Cohort N = 35,391 Mortality	Duration of work in jobs with elevated EMF	RR 1.0 (0.7–1.5)	RR 1.2 (0.8–1.8)
Håkansson et al.[204]	Swedish twins responding to job questionnaire in 1967 or 1973	Cohort N = 27,790	Job exposure matrix	1.3 (0.9–1.9)	
Johansen et al.[205]	Male utility workers, employed between 1990 and 1993, followed 1974–1993	Cohort N = 24,056 Incidence	JEM based on measurements		SIR With Pacemakers 1.0 (0.6–1.5)
Håkansson et al.[204]	Swedish twins responding to job questionnaire in 1967 or 1973	Case-control from cohort: 27,790 Mortality	Job exposure matrix	RR 1.3 (0.9–1.9)	
Sorahan et al.[206]	Utility workers, employed between 1973 and 1982, followed to 1997	Cohort N = 79,972 Mortality	Duration of work in jobs and locations with elevated EMF	RR 1.0 (0.9–1.2)	RR 0.9 (0.7–1.2)
Ahlbom et al.[207]	Male population of Stockholm 1992–1993	Case-control; 695/1,133 Incidence	Job titles, job exposure matrix	RR 0.6 (0.4–0.9)	

(Continued)

TABLE 13.6 (*Continued*)

Epidemiologic Studies of Cardiovascular Disease in Relation to EMF

Reference	Study Population	Study Design	Exposure	RR (95% CI) High Category AMI	RR (95% CI) High Category CHD
Mezei et al.[208]	Sample of deaths in United States 1986 and 1993, Controls other causes except ALS, CNN, lymphopoietic cancers	Case-control 2,992/34,891 Mortality	Longest job from interview with proxy	OR 1.0 (0.8–1.2)	OR 1.1 (0.9–1.4)
Röösli et al.[209]	Swiss railway workers between 1972 and 2002	Cohort N = 20,141	JEM based on measurements	HR 1.1 (0.6–2.0)	HR 1.0 (0.8–1.2)
Cooper et al.[210]	Workers in the U.S. between 1979 and 1981	Cohort N = 307,012 Mortality	Job exposure matrix	HR 1.0 (0.9–1.1)	HR 1.0 (0.8–1.2)
Koeman et al.[211]	Electric utility workers in the Netherlands	Cohort N = 120,852	Job exposure matrix and questionnaire	HR 1.0 (0.9–1.2)	HR 1.0 (0.87–1.16)

AMI, acute myocardial infarction; CHD, coronary heart disease.

based study, and controlled for blood pressure, serum cholesterol, socioeconomic status, and cigarette smoking. This methodologically advanced study strengthens the conclusion of no effect of magnetic fields on acute cardiovascular disease. In another morbidity study, Haakanson et al.[204] observed an increased risk of AMI with high exposure, though nonsignificant.

Most of the cardiovascular studies have been based on mortality records as the measure of outcome, problematic for cardiovascular disease since drawing the distinction between acute and chronic disease is nuanced as, in many instances, acute cardiac events follow long-term cardiovascular changes. Finkelstein[212] questioned the use of death certificates for outcomes involving loss of autonomic cardiovascular control and pointed out that etiologic conclusions should not be drawn solely on studies which use cause of death on death certificates. A recent UK study identified inaccuracy in listing of cause of death on the death certificates and difficulties in differentiating between acute and chronic cardiac classification.[213]

Only two small and uninformative studies (Perry et al.[199] and Fazzo et al.[99]) have looked at cardiovascular risk and residential exposures: one study found no risk, while the other found a risk for all ischemic diseases or spectrum of heart disease caused by weak oxygen supply to the heart, which was not limited to the high-exposure group.

13.8.1 Summary Cardiovascular Disease

Despite a biologic hypothesis that was initially supported by an epidemiologic study, studies that followed showed no effect. Thus, the overall evidence speaks against an etiologic relation between occupational EMF exposure and cardiovascular disease (for detailed review, see Kheifets et al.[214]).

13.9 Neurological Diseases

As defined by WHO, neurological diseases affect the central and peripheral nervous system. These systems include the brain, spinal cord, cranial nerves, peripheral nerves, nerve roots, autonomic nervous system, neuromuscular junction, and muscles.

Neurodegenerative diseases are a type of neurologic disease, characterized by a loss of neuron structure or function.

13.9.1 Alzheimer's Disease and Dementia

Dementias cover a broad spectrum of cognitive-related diseases, including Alzheimer's disease. Tangles and plaques in the brain typify Alzheimer's disease, the most common dementia. Alzheimer's disease is characterized clinically by progressive loss of memory and other cognitive abilities (e.g., language, attention). Its onset is thought to be heralded by a phase of mild cognitive impairment in which cognition is not normal but not severe enough to warrant a diagnosis of dementia. The exact duration of mild cognitive impairment is unclear, but is likely to last at least a few years. Many persons with Alzheimer's disease also develop motor, behavioral, and affective disturbances. In particular, parkinsonian signs, hallucinations, delusions, and depressive symptoms are present in half or more of persons with the disease.

Alzheimer's disease (a subset of dementia) parallels the trends observed for dementia overall. Dementia incidence usually increases beginning at the age of 70. Alzheimer's disease is classified by age of onset, early onset and late-age onset (>65 years), which has a recognized vascular component.[215] Late onset makes up about 95% of the cases. In 2014, there was an estimated 470,000 new Alzheimer's disease cases among persons aged 65 years or more.[216] However, Alzheimer's is considered a spectrum of diseases with respect to diagnostic criteria. Alzheimer's disease epidemiology remains challenging due to disease recognition, stemming from symptom subtleties experienced by patients to ensuing diagnostic challenges encountered by clinicians.

A notable weakness in neurodegenerative disease epidemiologic studies, particularly those of Alzheimer's disease and dementia, is case identification. In some studies, cases were identified in hospitals whereas in others on death certificates, which is particularly problematic because these diagnoses are often not reported as an underlying cause and are underrepresented as a contributing cause as well. In addition, changes in diagnostic criteria and disease duration make death records problematic for investigating relationships for Alzheimer's and Parkinson's diseases. Controls are often selected among patients with other diseases at the same hospitals or among friends or relatives of cases. Adding to the complexity, in some studies subjects with dementia are included as cases, while in others they are included as controls.

Alzheimer's and dementia residential EMF studies are few and largely uninformative (Table 13.7). A study from Turkey, while screened for cognitive impairment,[217] is cross-sectional and based on use of space and water heating. The Swiss mortality study reports no risk overall, but an increased risk for Alzheimer's for those who lived in the same residence close to power lines for at least 15 years (data not shown).[218] This finding was not confirmed by an incidence study of otherwise similar design in Denmark.[219]

When evaluated across all occupational studies, there appears to be no association for dementia (OR = 1.1, 95% CI: 0.96–1.1), but a weak association between estimated EMF exposure and Alzheimer's disease risk.[221] However, this result is influenced by the first

TABLE 13.7

Epidemiologic Studies of the Association between Alzheimer's Disease and Dementia and EMF

Reference	Study Population	Study Design	Exposure	High Category RR (95% CI)
Residential Studies				
Harmanci et al.[217]	Residents age ≥70 screened for cognitive impairment 1993–1997. Turkey	Cross sectional 57/127	Electrical heating house or water	AZ OR 2.8 (1.1–6.9)
Huss et al.[218]	≥30 y.o. with complete geocoded building, 2000–2005. Mortality. Switzerland	Cohort 4.7 M N = 9,758	Distance	0–50 m AZ HR 1.2 (0.4–1.9) Dem HR 1.2 (0.96–1.6)
Frei[219]	≥65 y.o.; 1994–2010 Cases discharge registry; controls population registry. Denmark	Case-control 20,575/11,3217	Distance	0–50 m AZ OR 1.0 (0.7–1.6) Dem OR 0.9 (0.7–1.2)
Meta-Analysis of Occupational studies				
Garcia et al.[220]	Occupational studies published 1995–2004	Meta-analysis of 14 studies	MF level	Case/control 2.0 (1.4–3.0) Cohort 1.6 (1.2–2.3)
Vergara et al.[221]	Occupational studies published 1983–2011	Meta-analysis of 20 studies	Occupation MF level	1.3 (1.2–1.4)

two studies,[222,223] which are likely affected by selection bias. The study populations are undefined in these studies and whether the controls were representative with respect to exposure of the population from which the cases originated cannot be determined. A meta-analysis of 20 studies found a small risk (OR = 1.3, 95% CI: 1.2–1.4) with the Alzheimer's risk largely limited to prevalence studies. However, reporting and publication bias seems as a likely explanation for this observation.[221] Since this meta-analysis, several occupational studies provide similar unremarkable results,[224–227] although one study suggested that the focus should be on severe cognitive dysfunction.[228]

13.9.2 Amyotrophic Lateral Sclerosis

ALS is characterized clinically by the progressive loss of function of both upper and lower motor neurons, painless muscle wasting and spasticity. Persons with ALS may develop cognitive and autonomic dysfunction. The disease is invariably fatal, thus use of death certificates for this outcome is adequate.[229] Among the motor neuron diseases, ALS is the most common.

The annual incidence of ALS is estimated around 1–2.5 per 100,000 people in Europe and North America.[230] The incidence of the disease, which is slightly higher among men than among women, sharply increases with age, reaching its peak in the seventh decade of life with an annual incidence rate of approximately 8–12 per 100,000.[231] Generally, ALS cases are classified into three major types: familial, sporadic, and the endemic cases of the Western Pacific. Familial cases, worldwide, comprise of about 5%–10% of ALS cases. Despite advances in our understanding of the role of genetic changes in the development of ALS, the etiology of the most common type, sporadic ALS, remains largely unknown. While a number of lifestyle-related (e.g., smoking, diet, exercise), environmental and occupational exposures (e.g., the Gulf War, military service, metals, solvents) have been hypothesized, the etiologic role of these factors remains unconfirmed.[230]

The earlier studies on ALS examined the possible etiology of electric shocks and ALS. After the first study in 1964 suggested a plausible relationship,[232] two subsequent studies from Japan, where the prevalence of electrical work (as recorded in the medical history) and of electrical shock was low, failed to provide any support for the hypothesis.[233]

More recently, five both incidence and mortality residential studies[97,218,219,234,235] based on distance or calculated fields did not find any risk of ALS (Table 13.8). A meta-analysis of 21 occupational studies found a small risk (OR = 1.3, 95% CI: 1.1–1.4), which was largely confined to associations based on occupations rather than associations for magnetic field measurements.[221]

Clearly, work in the utility industry, as well as in other electrical occupations, carries a risk of experiencing electric shocks; thus, shocks have been suggested as a possible confounder.[236] Four recent studies examined both magnetic fields and electric shocks based on JEMs[237–240] with inconsistent results.

In sum, there is modest epidemiological evidence to suggest that employment in electrical occupations may increase the risk of ALS; however, separating the increased risk due to receiving an electric shock from the increased exposure to EMFs is difficult.

TABLE 13.8

Epidemiologic Studies of the Association between Amyotrophic Lateral Sclerosis and EMF

Reference	Study Population	Study Design	Exposure	High Category RR (95% CI)
Residential Studies				
Huss et al.[218]	≥30 years old (y.o.) with complete geocoded building information, Switzerland	Cohort 4.7 M N = 759 Mortality	Distance	HR 0 cases
Marcilio et al.[97]	Death certificates; Controls other causes deaths, except those associated with MF. Brazil	Case-control 367/4,706 Mortality	Distance Calculated Fields	0–50 m 0.3 (0.1–1.1) >0.3 µT NR
Frei et al.[219]	≥20 y.o.; Cases discharge registry; controls population registry. Denmark	Case-control 2,990/14,996 Incidence	Distance	0–50 m 0.8 (0.3–1.9)
Seelen et al.[234]	Cases and controls from general practitioner roster 2006–2013. Netherlands	Case-control 1,139/2,864 Incidence	Distance to 50–150 kV	0–50 m 1.1 (0.4–2.8)
Vincenti et al.[235]	Cases from variety of sources controls residents in the provinces 1998–2011. Italy	Case-control 703/2,737 Incidence	Distance Calculated Fields	≥0.1 µT 0.7 (0.2–1.6)
Meta-Analysis of Occupational Studies				
Zhou et al.[241]	Occupational studies published 1980–2009	Meta-analysis of 17 studies	Occupation MF level	1.3 (1.0–1.6)
Vergara et al.[221]	Occupational studies published 1983–2011	Meta-analysis of 21 studies	Occupation MF level	1.3 (1.1–1.4)

13.9.3 Parkinson's Disease

Parkinson's disease is characterized clinically by progressive motor dysfunction, including bradykinesia, gait disturbance, rigidity, and tremor. Many persons with Parkinson's disease develop cognitive, behavioral, and autonomic signs. After Alzheimer's disease, Parkinson's disease is the second most common neurodegenerative disease. Involving cell loss in the neural pathway of the *substantia nigra* and presence of Lewy bodies, Parkinson's disease causes uncontrolled body tremors.

Reported age-adjusted yearly incidence rates range from 8 to 18 per 100,000.[242] Most studies reported prevalence range of 100–300 per 100,000.[243] Parkinson's disease is rare prior to the age of 50, but its prevalence increases with age.

Of the neurodegenerative diseases that have been considered, Parkinson's disease has received the least attention in epidemiology (Table 13.9). Two residential studies, one on incidence and one on mortality, based on distance to overhead lines did not find any risk of Parkinson's disease.[218,219]

Occupation has been considered as a possible cause of Parkinson's disease in several studies.[245–250] Two meta-analyses of occupational studies[221,244] found no risk (OR = 0.97, 95% CI: 0.9–1.0) for either occupations or magnetic field levels. A study,[226] published since meta-analysis and mentioned earlier, reports an (OR = 0.9, 95% CI: 0.6–1.3), for exposures $\geq 1.0\,\mu T$ (data not shown).

Parkinson's appears to be unrelated to either electric occupations or residential and occupational magnetic fields.

13.9.4 Epilepsy and Other Neurodegenerative Diseases

Epilepsy, characterized by recurrent, unprovoked seizures, is a common chronic neurologic disorder affecting persons of all ages.[251] A recent systematic review of 48 incidence studies found an incidence rate of 61.44 per 100,000 person-years.[252] Multiple sclerosis occurs when the immune system attacks the myelin of the nerve cells, impacting persons at ages 30–40 years. The incidence and prevalence rates published vary considerably. No

TABLE 13.9

Epidemiologic Studies of the Association between Parkinson's and EMF

Reference	Study Population	Study Design	Exposure	High Category RR (95% CI)
Residential Studies				
Huss et al.[218]	≥30 years old (y.o.) with complete geocoded building information, Switzerland	Cohort 4.7 M Cases 6,994 Mortality	Distance	HR 0.9 (0.5–1.6)
Frei et al.[219]	≥20 y.o.; Cases discharge registry; controls population registry. Denmark	Case-control 16,925/90,060 Incidence	Distance	0–50 m 1.1 (0.8–1.6)
Meta-Analysis of Occupational Studies				
Vergara et al.[221]	Occupational studies published 1983–2011	Meta-analysis of 18 studies	Occupation MF level	1.0 (0.9–1.0)
Huss et al.[244]	Occupational studies published 1998–2015	Meta-analysis of 11 studies	MF level	1.1 (0.98–1.1)

residential studies and only few occupational studies have examined epilepsy and multiple sclerosis among other neurodegenerative diseases.

Feychting et al.[247] found no increased risk multiple sclerosis or epilepsy for either men or women. Håkansson et al.[204] also found no increased risk for multiple sclerosis and they observed a decreased risk for epilepsy. A meta-analysis of five occupational studies found no risk of MS (OR = 1.0, 95% CI: 0.9–1.2).[221] On the other hand, a group of researchers from Denmark found an increased risk of epilepsy in the cohort of people who survived an electric accident (Standard Hospitalization Ratio = 1.5; 95% CI: 1.1–1.9).[253] The same group reported an increased risk of both multiple sclerosis and epilepsy in the Danish utility work cohort for those with the highest occupational ELF-MF exposure.[226] At this time, the literature is too sparse and heterogeneous to warrant any inference.

13.9.5 Summary Neurologic Diseases

Few EMF studies on multiple sclerosis and epilepsy exist to evaluate the evidence. There is no evidence linking EMF and Parkinson's disease and only very weak evidence to suggest that they affect Alzheimer's disease. Better studies of Alzheimer's are warranted. The evidence that people employed in electrical occupations have an increased risk of developing ALS is substantial, perhaps because such employees have an increased risk of experiencing an electric shock rather than any long-term exposure to the fields per se. Studies of ALS that can distinguish between electric shocks and magnetic fields, including pooled analysis of such studies, are needed.

13.10 Depression and Suicide

13.10.1 Depression

There have been few studies on depression and EMF (see Table 13.10). Depression is a common disorder, but its prevalence across the globe varies widely due to variable thresholds for recording, which ranges from major depressive episodes to major depressive disorders.[254] The early studies on the effects of EMF on depression did not use validated scales for identification of depressive symptoms,[199,255] hence limiting the inference.[256] A number of recent studies, however, have used validated depression scales. Although one of these studies demonstrated an association between proximity to power lines and depression,[257] another study of similar design[258,259] did not provide support for an association. A third study[206] was largely negative, but reported increased risk based on distance and calculated fields for severe depression, albeit based on very small numbers. Similarly, Savitz et al.[260] in the only occupational study, did not find an association in their study of U.S. veterans. In sum, the findings on depressive symptoms and EMF are largely inconsistent.

13.10.2 Suicide

Two early studies, based on the same population and relating residential EMF exposure and suicide, showed that cases came from homes in closer proximity to power lines and/or with significantly higher exposure levels than controls,[262,263] while another residential study did not report any risk.[89] Occupational studies used job titles and estimated fields,[145,200,201,264–268] with some identifying small and at times significant risks and at times

TABLE 13.10

Epidemiologic Studies on Depression and EMF

Reference	Study Population	Study Design	Exposure	High Category RR (95% CI)
Residential Studies				
Dowson et al.[255]	Living near 132 kV line and those living 3 miles away	Cross-sectional N = 226	Distance	Association between depression and distance
Perry et al.[199]	Hospital discharge with depression; controls from electoral list	Case-control N = 359	Front door Measurements	Average Cases = 0.23 μT Controls = 0.21 μT
Poole et al.[257]	Residents near Rights of Way CES-D[a] Scale	Cross-sectional N = 382	Distance	Near vs. Far 2.8 (1.6–5.1)
McMahon et al.[258]	Sample of homes near a PL and one block away. CES-D	Cross-sectional N = 152	Measurements at front door	Near vs. Far 0.9 (0.5–1.9)
Verkasalo et al.[259]	Finnish Twin Cohort Study with response to Beck Depression Inventory (BDI)	Cross-sectional N = 12,063	Distance Calculated fields	No difference in mean BDI by distance or high fields
Beale et al.[261]	Persons living near PL General Health Questionnaire GHQ including depression	Cross-sectional N = 540	Time-weighted average (TWA) based on measurements	Significant increase in somatic symp. anxiety, depression
Occupational Studies				
Savitz et al.[260]	Male United States veterans. The DX Interview Schedule & Minn. Personality Inventory	Cross-sectional N = 4,044	Present job and duration	Electrical worker 1.0 (0.5–1.7)

[a] Center for Epidemiologic Studies-Depression Scale.

significant deficit, particularly for selected occupations. See Table 13.11 for details on these studies. In sum, the data on suicide and EMF are inconsistent, but sparse.

13.11 Reproductive Outcomes

13.11.1 Maternal Exposure

13.11.1.1 Residential Exposure

Residential EMF exposures have also been studied for possible association with reproductive outcomes, including pregnancy loss (spontaneous abortion or miscarriage) and stillbirth (Table 13.12), neonatal outcomes, such as fetal growth (Table 13.13) and birth defects (Table 13.14).

Studies using wire codes or proximity to power lines as an EMF exposure proxy have suggested no association.[270–274] Studies that have used spot or front door measurements have shown mixed results. One study using spot measurements taken at the front door

TABLE 13.11

Epidemiologic Studies on Suicide and EMF

Reference	Study Population	Study Design	Exposure	High Category RR (95% CI)
Residential Studies				
Reichmanis et al.[263] and Perry et al.[262]	Suicide cases and controls in England	Case-control N = 589	Distance Home measurements	Higher estimated and measured fields at case homes
McDowall[89]	Persons resident in the vicinity of transmission facilities	SMR N = 8	Distance	0.75 (non-significant)
Occupational Studies				
Baris and Armstrong[264]	Mortality in utility workers 1970–1972 and 1979–1983. United Kingdom	Proportional mortality study N = 495	Job titles on death certificates	PMR 1970–1972: 89 (75–104) PMR 1979–1983: 102 (91–113)
Baris et al.[200,265]	Utility workers. mortality. Controls: 1% sample of cohort	Case-control 49/215	Job exposure matrix Electrical workers	OR ≥1.56 µT 1.4 (0.4–5.0)
Kelsh and Sahl[145]	Utility workers, employed between 1960 and 1991. United States	Cohort N = 40,335	Occupational categories	SMR 0.6 (0.5–0.7)
Johansen and Olsen[201]	Male utility employees 1974–1993; mortality registry	Cohort N = 21,236	Job exposure matrix ≥0.1 µT	SMR 1.4 (non-significant)
van Winjgaarden[266]	Male electric utility workers Mortality. United States	Nested CC 536/5,348	Jobs and JEM	≥3 µT-years 1.3 (0.9–2.0)
Jarvholm et al.[267]	Swedish electricians from 1971 to 1997; Mortality	Cohort N = 95	Occupational exposure	SMR 0.6 (0.5–0.7)
van Winjgaarden[269]	Workers death certificate files for the years 1991–1992. United States	Case-control 11,707/132,771	Usual occupation and industry	OR 1.3 (1.2–1.4)
Nichols and Sorahan[268]	UK Utility workers, employed between 1973 and 1982, Mortality	Cohort/ N = 72,889	First job Males	SMR 79 (69–92)

suggested an association between early pregnancy loss and front door fields of above 0.63 µT.[275] Although spot measurements have been shown to be correlated with personal exposure, there is potential for large exposure misclassification.[276] Another study found no association with spot bedroom measurement and pregnancy loss,[273] while two studies showed some risk but with very low exposures and/or unclear results.[277,278]

A prospective study found no association between TWA personal measures and spontaneous abortion.[271] There was, however, a significantly increased risk (OR = 1.8, 95%

TABLE 13.12

Epidemiological Studies on EMF Exposure and Miscarriage

Reference	Study Population	Study Design	Exposure	High Category RR (95% CI)
Residential Studies				
Juutilainen et al.[275]	Work and Fertility Study Early pregnancy loss	Case-control 89/102	Spot measurement	≥0.63 μT 5.1 (1.0–26)
Savitz and Ananth[273]	Cases: <15 years old (y.o.). Controls: random digit dialing (RDD). Denver, Colorado. Sibling analysis	Case-control WC—78/78 MF—42/73	Wire code Spot bedroom measurement	HCC 0.7 (0.3–1.8) ≥0.2 μT 0.8 (0.3–2.3)
Belanger et al.[274]	Women in obstetric practices health maintenance organizations	Prospective N = 2,967	Wire code	VHCC 0.4 (0.2–1.1)
Li et al.[271]	Pregnant women within northern California Kaiser Permanente medical care system	Prospective cohort N = 969	Personal TWA	≥0.3 μT 1.2 (0.7–2.2) ≥1.6 μT 1.8 (1.2–2.7)
Lee et al.[270]	Members of the northern California Kaiser Permanente medical care system'	Nested case–control 155/509 Cohort N = 3402 With measurement N = 219	Wire code Personal TWA Wire code Personal TWA	VHCC 1.2 (0.7–2.1) ≥0.128 μT 1.7 (0.9–3.2) VHCC 0 cases ≥0.2 μT 1.9 (0.6–6.1)
Auger et al.[279]	Still births, 1998–2007. Quebec City	Cohort N = 2033	Distance based on postal code	<25 m 1.4 (0.9–2.4)
Shamsi et al.[278]	Cases Miscarriage <14 weeks Controls pregnancies same hospital	Case-control 58/58	Measurements Method unclear	Not stated 1.9 (1.4–2.5)
Wang et al.[277]	Pregnant women living in two towns of China	Prospective N = 413	Front door measurement	≥0.1 μT 1.4 (0.6–3.1)
Sadeghi et al.[280]	Still births, 2013–2014. Babol, Iran	Unclear 20/8	Distance to power line	<600 0.8 (0.9–7.7)
Meta-Analysis of Video Display Terminal (VDT) Studies				
Parazzini et al.[281]	Mostly self reported VDT work in pregnant women	Meta-analysis of seven studies	Average hours/week	1.0 (0.9–1.0)

CI: 1.2–2.7) when maximum exposure above 1.6 μT was used as the exposure metric of interest. In the same year, a nested case-control study using personal exposure measurements[270] showed that TWA magnetic fields were not associated with miscarriage, but there were in fact statistically significant dose response trends for two different exposure metrics, maximum exposure, and magnetic field rate-of-change. In the theory, women with healthy pregnancies may be less active due to "morning sickness" and thus less likely to encounter magnetic field sources. This premise formed a hypothesis proposed that physical activity may be a potential confounder explaining both of these studies.[290]

TABLE 13.13

Epidemiological Studies on Residential EMF Exposure and Fetal Growth

Reference	Study Population	Study Design	Exposure	High Category RR (95% CI)	
				Low Birth Weight	Growth Retardation
Residential Studies					
Savitz and Ananth[273]	Cases: <15 years old (y.o.). Controls: random digit dialing. Denver, Colorado. Sibling analysis	Case-control WC—78/78 MF—42/73	Wire code Spot bedroom measurement	HCC 0.7 (0.2–2.3) ≥0.2 µT 0.3 (0.0–2.4)	
Bracken et al.[282]	Women in obstetric practices health maintenance organizations	Prospective Cohort N = 2,967	Wire code Personal TWA 7 day	VHCC 0.8 (0.3–2.1) ≥0.2 µT 1.4 (0.3–6.1)	VHCC 0.8 (0.4–1.6) ≥0.2 µT 1.2 (0.4–3.1)
Auger et al.[272]	Live singleton births from Montreal and Quebec City	Cohort N = 705,020	Distance based on postal code	<50 m 1.0 (0.9–1.0)	<50 m 1.1 (1.0–1.1)
de Vocht et al.[283]	Mothers of children born Perinatal Survey Unit, United Kingdom	Cohort N = 140,356	Distance incl. underground	≤50 m 1.4 (0.6–3.1)	≤50 m 1.3 (0.6–2.8)
Mahram et al.[284]	Women residing near and far from lines Qazvin, Iran	Cohort 222 + 158	Map of area measurements	No difference in BW p = 0.54	
Eskelinen et al.[285]	Children born at Kuopio University Hospital Finland	Prospective N = 373	Home spot measurement		≥0.3 µT 1.1 (0.2–5.1)
Meta-Analysis of VDT Studies					
Parazzini 1.0 (0.9–1.2) et al.[281]	Self-reported VDT work in pregnant women	Meta of two studies	Average hours/ week	1.0 (0.9–1.2)	

Studies of low birth weight or intrauterine growth retardation and wire codes and distance are all negative[272,273,282] (Table 13.13), except for a UK record-based study[283] which is suggestive of reduced birth weight for mothers residing within 50 m of lines. One study[291] used personal measurements of women post-planned abortion and found that bud length, an indicator of embryonic development (but not sac length and apoptosis levels), was inversely associated with magnetic field exposure ≥0.082 µT (OR = 3.95, 95% CI: 1.1–14.2) (data not shown). In a large prospective study using personal measurements, there was no association between exposure to time-weighted fields above 0.2 µT and low birth weight or

TABLE 13.14

Epidemiological Studies on EMF Exposure and Congenital Malformations

Residential Studies				
Robert et al.[286]	Cases from population-based registry. Birth certificate controls. France	Case-control 151/302	Distance to power line	≤50 m 1.3 (0.5–3.2)
Malagoli et al.[287]	Women residing in Reggio Emilia, northern Italy	Case-control 288/288	Modeled exposure	≥0.4 µT 0.7 (0.1–8.1)
Blaasas et al.[288,289]	Medical birth registry matched for sex, year, and municipality. Norway	Case-control 465/930	Calculated fields	≥0.1 µT 0.9 (0.8–1.0)
Mahram et al.[284]	Women residing near and far from lines. Qazvin, Iran	Cohort N = 222 and 158	Map of area measurements	6/3 p = 0.637
Sadeghi et al.[280]	Live births, 2013–2014. Babol, Iran	Unclear 20/8	Distance to power line	<600 m 5.0 (1.5–16.8)
Meta-Analysis of Video Display Terminal (VDT) Studies				
Parazzini et al.[281]	Self-reported VDT work in pregnant women	Meta-analysis of five studies	VDT average hours/week	1.0 (0.9–1.2)

intrauterine growth retardation.[282] Similarly, other measurement studies did not support an association.[284,285]

Finally, overall birth defects were not associated with distance or calculated fields,[286] except for one study, with unclear and problematic methodology and crude distance categorization (<600 m) which included mainly subjects with low exposure,[280] as fields approach background within 100–200 m depending on the size and design of the line. Sporadic findings for specific birth defects have been identified in some studies, but there is no specificity for any of the findings.

13.11.1.2 Electric Blankets and Heated Beds

Electric blankets and heated beds can be a major source of ELF EMF; it is estimated that exposure from waterbeds can be up to 0.5 µT and electric blankets produce fields up to 2.2 µT.[282,292,293]

The findings of the studies on electric blankets or heated beds and reproductive health effects have been mostly negative[294–296] (data not shown). Furthermore, a related outcome, urinary tract anomalies, has also been shown to be unrelated to EMF exposure from such electric devices, except, perhaps in women with a history of subfertility.[297] These studies were retrospective and assessment of exposure was usually based on self-reported data on the use of heated beds. Several prospective studies of miscarriages and growth that followed,[274,282,298] identified some risks for some high-exposure groups, but with different results for blankets and waterbeds. This difference might be explained by higher magnetic field exposures, or higher thermal stress from electric blankets. Note that most of the blankets have since been redesigned to produce low magnetic fields.

13.11.1.3 Occupational Exposure Including Video Display Terminals

Video display terminals (VDTs) emit both ELF EMF as well as higher frequencies of up to 100 kHz. The average exposure to a VDT user was typically low (around 0.1 µT) and VDTs are no longer widely used. The health risks associated with use of such devices, particularly adverse birth outcomes during pregnancy have been examined in several studies.[275,299–301] For the most part, studies have not shown increased risks for spontaneous abortion, low birth weight, pre-term delivery, intrauterine growth retardation, or congenital abnormalities. As a result, a meta-analysis of VDT studies[281] did not report risk with any of the outcomes. One population-based study in Norway assigned parental occupational exposure to ELF-MF, based on jobs captured in a census and linked to a JEM, and found no association with overall birth defects, but risk for selected disorders of the CNS.[302]

13.11.2 Paternal Exposure

13.11.2.1 Sperm Quality and Infertility

The earliest study described by Buiatti et al.[303] found persons with infertility were more likely to report radioelectric work than controls. Similarly, fertility difficulties were observed among the offspring of high-voltage switchyard workers.[304] However, Gracia et al.[305] reported no association between infertility and exposure to electromagnetic fields, and Lunsberg et al.[306] observed no association between job titles with high EMF exposure and semen abnormalities. Based on a Chinese case-control study of men recruited in a sperm bank, Li et al.[307] report an increased risk of poor semen quality (adjusted OR = 2.0, 95% CI: 1–4) for exposures ≥0.16 µT. Suggestions of an association between EMF exposure and decreased male to female ratio in the offspring have also been made.[308,309]

13.11.2.2 Pregnancy Outcomes

Paternal magnetic field exposure has also been studied in relation to adverse reproductive outcomes. There was no raised risk of abnormal birth outcome among offspring of power-industry workers.[310] An excess of birth defects was observed among children of fathers who were electronic equipment operators[311] and among the offspring of high-voltage switchyard workers,[304] but the data are sparse and methodologically weak.

13.11.3 Summary of Reproductive Outcomes

There is some evidence for increased miscarriage risk associated with high residential EMF exposure; however, methodologic problems make interpretation of these studies difficult.[312] In particular, they are difficulties in studying EMF exposure levels similar to background levels, capturing early miscarriages, and reporting accurate information free from recall bias. There is little evidence of increased risks of adverse reproductive outcomes other than miscarriage, albeit good data are lacking.[5] The results of the studies on paternal ELF-EMF exposure and adverse reproductive outcomes are unconvincing.

13.12 Childhood Asthma

Asthma is the most common non-communicable disease among children and often poses a significant health burden.[313] Like other chronic inflammatory diseases, asthma and allergic diseases result from interactions between genetic background, the immune system, and environmental factors. The exposure to various environmental factors depends on lifestyles, which have changed greatly during the last few decades, and may affect the immune system through changes in the microbiome and epigenetic factors.[314,315]

Beale et al. conducted a cross-sectional study to examine the relationship between the ELF-MF exposure of adults in their homes and prevalence of immune-related and other chronic illnesses.[316] In this small study, based on self-reporting, significantly elevated ORs were observed at higher exposure levels for asthma. Employing a better design, using a Northern California cohort from a previously referenced study of miscarriages, but using different exposure cutpoints, Li et al. reported an increased risk of asthma in children whose mothers were exposed to higher levels of measured MF during pregnancy,[317] hazard ratio (HR) = 1.7 (95% CI: 0.9–3.3) for medium exposure (≥0.03–0.2 µT) and 3.5 (95% CI: 1.7–7.4) for the highest exposure (above 0.2 µT) for "definitive" asthma diagnosis. A stronger association was observed in a subset of children whose mothers had a history of asthma, but a weaker association was seen among the suspected asthma cases. In a Danish National Birth Cohort study based on 92,675 singleton births and calculated fields, Sudan et al.[318] did not find evidence that residential exposure to MF during pregnancy or early childhood increased the risk of childhood asthma: for definitive cases at any non-zero exposure, the HR was 0.7 (95% CI: 0.3–1.9) and for those exposed to ≥0.2 µT, the HR was 0.4 (95% CI: 0.1–2.9).

On the balance, it seems unlikely that residential magnetic fields are related to asthma.

13.13 Discussion

13.13.1 Challenges

Consistent epidemiologic evidence carries a good deal of weight when considering the potential health effects of EMF. Consistency in results may reveal key clues, since epidemiologic studies of EMF are difficult to design, conduct, and interpret for a number of methodologic reasons. In addition to the usual methodologic complexities of designing and carrying out almost any high-quality epidemiologic investigation, studying effects of EMF exposure poses unique and substantial difficulties. The challenges that arise relate to three main attributes of epidemiologic studies: assessment of exposure, outcome (disease), and interpretation of findings.

13.13.2 Exposure

An expected major weakness of epidemiologic studies is EMF exposure assessment. Several factors make assessment of EMF exposure more difficult than assessment of many other environmental exposures. Magnetic fields are variable in time and space and our understanding of the contributions of the multitude of different sources to total exposure is limited. EMF exposure is ubiquitous, but neither detectable nor memorable in most circumstances. The difficulties in exposure assessment are further exacerbated by the retrospective nature of most EMF epidemiologic research, as many of diseases are rare and have long latency periods. To quantify past unnoticed and unmeasured exposure, epidemiologists rely on surrogate measurements or indicators of exposure. The surrogates used to study EMF have included wire codes, occupational job titles, surveys regarding appliance use and present day measurements. Further, some studies must rely on information provided by proxy respondents, especially for cancer and Alzheimer's diseases, if the study subject has died or has been incapacitated.

Although occupational exposures are generally much higher than exposures encountered elsewhere, they are usually fleeting. The "highly exposed" worker generally encounters high fields not for hours, but for seconds or minutes at a time while working. When we consider EMF exposure integrated over a 24 h time period, the brevity of high exposures in most work places (often minutes to hours) and in non-occupational environments combine to obscure the distinctions between the supposedly "highly exposed" occupational groups and the general population. Thus, the relative separation between high- and low-exposure groups may be insufficient to detect an effect of EMF exposure if we rely on time-weighted averages.

Because EMF exposures are complex, numerous parameters have been used to characterize them including transients, harmonic content, resonance conditions, peak values, as well as various average levels. It is unknown which of these parameters or what combinations of parameters, if any, are biologically relevant. If there were a known biological mechanism of interaction for carcinogenesis, critical parameters of exposure, including the relevant period or timing of exposure, it might be possible to identify and measure these parameters in the studies. Because EMF is commonplace with almost no single person unexposed, epidemiologists are faced with the challenge of assessing exposure and separating the more exposed from the less exposed rather than from unexposed. There is also a considerable degree of variability in both short- and long-term exposures which are influenced by the variability in exposure over space and can differ between occupational versus household exposure.

All of these difficulties with EMF exposure assessment are likely to lead to substantial exposure misclassification which is likely, in turn, to interfere with detection of an association between exposure and disease (if indeed such an association exists). In particular, if the true association is small or moderate in magnitude, it may be difficult to detect with this amount of measurement error.

13.13.3 Outcome

Leukemias and malignant brain tumors have received the most attention in both residential and occupational EMF studies. While they are the most common childhood malignancies, in absolute terms they still are quite rare, and even relatively rarer in adults. Thus, a major challenge in EMF epidemiology is the small number of cases available in any given study and the necessity for retrospective study designs, as well as pooled or meta-analysis. Furthermore, the etiologies of these diseases are poorly understood making a search for confounding as an explanation for any observed association difficult.

EMF does not appear to be genotoxic, but biological evidence suggests that it might influence cellular function and proliferation. Therefore, it could act as a promoter, growth enhancer, or co-carcinogen. Epidemiologic studies that attempt to consider such secondary events are rare and methodologic developments in this area are needed.

13.13.4 Interpretation

Five circumstances make interpretation of the role of EMF in the development of disease challenging: (1) large exposure misclassification, (2) difficulties in the appraisal of small risks, (3) inconsistencies among and within studies, (4) lack of knowledge of other risk factors for some diseases that may be potential confounding variables, and (5) lack of biological mechanism that can be operating at low levels of exposure.

Small risks are notoriously hard to evaluate, both because of the lack of precision to distinguish a small risk from no risk, and because small risks are more vulnerable to subtle confounding and biases that can go undetected. Study quality remains an important consideration in evaluating epidemiologic evidence of EMF. The quality of some studies has improved in a number of important ways. However, earlier studies, many of which were fraught with methodologic difficulties, still represent a substantial proportion of available evidence. Unfortunately, a number of methodologically problematic studies have been also published in recent years. Any attempt to summarize the available evidence, whether narrative or meta-analytic in its approach, must explicitly consider study date and study design elements to arrive at a summary risk estimate that is not unduly influenced by less well-done studies. Given the difficulties with EMF exposure assessment and the other methodological difficulties outlined above, many results of EMF studies are unsurprisingly inconsistent. Nevertheless, an assessment of the internal and external consistency of studies is paramount to our understanding of the underlying risks.

Another impediment to a clear interpretation of these epidemiologic studies is the absence of a dose-response (exposure-response) relationship. Distortion of the underlying dose-response relationship by substantial exposure misclassification,[319] or by a nonmonotonic relationship between exposure and disease, has been offered as potential explanation. However, both possibilities remain speculative. A well-characterized and reproducible relationship between the most relevant aspect of exposure and disease is needed for the association to be scientifically acceptable.

13.13.5 Advances

Despite many difficulties and challenges of epidemiologic studies of EMF, much progress has been made; for many of the more common diseases once thought influenced by EMF exposure the issue is now considered resolved. For example, investigations of cardiovascular disease were driven by a biologically based hypothesis initially confirmed by an epidemiologic study. Due to high rates of disease under study and relatively common exposure, it had a potential to be of great public-health importance. Epidemiologic studies with rigorous and varied designs that followed showed no effect. Thus, this line of research represents an interesting case study of a scientific inquiry which, despite numerous methodologic difficulties inherent in research on health effects of low-level environmental exposures, has been successfully resolved through continued generation of informative if not definitive studies.

13.14 Conclusions

Overall, with close to four decades of epidemiologic investigation on the relation of EMF and the risk of various diseases, we have learned a great deal and have been reassured that EMF is not involved in many diseases. However, there remain a number of uncertainties.

The strength of epidemiologic evidence varies for the different diseases that have been investigated.

Among all the outcomes evaluated in EMF epidemiological studies, the strongest evidence of an association in relation to residential exposures above 0.3–0.4 μT is for childhood leukemia. Further study is certainly warranted, but only if investigations are of high methodological quality, of sufficient size and with sufficient numbers of highly exposed subjects, and must include appropriate exposure groups and validated exposure assessment.

Particularly for childhood leukemia, few insights can be gained from further repetition of investigation of risks at moderate and low exposure levels, unless such studies can be designed to test specific hypotheses, such as selection bias or aspects of exposure not previously captured.

For brain tumors in children, for both leukemia and brain tumors in adults, for other cancers, and for various other endpoints such as suicide and depression, the epidemiologic literature taken as a whole, while not definitive, does not present any clear evidence of an association. Further work on neurodegenerative diseases, particularly ALS, is warranted as current evidence indicates a potential association. New neurodegenerative disease studies should improve upon the current evidence, which have numerous methodological limitations.

Investigations of certain other major diseases, such as breast cancer and cardiovascular disease, although initially biologically driven, did not confirm biological hypotheses or early positive studies. There is good evidence that these diseases are not associated with EMF exposure. *De novo* studies or meta-analysis of birth weight and miscarriages, as well as of the potential role of parental EMF exposure in childhood cancer could be informative.

References

1. IARC. *Non-Ionizing Radiation, Part 1: Static and Extremely Low-Frequency (ELF) Electric and Magnetic Fields.* (International Agency for Research on Cancer, 2002).
2. National Institute of Environmental Health Sciences (NIEHS). *NIEHS Report on Health Effects from Exposure to Power-Line Frequency Electric and Magnetic Fields.* (National Institute of Environmental Health Sciences, National Institutes of Health, 1999).
3. National Radiological Protection Board (NRPB). Health effects from radiofrequency electromagnetic fields. Report No. 14. (National Radiological Protection Board, 2003).
4. National Research Council (NRC). *Possible Health Effects of Exposure to Residential Electric and Magnetic Field.* (National Research Council, National Academy Press, 1997).
5. *Environmental Health Criteria Document on Extremely Low Frequency Fields.* (World Health Organization, Geneva, 2007).
6. Bracken, T., Kheifets, L. & Sussman, S. Exposure assessment for power frequency electric and magnetic fields (EMF) and its application to epidemiologic studies. *J Expo Anal Environ Epidemiol* 3, 1–22 (1993).
7. Wertheimer, N. & Leeper, E. Electrical wiring configurations and childhood cancer. *Am J Epidemiol* 109, 273–284 (1979).
8. Wertheimer, N. & Leeper, E. Adult cancer related to electrical wires near the home. *Int J Epidemiol* 11, 345–355 (1982).
9. Savitz, D., Wachtel, H., Barnes, F., John, E. & Tvrdik, J. Case-control study of childhood cancer and exposure to 60-Hz magnetic fields. *Am J Epidemiol* 128, 21–38 (1988).
10. Friedman, D.R et al., Childhood exposure to magnetic fields: Residential area measurements compared to personal dosimetry. Epidemiology 7(2), 151–155 (1996).
11. Fulton, J., Cobb, S., Preble, L., Leone, L. & Forman, E. Electrical wiring configurations and childhood leukemia in Rhode Island. *Am J Epidemiol* 111, 292–296 (1980).
12. Tomenius, L. 50-Hz electromagnetic environment and the incidence of childhood tumors in Stockholm County. *Bioelectromagnetics* 7, 191–207 (1986).
13. Myers, A., Clayden, A., Cartwright, R. & Cartwright, S. Childhood cancer and overhead powerlines: a case-control study. *Br J Cancer* 62, 1008–1014 (1990).

14. London, S. et al., Exposure to residential electric and magnetic fields and risk of childhood leukemia. *Am J Epidemiol* **134**, 923–937 (1991).

15. Feychting, M. & Ahlbom, A. Magnetic fields and cancer in children residing near Swedish high-voltage power lines. *Am J Epidemiol* **138**, 467–481 (1993).

16. Verkasalo, P. et al., Risk of cancer in Finnish children living close to power lines. *BMJ* **307**, 895–899 (1993).

17. Coghill, R.W., Steward, J. & Philips, A. Extra low frequency electric and magnetic fields in the bedplace of children diagnosed with leukaemia: a case-control study. *Eur J Cancer Prev* **5**, 153–158 (1996).

18. Tynes, T. & Haldorsen, T. Electromagnetic fields and cancer in children residing near Norwegian high-voltage power lines. *Am J Epidemiol* **145**, 219–226 (1997).

19. Fajardo-Gutierrez, A. et al., [Residence close to high-tension electric power lines and its association with leukemia in children]. *Bol Med Hosp Infant Mex* **50**, 32–38 (1993).

20. Petridou, E. et al., Electrical power lines and childhood leukemia: a study from Greece. *Int J Cancer* **73**, 345–348 (1997).

21. Linet, M. et al., Residential exposure to magnetic fields and acute lymphoblastic leukemia in children. *N Eng J Med* **337**, 1–7 (1997).

22. Michaelis, J. et al., Childhood leukemia and electromagnetic fields: results of a population-based case-control study in Germany. *Cancer Causes Control* **8**, 167–174 (1997).

23. Dockerty, J., Elwood, J., Skegg, D. & Herbison, G. Electromagnetic field exposures and childhood cancers in New Zealand. *Cancer Causes Control* **9**, 299–309 (1998).

24. Lin, R.S. & Lee, W.C. Risk of childhood leukemia in areas passed by high power lines. *Rev Environ Health* **10**, 97–103 (1994).

25. Li, C.Y., Lee, W.C. & Lin, R.S. Risk of leukemia in children living near high-voltage transmission lines. *J Occup Environ Med* **40**, 144–147 (1998).

26. McBride, M. et al., Power-frequency electric and magnetic fields and risk of childhood leukemia in Canada. *Am J Epidemiol* **149**, 831–842 (1999).

27. Green, L. et al., A case-control study of childhood leukemia in Southern Ontario, Canada, and exposure to magnetic fields in residences. *Int J Cancer* **82**, 161–170 (1999).

28. Green, L.M. et al., Childhood leukemia and personal monitoring of residential exposures to electric and magnetic fields in Ontario, Canada. *Cancer Causes Control* **10**, 233–243 (1999).

29. UK Childhood Cancer Study Investigators. The United Kingdom Childhood Cancer Study: objectives, materials and methods. *Br J Cancer* **85**(5), 1073–1102 (2000).

30. UK Childhood Cancer Study Investigators. Childhood cancer and residential proximity to power lines. *Br J Cancer* **83**, 1573–1580, doi:10.1054/bjoc.2000.1550 (2000).

31. Bianchi, N. et al., Overhead electricity power lines and childhood leukemia: a registry-based, case-control study. *Tumori* **86**, 195–198 (2000).

32. Schuz, J. et al., Extremely low frequency magnetic fields in residences in Germany. Distribution of measurements, comparison of two methods for assessing exposure, and predictors for the occurrence of magnetic fields above background level. *Radiat Environ Biophys* **39**, 233–240 (2000).

33. Mizoue, T. et al., Residential proximity to high-voltage power lines and risk of childhood hematological malignancies. *J Epidemiol* **14**, 118–123 (2004).

34. Perez C.B., Pineiro R.G. & N.T., D. Campos electromagneticos de baja frecuencia y leucemia infantil en Ciudad de La Habana. *Cubana Hig Epidemiol* **43**, 1–10 (2005).

35. Kabuto, M. et al., Childhood leukemia and magnetic fields in Japan: a case-control study of childhood leukemia and residential power-frequency magnetic fields in Japan. *Int J Cancer* **119**, 643–650, doi:10.1002/ijc.21374 (2006).

36. Mejia-Arangure, J.M. et al., Magnetic fields and acute leukemia in children with Down syndrome. *Epidemiology* **18**, 158–161, doi:10.1097/01.ede.0000248186.31452.be (2007).

37. Feizi, A.A. & Arabi, M.A. Acute childhood leukemias and exposure to magnetic fields generated by high voltage overhead power lines - a risk factor in Iran. *Asian Pac J Cancer Prev* **8**, 69–72 (2007).

38. Yang, Y. et al., Case-only study of interactions between DNA repair genes (hMLH1, APEX1, MGMT, XRCC1 and XPD) and low-frequency electromagnetic fields in childhood acute leukemia. *Leuk Lymphoma* **49**, 2344–2350, doi:10.1080/10428190802441347 (2008).

39. Malagoli, C. et al., Risk of hematological malignancies associated with magnetic fields exposure from power lines: a case-control study in two municipalities of northern Italy. *Environ Health* **9**, 16, doi:10.1186/1476-069X-9-16 (2010).

40. Sohrabi, M.R., Tarjoman, T., Abadi, A. & Yavari, P. Living near overhead high voltage transmission power lines as a risk factor for childhood acute lymphoblastic leukemia: a case-control study. *Asian Pac J Cancer Prev* **11**, 423–427 (2010).

41. Does, M. et al., Exposure to electrical contact currents and the risk of childhood leukemia. *Radiat Res* **175**, 390–396, doi:10.1667/RR2357.1 (2011).

42. Wunsch-Filho, V. et al., Exposure to magnetic fields and childhood acute lymphocytic leukemia in Sao Paulo, Brazil. *Cancer Epidemiol* **35**, 534–539, doi:10.1016/j.canep.2011.05.008 (2011).

43. Jirik, V., Pekarek, L., Janout, V. & Tomaskova, H. Association between childhood leukaemia and exposure to power-frequency magnetic fields in Middle Europe. *Biomed Environ Sci* **25**, 597–601, doi:10.3967/0895-3988.2012.05.015 (2012).

44. Sermage-Faure, C. et al., Childhood leukaemia close to high-voltage power lines–the Geocap study, 2002–2007. *Br J Cancer* **108**, 1899–1906, doi:10.1038/bjc.2013.128 (2013).

45. Abdul Rahman, H.I., Shah, S.A., Alias, H. & Ibrahim, H.M. A case-control study on the association between environmental factors and the occurrence of acute leukemia among children in Klang Valley, Malaysia. *Asian Pac J Cancer Prev* **9**, 649–652 (2008).

46. Ba Hakim, A.S., Abd Rahman, N.B., Mokhtar, M.Z., Said, I.B. & Hussain, H. in *IEEE Conference on Biomedical Engineering and Sciences (IECBES), 2014*, 710–714 (IEEE, 2014).

47. Pedersen, C. et al., Distance from residence to power line and risk of childhood leukemia: a population-based case-control study in Denmark. *Cancer Causes Control* **25**, 171–177, doi:10.1007/s10552-013-0319-5 (2014).

48. Pedersen, C., Johansen, C., Schuz, J., Olsen, J.H. & Raaschou-Nielsen, O. Residential exposure to extremely low-frequency magnetic fields and risk of childhood leukaemia, CNS tumour and lymphoma in Denmark. *Br J Cancer* **113**, 1370–1374, doi:10.1038/bjc.2015.365 (2015).

49. Bunch, K.J., Keegan, T.J., Swanson, J., Vincent, T.J. & Murphy, M.F. Residential distance at birth from overhead high-voltage powerlines: childhood cancer risk in Britain 1962–2008. *Br J Cancer* **110**, 1402–1408, doi:10.1038/bjc.2014.15 (2014).

50. Bunch, K.J., Swanson, J., Vincent, T.J. & Murphy, M.F. Epidemiological study of power lines and childhood cancer in the UK: further analyses. *J Radiol Prot* **36**, 437–455, doi:10.1088/0952-4746/36/3/437 (2016).

51. Salvan, A., Ranucci, A., Lagorio, S. & Magnani, C. Childhood leukemia and 50 Hz magnetic fields: findings from the Italian SETIL case-control study. *Int J Environ Res Public Health* **12**, 2184–2204, doi:10.3390/ijerph120202184 (2015).

52. Crespi, C.M. et al., Childhood leukaemia and distance from power lines in California: a population-based case-control study. *Br J Cancer* **115**, 122–128, doi:10.1038/bjc.2016.142 (2016).

53. Kheifets, L., Swanson, J., Yuan, Y., Kusters, C. & Vergara, X. Comparative analyses of studies of childhood leukemia and magnetic fields, radon and gamma radiation. *J Radiol Prot* **37**, 459–491, doi:10.1088/1361-6498/aa5fc7 (2017).

54. Greenland, S., Sheppard, A.R., Kaune, W.T., Poole, C. & Kelsh, M.A. A pooled analysis of magnetic fields, wire codes, and childhood leukemia. Childhood Leukemia-EMF Study Group. *Epidemiology* **11**, 624–634 (2000).

55. Ahlbom, A. et al., A pooled analysis of magnetic fields and childhood leukaemia. *Br J Cancer* **83**, 692–698 (2000).

56. Kheifets, L. et al., Pooled analysis of recent studies on magnetic fields and childhood leukaemia. *Br J Cancer* **103**, 1128–1135, doi:10.1038/sj.bjc.6605838 (2010).

57. Olsen, J., Nielsen, A. & Schulgen, G. Residence near high voltage facilities and risk of cancer in children. *BMJ* **307**, 891–895 (1993).

58. Ebi, K.L., Kheifets, L.I., Pearson, R.L. & Wachtel, H. Description of a new computer wire coding method and its application to evaluate potential control selection bias in the Savitz et al., childhood cancer study. *Bioelectromagnetics* **21**, 346–353 (2000).

59. Kheifets, L.I., Kavet, R. & Sussman, S.S. Wire codes, magnetic fields, and childhood cancer. *Bioelectromagnetics* **18**, 99–110 (1997).

60. Greenland, S., Fischer, H.J. & Kheifets, L. Methods to explore uncertainty and bias introduced by job exposure matrices. *Risk Anal* **36**, 74–82, doi:10.1111/risa.12438 (2016).

61. Kelsh, M.A., Kheifets, L. & Smith, R. The impact of work environment, utility, and sampling design on occupational magnetic field exposure summaries. *Aihaj* **61**, 174–182 (2000).

62. Bowman, J.D., Touchstone, J.A. & Yost, M.G. A population-based job exposure matrix for power-frequency magnetic fields. *J Occup Environ Hyg* **4**, 715–728, doi:10.1080/15459620701528001 (2007).

63. Renew, D.C., Cook, R.F. & Ball, M.C. A method for assessing occupational exposure to power-frequency magnetic fields for electricity generation and transmission workers. *J Radiol Prot* **23**, 279–303 (2003).

64. Coble, J.B. et al., Occupational exposure to magnetic fields and the risk of brain tumors. *Neuro Oncol* **11**, 242–249, doi:10.1215/15228517-2009-002 (2009).

65. Fischer, H.J. et al., Developing a job-exposure matrix with exposure uncertainty from expert elicitation and data modeling. *J Expo Sci Environ Epidemiol* **27**, 7–15, doi:10.1038/jes.2015.37 (2017).

66. Mezei, G. & Kheifets, L. Selection bias and its implications for case-control studies: a case study of magnetic field exposure and childhood leukaemia. *Int J Epidemiol* **35**, 397–406, doi:10.1093/ije/dyi245 (2006).

67. Draper, G., Vincent, T., Kroll, M.E. & Swanson, J. Childhood cancer in relation to distance from high voltage power lines in England and Wales: a case-control study. *BMJ* **330**, 1290, doi:10.1136/bmj.330.7503.1290 (2005).

68. Forssen, U.M., Ahlbom, A. & Feychting, M. Relative contribution of residential and occupational magnetic field exposure over twenty-four hours among people living close to and far from a power line. *Bioelectromagnetics* **23**, 239–244 (2002).

69. Greenland, S. & Kheifets, L. Leukemia attributable to residential magnetic fields: results from analyses allowing for study biases. *Risk Anal* **26**, 471–482, doi:10.1111/j.1539-6924.2006.00754.x (2006).

70. IARC. Globocan 2000: Cancer Incidence, Mortality and Prevalence Worldwide, www-dep.iarc.fr/globocan/globocan.html (2000).

71. Steliarova-Foucher, E. et al., Geographical patterns and time trends of cancer incidence and survival among children and adolescents in Europe since the 1970s (the ACCISproject): an epidemiological study. *Lancet* **364**, 2097–2105 (2004).

72. Mezei, G. & Kheifets, L. Clues to the possible viral etiology of childhood leukemia. *Technology* **9**, 3–14 (2002).

73. Poole, C. Greenland, S. Luetters, C. & Mezei, G. Childhood leukemia and socioeconomic status: A systematic review. (Submitted for publication).

74. Kheifets, L. & Shimkhada, R. Childhood leukemia and EMF: review of the epidemiologic evidence. *Bioelectromagnetics* (forthcoming).

75. Dockerty, J., Elwood, J., Skegg, D. & Herbison, G. Electromagnetic field exposures and childhood leukemia in New Zealand. *Lancet* **354**, 1967–1968 (1999).

76. Kabuto, M. et al., A Japanese case-control study of childhood leukaemia and residential power-frequency magnetic fields. Unpublished (2002).

77. Schuz, J., Grigat, J., Brinkmann, K. & Michaelis, J. Residential magnetic fields as a risk factor for childhood acute leukaemia: results from a German population-based case-control study. *Int J Cancer* **91**, 728–735 (2001).

78. Hatch, E. et al., Association between childhood acute lymphoblastic leukemia and use of electrical appliances during pregnancy and childhood. *Epidemiology* **9**, 234–245 (1998).

79. Savitz, D.A. & Chen, J.H. Parental occupation and childhood cancer: review of epidemiologic studies. *Environ Health Perspect* **88**, 325–337 (1990).

80. Kheifets, L., Renew, D., Sias, G. & Swanson, J. Extremely low frequency electric fields and cancer: assessing the evidence. *Bioelectromagnetics* **31**, 89–101, doi:10.1002/bem.20527 (2010).

81. Su, L. et al., Associations of parental occupational exposure to extremely low-frequency magnetic fields with childhood leukemia risk. *Leuk Lymphoma* **57**, 2855–2862, doi:10.3109/10428194.2016.1165812 (2016).

82. Foliart, D.E. et al., Magnetic field exposure and long-term survival among children with leukaemia. *Br J Cancer* **94**, 161–164, doi:10.1038/sj.bjc.6602916 (2006).

83. Svendsen, A.L., Weihkopf, T., Kaatsch, P. & Schuz, J. Exposure to magnetic fields and survival after diagnosis of childhood leukemia: a German cohort study. *Cancer Epidemiol Biomarkers Prev* **16**, 1167–1171, doi:10.1158/1055-9965.EPI-06-0887 (2007).

84. Schuz, J. et al., Extremely low-frequency magnetic fields and survival from childhood acute lymphoblastic leukemia: an international follow-up study. *Blood Cancer J* **2**, e98, doi:10.1038/bcj.2012.43 (2012).

85. Schuz, J. et al., Nighttime exposure to electromagnetic fields and childhood leukemia: an extended pooled analysis. *Am J Epidemiol* **166**, 263–269, doi:10.1093/aje/kwm080 (2007).

86. Kheifets, L., Afifi, A.A. & Shimkhada, R. Public health impact of extremely low-frequency electromagnetic fields. *Environ Health Perspect* **114**, 1532–1537 (2006).

87. Kheifets, L., Afifi, A., Monroe, J. & Swanson, J. Exploring exposure–response for magnetic fields and childhood leukemia. *J Expo Sci Environ Epidemiol* **21**, 625–633, doi:10.1038/jes.2010.38 (2011).

88. Coleman, M.P., Bell, C.M., Taylor, H.L. & Primic-Zakelj, M. Leukaemia and residence near electricity transmission equipment: a case-control study. *Br J Cancer* **60**, 793–798 (1989).

89. McDowall, M.E. Mortality of persons resident in the vicinity of electricity transmission facilities. *Br J Cancer* **53**, 271–279 (1986).

90. Schreiber, G.H., Swaen, G.M., Meijers, J.M., Slangen, J.J. & Sturmans, F. Cancer mortality and residence near electricity transmission equipment: a retrospective cohort study. *Int J Epidemiol* **22**, 9–15 (1993).

91. Youngson, J.H., Clayden, A.D., Myers, A. & Cartwright, R.A. A case/control study of adult haematological malignancies in relation to overhead powerlines. *Br J Cancer* **63**, 977–985 (1991).

92. Feychting, M. & Ahlbom, A. Magnetic fields, leukemia, and central nervous system tumors in Swedish adults residing near high-voltage power lines. *Epidemiology* **5**, 501–509 (1994).

93. Severson, R.K. et al., Acute nonlymphocytic leukemia and residential exposure to power frequency magnetic fields. *Am J Epidemiol* **128**, 10–20 (1988).

94. Verkasalo, P.K. Magnetic fields and leukemia--risk for adults living close to power lines. *Scand J Work Environ Health* **22 Suppl 2**, 1–56 (1996).

95. Li, C.Y., Theriault, G. & Lin, R.S. Residential exposure to 60-Hertz magnetic fields and adult cancers in Taiwan. *Epidemiology* **8**, 25–30 (1997).

96. Lowenthal, R.M., Tuck, D.M. & Bray, I.C. Residential exposure to electric power transmission lines and risk of lymphoproliferative and myeloproliferative disorders: a case-control study. *Intern Med J* **37**, 614–619, doi:10.1111/j.1445-5994.2007.01389.x (2007).

97. Marcilio, I., Gouveia, N., Pereira Filho, M.L. & Kheifets, L. Adult mortality from leukemia, brain cancer, amyotrophic lateral sclerosis and magnetic fields from power lines: a case-control study in Brazil. *Rev Bras Epidemiol* **14**, 580–588 (2011).

98. Elliott, P. et al., Adult cancers near high-voltage overhead power lines. *Epidemiology* **24**, 184–190, doi:10.1097/EDE.0b013e31827e95b9 (2013).

99. Fazzo, L. et al., Morbidity experience in populations residentially exposed to 50 Hz magnetic fields: methodology and preliminary findings of a cohort study. *Int J Occup Environ Health* **15**, 133–142, doi:10.1179/oeh.2009.15.2.133 (2009).

100. Feychting, M., Forssen, U. & Floderus, B. Occupational and residential magnetic field exposure and leukemia and central nervous system tumors. *Epidemiology* **8**, 384–389 (1997).

101. Kheifets, L.I. et al., Comparative analyses of the studies of magnetic fields and cancer in electric utility workers: studies from France, Canada, and the United States. *Occup Environ Med* **56**, 567–574 (1999).

102. Kheifets, L., Monroe, J., Vergara, X., Mezei, G. & Afifi, A.A. Occupational electromagnetic fields and leukemia and brain cancer: an update to two meta-analyses. *J Occup Environ Med* **50**, 677–688, doi:10.1097/JOM.0b013e3181757a27 (2008).

103. Preston-Martin, S., Peters, J.M., Yu, M.C., Garabrant, D.H. & Bowman, J.D. Myelogenous leukemia and electric blanket use. *Bioelectromagnetics* **9**, 207–213 (1988).

104. Lovely, R.H. et al., Adult leukemia risk and personal appliance use: a preliminary study. *Am J Epidemiol* **140**, 510–517 (1994).

105. Sussman, S.S. & Kheifets, L.I. Re: "Adult leukemia risk and personal appliance use: a preliminary study". *Am J Epidemiol* **143**, 743–744 (1996).

106. Kheifets, L.I., Afifi, A.A., Buffler, P.A., Zhang, Z.W. & Matkin, C.C. Occupational electric and magnetic field exposure and leukemia. A meta-analysis. *J Occup Environ Med* **39**, 1074–1091 (1997).

107. Linet, M.S., Ries, L.A., Smith, M.A., Tarone, R.E. & Devesa, S.S. Cancer surveillance series: recent trends in childhood cancer incidence and mortality in the United States. *J Natl Cancer Inst* **91**, 1051–1058 (1999).

108. Johnson, K.J. et al., Childhood brain tumor epidemiology: a brain tumor epidemiology consortium review. *Cancer Epidemiol Biomarkers Prev* **23**, 2716–2736, doi:10.1158/1055-9965.EPI-14-0207 (2014).

109. Lin, R.S.L.P.Y. An epidemiologic study of childhood cancer in relation to residential exposure to electromagnetic fields. (Abstract). Presented at: *The DOE-EPRI Contractor's Review Meeting*, Portland, Oregon, US (1994).

110. Preston-Martin, S. et al., Los Angeles study of residential magnetic fields and childhood brain tumors. *Am J Epidemiol* **143**, 105–119 (1996).

111. Preston-Martin, S., Gurney, J.G., Pogoda, J.M., Holly, E.A. & Mueller, B.A. Brain tumor risk in children in relation to use of electric blankets and water bed heaters. Results from the United States West Coast Childhood Brain Tumor Study. *Am J Epidemiol* **143**, 1116–1122 (1996).

112. Schuz, J., Kaletsch, U., Kaatsch, P., Meinert, R. & Michaelis, J. Risk factors for pediatric tumors of the central nervous system: results from a German population-based case-control study. *Med Pediatr Oncol* **36**, 274–282, doi:10.1002/1096-911X(20010201)36:2<274::AID-MPO1065>3.0.CO;2-D (2001).

113. Kroll, M.E., Swanson, J., Vincent, T.J. & Draper, G.J. Childhood cancer and magnetic fields from high-voltage power lines in England and Wales: a case-control study. *Br J Cancer* **103**, 1122–1127, doi:10.1038/sj.bjc.6605795 (2010).

114. Saito, T. et al., Power-frequency magnetic fields and childhood brain tumors: a case-control study in Japan. *J Epidemiol* **20**, 54–61 (2010).

115. Gurney, J.G. et al., Childhood brain tumor occurrence in relation to residential power line configurations, electric heating sources, and electric appliance use. *Am J Epidemiol* **143**, 120–128 (1996).

116. Savitz, D.A., John, E.M. & Kleckner, R.C. Magnetic field exposure from electric appliances and childhood cancer. *Am J Epidemiol* **131**, 763–773 (1990).

117. McCredie, M., Maisonneuve, P. & Boyle, P. Perinatal and early postnatal risk factors for malignant brain tumours in New South Wales children. *Int J Cancer* **56**, 11–15 (1994).

118. Hug, K., Grize, L., Seidler, A., Kaatsch, P. & Schuz, J. Parental occupational exposure to extremely low frequency magnetic fields and childhood cancer: a German case-control study. *Am J Epidemiol* **171**, 27–35, doi:10.1093/aje/kwp339 (2010).

119. Bunin, G.R., Ward, E., Kramer, S., Rhee, C.A. & Meadows, A.T. Neuroblastoma and parental occupation. *Am J Epidemiol* **131**, 776–780 (1990).

120. Johnson, C.C. & Spitz, M.R. Childhood nervous system tumours: an assessment of risk associated with paternal occupations involving use, repair or manufacture of electrical and electronic equipment. *Int J Epidemiol* **18**, 756–762 (1989).

121. Nasca, P.C. et al., An epidemiologic case-control study of central nervous system tumors in children and parental occupational exposures. *Am J Epidemiol* **128**, 1256–1265 (1988).
122. Spitz, M.R. & Johnson, C.C. Neuroblastoma and paternal occupation. A case-control analysis. *Am J Epidemiol* **121**, 924–929 (1985).
123. Wilkins, J.R., 3rd & Hundley, V.D. Paternal occupational exposure to electromagnetic fields and neuroblastoma in offspring. *Am J Epidemiol* **131**, 995–1008 (1990).
124. Wilkins, J.R., 3rd & Koutras, R.A. Paternal occupation and brain cancer in offspring: a mortality-based case-control study. *Am J Ind Med* **14**, 299–318 (1988).
125. Pearce, M.S., Hammal, D.M., Dorak, M.T., McNally, R.J. & Parker, L. Paternal occupational exposure to electro-magnetic fields as a risk factor for cancer in children and young adults: a case-control study from the North of England. *Pediatr Blood Cancer* **49**, 280–286, doi:10.1002/pbc.21021 (2007).
126. Li, P., McLaughlin, J. & Infante-Rivard, C. Maternal occupational exposure to extremely low frequency magnetic fields and the risk of brain cancer in the offspring. *Cancer Causes Control* **20**, 945–955, doi:10.1007/s10552-009-9311-5 (2009).
127. Feingold, L., Savitz, D.A. & John, E.M. Use of a job-exposure matrix to evaluate parental occupation and childhood cancer. *Cancer Causes Control* **3**, 161–169 (1992).
128. Ali, R. et al., A case-control study of parental occupation, leukemia, and brain tumors in an industrial city in Taiwan. *J Occup Environ Med* **46**, 985–992 (2004).
129. Kheifets, L. et al., A pooled analysis of extremely low-frequency magnetic fields and childhood brain tumors. *Am J Epidemiol* **172**, 752–761, doi:10.1093/aje/kwq181 (2010).
130. Baldi, I. et al., Occupational and residential exposure to electromagnetic fields and risk of brain tumors in adults: a case-control study in Gironde, France. *Int J Cancer* **129**, 1477–1484, doi:10.1002/ijc.25765 (2011).
131. Verkasalo, P.K., Pukkala, E., Kaprio, J., Heikkila, K.V. & Koskenvuo, M. Magnetic fields of high voltage power lines and risk of cancer in Finnish adults: nationwide cohort study. *BMJ* **313**, 1047–1051 (1996).
132. Wrensch, M., Yost, M., Miike, R., Lee, G. & Touchstone, J. Adult glioma in relation to residential power frequency electromagnetic field exposures in the San Francisco Bay area. *Epidemiology* **10**, 523–527 (1999).
133. Klaeboe, L., Blaasaas, K.G., Haldorsen, T. & Tynes, T. Residential and occupational exposure to 50-Hz magnetic fields and brain tumours in Norway: a population-based study. *Int J Cancer* **115**, 137–141, doi:10.1002/ijc.20845 (2005).
134. Loomis, D.P. Cancer of breast among men in electrical occupations. *Lancet* **339**, 1482–1483 (1992).
135. Ryan, P., Lee, M.W., North, B. & McMichael, A.J. Risk factors for tumors of the brain and meninges: results from the Adelaide Adult Brain Tumor Study. *Int J Cancer* **51**, 20–27 (1992).
136. Kheifets, L.I., Afifi, A.A., Buffler, P.A. & Zhang, Z.W. Occupational electric and magnetic field exposure and brain cancer: a meta-analysis. *J Occup Environ Med* **37**, 1327–1341 (1995).
137. Kheifets, L.I. Electric and magnetic field exposure and brain cancer: a review. *Bioelectromagnetics* **Suppl 5**, S120–S131 (2001).
138. Armstrong, B. et al., Association between exposure to pulsed electromagnetic fields and cancer in electric utility workers in Quebec, Canada, and France. *Am J Epidemiol* **140**, 805–820 (1994).
139. Beall, C., Delzell, E., Cole, P. & Brill, I. Brain tumors among electronics industry workers. *Epidemiology* **7**, 125–130 (1996).
140. Fear, N.T., Roman, E., Carpenter, L.M., Newton, R. & Bull, D. Cancer in electrical workers: an analysis of cancer registrations in England, 1981–87. *Br J Cancer* **73**, 935–939 (1996).
141. Heineman, E.F., Gao, Y.T., Dosemeci, M. & McLaughlin, J.K. Occupational risk factors for brain tumors among women in Shanghai, China. *J Occup Environ Med* **37**, 288–293 (1995).
142. Harrington, J.M., McBride, D.I., Sorahan, T., Paddle, G.M. & van Tongeren, M. Occupational exposure to magnetic fields in relation to mortality from brain cancer among electricity generation and transmission workers. *Occup Environ Med* **54**, 7–13 (1997).

143. Guenel, P., Nicolau, J., Imbernon, E., Chevalier, A. & Goldberg, M. Exposure to 50-Hz electric field and incidence of leukemia, brain tumors, and other cancers among French electric utility workers. *Am J Epidemiol* **144**, 1107–1121 (1996).

144. Kaplan, S., Etlin, S., Novikov, I. & Modan, B. Occupational risks for the development of brain tumors. *Am J Ind Med* **31**, 15–20 (1997).

145. Kelsh, M.A. & Sahl, J.D. Mortality among a cohort of electric utility workers, 1960–1991. *Am J Ind Med* **31**, 534–544 (1997).

146. Miller, R.D., Neuberger, J.S. & Gerald, K.B. Brain cancer and leukemia and exposure to power-frequency (50- to 60-Hz) electric and magnetic fields. *Epidemiol Rev* **19**, 273–293 (1997).

147. Johansen, C. & Olsen, J.H. Risk of cancer among Danish utility workers--a nationwide cohort study. *Am J Epidemiol* **147**, 548–555 (1998).

148. Cocco, P., Dosemeci, M. & Heineman, E.F. Occupational risk factors for cancer of the central nervous system: a case-control study on death certificates from 24 U.S. states. *Am J Ind Med* **33**, 247–255 (1998).

149. Rodvall, Y. et al., Occupational exposure to magnetic fields and brain tumours in central Sweden. *Eur J Epidemiol* **14**, 563–569 (1998).

150. Sahl, J.D., Kelsh, M.A. & Greenland, S. Cohort and nested case-control studies of hematopoietic cancers and brain cancer among electric utility workers. *Epidemiology* **4**, 104–114 (1993).

151. Theriault, G. et al., Cancer risks associated with occupational exposure to magnetic fields among electric utility workers in Ontario and Quebec, Canada, and France: 1970–1989. *Am J Epidemiol* **139**, 550–572 (1994).

152. Savitz, D.A. & Loomis, D.P. Magnetic field exposure in relation to leukemia and brain cancer mortality among electric utility workers. *Am J Epidemiol* **141**, 123–134 (1995).

153. Turner, M.C. et al., Occupational exposure to extremely low-frequency magnetic fields and brain tumor risks in the INTEROCC study. *Cancer Epidemiol Biomarkers Prev* **23**, 1863–1872, doi:10.1158/1055-9965.EPI-14-0102 (2014).

154. Globocan. Estimated Cancer Incidence Mortality and Incidence worldwide in 2012, http://globocan.iarc.fr/Pages/fact_sheets_cancer.aspx (2012).

155. Stevens, R.G. Electric power use and breast cancer: a hypothesis. *Am J Epidemiol* **125**, 556–561 (1987).

156. Coogan, P.F. & Aschengrau, A. Exposure to power frequency magnetic fields and risk of breast cancer in the Upper Cape Cod Cancer Incidence Study. *Arch Environ Health* **53**, 359–367, doi:10.1080/00039899809605722 (1998).

157. Feychting, M., Forssen, U., Rutqvist, L.E. & Ahlbom, A. Magnetic fields and breast cancer in Swedish adults residing near high-voltage power lines. *Epidemiology* **9**, 392–397 (1998).

158. Kliukiene, J., Tynes, T. & Andersen, A. Residential and occupational exposures to 50-Hz magnetic fields and breast cancer in women: a population-based study. *Am J Epidemiol* **159**, 852–861 (2004).

159. Davis, S., Mirick, D.K. & Stevens, R.G. Residential magnetic fields and the risk of breast cancer. *Am J Epidemiol* **155**, 446–454 (2002).

160. London, S.J. et al., Residential magnetic field exposure and breast cancer risk: a nested case-control study from a multiethnic cohort in Los Angeles County, California. *Am J Epidemiol* **158**, 969–980 (2003).

161. Schoenfeld, E.R. et al., Electromagnetic fields and breast cancer on Long Island: a case-control study. *Am J Epidemiol* **158**, 47–58 (2003).

162. Chen, Q. et al., A meta-analysis on the relationship between exposure to ELF-EMFs and the risk of female breast cancer. *PLoS One* **8**, e69272, doi:10.1371/journal.pone.0069272 (2013).

163. Sun, J.W. et al., Electromagnetic field exposure and male breast cancer risk: a meta-analysis of 18 studies. *Asian Pac J Cancer Prev* **14**, 523–528 (2013).

164. Forssen, U.M., Feychting, M., Rutqvist, L.E., Floderus, B. & Ahlbom, A. Occupational and residential magnetic field exposure and breast cancer in females. *Epidemiology* **11**, 24–29 (2000).

165. Vena, J.E. et al., Risk of premenopausal breast cancer and use of electric blankets. *Am J Epidemiol* **140**, 974–979 (1994).

166. Vena, J.E., Graham, S., Hellmann, R., Swanson, M. & Brasure, J. Use of electric blankets and risk of postmenopausal breast cancer. *Am J Epidemiol* **134**, 180–185 (1991).
167. Guenel, P., Raskmark, P., Andersen, J.B. & Lynge, E. Incidence of cancer in persons with occupational exposure to electromagnetic fields in Denmark. *Br J Ind Med* **50**, 758–764 (1993).
168. Kelsh, M.A. & Sahl, J.D. Sex differences in work-related injury rates among electric utility workers. *Am J Epidemiol* **143**, 1050–1058 (1996).
169. Vagero, D., Ahlbom, A., Olin, R. & Sahlsten, S. Cancer morbidity among workers in the telecommunications industry. *Br J Ind Med* **42**, 191–195 (1985).
170. Vagero, D. & Olin, R. Incidence of cancer in the electronics industry: using the new Swedish Cancer Environment Registry as a screening instrument. *Br J Ind Med* **40**, 188–192 (1983).
171. Loomis, D.P., Savitz, D.A. & Ananth, C.V. Breast cancer mortality among female electrical workers in the United States. *J Natl Cancer Inst* **86**, 921–925 (1994).
172. Cantor, K.P., Stewart, P.A., Brinton, L.A. & Dosemeci, M. Occupational exposures and female breast cancer mortality in the United States. *J Occup Environ Med* **37**, 336–348 (1995).
173. Kheifets, L.I. & Matkin, C.C. Industrialization, electromagnetic fields, and breast cancer risk. *Environ Health Perspect* **107 Suppl 1**, 145–154 (1999).
174. Guberan, E., Usel, M., Raymond, L., Tissot, R. & Sweetnam, P.M. Disability, mortality, and incidence of cancer among Geneva painters and electricians: a historical prospective study. *Br J Ind Med* **46**, 16–23 (1989).
175. Milham, S., Jr. Mortality in workers exposed to electromagnetic fields. *Environ Health Perspect* **62**, 297–300 (1985).
176. Pearce, N., Reif, J. & Fraser, J. Case-control studies of cancer in New Zealand electrical workers. *Int J Epidemiol* **18**, 55–59 (1989).
177. Spinelli, J.J., Band, P.R., Svirchev, L.M. & Gallagher, R.P. Mortality and cancer incidence in aluminum reduction plant workers. *J Occup Med* **33**, 1150–1155 (1991).
178. Tornqvist, S., Norell, S., Ahlbom, A. & Knave, B. Cancer in the electric power industry. *Br J Ind Med* **43**, 212–213 (1986).
179. Demers, P.A. et al., Occupational exposure to electromagnetic fields and breast cancer in men. *Am J Epidemiol* **134**, 340–347 (1991).
180. Floderus, B., Tornqvist, S. & Stenlund, C. Incidence of selected cancers in Swedish railway workers, 1961–79. *Cancer Causes Control* **5**, 189–194 (1994).
181. Matanoski, G.M., Elliott, E.A., Breysse, P.N. & Lynberg, M.C. Leukemia in telephone linemen. *Am J Epidemiol* **137**, 609–619 (1993).
182. Tynes, T. & Andersen, A. Electromagnetic fields and male breast cancer. *Lancet* **336**, 1596 (1990).
183. Cammarano, G., Crosignani, P., Berrino, F. & Berra, G. Cancer mortality among workers in a thermoelectric power plant. *Scand J Work Environ Health* **10**, 259–261 (1984).
184. Sorahan, T. Cancer incidence in UK electricity generation and transmission workers, 1973–2008. *Occup Med (Lond)* **62**, 496–505, doi:10.1093/occmed/kqs152 (2012).
185. Grundy, A. et al., Occupational exposure to magnetic fields and breast cancer among Canadian men. *Cancer Med* **5**, 586–596, doi:10.1002/cam4.581 (2016).
186. Koeman, T. et al., Occupational extremely low-frequency magnetic field exposure and selected cancer outcomes in a prospective Dutch cohort. *Cancer Causes Control* **25**, 203–214, doi:10.1007/s10552-013-0322-x (2014).
187. Tynes, T., Klaeboe, L. & Haldorsen, T. Residential and occupational exposure to 50 Hz magnetic fields and malignant melanoma: a population based study. *Occup Environ Med* **60**, 343–347 (2003).
188. Asanova, T.P. & Rakov, A.N. [Health conditions of workers exposed to electric fields of open switchboard installations of 400–500 kv. (Preliminary report)]. *Gig Tr Prof Zabol* **10**, 50–52 (1966).
189. Baroncelli, P. et al., A health examination of railway high-voltage substation workers exposed to ELF electromagnetic fields. *Am J Ind Med* **10**, 45–55 (1986).
190. Sastre, A., Cook, M.R. & Graham, C. Nocturnal exposure to intermittent 60 Hz magnetic fields alters human cardiac rhythm. *Bioelectromagnetics* **19**, 98–106 (1998).

191. Dekker, J.M. et al., Heart rate variability from short electrocardiographic recordings predicts mortality from all causes in middle-aged and elderly men. The Zutphen Study. *Am J Epidemiol* **145**, 899–908 (1997).

192. Liao, D. et al., Cardiac autonomic function and incident coronary heart disease: a population-based case-cohort study. The ARIC Study. Atherosclerosis Risk in Communities Study. *Am J Epidemiol* **145**, 696–706 (1997).

193. Martin, G.J. et al., Heart rate variability and sudden death secondary to coronary artery disease during ambulatory electrocardiographic monitoring. *Am J Cardiol* **60**, 86–89 (1987).

194. Kleiger, R.E., Miller, J.P., Bigger, J.T., Jr. & Moss, A.J. Decreased heart rate variability and its association with increased mortality after acute myocardial infarction. *Am J Cardiol* **59**, 256–262 (1987).

195. Lombardi, F. et al., Heart rate variability as an index of sympathovagal interaction after acute myocardial infarction. *Am J Cardiol* **60**, 1239–1245 (1987).

196. Vaishnav, S. et al., Relation between heart rate variability early after acute myocardial infarction and long-term mortality. *Am J Cardiol* **73**, 653–657 (1994).

197. Malik, M., Farrell, T. & Camm, A.J. Circadian rhythm of heart rate variability after acute myocardial infarction and its influence on the prognostic value of heart rate variability. *Am J Cardiol* **66**, 1049–1054 (1990).

198. Savitz, D.A., Liao, D., Sastre, A., Kleckner, R.C. & Kavet, R. Magnetic field exposure and cardiovascular disease mortality among electric utility workers. *Am J Epidemiol* **149**, 135–142 (1999).

199. Perry, S., Pearl, L. & Binns, R. Power frequency magnetic field; depressive illness and myocardial infarction. *Public Health* **103**, 177–180 (1989).

200. Baris, D., Armstrong, B.G., Deadman, J. & Theriault, G. A mortality study of electrical utility workers in Quebec. *Occup Environ Med* **53**, 25–31 (1996).

201. Johansen, C. & Olsen, J.H. Mortality from amyotrophic lateral sclerosis, other chronic disorders, and electric shocks among utility workers. *Am J Epidemiol* **148**, 362–368 (1998).

202. van Wijngaarden, E., Savitz, D.A., Kleckner, R.C., Kavet, R. & Loomis, D. Mortality patterns by occupation in a cohort of electric utility workers. *Am J Ind Med* **40**, 667–673 (2001).

203. Sahl, J. et al., Occupational magnetic field exposure and cardiovascular mortality in a cohort of electric utility workers. *Am J Epidemiol* **156**, 913–918 (2002).

204. Hakansson, N., Gustavsson, P., Sastre, A. & Floderus, B. Occupational exposure to extremely low frequency magnetic fields and mortality from cardiovascular disease. *Am J Epidemiol* **158**, 534–542 (2003).

205. Johansen, C. et al., Risk of severe cardiac arrhythmia in male utility workers: a nationwide danish cohort study. *Am J Epidemiol* **156**, 857–861 (2002).

206. Sorahan, T. & Nichols, L. Mortality from cardiovascular disease in relation to magnetic field exposure: findings from a study of UK electricity generation and transmission workers, 1973–1997. *Am J Ind Med* **45**, 93–102 (2004).

207. Ahlbom, A. et al., Occupational magnetic field exposure and myocardial infarction incidence. *Epidemiology* **15**, 403–408 (2004).

208. Mezei, G. et al., Occupational magnetic field exposure, cardiovascular disease mortality, and potential confounding by smoking. *Ann Epidemiol* **15**, 622–629, doi:10.1016/j.annepidem.2004.12.013 (2005).

209. Roosli, M., Egger, M., Pfluger, D. & Minder, C. Cardiovascular mortality and exposure to extremely low frequency magnetic fields: a cohort study of Swiss railway workers. *Environ Health* **7**, 35, doi:10.1186/1476-069X-7-35 (2008).

210. Cooper, A.R. et al., A population-based cohort study of occupational exposure to magnetic fields and cardiovascular disease mortality. *Ann Epidemiol* **19**, 42–48, doi:10.1016/j.annepidem.2008.10.001 (2009).

211. Koeman, T. et al., Occupational exposure to extremely low-frequency magnetic fields and cardiovascular disease mortality in a prospective cohort study. *Occup Environ Med* **70**, 402–407, doi:10.1136/oemed-2012-100889 (2013).

212. Finkelstein, M.M. Re: "Magnetic field exposure and cardiovascular disease mortality among electric utility workers". *Am J Epidemiol* **150**, 1258–1259 (1999).
213. Mant, J. et al., Clinicians didn't reliably distinguish between different causes of cardiac death using case histories. *J Clin Epidemiol* **59**, 862–867, doi:10.1016/j.jclinepi.2005.11.021 (2006).
214. Kheifets, L. et al., Extremely low-frequency magnetic fields and heart disease. *Scand J Work Environ Health* **33**, 5–12 (2007).
215. Reitz, C., Brayne, C. & Mayeux, R. Epidemiology of Alzheimer disease. *Nat Rev Neurol* **7**, 137–152, doi:10.1038/nrneurol.2011.2 (2011).
216. Alzheimer's Association. 2014 Alzheimer's disease facts and figures. *Alzheimers Dement* **10**, e47–e92 (2014).
217. Harmanci, H. et al., Risk factors for Alzheimer disease: a population-based case-control study in Istanbul, Turkey. *Alzheimer Dis Assoc Disord* **17**, 139–145 (2003).
218. Huss, A., Spoerri, A., Egger, M. & Roosli, M. Residence near power lines and mortality from neurodegenerative diseases: longitudinal study of the Swiss population. *Am J Epidemiol* **169**, 167–175, doi:10.1093/aje/kwn297 (2009).
219. Frei, P. et al., Residential distance to high-voltage power lines and risk of neurodegenerative diseases: a Danish population-based case-control study. *Am J Epidemiol* **177**, 970–978, doi:10.1093/aje/kws334 (2013).
220. Garcia, A.M., Sisternas, A. & Hoyos, S.P. Occupational exposure to extremely low frequency electric and magnetic fields and Alzheimer disease: a meta-analysis. *Int J Epidemiol* **37**, 329–340, doi:10.1093/ije/dym295 (2008).
221. Vergara, X. et al., Occupational exposure to extremely low-frequency magnetic fields and neurodegenerative disease: a meta-analysis. *J Occup Environ Med* **55**, 135–146, doi:10.1097/JOM.0b013e31827f37f8 (2013).
222. Sobel, E., Dunn, M., Davanipour, Z., Qian, Z. & Chui, H.C. Elevated risk of Alzheimer's disease among workers with likely electromagnetic field exposure. *Neurology* **47**, 1477–1481 (1996).
223. Sobel, E. et al., Occupations with exposure to electromagnetic fields: a possible risk factor for Alzheimer's disease. *Am J Epidemiol* **142**, 515–524 (1995).
224. Sorahan, T. & Mohammed, N. Neurodegenerative disease and magnetic field exposure in UK electricity supply workers. *Occup Med (Lond)* **64**, 454–460, doi:10.1093/occmed/kqu105 (2014).
225. Koeman, T. et al., Occupational exposures and risk of dementia-related mortality in the prospective Netherlands Cohort Study. *Am J Ind Med* **58**, 625–635, doi:10.1002/ajim.22462 (2015).
226. Pedersen, C. et al., Occupational exposure to extremely low-frequency magnetic fields and risk for central nervous system disease: an update of a Danish cohort study among utility workers. *Int Arch Occup Environ Health*, doi:10.1007/s00420-017-1224-0 (2017).
227. Davanipour, Z., Tseng, C.C., Lee, P.J. & Sobel, E. A case-control study of occupational magnetic field exposure and Alzheimer's disease: results from the California Alzheimer's Disease Diagnosis and Treatment Centers. *BMC Neurol* **7**, 13, doi:10.1186/1471-2377-7-13 (2007).
228. Davanipour, Z., Tseng, C.C., Lee, P.J., Markides, K.S. & Sobel, E. Severe cognitive dysfunction and occupational extremely low frequency magnetic field exposure among elderly Mexican Americans. *Br J Med Med Res* **4**, 1641–1662, doi:10.9734/BJMMR/2014/7317 (2014).
229. Chio, A., Magnani, C., Oddenino, E., Tolardo, G. & Schiffer, D. Accuracy of death certificate diagnosis of amyotrophic lateral sclerosis. *J Epidemiol Community Health* **46**, 517–518 (1992).
230. Al-Chalabi, A. & Hardiman, O. The epidemiology of ALS: a conspiracy of genes, environment and time. *Nat Rev Neurol* **9**, 617–628, doi:10.1038/nrneurol.2013.203 (2013).
231. McGuire, V.N.L.M. in *Amyotrophic Lateral Sclerosis* (eds. H. Mitsumoto; S. Przedborski; P.H. Gordon) 17–41 (Taylor & Francis, 2006).
232. Haynal A. & Regli F. Zusammenhang der amyotrophischen lateralsclerose mit gehäufter elektrotraumata. *Confinia Neurologica* **24**, 189–198 (1964).
233. Kondo, K. & Tsubaki, T. Case-control studies of motor neuron disease: association with mechanical injuries. *Arch Neurol* **38**, 220–226 (1981).
234. Seelen, M. et al., Residential exposure to extremely low frequency electromagnetic fields and the risk of ALS. *Neurology* **83**, 1767–1769, doi:10.1212/WNL.0000000000000952 (2014).

235. Vinceti, M. et al., Magnetic fields exposure from high-voltage power lines and risk of amyotrophic lateral sclerosis in two Italian populations. *Amyotroph Lateral Scler Frontotemporal Degener* **18**, 1–7, doi:10.1080/21678421.2017.1332078 (2017).

236. Kheifets, L. et al., Future needs of occupational epidemiology of extremely low frequency electric and magnetic fields: review and recommendations. *Occup Environ Med* **66**, 72–80, doi:10.1136/oem.2007.037994 (2009).

237. Vergara, X., Mezei, G. & Kheifets, L. Case-control study of occupational exposure to electric shocks and magnetic fields and mortality from amyotrophic lateral sclerosis in the US, 1991–1999. *J Expo Sci Environ Epidemiol* **25**, 65–71, doi:10.1038/jes.2014.39 (2015).

238. Huss, A., Spoerri, A., Egger, M., Kromhout, H. & Vermeulen, R. Occupational exposure to magnetic fields and electric shocks and risk of ALS: the Swiss National Cohort. *Amyotroph Lateral Scler Frontotemporal Degener* **16**, 80–85, doi:10.3109/21678421.2014.954588 (2015).

239. Fischer, H. et al., Occupational exposure to electric shocks and magnetic fields and amyotrophic lateral sclerosis in Sweden. *Epidemiology* **26**, 824–830, doi:10.1097/EDE.0000000000000365 (2015).

240. Koeman, T. et al., Occupational exposure and amyotrophic lateral sclerosis in a prospective cohort. *Occup Environ Med* **74**, 578–585, doi:10.1136/oemed-2016-103780 (2017).

241. Zhou, H., Chen, G., Chen, C., Yu, Y. & Xu, Z. Association between extremely low-frequency electromagnetic fields occupations and amyotrophic lateral sclerosis: a meta-analysis. *PLoS One* **7**, e48354, doi:10.1371/journal.pone.0048354 (2012).

242. de Lau, L.M. & Breteler, M.M. Epidemiology of Parkinson's disease. *Lancet Neurol* **5**, 525–535, doi:10.1016/S1474-4422(06)70471-9 (2006).

243. Wirdefeldt, K., Adami, H.O., Cole, P., Trichopoulos, D. & Mandel, J. Epidemiology and etiology of Parkinson's disease: a review of the evidence. *Eur J Epidemiol* **26 Suppl 1**, S1–S58, doi:10.1007/s10654-011-9581-6 (2011).

244. Huss, A., Koeman, T., Kromhout, H. & Vermeulen, R. Extremely low frequency magnetic field exposure and Parkinson's disease—A systematic review and meta-analysis of the data. *Int J Environ Res Public Health* **12**, 7348–7356, doi:10.3390/ijerph120707348 (2015).

245. Savitz, D.A., Loomis, D.P. & Tse, C.K. Electrical occupations and neurodegenerative disease: analysis of U.S. mortality data. *Arch Environ Health* **53**, 71–74, doi:10.1080/00039899809605691 (1998).

246. Savitz, D.A., Checkoway, H. & Loomis, D.P. Magnetic field exposure and neurodegenerative disease mortality among electric utility workers. *Epidemiology* **9**, 398–404 (1998).

247. Feychting, M., Jonsson, F., Pedersen, N.L. & Ahlbom, A. Occupational magnetic field exposure and neurodegenerative disease. *Epidemiology* **14**, 413–419; discussion 427–418 (2003).

248. Wechsler, L.S., Checkoway, H., Franklin, G.M. & Costa, L.G. A pilot study of occupational and environmental risk factors for Parkinson's disease. *Neurotoxicology* **12**, 387–392 (1991).

249. Noonan, C.W., Reif, J.S., Yost, M. & Touchstone, J. Occupational exposure to magnetic fields in case-referent studies of neurodegenerative diseases. *Scand J Work Environ Health* **28**, 42–48 (2002).

250. Hakansson, N., Gustavsson, P., Johansen, C. & Floderus, B. Neurodegenerative diseases in welders and other workers exposed to high levels of magnetic fields. *Epidemiology* **14**, 420–426; discussion 427–428, doi:10.1097/01.EDE.0000078446.76859.c9 (2003).

251. Banerjee, T.K. et al., Epidemiology of epilepsy and its burden in Kolkata, India. *Acta Neurol Scand* **132**, 203–211, doi:10.1111/ane.12384 (2015).

252. Fiest, K.M. et al., Prevalence and incidence of epilepsy: a systematic review and meta-analysis of international studies. *Neurology* **88**, 296–303, doi:10.1212/WNL.0000000000003509 (2017).

253. Grell, K., Meersohn, A., Schuz, J. & Johansen, C. Risk of neurological diseases among survivors of electric shocks: a nationwide cohort study, Denmark, 1968–2008. *Bioelectromagnetics* **33**, 459–465, doi:10.1002/bem.21705 (2012).

254. Kessler, R.C. & Bromet, E.J. The epidemiology of depression across cultures. *Annu Rev Public Health* **34**, 119–138, doi:10.1146/annurev-publhealth-031912-114409 (2013).

255. Dowson, D.I., Lewith, G.T., Campbell, M., Mullee, M.A. & Brewster, L.A. Overhead high-voltage cables and recurrent headache and depressions. *Practitioner* **232**, 435–436 (1988).

256. International Commission on Non-Ionizing Radiation Protection (ICNIRP). *Exposure to Static and Low Frequency Electromagnetic Fields, Biological Effects and Health Consequences (0–100 kHz).* (ICNRP Publications, 2003).

257. Poole, C. et al., Depressive symptoms and headaches in relation to proximity of residence to an alternating-current transmission line right-of-way. *Am J Epidemiol* **137**, 318–330 (1993).

258. McMahan, S., Ericson, J. & Meyer, J. Depressive symptomatology in women and residential proximity to high-voltage transmission lines. *Am J Epidemiol* **139**, 58–63 (1994).

259. Verkasalo, P.K. et al., Magnetic fields of transmission lines and depression. *Am J Epidemiol* **146**, 1037–1045 (1997).

260. Savitz, D.A., Boyle, C.A. & Holmgreen, P. Prevalence of depression among electrical workers. *Am J Ind Med* **25**, 165–176 (1994).

261. Beale, I.L., Pearce, N.E., Conroy, D.M., Henning, M.A. & Murrell, K.A. Psychological effects of chronic exposure to 50 Hz magnetic fields in humans living near extra-high-voltage transmission lines. *Bioelectromagnetics* **18**, 584–594 (1997).

262. Perry, F.S., Reichmanis, M., Marino, A.A. & Becker, R.O. Environmental power-frequency magnetic fields and suicide. *Health Phys* **41**, 267–277 (1981).

263. Reichmanis, M., Perry, F.S., Marino, A.A. & Becker, R.O. Relation between suicide and the electromagnetic field of overhead power lines. *Physiol Chem Phys* **11**, 395–403 (1979).

264. Baris, D. & Armstrong, B. Suicide among electric utility workers in England and Wales. *Br J Ind Med* **47**, 788–789 (1990).

265. Baris, D., Armstrong, B.G., Deadman, J. & Theriault, G. A case cohort study of suicide in relation to exposure to electric and magnetic fields among electrical utility workers. *Occup Environ Med* **53**, 17–24 (1996).

266. van Wijngaarden, E., Savitz, D.A., Kleckner, R.C., Cai, J. & Loomis, D. Exposure to electromagnetic fields and suicide among electric utility workers: a nested case-control study. *Occup Environ Med* **57**, 258–263 (2000).

267. Jarvholm, B. & Stenberg, A. Suicide mortality among electricians in the Swedish construction industry. *Occup Environ Med* **59**, 199–200 (2002).

268. Nichols, L. & Sorahan, T. Mortality of UK electricity generation and transmission workers, 1973–2002. *Occup Med (Lond)* **55**, 541–548, doi:10.1093/occmed/kqi157 (2005).

269. van Wijngaarden, E. An exploratory investigation of suicide and occupational exposure. *J Occup Environ Med* **45**, 96–101 (2003).

270. Lee, G.M., Neutra, R.R., Hristova, L., Yost, M. & Hiatt, R.A. A nested case-control study of residential and personal magnetic field measures and miscarriages. *Epidemiology* **13**, 21–31 (2002).

271. Li, D.K. et al., A population-based prospective cohort study of personal exposure to magnetic fields during pregnancy and the risk of miscarriage. *Epidemiology* **13**, 9–20 (2002).

272. Auger, N., Joseph, D., Goneau, M. & Daniel, M. The relationship between residential proximity to extremely low frequency power transmission lines and adverse birth outcomes. *J Epidemiol Community Health* **65**, 83–85, doi:10.1136/jech.2009.097709 (2011).

273. Savitz, D.A. & Ananth, C.V. Residential magnetic fields, wire codes, and pregnancy outcome. *Bioelectromagnetics* **15**, 271–273 (1994).

274. Belanger, K. et al., Spontaneous abortion and exposure to electric blankets and heated water beds. *Epidemiology* **9**, 36–42 (1998).

275. Juutilainen, J., Matilainen, P., Saarikoski, S., Laara, E. & Suonio, S. Early pregnancy loss and exposure to 50-Hz magnetic fields. *Bioelectromagnetics* **14**, 229–236 (1993).

276. Eskelinen, T., Keinanen, J., Salonen, H. & Juutilainen, J. Use of spot measurements for assessing residential ELF magnetic field exposure: a validity study. *Bioelectromagnetics* **23**, 173–176 (2002).

277. Wang, Q. et al., Residential exposure to 50 Hz magnetic fields and the association with miscarriage risk: a 2-year prospective cohort study. *PLoS One* **8**, e82113, doi:10.1371/journal.pone.0082113 (2013).

278. Shamsi Mahmoudabadi, F., Ziaei, S., Firoozabadi, M. & Kazemnejad, A. Exposure to extremely low frequency electromagnetic fields during pregnancy and the risk of spontaneous abortion: a case-control study. *J Res Health Sci* **13**, 131–134 (2013).

279. Auger, N., Park, A.L., Yacouba, S., Goneau, M. & Zayed, J. Stillbirth and residential proximity to extremely low frequency power transmission lines: a retrospective cohort study. *Occup Environ Med* **69**, 147–149, doi:10.1136/oemed-2011-100031 (2012).

280. Sadeghi, T. et al., Preterm birth among women living within 600 meters of high voltage overhead Power Lines: a case-control study. *Rom J Intern Med* **55**, 145–150, doi:10.1515/rjim-2017-0017 (2017).

281. Parazzini, F., Luchini, L., La Vecchia, C. & Crosignani, P.G. Video display terminal use during pregnancy and reproductive outcome–a meta-analysis. *J Epidemiol Community Health* **47**, 265–268 (1993).

282. Bracken, M.B. et al., Exposure to electromagnetic fields during pregnancy with emphasis on electrically heated beds: association with birthweight and intrauterine growth retardation. *Epidemiology* **6**, 263–270 (1995).

283. de Vocht, F., Hannam, K., Baker, P. & Agius, R. Maternal residential proximity to sources of extremely low frequency electromagnetic fields and adverse birth outcomes in a UK cohort. *Bioelectromagnetics* **35**, 201–209, doi:10.1002/bem.21840 (2014).

284. Mahram, M. & Ghazavi, M. The effect of extremely low frequency electromagnetic fields on pregnancy and fetal growth, and development. *Arch Iran Med* **16**, 221–224, doi:013164/AIM.006 (2013).

285. Eskelinen, T. et al., Maternal exposure to extremely low frequency magnetic fields: association with time to pregnancy and foetal growth. *Environ Int* **94**, 620–625, doi:10.1016/j.envint.2016.06.027 (2016).

286. Robert, E., Harris, J.A., Robert, O. & Selvin, S. Case-control study on maternal residential proximity to high voltage power lines and congenital anomalies in France. *Paediatr Perinat Epidemiol* **10**, 32–38 (1996).

287. Malagoli, C. et al., Maternal exposure to magnetic fields from high-voltage power lines and the risk of birth defects. *Bioelectromagnetics* **33**, 405–409 (2012).

288. Blaasaas, K.G., Tynes, T. & Lie, R.T. Residence near power lines and the risk of birth defects. *Epidemiology* **14**, 95–98, doi:10.1097/01.EDE.0000036699.57059.BA (2003).

289. Blaasaas, K.G., Tynes, T. & Lie, R.T. Risk of selected birth defects by maternal residence close to power lines during pregnancy. *Occup Environ Med* **61**, 174–176 (2004).

290. Savitz, D.A. Magnetic fields and miscarriage. *Epidemiology* **13**, 1–4 (2002).

291. Su, X.J. et al., Correlation between exposure to magnetic fields and embryonic development in the first trimester. *PLoS One* **9**, e101050, doi:10.1371/journal.pone.0101050 (2014).

292. Florig, H.K. & Hoburg, J.F. Power-frequency magnetic fields from electric blankets. *Health Phys* **58**, 493–502 (1990).

293. Kaune, W.T., Stevens, R.G., Callahan, N.J., Severson, R.K. & Thomas, D.B. Residential magnetic and electric fields. *Bioelectromagnetics* **8**, 315–335 (1987).

294. Dlugosz, L. et al., Congenital defects and electric bed heating in New York State: a register-based case-control study. *Am J Epidemiol* **135**, 1000–1011 (1992).

295. Milunsky, A. et al., Maternal heat exposure and neural tube defects. *JAMA* **268**, 882–885 (1992).

296. Shaw, G.M., Nelson, V., Todoroff, K., Wasserman, C.R. & Neutra, R.R. Maternal periconceptional use of electric bed-heating devices and risk for neural tube defects and orofacial clefts. *Teratology* **60**, 124–129, doi:10.1002/(SICI)1096-9926(199909)60:3<124::AID-TERA6>3.0.CO;2-D (1999).

297. Li, D.K., Checkoway, H. & Mueller, B.A. Electric blanket use during pregnancy in relation to the risk of congenital urinary tract anomalies among women with a history of subfertility. *Epidemiology* **6**, 485–489 (1995).

298. Lee, G.M., Neutra, R.R., Hristova, L., Yost, M. & Hiatt, R.A. The use of electric bed heaters and the risk of clinically recognized spontaneous abortion. *Epidemiology* **11**, 406–415 (2000).

299. Brent, R.L., Gordon, W.E., Bennett, W.R. & Beckman, D.A. Reproductive and teratologic effects of electromagnetic fields. *Reprod Toxicol* **7**, 535–580 (1993).

300. Delpizzo, V. Epidemiological studies of work with video display terminals and adverse pregnancy outcomes (1984–1992). *Am J Ind Med* **26**, 465–480 (1994).

301. Shaw, G.M. & Croen, L.A. Human adverse reproductive outcomes and electromagnetic field exposures: review of epidemiologic studies. *Environ Health Perspect* **101 Suppl 4**, 107–119 (1993).

302. Blaasaas, K.G., Tynes, T., Irgens, A. & Lie, R.T. Risk of birth defects by parental occupational exposure to 50 Hz electromagnetic fields: a population based study. *Occup Environ Med* **59**, 92–97 (2002).

303. Buiatti, E. et al., Risk factors in male infertility: a case-control study. *Arch Environ Health* **39**, 266–270 (1984).

304. Nordstrom, S., Birke, E. & Gustavsson, L. Reproductive hazards among workers at high voltage substations. *Bioelectromagnetics* **4**, 91–101 (1983).

305. Gracia, C.R., Sammel, M.D., Coutifaris, C., Guzick, D.S. & Barnhart, K.T. Occupational exposures and male infertility. *Am J Epidemiol* **162**, 729–733, doi:10.1093/aje/kwi269 (2005).

306. Lundsberg, L.S., Bracken, M.B. & Belanger, K. Occupationally related magnetic field exposure and male subfertility. *Fertil Steril* **63**, 384–391 (1995).

307. Li, D.K. et al., Exposure to magnetic fields and the risk of poor sperm quality. *Reprod Toxicol* **29**, 86–92, doi:10.1016/j.reprotox.2009.09.004 (2010).

308. Irgens, A., Kruger, K., Skorve, A.H. & Irgens, L.M. Male proportion in offspring of parents exposed to strong static and extremely low-frequency electromagnetic fields in Norway. *Am J Ind Med* **32**, 557–561 (1997).

309. Mubarak, A.A. & Mubarak, A.A. Does high voltage electricity have an effect on the sex distribution of offspring? *Hum Reprod* **11**, 230–231 (1996).

310. Tornqvist, S. Paternal work in the power industry: effects on children at delivery. *J Occup Environ Med* **40**, 111–117 (1998).

311. Schnitzer, P.G., Olshan, A.F. & Erickson, J.D. Paternal occupation and risk of birth defects in offspring. *Epidemiology* **6**, 577–583 (1995).

312. Lewis, R.C. et al., Exposure to power-frequency magnetic fields and the risk of infertility and adverse pregnancy outcomes: update on the human evidence and recommendations for future study designs. *J Toxicol Environ Health B Crit Rev* **19**, 29–45, doi:10.1080/10937404.2015.1134370 (2016).

313. Zar, H.J. & Ferkol, T.W. The global burden of respiratory disease—Impact on child health. *Pediatr Pulmonol* **49**, 430–434, doi:10.1002/ppul.23030 (2014).

314. Harb, H., Alashkar Alhamwe, B., Garn, H., Renz, H. & Potaczek, D.P. Recent developments in epigenetics of pediatric asthma. *Curr Opin Pediatr* **28**, 754–763, doi:10.1097/MOP.0000000000000424 (2016).

315. Platts-Mills, T.A. The allergy epidemics: 1870–2010. *J Allergy Clin Immunol* **136**, 3–13, doi:10.1016/j.jaci.2015.03.048 (2015).

316. Beale, I.L.P., N.E.; Booth, R.J.; Heriot, S.A. Association of health problems with 50-Hz magnetic fields in human adults living near power transmission lines. *ACNEM* **20**, 9–12, 15, 30 (2001).

317. Li, D.-K., Chen, H. & Odouli, R. Maternal exposure to magnetic fields during pregnancy in relation to the risk of asthma in offspring. *Arch Pediatr Adolesc Med* **165**, 945–950, doi:10.1001/archpediatrics.2011.135 (2011).

318. Sudan, M. et al., Re-examining the association between residential exposure to magnetic fields from power lines and childhood asthma in the Danish National Birth Cohort. *PLoS One* **12**, e0177651, doi:10.1371/journal.pone.0177651 (2017).

319. Dosemeci, M., Wacholder, S. & Lubin, J.H. Does nondifferential misclassification of exposure always bias a true effect toward the null value? *Am J Epidemiol* **132**, 746–748 (1990).

14

HF Epidemiologic Studies

Maria Feychting
Karolinska Institute

Martin Röösli
University of Basel

Joachim Schüz
International Agency for Research on Cancer

CONTENTS

14.1 Introduction

Before the introduction of mobile phone technology in the 1980s, exposures to radio frequency (RF) fields in the general population were rare and mostly limited to the very low fields from radio and television transmitters and a few occupational settings. Handheld mobile phones were introduced toward the end of the 1980s, and since then the number of people exposed to low-level RF fields has increased tremendously. The rapid increase in mobile phone use and other wireless technologies has led to a growing concern among the public about potential harmful effects of these exposures.

The scientifically established mechanism for interaction between RF fields and the human body is heating, and current exposure guidelines are set to protect from excessive heating of tissue [1,2]. For exposure levels below these guidelines, there is no generally accepted mechanism by which RF fields might cause health effects such as cancer or different types of symptoms. This chapter will review the epidemiological evidence regarding potential health effects of exposure to RF fields below current guidelines that cannot cause substantial heating of tissue.

14.2 General Aspects of Epidemiology

Epidemiological studies are important in health risk assessment; they study the effects of exposures under real circumstances and in the relevant host (humans) [3]. However, as for health risk assessment of long-term exposure, they are mostly observational, epidemiological studies also have some limitations; the most frequently discussed are the possibility of confounding, exposure misclassification, and selection bias. These problems can be handled more or less successfully, depending on how the study is designed and conducted. Generally, a cohort study with exposure information collected prior to disease occurrence or independently of study subjects is regarded as the superior study design, as it minimizes differential exposure misclassification, i.e., misclassification that is dependent on the disease and can lead to biased risk estimates. In studies of rare outcomes, however, very large cohorts are required, which limits the possibility to collect a very detailed exposure history. Further, the correlation between exposure to RF fields and the usage of various applications may be low to moderate and depend on many unknown contextual factors. Therefore, non-differential exposure misclassification can be a problem in cohort studies. Non-differential exposure misclassification can dilute risk estimates, should a true effect exist, and make it difficult to detect modest risk increases. In a cohort study, selection bias can be minimized if follow-up of the study participants can be achieved through population based health data registers.

In a case-control study, all cases of the disease should be identified from a defined population, and a sample of controls free from the disease randomly selected to represent the exposure distribution in this defined population. Generally, exposure information is collected after the occurrence of the disease. This makes case-control studies more prone to differential exposure misclassification, unless this information can be collected independently of study participants. Usually, however, exposure information in a case-control study is collected from cases and controls through questionnaires or interviews, relying on the participants' ability to correctly remember their past exposures many years back in time. If cases and controls differ in their ability to remember their exposures, differential exposure misclassification may occur, i.e., recall bias. A validation study comparing self-report with mobile phone operator data among participants of a multinational case-control study on mobile phone use and brain tumors (Interphone study), found that brain tumor patients tended to overestimate their mobile phone use more than controls for periods in the distant past [4], which could lead to an overestimation of the effect or spurious associations. In a case-control study, selection bias may occur if the population that generated the cases is not available for random sampling, i.e., in the absence of a population register. In such a situation, controls may be selected among other patients at the hospital, friends, or neighbors, raising questions as to their representativeness. Selection bias may also be caused by non-participation, if the likelihood of participation is related to both the exposure and the disease. Such selection bias through non-participation was identified in the above-mentioned Interphone study insofar that among controls regular mobile phone users turned out to be under-represented, as was found with the use of short non-responder questionnaires, thereby creating a spurious inverse association with regular mobile phone use [5].

A third study design, cross-sectional studies, has generally all the limitations of a case-control study; in addition to this, it is based on prevalent cases of the disease, which makes it difficult to distinguish between cause and effect, as the time sequence of events cannot be determined. Cross-sectional studies are justified when investigating prevalent outcomes in relation to time invariant exposure.

Confounding can occur when a risk factor other than the studied exposure is related to both the exposure and the disease. To completely explain an observed association, in the sense that the confounder rather than the exposure can be considered as the cause of the association, a confounder needs to be strongly related to the exposure and at the same time have an association with the disease that is considerably stronger than the observed association between the studied exposure and the disease. As long as information has been collected about exposure to potential confounding factors, adjustments can be made in the analyses to reduce the effect of the confounders.

14.3 Exposure Sources

The general population is exposed to different sources of RF fields, but most common in the everyday environment are wireless communication applications such as mobile and cordless phones, broadcasting, or WLAN/WIFI. For these sources, a basic distinction must be made between devices used close to the body, resulting in a near field exposure situation, and sources, which operate away from the body, such as fixed site transmitters (far field or environmental exposure). RF from near field sources is coupling to the body and thus specific absorption rate (SAR, W/kg tissue weight) is most relevant exposure metric. For far field sources incident electrical field fields (V/m) or power flux density (W/m²) are the most common quantities to quantify exposure. Output power of fixed site transmitters is typically much higher than for devices operating close to the body. However, electric field strength decreases rapidly with distance (~1/x), which typically results in relatively low whole body exposure from environmental sources in contrast to much higher but highly localized exposure from devices operation close to body. A systematic review of measurement studies conducted in Europe between 2000 and 2015 concluded that typical exposure levels in homes are in the range of 0.1–0.4 V/m [6]. Outdoor levels in inhabited areas are mostly in the range of 0.3–0.7 V/m, and exposure levels in crowded public transportations are mainly around 0.5–1.0 V/m.

It is not trivial to compare environmental RF exposure with absorbed radiation from devices operating close to the body since this needs dosimetric calculations. For an average mobile and cordless phone user (5 min calling and 1 h internet use per day), approximately 90% of all RF absorbed by the body originates from near field sources [7]. For body parts closer to the emitting devices like the brain when calling, contribution from near field sources is even higher.

Beside wireless communication, RF exposure occurs in various industries, military, and medical facilities, for instance from RF PVC welding machines, plasma etching, radar systems, diathermy, or MRI, all operating at different frequencies. A few occupational studies have been conducted in these workers.

In epidemiological studies, exact measurement of RF fields is often not possible, as the measurement methods are too laborious and costly for large study populations, and it is most often past exposures that count when investigating occurrence of today's diseases. Hence, exposure proxies were developed and improved over time, with those being applicable are those shown in validation studies to have sufficient correlation between the proxy and measured values. For earlier studies of mobile phone use, cumulative call time was shown to be a good predictor of exposure [8], but with more recent technologies this becomes more questionable due to the lower output power of the handset compared to environmental sources, the use of various networks with different power adaption of mobile phones, and the changing usage patterns of holding the phone less to your head but watching the screen. Exposure from environmental sources was more difficult to predict as distance from transmitter worked only for some types of major broadcast towers serving very large areas [9], but not for instance for mobile phone base stations [10]. Prediction of exposure from RF modeling has since then been a research field of its own [11].

14.4 Cancer

14.4.1 Brain Tumors and Mobile Phone Use

Mobile phone use is an important source of localized RF exposure to the head when the phone is held to the ear. Therefore, epidemiologic research on the potential carcinogenicity of RF fields from mobile phones has mainly focused on tumors in the head, primarily brain tumors (glioma, meningioma, and acoustic neuroma). The number of studies in this area has increased considerably during the last decades, and several national and international bodies regularly review the scientific evidence, for example the European Union Scientific Committee on Emerging and Newly Identified Health Risks (SCENIHR), Public Health England, and The Health Council of The Netherlands [12–14]. In 2011, the International Agency for Research on Cancer (IARC) classified RF fields as possibly carcinogenic to humans, based on limited evidence in humans from epidemiological case-control studies of mobile phone use and limited evidence from animal studies [15]. The Public Health England independent advisory group on non-ionizing radiation concluded in 2012 that the evidence was accumulating "in the direction toward no material effect of exposure" [12]. Based on additional evidence, SCENIHR noted in 2015 that the evidence for an effect on glioma had become weaker since the IARC evaluation [14], and the Health Council of the Netherlands concluded in 2016 that it is "unlikely that exposure to radiofrequency fields, which is associated with the use of mobile telephones, causes cancer" [13].

Different indicators of RF exposure from mobile phones have been used in the epidemiological studies, as introduced above. The most commonly used exposure estimate has been time since first starting to use a mobile phone, allowing consideration of different induction periods, but with no information on exposure intensity. To also take the amount of mobile phone use into account, case-control studies have included questions about the number and duration of calls, and constructed summary exposure estimates such as cumulative hours of use throughout the user's lifetime and cumulative number of calls.

Most of the epidemiological studies have not indicated an increased risk of glioma, meningioma, or acoustic neuroma associated with time since first mobile phone use. None of the cohort studies with prospectively collected exposure information have found indications of an increased risk, including exposure durations of more than 13 years among >350,000 mobile phone subscribers in Denmark [16,17], and more than 10 years among almost 800,000 women in the UK [18,19]. Most case-control studies also do not report associations with time since first use, including also studies that cover more than 10 years duration of mobile phone use; for a detailed review, see for example references [12,14]. Time since first starting mobile phone use is a rather crude measure of exposure, as it does not take amount of phone use into consideration. The cohort studies have not had access to information about amount of mobile phone use [16,17] or used only a crude measure, daily use, which was not related to tumor risk [18]. The amount of phone use is available in most of the case-control studies, but relies on retrospective self-report, vulnerable to recall bias. Again, many case-control studies have not observed associations between amount of mobile phone use and brain tumor risk [14,15], but there are some exceptions. The Interphone study, a 13 country international collaborative case-control study, observed an increased risk of glioma in the 10th decile of cumulative hours of phone use (≥1640 h) compared to non-regular users (OR=1.40; 95% CI 1.03–1.89), whereas no trend in risk was observed over the first nine exposure categories, and the OR in the 9th decile (735–1639 h) was 0.71 (95% CI 0.53–0.96), one of the lowest risk estimates observed [20]. A similar pattern of results was observed for acoustic neuroma [21], while for meningioma, the OR was 1.15 (95% CI 0.81–1.62) in the 10th decile and 0.76 (0.54–1.08) in the 9th decile. A much smaller French study reported an increased risk of both glioma and meningioma among the heaviest mobile phone users [22], defined as ≥896 cumulative hours, an amount of use that essentially captures both the 9th and 10th deciles in the Interphone study [20]. In addition, the risk estimates were considerably higher than in the Interphone study; OR = 2.89 (95% CI 1.41–5.93) for glioma and 2.57 (95% CI 1.02–6.44) for meningioma; thus, these findings are not compatible with the results of the Interphone study, nor with observed incidence trends (see below).

A series of case-control studies in Sweden found risk increases after only a few years of mobile phone use and also reported increased risks starting with relatively low amounts of mobile phone use [23,24]. Categorizing cumulative hours of phone use into quartiles, this group observed increased risks of glioma and acoustic neuroma in all four quartiles of use compared to non-users, with 30% higher risk of glioma and 60% higher risk of acoustic neuroma after a total of 1–122 h of mobile phone use. In the 25% of mobile phone users who had used the mobile phone the most (>1,486 h), an OR of 2.2 (95% CI 1.7–2.9) for glioma and 2.6 (95% CI 1.5–4.4) for acoustic neuroma was observed.

These last results appear implausible for several reasons. First, they report raised risk estimates already after a short exposure duration, e.g., within 5 years since starting mobile phone use for glioma and acoustic neuroma [24,25]. Acoustic neuroma is a slow-growing tumor, likely to have been present several years before being diagnosed, making it likely that tumors were already present when short-term users started their mobile phone use [26]. In addition, the highest glioma risk estimate was reported for persons who started to use a mobile phone before they turned 20-years old (the odds ratio (OR) was 1.80; 95% CI 1.2–2.8) [24]. None of these results are compatible with incidence trends for these tumors from simulation studies, which have modeled the expected change in glioma incidence over time under assumptions that mobile phone use increases the risk of glioma as reported by a few case-control studies, and compared this to observed incidence rates [27,28]. They have demonstrated that risk increases after a few years and up to more than 10 years of mobile phone use are incompatible with the observed, stable, incidence trends.

Taking all the evidence together, it is safe to conclude that moderate use of mobile phones does not pose an increased risk of brain tumors. For heavy mobile phone use or very rare tumor types, few and inconsistent data are available, and a modest risk increase cannot be entirely excluded, although it is becoming less likely with accumulating years of not seeing any increase in the incidence rates for glioma and acoustic neuroma. For glioma, a usually fast-growing tumor, observation time is believed to be sufficiently long, and glioma incidence rates worldwide are still stable in the age groups of most frequent mobile phone use [27–30]. Acoustic neuroma is a slow-growing tumor, and one would not expect an effect on the tumor occurrence after a short latency period. While this makes observed risk increases for acoustic neuroma implausible and likely to be the result of bias, there is a lack of high quality data with a sufficiently long induction period.

Fewer studies were conducted on other tumors. Among those were salivary gland tumors, pituitary gland tumors, leukemia, uveal, and skin melanoma, and non-Hodgkin lymphoma, for which RF exposure from mobile phone may be relevant. However, these studies provided little indications for an effect [14,15].

14.4.2 Cancer and Environmental RF Fields

Members of the public are concerned about RF fields from transmitters due to the involuntary nature of exposure, even though exposure levels are lower than those to the head from using a mobile phone. Several cancer clusters have been reported in the vicinity of individual transmitters, but those are not informative since, due to the large numbers of transmitters and to cancer being a relatively common disease, a large number of those clusters are expected to occur by chance. No single in-depth investigation of any such cluster has provided additional insight into the causes of its occurrence. Several population based studies looked at childhood cancer in relation to calculated field strengths from high output power radio and TV broadcast transmitters [31,32] and in relation to mobile phone base stations [33]. These found some evidence against an association between childhood leukemia and brain tumors related to exposure, based on altogether large numbers of children. Less systematic studies have been conducted for adult cancers.

14.5 Neurodegenerative Disease

Risk of neurodegenerative disease was studied in relation to extremely low-frequency electric and magnetic fields, mainly at the workplace, but much less often for RF fields. In a Danish cohort study, for neurodegenerative disease, hospitalizations for a variety of diseases occurring before the end of 2002 among 420,000 subscribers of a mobile phone were compared to the number of hospitalizations observed in the remaining general public (approximately 3.6 million Danes) during the same time period [34]. Overall, the number of subscriber hospitalizations for Alzheimer's disease was statistically significantly lower than expected from the respective rates of the general population. No association was seen for amyotrophic lateral sclerosis (ALS). Significantly lower rates of hospitalizations were also observed for vascular dementia and Parkinson's disease. The reduced rates of patients with Alzheimer's disease or Parkinson's disease seen following a short subscription time is likely to be reversed causation, i.e., that persons with early symptoms of those diseases were less likely to subscribe for a mobile phone. Interestingly, a reduced relative risk estimate for Alzheimer's disease but not Parkinson's disease was also seen among those subscribers who had their mobile phone for 10+ years, which is unlikely to be solely attributable to such prodromal symptoms. No association was seen with multiple sclerosis, but presenting symptoms differed between mobile phone subscribers and the comparison group [35]. Mobile phone subscribers had more hospitalizations for migraine, but reverse causation may be an explanation [34].

14.6 Symptoms, Behavior, and Cognitive Functions

A part of the population attributes non-specific symptoms such as sleep disorders, headache, and sensation of prickling and concentration difficulties to RF-EMF exposure in the everyday environment. Such self-attribution of symptoms to EMF is called electromagnetic hypersensitivity (EHS) or idiopathic environmental intolerance attributed to electromagnetic fields (IEI-EMF) [36]. Prevalence varies considerably between different studies and lies mostly between 1% and 15% [37]. Randomized, double blind provocation studies in well controlled laboratory conditions could not reveal any individual who reacts to RF fields below regulatory limits within a few minutes [38] or who were able to detect presence and absence of RF fields [39], although many individuals state an ability to do so [40]. However, several studies documented that nocebo is relevant in this context, meaning that people immediately react if they are convinced they are exposed to RF fields regardless of the true exposure status [38,41].

Long-term consequences of RF fields on health related quality of life needs to be investigated by observational epidemiological studies. Since EHS individuals are avoiding RF exposure, causal inference from observational research in this collective is problematic and most studies have been conducted in the general population. In relation to far field sources various early studies were of cross-sectional design and did not find indications for impaired health related quality of life if they used objective exposure measures [42]. These findings have been confirmed by recent longitudinal studies [43–47]. With respect to close-to-body sources, several studies reported associations, mainly for headache, in relation to self-reported mobile phone use [48–52]. However, reverse causality, selection bias, differential exposure misclassification and residual confounding is a concern for many of these findings and could not be confirmed in a study using objective operator recorded mobile phone use [44].

Mobile phone use has become an integral part of daily activities in children and adolescents, and thus potential effects from RF fields in this collective have received increased attention recently. Several studies found indications that quality of life and mental health is associated with certain aspects of mobile phone use, such as night-time use [53–57]. However, the few studies attempting to disentangle the various exposure aspects of mobile phone use provide little evidence that RF exposure is relevant in this context [58]. Similar conclusions can be drawn from various studies observing associations between behavioral problems and mobile phone use of children or adolescents [59,60]. Several birth cohort studies also reported an association of maternal mobile phone use during pregnancy and behavioral problems including attention deficits in their offspring during childhood [61]. However, it is unlikely and has not yet been proven that duration of maternal mobile phone use is correlated with RF exposure of fetuses and thus, confounding is a plausible explanation for the observed associations.

Numerous randomized, double blind human experimental studies addressed acute effects of RF fields on cognitive function and brain physiology with inconsistent findings for cognitive functions and fairly consistent effects on the electroencephalogram (EEG) during night [62,63]. Epidemiological research addressing long-term effects is scarce with sporadic associations reported for cognitive functions [60,64–68]. But again, disentangling RF exposure from other aspects of mobile phone use and its consequences for cognitive function is challenging and the underlying causal pattern of observed associations remains uncertain.

In relation to mobile phone use, reverse causality is of concern, which means that subjective health status and also behavioral problems may affect the amount of mobile phone use and not vice versa. For instance, the decision to use a mobile phone may depend on the cognitive performance (in the form of reverse causality). This is expected to be particularly relevant for the uptake of mobile phone use in the elderly generation. It is also conceivable that using a mobile phone might have a training effect on cognitive performance, independent of any radiation effect. Further, some common latent variables (confounders) may affect both quality of life and use of mobile phone or other life-style related RF-EMF sources (cordless phones, WLAN). Further, these mobile phone studies almost exclusively rely on self-reported exposure data, which makes them vulnerable to reporting bias or nocebo effects, especially since the outcomes are also self-reported. The nocebo effect is the inverse of the placebo effect and means that adverse symptoms occur due to expectations (e.g., due to concerns). Human experimental research has consistently demonstrated the occurrence of nocebo phenomena in EMF research [38,39]. With respect to far-field sources, exposure assessment is a challenge. The first studies used self-reported distance to the closest base-station as an exposure proxy, but it is now well established that such an exposure measure is not correlated to RF exposure and likely to be biased [10,11]. This is due to the fact that persons who are worried about base stations tend to underestimate the distance compared to persons without such worries [69]. Selection bias, reporting bias and nocebo phenomena are of concern if people are aware of their exposure status, which is typically the case for large transmitters where exposure levels tend to be associated with distance to the source [70,71]. For measured RF fields from base stations and other small transmitters, exposure pattern is more complex and thus exposure is not related to distance [10], making nocebo and reporting bias in general less of a problem. Conversely, this implies that associations between distance to such sources and symptoms cannot be due to RF exposure. A particular challenge for studies dealing with environmental RF is the fact that these sources contribute only minimally to overall cumulative RF exposure compared to RF from devices used close to body. However, the latter is not considered in many of these environmental RF studies, which is expected to produce substantial exposure misclassification. Reverse causality is expected to play a minor role for these studies on far-field EMF sources since they are not related to life style.

14.7 Conclusions

Most epidemiological studies were conducted on the possible relationship between the use of mobile phones and the risk of different types of both benign as well as malignant brain tumors. Two large-scale cohort studies and the most comprehensive multinational case-control study, including various validation studies, are consistent insofar that they showed no association with up to around 15 years of use or moderate use of mobile phones. While the cohort studies showed no effect overall, the case-control study showed a modest ~40% risk increase for glioma and acoustic neuroma among the very heaviest users, an effect that may have been missed by the cohorts due to their cruder exposure assessment. Incidence time trends from the Nordic countries, the United States, Australia, and the United Kingdom add to the evidence against any major effect. Some case-control studies reporting large effects are incompatible with the lack of any resulting epidemic of the diseases, therefore their effect estimates appear to be massively inflated and the studies are noninformative for any health risk assessment. Fewer studies are available for other cancers or for neurodegenerative disease. RF fields from transmitters have been only systematically studied for childhood cancer, with several large-scale studies not finding an association. There is no convincing evidence that RF exposure is related to any symptoms, behavior, and cognitive functions, with the nocebo effect as the most likely explanation for some of the positive symptom findings and confounding as the most likely explanation for behavioral effects. Few data are available on long-term consequences from the technologies, as exposure of large segments of the population remains a relatively recent phenomenon. From the epidemiological side, surveillance studies such as prospective cohorts are therefore indicated, which follow developments in a changing world of exposure and have the ability to address a variety of outcomes; the largest ongoing study in this regard is the multinational cohort Cosmos [72,73].

References

1. ICNIRP. Guidelines for limiting exposure to time-varying electric, magnetic, and electromagnetic fields (up to 300 GHz). International Commission on Non-Ionizing Radiation Protection. *Health Phys* 1998; 74(4):494–522.
2. IEEE. Std C95.1–2005. IEEE standard for safety levels with respect to human exposure to radio frequency electromagnetic fields, 100 kHz-300 GHz. 2005.
3. Schüz J, Berg-Beckhoff G, Schlehofer B, Blettner M. The role of epidemiology in cancer risk assessment of non-ionising radiation. In: Obe G, Jandrig B, Marchant GE, Schütz H, Wiedemann PM (Eds.) *Cancer Risk Evaluation: Methods and Trends*. Weinheim: Wiley-Blackwell; 2011.
4. Vrijheid M, Armstrong BK, Bedard D, Brown J, Deltour I, Iavarone I, et al., Recall bias in the assessment of exposure to mobile phones. *J Expo Sci Environ Epidemiol* 2009; 19(4):369–381.
5. Vrijheid M, Richardson L, Armstrong BK, Auvinen A, Berg G, Carroll M, et al., Quantifying the impact of selection bias caused by nonparticipation in a case-control study of mobile phone use. *Ann Epidemiol* 2009; 19:33–41.
6. Sagar S, Dongus D, Schoeni A, Roser K, Eeftens M, Struchen B, et al., Radiofrequency electromagnetic field exposure in everyday microenvironments in Europe: A systematic literature review. *J Expo Science Environ Epidemiol* 2017; 28(2):147–160. DOI:10.1038/jes.2017.13.
7. Roser K, Schoeni A, Struchen B, Zahner M, Eeftens M, Fröhlich J, et al., Personal radiofrequency electromagnetic field exposure measurements in Swiss adolescents. *Environ Int* 2017; 99:303–314. DOI:10.1016/j.envint.2016.12.008.
8. Vrijheid M, Cardis E, Armstrong BK, Auvinen A, Berg G, Blaasaas KG, et al., Validation of short term recall of mobile phone use for the Interphone study. *Occup Environ Med* 2006; 63:237–243.
9. Schmiedel S, Brüggemeyer H, Philipp J, Wendler J, Merzenich H, Schüz J. An evaluation of exposure metrics in an epidemiologic study on radio and television broadcast transmitters and the risk of childhood leukemia. *Bioelectromagnetics* 2009; 30:81–91.
10. Frei P, Mohler E, Bürgi A, Fröhlich J, Neubauer G, Braun-Fahrländer C, et al., Classification of personal exposure to radio frequency electromagnetic fields (RF-EMF) for epidemiological research: Evaluation of different exposure assessment methods. *Environ Int* 2010; 36(7):714–720.
11. Neubauer G, Feychting M, Hamnerius Y, Kheifets L, Kuster N, Ruiz I, et al., Feasibility of future epidemiological studies on possible health effects of mobile phone base stations. *Bioelectromagnetics* 2007; 28:224–230.
12. AGNIR. Health effects from radiofrequency electromagnetic fields. Report from the Independent Advisory Group on Non-Ionising Radiation. Documents of the Health Protection Agency, Radiation, Chemical and Environmental Hazards. RCE 20, Health Protection Agency, UK. 2012.

13. Health Council of the Netherlands. Mobile phones and cancer. Part 3. Update and overall conclusions from epidemiological and animal studies. No. 2016/06, The Hague. 2016.

14. SCENIHR. Scientific Committee on Emerging and newly identified health risks: Potential health effects of exposure to electromagnetic fields (EMF): http://ec.europa.eu/health/scientific_committees/emerging/docs/scenihr_o_041.pdf, Accessed 15 Aug 2015. 2015.

15. International Agency for Research on Cancer (IARC). *Non-Ionizing Radiation. Part 2, Radiofrequency Electromagnetic Fields. IARC Monographs on the Evaluation of Carcinogenic Risks to Humans.* Lyon: International Agency for Research on Cancer; 2013.

16. Frei P, Poulsen AH, Johansen C, Olsen JH, Steding-Jessen M, Schüz J. Use of mobile phones and risk of brain tumours: update of Danish cohort study. *BMJ* 2011; 343:d6387.

17. Schüz J, Steding-Jessen M, Hansen S, Stangerup SE, Caye-Thomasen P, Poulsen AH, et al., Long-term mobile phone use and the risk of vestibular schwannoma: a Danish nationwide cohort study. *Am J Epidemiol* 2011; 174(4):416–422.

18. Benson VS, Pirie K, Schüz J, Reeves GK, Beral V, Green J. Mobile phone use and risk of brain neoplasms and other cancers: prospective study. *Int J Epidemiol* 2013; 42(3):792–802.

19. Benson VS, Pirie K, Schüz J, Reeves GK, Beral V, Green J. Authors' response to: The case of acoustic neuroma: comment on mobile phone use and risk of brain neoplasms and other cancers. *Int J Epidemiol* 2013; 43(1):275. DOI:10.1093/ije/dyt186.

20. Interphone Study Group. Brain tumour risk in relation to mobile telephone use: results of the INTERPHONE international case-control study. *Int J Epidemiol* 2010; 39(3):675–694.

21. Interphone Study Group. Acoustic neuroma risk in relation to mobile telephone use: results of the INTERPHONE international case-control study. *Cancer Epidemiol* 2011; 35(5):453–464.

22. Coureau G, Bouvier G, Lebailly P, Fabbro-Peray P, Gruber A, Leffondre K, et al., Mobile phone use and brain tumours in the CERENAT case-control study. *Occup Environ Med* 2014; 71(7):514–522. DOI:10.1136/oemed–2013-101754.

23. Hardell L, Carlberg M, Soderqvist F, Mild KH. Case-control study of the association between malignant brain tumours diagnosed between 2007 and 2009 and mobile and cordless phone use. *Int J Oncol* 2013; 43(6):1833–1845.

24. Hardell L, Carlberg M. Mobile phone and cordless phone use and the risk for glioma - Analysis of pooled case-control studies in Sweden, 1997–2003 and 2007–2009. *Pathophysiology* 2015; 22(1):1–13.

25. Hardell L, Carlberg M, Soderqvist F, Mild KH. Pooled analysis of case-control studies on acoustic neuroma diagnosed 1997–2003 and 2007–2009 and use of mobile and cordless phones. *Int J Oncol* 2013; 43(4):1036–1044.

26. Thomsen J, Tos M. Acoustic neuroma: clinical aspects, audiovestibular assessment, diagnostic delay, and growth rate. *Am J Otol* 1990; 11(1):12–19.

27. Deltour I, Auvinen A, Feychting M, Johansen C, Klaeboe L, Sankila R, et al., Mobile phone use and incidence of glioma in the Nordic countries 1979–2008: consistency check. *Epidemiology* 2012; 23(2):301–307.

28. Little MP, Rajaraman P, Curtis RE, Devesa SS, Inskip PD, Check DP, et al., Mobile phone use and glioma risk: comparison of epidemiological study results with incidence trends in the United States. *BMJ* 2012; 344:e1147.

29. Larjavaara S, Feychting M, Sankila R, Johansen C, Klaeboe L, Schüz J, et al., Incidence trends of vestibular schwannomas in Denmark, Finland, Norway and Sweden in 1987–2007. *Br J Cancer* 2011; 105(7):1069–1075.

30. Chapman S, Azizi L, Luo Q, Sitas F. Has the incidence of brain cancer risen in Australia since the introduction of mobile phones 29 years ago? *Cancer Epidemiol* 2016; 42:199–205.

31. Schüz J, Ahlbom A. Exposure to electromagnetic fields and the risk of childhood leukaemia: a review. *Radiat Prot Dosimetry* 2008; 132:202–211.

32. Hauri DD, Spycher B, Huss A, Zimmermann F, Grotzer M, von der Weid N, et al., Exposure to radio-frequency electromagnetic fields from broadcast transmitters and risk of childhood cancer: a census-based cohort study. *Am J Epidemiol* 2014; 179(7):843–851.

33. Elliott P, Toledano MB, Bennett J, Beale L, de Hoogh K, Best N, Briggs DJ. Mobile phone base stations and early childhood cancers: case-control study. *BMJ* 2010; 340:c3077.

34. Schüz J, Waldemar G, Olsen JH, Johansen C. Risk for central nervous system diseases among mobile phone subscribers: a Danish retrospective cohort study. *PLoS One* 2009; 4:e4389.
35. Poulsen AH, Stenager E, Johansen C, Bentzen J, Friis S, Schüz J. Mobile phones and Multiple sclerosis – a nationwide cohort study in Denmark. *PLoS One* 2012; 7:e34453.
36. WHO. Fact sheet 296: Electromagnetic fields and public health - Electromagnetic Hypersensitivity. www.who.int/mediacentre/factsheets/fs296/en/index.html. Accessed 3 Aug, 2017. 2005.
37. Baliatsas C, Van Kamp I, Lebret E, Rubin GJ. Idiopathic environmental intolerance attributed to electromagnetic fields (IEI-EMF): A systematic review of identifying criteria. *BMC Public Health* 2012; 12:643.
38. Rubin GJ, Nieto-Hernandez R, Wessely S. Idiopathic environmental intolerance attributed to electromagnetic fields (formerly 'electromagnetic hypersensitivity'): An updated systematic review of provocation studies. *Bioelectromagnetics* 2011; 31(1):1–11.
39. Röösli M. Radiofrequency electromagnetic field exposure and non-specific symptoms of ill health: A systematic review. *Environ Res* 2008; 107(2):277–287.
40. Röösli M, Moser M, Baldinini Y, Meier M, Braun-Fahrländer C. Symptoms of ill health ascribed to electromagnetic field exposure—a questionnaire survey. *Int J Hyg Environ Health* 2004; 207(2):141–150.
41. Baliatsas C, Van Kamp I, Bolte J, Schipper M, Yzermans J, Lebret E Non-specific physical symptoms and electromagnetic field exposure in the general population: Can we get more specific? A systematic review. *Environ Int* 2012; 41:15–28.
42. Röösli M, Frei P, Mohler E, Hug K. Systematic review on the health effects of exposure to radiofrequency electromagnetic fields from mobile phone base stations. *Bull World Health Organ* 2010; 88(12):887–896.
43. Baliatsas C, van Kamp I, Bolte J, Kelfkens G, van Dijk C, Spreeuwenberg P, et al., Clinically defined non-specific symptoms in the vicinity of mobile phone base stations: A retrospective before-after study. *Sci Total Environ* 2016; 565:714–720.
44. Frei P, Mohler E, Braun-Fahrländer C, Fröhlich J, Neubauer G, Röösli M. Cohort study on the effects of everyday life radio frequency electromagnetic field exposure on non-specific symptoms and tinnitus. *Environ Int* 2012; 38(1):29–36.
45. Schoeni A, Roser K, Bürgi A, Röösli M. Symptoms in Swiss adolescents in relation to exposure from fixed site transmitters: A prospective cohort study. *Environ Health* 2016; 15(1):77.
46. Martens AL, Slottje P, Timmermans DRM, Kromhout H, Reedijk M, Vermeulen RCH, et al., Modeled and perceived exposure to radiofrequency electromagnetic fields from mobile-phone base stations and the development of symptoms over time in a general population cohort. *Am J Epidemiol* 2017; 186(2):210–219.
47. Mohler E, Frei P, Braun-Fahrländer C, Fröhlich J, Röösli M. Exposure to radiofrequency electromagnetic fields and sleep quality: A prospective cohort study. *PLoS One* 2012; 7(5): e37455.
48. Chia SE, Chia HP, Tan JS. Prevalence of headache among handheld cellular telephone users in Singapore: A community study. *Environ Health Perspect* 2000; 108(11):1059.
49. Cho YM, Lim HJ, Jang H, Kim K, Choi JW, Shin C, et al., A follow-up study of the association between mobile phone use and symptoms of ill health. *Environ Health Toxicol* 2016; 32:e2017001.
50. Cho YM, Lim HJ, Jang H, Kim K, Choi JW, Shin C, et al., A cross-sectional study of the association between mobile phone use and symptoms of ill health. *Environ Health Toxicol* 2016; 31:e2016022.
51. Oftedal G, Wilen J, Sandstrom M, Mild KH. Symptoms experienced in connection with mobile phone use. *Occup Med Lond* 2000; 50(4):237.
52. Thomee S, Harenstam A, Hagberg M. Mobile phone use and stress, sleep disturbances, and symptoms of depression among young adults—a prospective cohort study. *BMC Public Health* 2011; 11:66.
53. Schoeni A, Roser K, Röösli M. Symptoms and cognitive functions in adolescents in relation to mobile phone use during night. *PLoS One* 2015; 10(7):e0133528.
54. Van den Bulck J. Adolescent use of mobile phones for calling and for sending text messages after lights out: Results from a prospective cohort study with a one-year follow-up. *Sleep* 2007; 30(9):1220–1223.

55. Söderqvist F, Carlberg M, Hardell L. Use of wireless telephones and self-reported health symptoms: A population-based study among Swedish adolescents aged 15–19 years. *Environ Health* 2008; 7:18.

56. Redmayne M, Smith E, Abramson MJ. The relationship between adolescents' well-being and their wireless phone use: A cross-sectional study. *Environ Health* 2013; 12:90.

57. Huss A, van Eijsden M, Guxens M, Beekhuizen J, van Strien R, Kromhout H, et al., Environmental radiofrequency electromagnetic fields exposure at home, mobile and cordless phone use, and sleep problems in 7-year-old children. *PLoS One* 2015; 10(10):e0139869.

58. Schoeni A, Roser K, Röösli M. Symptoms and the use of wireless communication devices: A prospective cohort study in Swiss adolescents. *Environ Res* 2017; 154:275–283.

59. Divan HA, Kheifets L, Obel C, Olsen J. Cell phone use and behavioural problems in young children. *J Epidemiol Community Health.* 2012; 66(6):524–529.

60. Roser K, Schoeni A, Röösli M. Mobile phone use, behavioural problems and concentration capacity in adolescents: A prospective study. *Int J Hygiene Environ Health* 2016; 219(8):759–769. DOI:10.1016/j.ijheh.2016.08.007.

61. Birks L, Guxens M, Papadopoulou E, Alexander J, Ballester F, Estarlich M, et al., Maternal cell phone use during pregnancy and child behavioral problems in five birth cohorts. *Environ Int* 2017; 104:122–131.

62. Regel SJ, Achermann P. Cognitive performance measures in bioelectromagnetic research—critical evaluation and recommendations. *Environ Health* 2011; 10(1):10.

63. Kwon MS, Hamalainen H. Effects of mobile phone electromagnetic fields: Critical evaluation of behavioral and neurophysiological studies. *Bioelectromagnetics* 2011; 32(4):253–272.

64. Abramson MJ, Benke GP, Dimitriadis C, Inyang IO, Sim MR, Wolfe RS, et al., Mobile telephone use is associated with changes in cognitive function in young adolescents. *Bioelectromagnetics* 2009; 30(8):678–686.

65. Guxens M, Vermeulen R, van Eijsden M, Beekhuizen J, Vrijkotte TG, van Strien RT, et al., Outdoor and indoor sources of residential radiofrequency electromagnetic fields, personal cell phone and cordless phone use, and cognitive function in 5–6 years old children. *Environ Res* 2016; 150:364–374.

66. Redmayne M, Smith CL, Benke G, Croft RJ, Dalecki A, Dimitriadis C, et al., Use of mobile and cordless phones and cognition in Australian primary school children: A prospective cohort study. *Environ Health* 2016; 15:26.

67. Thomas S, Benke B, Dimitriadis C. Use of mobile phones and changes in cognitive function in adolescents. *Occup Environ Med* 2010; 67(12):861–866.

68. Schoeni A, Roser K, Röösli M. Memory performance, wireless communication and exposure to radiofrequency electromagnetic fields: A prospective cohort study in adolescents. *Environ Int* 2015; 85:343–351.

69. Blettner M, Schlehofer B, Breckenkamp J, Kowall B, Schmiedel S, Reis U, et al., Mobile phone base stations and adverse health effects: A population-based cross-sectional study in Germany. *Occup Environ Med* 2009; 66:118–123.

70. Abelin T., Altpeter E., Röösli M. Sleep disturbances in the vicinity of the short-save broadcast transmitter. *Schwarzenburg. Somnologie,* 2005; 9:203–209.

71. Preece AW, Georgiou AG, Dunn EJ, Farrow SC. Health response of two communities to military antennae in Cyprus. *Occup Environ Med* 2007; 64(6):402–408.

72. Schüz J, Elliott P, Auvinen A, Kromhout H, Poulsen AH, Johansen C, et al., An international prospective cohort study of mobile phone users and health (Cosmos): Design considerations and enrolment. *Cancer Epidemiol* 2011; 35:37–43.

73. Toledano MB, Auvinen A, Tettamanti G, Cao Y, Feychting M, Ahlbom A, et al., An international prospective cohort study of mobile phone users and health (COSMOS): Factors affecting validity of self-reported mobile phone use. *Int J Hyg Environ Health* 2018; 221(1):1–8.

15

Behavioral and Cognitive Effects of Electromagnetic Field Exposure

Andrew W. Wood
Swinburne University of Technology
RMIT University

Sarah P. Loughran
University of Wollongong

CONTENTS

15.1 Introduction

This chapter will consider effects that electromagnetic fields (EMFs), in the frequency range up to 300 GHz and including static fields, can and do have on behavior and cognition. Although the focus is on effects in humans, where relevant, we will also consider effects on animal species. If the effects are an impairment, then the significance in terms of reduced efficiency in cognitive tasks (such as decision-making, recall of vital information, alteration of eye-hand coordination or distraction) can all lead to potentially hazardous situations if high precision is called for in these tasks. For example, specialist surgeons now routinely operate within the bore of magnetic resonance imaging (MRI) magnets and are exposed to a variety of strong magnetic fields. It is essential to assess possible influences on performance.

The status of the bioeffects reviewed in this chapter varies widely. At one end of this range, there are those effects for which there is sufficient experimental evidence from a variety of investigations, backed up with credible biophysical mechanisms to afford them the status of established science. At the other end, there are those for which the evidence is incomplete or conflicting and the biophysical mechanism either completely lacking or unconvincing (at least, to the majority of scientists working in the area). The bioeffects considered can also be divided firstly into those resulting from possible effects on *sensory* systems (such as magneto- and electro-sensation) and secondly into those following on from "direct" stimulation of the central nervous system (CNS) or peripheral nervous system (PNS). In cases where cognitive processes are affected by blood-borne hormones, possible EMF effects on secretion patterns will also be included. Finally, there is a proportion of the population which attributes a cluster of diverse and debilitating symptoms (some behavioral) to being exposed to EMFs. The strength and coherence of evidence for this "self-ascribed electro-hypersensitivity" or "idiopathic environmental intolerance attributed to EMF" (IEI-EMF) will also be reviewed.

15.2 Exposure to Static Fields

Humans are chronically exposed to the Earth's (static) magnetic field, of around 50 µT, but are occasionally exposed to fields up to 8 T in diagnostic MRI facilities. Likewise, before thunderstorms, humans are exposed to static electric fields of up to 40 kV/m (WHO 2007) and will occasionally experience spark discharges from car doors or items of furniture. For a spark to form, a field in excess of 3 MV/m must exist for "dielectric breakdown" to occur. Since spark discharges constitute an annoyance, and because performance could be affected due to the surprise element, the avoidance of these form part of the formulation of basic restrictions for ac power delivery exposures. Since spark discharges are also associated with dc power systems, behavioral effects of static electric fields are dealt with in this section.

15.2.1 Static Electric Field Exposures

The effects of strong static electric fields on the human body are summarized in Karipids (2017). The spark discharges just referred to can arise from contact with nearby isolated conductors, which have accumulated charge by their position in the electric field. Alternatively, a person, when isolated from the ground, can accumulate a charge. This can give rise to a spark discharge when the person touches a grounded object (an example is someone working on a roof near to a dc transmission line touching a metal gutter or downpipe). Since the local electric field distribution is very sensitive to nearby objects, it is often hard to predict where and when these "microshocks" can occur. Sensations can vary from perception (via movement of skin hairs) through to pain and burn, depending on the magnitude of the field. Since these sensations can be unpleasant and unexpected, the main behavioral effects are aversion or overcompensation and the potential distraction can conceivably lead to poorer performance in precision tasks. Further analysis can be found in ICNIRP (2003), International Commission on Non-Ionizing Radiation Protection (2009), and Repacholi and Greenebaum (1999). Possible effects of environmentally relevant static electric fields on humans and vertebrates have recently been reviewed (Petri et al. 2017), with an overall conclusion that any effects on physiological functions are a consequence of hair and skin sensations.

15.2.2 Electroreception

In terms of predatory behavior of certain fish species, the ability to sense electric fields is particularly important. For example, electroreceptors in elasmobranch fish are able to sense static fields of 5×10^{-7} V/m (Kalmijn 2000). Many species are able to detect prey on based on disturbances in the electric fields sensed, but the so-called "electric fish" such as the rays and gymnotid fish, are able to stun prey via electric organ discharge (see Scheich (1983) for a review). More recent work has shown that in addition to vertebrate fish, invertebrate crayfish also possess electrosensory ability (Patullo and Macmillan 2010). In fact, among mammals, platypuses (Pettigrew 1999) and dolphins (Czech-Damal et al. 2012) show electroreception, with the former using flicking motion of the bill (on which the receptors reside) to create directional and distance information. Electroreception appears to rely on specialized, modified, hair cells at the bottom of deep pits (ampullae), filled with either conductive gel (as in the case of ampullae of Lorenzini) or "plug cells" (tuberous receptors). Those in the dolphin (which are closest to the human) are of the latter type and show sensitivity of around 5 mV/m, and the former show AC sensitivity up to 30 Hz. Humans do not appear to have any organs within the skin analogous to these electroreceptor organs.

The mechanism underlying the extreme sensitivity has been extensively researched, the amplification from μV changes in the ampulla epithelium to the mV changes required to modulate ion channel conductances (and hence neurotransmitter release) appears to be accomplished by a combination of effects. These include spatial and temporal integration of potential shifts and the phenomenon of opposing Ca^{++} and Cl^- channel characteristics, giving rise to oscillations in basal membrane voltage, in turn modulating neurotransmitter release (Lu and Fishman 1995a,b, Pickard 1988).

A number of investigators have studied animal behavior, using strong static electric field exposure, similar to that associated with high-voltage dc transmission systems. For example, Xu et al. (2016) studied the ability of mice to locate a hidden platform (Morris water maze) after several weeks of exposure to fields from actual power lines. When tested after 34 days of exposure, the mice exposed to the higher level of fields (9–22 kV/m) showed reduced ability to recall the location of the platform. However, no allowance was made for multiple comparisons, so this finding must be regarded as exploratory at this stage. At the highest field level, the fields induced within mouse tissue will be of the order of 20–50 nV/m (Polk and Postow 1996). Tissue fields of approximately 10^9 times this value are known to affect the growth of axons (McCaig et al. 2005) and occur naturally in the process of wound healing (Nuccitelli 2003). More recent work has suggested that charged polyamines could redistribute in impressed fields (above 100 V/m), which could then bind to proteins involved in the regulation of K^+ fluxes (Levin 2014a,b, Nakajima et al. 2015).

In humans, effects on the vestibular system have been demonstrated (Fitzpatrick et al. 1994). In this study, direct currents of >0.5 mA applied via electrodes 6–8 cm² in area proved sufficient to cause balance disruption. This represents a current density of the order of 1 A/m², which would induce a tissue electric field of ~5 V/m dc, assuming a mean conductivity of 0.2 S/m. This would require external electric fields in excess of 1 MV/m to induce internal fields of this magnitude. Magnetically induced vertigo, however, is caused by a different phenomenon and is discussed in the next section.

15.2.3 Effects of Static Magnetic Field Exposures

In medical imaging, humans are being exposed to progressively higher field strengths. Since functional MRI (fMRI) is increasingly used as a tool in experimental neuroscience, it is important to know whether the tool itself could be influencing the cognitive effects being studied. As indicated above, patients/participants are exposed to up to 8 T static fields with high time-varying spatial gradients (in addition to radiofrequency fields). An early study of cardiac and cognitive endpoints (Kangarlu et al. 1999) did not reveal any significant effects of 8 T for up to 3 h. Similarly, in a study of stray fields from a 7 T magnet affecting workers (de Vocht et al. 2007), no major effects on memory were noted, but effects on visual perception and hand-eye co-ordination were reported, at stray static fields above 1.6 T in magnitude. However, it was not possible to identify whether these changes were due to the static field, to time changing fields or switched gradient fields. In addition to discrete studies, there have been a number of reviews of possible cognitive effects of strong static MRI fields (Heinrich et al. 2011, Nolte et al. 1998, Weiss et al. 1992). The latter is a meta-analysis of seven studies, which although reporting a significant impairment in the category "neuropsychology" (combining reaction time; visual system; hand-eye coordination and working memory) also showed significant heterogeneity in the studies considered. The overall conclusion was that firm statements could not be made, and recommendations were made on possible improvements in study design. However, in the last few years, studies have tended to provide more clear-cut evidence and in particular have elucidated possible mechanisms.

In a recent study of 30 participants (van Nierop et al. 2012), significant changes in measures of attention and memory were obtained. This study was conducted in a double-blind design, using a tent to ensure participants were unaware of exposure status: in the sham condition relevant MRI-related sounds were played. There were also significant changes in spatial orientation, presumably related to sensations of vertigo and nystagmus. The estimates of trend (in % per T) are based only on three exposure conditions (0/0.5/1 T) so extrapolation to higher fields is also not warranted and adequate adjustments for multiple comparisons may not have been applied.

More recent studies (Mian et al. 2013, Mian et al. 2015) have investigated sensations of magnetic-field-associated vertigo linked to nystagmus induced by vestibular system. Other recent studies (Schaap et al. 2016) logged vertigo experienced by MRI workers and have found a clear association with probability of symptoms and high peak or TWA fields or dB/dt values. Approximately 8.5% of workers (in 22 out of 358 shifts) reported symptoms.

It is hard to disentangle the effects of field spatial gradients from movement of the person within a nonuniform field: the latter involves time rate of change of field and it thus an alternating current rather than a static field effect. Sensations are also confounded by noise and claustrophobia often suffered while within the bore of the magnet. It is thus unclear if we can assume that the effects on cognition (attention and memory) are a direct result of sensations of vertigo, nystagmus, and nausea (in other words, the vestibular system) rather than direct influences on brain cognitive processes.

Regarding mechanism for magnetically induced vertigo, it was previously thought that there needed to be relative motion or nonuniform fields in order to induce the effects just mentioned (Glover et al. 2007). More recent work (Roberts et al. 2011), however, has indicated that the force on the cupolas of the semicircular canals produced by the interaction of the ionic currents with the strong, steady magnetic fields *per se* is sufficient to produce mechanical distortion and hence sensations of rotation, triggering nystagmus. The Lorentz force is given by $\mathbf{B} \times \mathbf{L} \bullet \mathbf{I}$, where B is of the order of 7 T, L is the width of the semicircular canals (estimated to be 1 mm). The current I is the product of the 10–100 pA per cell and the total number of cells in the utricle. Assuming that this force is exerted over an estimated area of 10^{-6} m^2, this force gives rise to a pressure of up to 0.023 Pa, which is well above the reported nystagmus threshold of 10^{-4} Pa. There has been some discussion on whether the nystagmus experienced by persons lying in 7 T fields in a dark environment has the same mechanistic origin as perceptions of vertigo, because the two phenomena appear to be temporally and spatially discordant. Recent in-depth analysis presents strong arguments that they do have the same origin (Mian et al. 2015). More traditional tests of cognitive function, such as reaction times and cognitive task accuracies, appear to be unaffected by exposures associated with 3 T fMRI (Lepsien et al. 2012). Here, the comparison was between being with the bore of the magnet during standard fMRI procedures and with a period when the magnet was ramped down for a major hardware update. Thus, in addition to static field exposure, there was also switched gradient and RF field exposure in the "field on" condition. Since fMRI is often used to assess cognitive performance, it is crucial to fully investigate possible effects of fields on cognition. An earlier study (de Vocht et al. 2007) has already been referred to.

15.2.4 Magneto-Reception

The ability of organisms to detect the Earth's field and subtle changes in it can be found across all phyla (Johnsen and Lohmann 2005). The sensing is of two principal types: an inclination compass and a polarity compass (Wiltschko and Wiltschko 2012). There are at least three mechanisms involved in magneto-reception: the first of these is the interaction of magnetic fields with electroreceptors via the Lorentz force. Sharks and rays are able to detect changes in geomagnetic field by the electric field induced from ocean currents (which constitute a current of ions), flowing across lines of magnetic flux (this is known as the Hall effect, arising from the Lorentz force). The electrosensory apparatus of the fish then measures the Hall voltage, with the magnitude varying with the direction the animal is facing. This mechanism is of course only available to those organisms with highly developed electrosensory systems, such as those aquatic species already mentioned. Migrating birds are able to sense small variations on the Earth's field (Mouritsen and Hore 2012) and are widely understood to use magnetic field cues as well as well as other sensory inputs to aid migratory behavior, with an directional accuracy of 5° or better (Hore and Mouritsen 2016). In mammalian species, there is emerging evidence that cows, deer and foxes align preferentially with the N-S axis (Begall et al. 2013), the latter species showing preferential

N-E directed jumps to surprise prey. In addition, dogs have been shown to preferentially adopt a N-S alignment during the process of excretion (Hart et al. 2013).

The second of the three mechanisms mentioned above involves an interaction of the geomagnetic field with biogenic magnetite (Fe_3O_4) particles in the upper beak area of birds (Fleissner et al. 2003) and olfactory lamellae of fish (Diebel et al. 2000). There is evidence that an intact ophthalmic branch of the trigeminal nerve (V1) is required for the transfer of magnetic field information from the beak to brain processing regions. The precise sensory mechanism is unknown, but one hypothesis is that movement of these magnetite particles in the magnetic field causes changes in cell membrane morphology, via "tethering" arrangements between the particles and the membrane material, leading in turn to a change in ion currents (Winklhofer and Kirschvink 2010).

The third mechanism, which is gaining in acceptance (although precise details of the detection mechanism are still uncertain), involves geomagnetic field modulation in the rate of interconversion of radical pairs, very likely associated in some way with the retinal pigment cryptochrome (Hore and Mouritsen 2016, Johnsen and Lohmann 2005, Kattnig et al. 2016, Mouritsen 2012). Although the details of this mechanism are quite involved, some of the features are as follows: chemical reactions can produce pairs of fragments which each have an unpaired electron (a radical pair); the electrons in these pairs can interconvert from an initial state where both are spinning in the same direction (singlet) to states where they are opposed (triplet). The fraction of radicals in the triplet state fluctuates (with a rate determined by the magnetic field generated by the interaction between the unpaired electron and its nucleus), but this fluctuation is modulated by the value of the Earth's field (around 50 µT, which corresponds to a characteristic frequency, or Larmor frequency) of 1.4 MHz. Since the yield of reaction product (from both singlet and triplet states) is dependent on the direction of coupling of the Earth's field, this provides the basis for a magnetic compass, if the reaction product is linked to some feature of visual perception (such as hypothesized "bands" in the visual field). It is assumed that the radicals are generated within the cryptochrome molecule (or one closely associated with it) and that these molecules are aligned within the retinal photoreceptors (the cones in particular) (Hore and Mouritsen 2016). Since the spin system of radical pairs is somewhat isolated from the surroundings, the effect of external fields is not much influenced by thermal agitations. The latter point overcomes the criticism usually levelled at putative low-field effects, where the interaction energy from the field is far less than the intrinsic energy due to thermal vibrations (given by Boltzmann's constant k multiplied by the absolute temperature, which at room temperature is of the order of 10^{-21} J).

15.2.5 Human Behavior

Human sensory systems are incredibly sensitive. For example, the human auditory hair cells respond to movements of the order of 1 nm (Fettiplace and Hackney 2006) and the retinal receptors respond to a single photon of light (Rieke and Baylor 1998). These sensory systems involve exquisite cascades and tuning mechanisms, coupled to sources of metabolic energy to allow such sensitivity. On the other hand, humans appear not to be able to sense weak electric or magnetic fields directly in the same way that other animals do. Intense extremely low frequency (ELF) electric fields are sensed through motion of hairs on the skin and strong magnetic fields through the production of retinal phosphenes (see Section 15.3 for discussion of frequency range). These phenomena contribute to the setting of exposure guidelines. The consensus seems to be that humans are unable to orient towards magnetic North, although there is evidence from some controlled trials of an ability to do this with a p value of 0.005 (Baker 1989). On the other hand, human crypto-chrome, when transferred via transgenic means to fruit flies (*Drosophila*) confer upon these organisms the ability to respond to magnetic cues (Foley et al. 2011). Light sensitivity of the human visual system is also reported to be influenced by the direction and magnitude of external static geomagnetic-strength fields (Thoss and Bartsch 2003).

15.2.6 Magnetotactic Bacteria

Evidence emerged as early as the 1950s of the ability of bacteria in mud sediments to follow geomagnetic field lines in order to locate nutrients (Komeili 2012). The ability to orient to magnetic fields is linked to specialized phospholipid bilayer-bound organelles named magnetosomes. These contain single domain magnetic crystals of magnetite (Fe_3O_4) or greigite (Fe_3S_4). Up to 30 individual magnetosomes form into one or several chains aligned with the long axis of the organism. These behave like miniature compass needles, constraining the bacteria to swim along lines of geomagnetic flux. The formation of magnetosomes, the initiation and maturation of magnetic crystals, and the formation of chains all appear to be controlled by sequential expression of specific genes (Komeili 2012). However, since bacteria which have died are still able to orient to the field (Wiltschko and Wiltschko 2012), this effect cannot be linked to the organism's behavior, so will not be considered further.

15.3 Extremely Low Frequency (ELF) Fields

The extremely low frequency (ELF) range is usually taken from just above 0 Hz to a few kHz, to encompass the power frequencies (50/60 Hz) and harmonics. However, the World Health Organization has designated ELF to be between 0 and 300 Hz, intermediate frequencies (IF) between 300 Hz and 10 MHz and Radiofrequencies between 10 MHz and 300 GHz (http://www.who.int/peh-emf/about/WhatisEMF/en/). Since there are sparse data on cognitive effects associated with IF, the ELF range discussed in this chapter has been extended to 100 kHz, with RF extending above that.

Intense ELF electric fields give rise to sensation through motion of hairs on the skin and via the induction of sparks or "microshocks" from nearby conductors, in a similar manner as static electric fields as discussed above. In humans, strong ELF magnetic fields give rise to sensation through the production of retinal phosphenes or by induction of sufficiently high electric fields in tissue to produce nerve stimulation. These phenomena contribute to the setting of exposure guidelines. Since this chapter is concerned with possible cognitive or behavioral responses from field stimulation, these phenomena will be discussed in relation to these specific endpoints. However, there are reports of cognitive or behavioral effects arising from ELF field exposure at intensities well below the thresholds for the phenomena just mentioned, and by implication, below the exposure limits set in relevant guidelines (ICNIRP 2010, IEEE 2002).

15.3.1 ELF Electric Field Effects

The use of pulsed electric fields in treatment for a range of illnesses goes back to ancient Egypt and Greece, where electric fish such as skates and rays were kept in tanks, so that sufferers could experience the supposed healing effects of electric shocks (Finger and Piccolino 2011). The 18th century saw the application of newly developed spark genera-tors to the treatment of many disorders, including mental illness. The churchman John Wesley was one enthusiastic promoter of such treatments, on the grounds of it being avail-able at very small cost to disadvantaged members of the community (Bertucci 2006). The application of electric shocks to the scalp in the form of electroconvulsive therapy, or ECT, continues to this day as an effective treatment for intractable cases of Major Depression or other affective illnesses (Pagnin et al. 2004). Typically, currents of up to 0.8 A are applied as short (ms) pulses with a repetition rate between 25 and 100 Hz with a duration of up to 20 s (total charge transfer is limited to below 1 Coulomb) (Tiller and Lyndon 2003). This induces fields in brain tissue sufficiently high to cause neurostimulation (hence, convul-sions ensue, requiring premedication with muscle relaxants to prevent self-injury). The effects persist well after the application of these shocks, leading in many cases to a perma-nent improvement in condition.

Some workers in the electrical generation, transmission, and distribution industry experience relatively high electric (and magnetic) fields in the course of their business. These may lead to the "microshocks" referred to earlier. During the 1960s, there were Russian reports of association of electric field exposures with general health deficits (WHO 2007). The study of the effects of (occupational) electric fields on cognition is complicated by the possibility of distractions. In the case of "microshocks" the partici-pants react to the unexpected sensations and similarly for field-induced movement of skin hairs, even though less disconcerting. It is generally agreed that these fields are insufficient to cause direct neurostimulation of the CNS. Stollery (1986, 1987) subjected participants to simulated 50 Hz fields of approximately 36 kV/m (by applying currents of 0.5 mA to the scalp, with the feet connected to Earth). In a double-blind, counterbal-anced design, 38 pairs of male participants were given a battery of psychological tests over a 2-day period. Although no significant changes were reported for the majority of endpoints, the "exposed" group showed poorer response times in a syntactic reasoning test and felt less aroused at the end of the second day, compared to the "sham" group. It is not recorded whether participants were aware of sensations at the points of injection of current.

15.3.2 ELF Magnetic Field Effects

15.3.2.1 Effects of Strong Fields

The effect of bringing about a change in magnetic field in a medium is to induce an elec-tric field in that medium. High rates of time variations of magnetic field (dB/dt) can cause appreciable electric fields in tissue (and thus ionic currents in that tissue). If the dB/dt value is sufficiently high, resulting induced electric fields can be sufficient to depolarize nerve cells, producing action potentials, particularly in the cortex just below the skull (Ueno and Sekino 2015). Transcranial magnetic stimulation (TMS) involves delivering a rapidly changing magnetic field via insulated coils close to the scalp (Pascual-Leone et al. 2000, Walsh and Cowey 2000). TMS is considered further in Chapter 10 of this vol-ume. The coils are often in the form of a "figure of eight" but other configurations are also used. The threshold dB/dt for nerve stimulation is in excess of 20–30 T/s (in situ), and is often presented in the form of a single cycle of a sine wave. Clinical TMS machines are capable of producing over 1 T field amplitude with a single cycle of less than 1 ms. The maximum dB/dt can be estimated from $2\pi B/T = 2\pi(1.2)/(0.36 \times 10^{-3}) = 20$ kT/s, thus exceeding the notional threshold by a large margin. However, the effective amplitude of B decreases rapidly with distance from the coils, so within sensitive regions of the cortex the excitation threshold may be only just exceeded. Typically, stimulation over the motor cortex can elicit specific groups of motor nerves, for example, the adductor muscle of a specific finger. There can be more subtle behavioral and cognitive effects (Siebner et al. 2009) such as alterations of sensual perception (such as color perception and pattern discrimination) and cognitive effects such as visual information processing or motor execution. These are immediate consequences of temporary "virtual lesions" (due to specific regions of neural pathways being blocked because of certain nerve fibers being rendered refractory by TMS stimulation), but there are also longer aftereffects (Thut and Pascual-Leone 2010). The latter review, which included results from over 50 studies, highlights that although stimulation time is brief, aftereffects such as effects on learning or fatigue can persist for up to an hour. In fact, in situations where TMS is used therapeutically, for treatment of major depression (for example, Fitzgerald et al. 2009), the beneficial effects are thought to persist for many months, if not permanently. Although the fields concerned are many orders of magnitudes greater than those experienced by "electrical workers" or indeed members of the public, these studies serve to identify definite cognitive and behavioral effects occurring in humans once field levels are sufficiently high.

The currents elicited by TMS in the brain have similarities to those induced via the application of electrodes to the scalp in clinical techniques such as electroconvulsive therapy (ECT), transcranial direct-current stimulation (tDCS) (Nitsche et al. 2008), and deep brain stimulation (DBS) (Perlmutter and Mink 2006). Since these represent the direct application of current rather than the consequence of external electric fields, these were not included in the discussion of ELF electric field effects above. There have been a number of studies comparing the clinical effectiveness of TMS with ECT (Berlim et al. 2013) and also comparing the magnitudes and distributions of induced fields or current densities (Nadeem et al. 2003, Ueno and Sekino 2015). It needs remarking that although the clinical benefits of tDCS and DBS are yet to be established, neither of these involves the generation of action potentials, so the possibility of behavioral effects resulting from modest induced electric fields, below those leading to such action-potential related phenomena as retinal phosphenes and neurostimulation, needs careful consideration.

In a series of experiments investigating retinal magnetophosphenes, the researchers noted that "virtually all volunteers noted tiredness and some reported headaches after the experiment" (Lovsund et al. 1980). In addition, some reported afterimages and spasms of eye muscles. It is not clear whether this was purely a consequence of the increased concentration necessary to report the phenomenon, but there appears to be a link between the specialized "ribbon synapses" in the retina to similar structures in electrosensory receptors (Sterling and Matthews 2005). They also appear to be abundant in the hippocampus, which has a key function in memory formation (Singer et al. 2004). There are still some unanswered questions on the precise transduction mechanism (and hence whether effects on memory might be likely) but ongoing work by the London, Ontario group is intending to elucidate this. The switched gradient fields in MRI investigations produce time rates of change of magnetic field (dB/dt) sufficiently high to cause peripheral nerve stimulation, with effective frequency in the ELF range (typically around 500 Hz). Some of the studies referred to in the static magnetic field section would have also included additional switched gradient field exposure, but since the overall conclusion seems to be that field-related cognitive effects in fMRI are of little consequence, these do not need further consideration.

15.3.2.2 Effects of Weak Fields on Humans

ELF standards for human safety are designed to prevent the simulation of nerves by tissue electric fields induced by time-varying magnetic fields (WHO 2007). The general public limit of 0.2 and 0.24 mT at 50 and 60 Hz, respectively, correspond to tissue fields of approximately 7 mV/m, which offers a significant margin of safety when compared to the best estimates of retinal magnetophosphenes, which are induced by tissue fields of 100 mV/m or more. It is rare for the general public to encounter environmental power frequency fields above 0.03 mT at these frequencies (ICNIRP 2010). Controlled testing of human behavioral or cognitive effects of weak ELF fields has been mainly carried out in laboratory rather than environmental settings, with the fields carefully calibrated and delivered in a "double-blind" manner (where neither the participants nor the experimenters directly dealing with the participants or the data analysis have been aware of the times of actual exposure). Most of the testing has involved comparisons of responses during real exposure with that during "sham" exposure, and in many cases, the same participants have been tested in both orders (real then sham: sham then real) in order to compensate for "practice effects." Measures can be categorized into two types: neurophysiological and electrophysiological testing. The first requires participants to perform sensorineural or cognitive tasks, usually responding to computer-delivered tests, in which speed and accuracy of responses are often the quantitative measures. The second involves recording of brain electrical activity from several electrodes placed in standard positions on the scalp (the electroencephalogram or EEG). This activity can either be spontaneous (in which the participant merely relaxes, usually with eyes shut), or evoked, in which a visual, auditory, or cognitive task is presented, and the time course of the EEG activity in the time immediately following the presentation of the stimulus is recorded and analyzed. The latter analysis quantifies certain features in the EEG signal following the moment of stimulus presentation related to the brain processing the information presented in the stimulus. Since these features are often buried in noise, repeated presentation of identical or similar stimuli, with averaging of the time-course of responses, is usually performed to improve signal to noise ratio.

The design and outcomes of more recent experiments involving neuropsychological testing are summarized in Table 15.1. The magnetic intensities have varied between 10 and 3,000 μT (0.01–3 mT), and although most have been at or near power frequencies, static fields have also been tested. There have also been several different orientations and types of polarization of the fields. Of the outcomes, four studies report significant improvements and six studies report significant decrements in performance, while the other 10 studies report no significant changes. Ignoring the frequency used, the geometric mean exposures for the three groups are 45 μT for improvement, 110 μT for detriment and 228 μT for no effect, with Standard Deviations almost completely overlapping. Thus no clear "dose-response" characteristic emerges and since the reported changes are in both directions, there is little that can be concluded about effects on human behavior. This of course does not rule out the possibility of specific ranges in frequency or intensity being biologically active, but the emerging pattern is certainly not one of consistency.

Turning now to experiments involving neurophysiological, or to be more precise, EEG measurements, there are at least 20 to consider. These are summarized in Table 15.2. Most of these report significant changes in EEG responses, but in view of the widely disparate exposure conditions, the possibility of electrode "pickup" of the impressed fields and the lack of consistency of significant changes found, it is again difficult to form definitive conclusions. It is also of note that for the Shreveport experiments, there may be false positives arising from the way a "response" is gauged, since it relies on identifying recurrence

TABLE 15.1

Human Volunteer Experiments Involving ELF Exposure with Behavioral Measurements

Author, Year	Number of Participants	Type of Coils	Orientation	Frequency	Field Strength(s) (μT)	Duration and Intermittency of Exposure	Measures	Outcomes (Effects of Exposure)	Notes
Midwest Research Institute									
Graham et al. (1987)	12, DB, RM	Hmhz	T and C	60	20	?3 h × 2	Psychometric test battery	Fewer errors on Choice Reaction Time	
Cook et al. (1992)	18, DB, RM	Hmhz	Circularly polarized, axis aligned with GMF horizontal component	60	20	3 h × 2	As above, with physiological measures	As above	
Cook et al. (1992)	12, DB, RM	Hmhz	As above, with E-field T	60	20, but with additional Electric field (9 kV/m)	3 h × 2	As above	As above, but failed to reach significance	
Graham et al. (1994)	3 groups of 18, DB	Hmhz	As above	60	Low: 10, with 6 kV/m; Med: 20, with 9 kV/k; High: 30 with 12 kV/m	6 h × 2	As above	For the L group, slower Reaction Time and accuracy (on time estimation task)	
St Petersburg/Umea									
Lyskov et al. (1993b)	14, ?DB, RM	Hmhz	Head, S	45	1,260	I, 1 s on/off, for 15 min	Reaction Time and target-deletion task	No clear effects	Practice effect possible. N.B. some EEG data collected (see also Table 15.2)
Lyskov et al. (1994)	10 sham, 10 exposed	Hmhz	? Head, S	45	1,260	I, 120 min	Battery of tests given 8 times	Reaction time for Choice Reaction Time and Sequence Search increased (poorer)	

(Continued)

TABLE 15.1 (Continued)

Human Volunteer Experiments Involving ELF Exposure with Behavioral Measurements

Author, Year	Number of Participants	Type of Coils	Orientation	Frequency	Field Strength(s) (μT)	Duration and Intermittency of Exposure	Measures	Outcomes (Effects of Exposure)	Notes
New Zealand									
Podd et al. (1995)	12, DB, RM	Hmhz	S	0.1; 0.2	1,100	C, 300 s	Reaction Time to visual stimulus	No effects	
Podd et al. (1995)	24, DB, RM	Hmhz	Perpendicular or parallel to GMF	0.2; 43	100	C, ?300s	Reaction Time to visual stimulus	No effects	43 Hz is Cyclotron resonance frequency
Whittington et al. (1996)	101, DB, RM	Hmhz	Parallel to GMF	50	100	I, 1 s on/off for 9 min	Visual duration discrimination	Reduced RT (improvement)	
Kazantzis et al. (1998)	99, 2 occasions, DB, RM	Hmhz	S	50	100	I, 1 s on/off, for 7.9 min	Visual duration discrimination	Improvement at highest difficulty level, with F > M	
Podd et al. (2002)	80, 2 groups, DB	Hmhz	S	50	100	I, 1 s on/off, for 11 min	Visual duration discrimination, shape recognition task	No changes in RT or accuracy for discrimination task, but decrement in performance in recognition task *following* exposure.	
Liege, Belgium									
Crasson et al. (1996)	21, 3 occasions	Hlmt	Aligned with GMF	50	100	C vs I, 15 s on/off for 30 min	Attention and memory tests	No significant effects	
Crasson et al. (1999)	18 (of previous cohort of 21), DB, RM	Hlmt	Aligned with GMF	50	100	C vs I, 15 s on/off for 30 min	Selective attention tests	RT increased significantly (for oddball paradigm test)	detriment

(Continued)

TABLE 15.1 (*Continued*)

Human Volunteer Experiments Involving ELF Exposure with Behavioral Measurements

Author, Year	Number of Participants	Type of Coils	Orientation	Frequency	Field Strength(s) (μT)	Duration and Intermittency of Exposure	Measures	Outcomes (Effects of Exposure)	Notes
Delhez et al. (2004)	32, 3 occasions, DB, RM	Hlmt	T	50	20, 400	C, 55 min	Battery of tests	No effects	
Crasson and Legros (2005)	18, DB, RM	Hlmt	aligned with GMF	50	100	C, 30 min	Battery of tests	No effects	
Nevelsteen et al. (2007)	74 in 5 groups	Hlmt	T	50	400	C, 30 min	Mood, vigilance, Physiological	No effects	Clinical subjects: some deception: effects of + and – information prior also tested
Bristol, United Kingdom									
Preece et al. (1998)	16, DB, RM	Lee-Whiting coils	Head, sagittal	50 or static	600 in either case	C, duration of tests	Battery of 10 tests	Poorer accuracy in attentional task	overall deterioration in memory
Melbourne, Australia									
Keetley et al. (2001)	30, DB, RM	Hmhz	Circularly polarised, sagittal and coronal, whole body	50	28 resultant	C, 50 min	Battery of 6 tests (10 measures)	Impairment of verbal recall after interference, decrease in performance in 'Trail-Making Task'	

(*Continued*)

TABLE 15.1 (Continued)

Human Volunteer Experiments Involving ELF Exposure with Behavioral Measurements

Author, Year	Number of Participants	Type of Coils	Orientation	Frequency	Field Strength(s) (μT)	Duration and Intermittency of Exposure	Measures	Outcomes (Effects of Exposure)	Notes
Ibaraki, Japan									
Kurokawa et al. (2003)	20, ?SB, RM	Hmhz	Circularly polarised, sagittal and coronal, whole body	50	20 resultant	C, 55 min	Battery of 4 tests	No effects	
London, Ontario									
Corbacio et al. (2011)	99, DB, RM	Hmhz	Sagittal	60	3,000	C, 30 min × 2	Battery of 10 tests	No clear effects	Practice effects noted

Key:

Design: DB: Double-blind; RM: Repeated Measures (i.e each participants underwent all treatments, after a suitable wash-out period).
Type of coils: Hmhz: Helmholtz coils; Coax: Coaxial coils; Hlmt: Helmet coils; VDT: Visual Display Terminal.
Orientation: S: Sagittal (L to R); C: Coronal (Front to back); T: Transverse (up and down); GMF: parallel to Geomagnetic field.
Duration/intermittency of exposure: I: Intermittent; C: Continuous.

TABLE 15.2

Human Volunteer Experiments Involving ELF Exposure with Electrophysiological Measurements

Author, Year	Number of Participants	Type of Coils	Orientation	Frequency	Field Strength(s) (µT)	Duration and Intermittency of Exposure	Measures	Outcomes (Effects) of Exposure	Notes
Shreveport, LA									
Bell et al. (1991)	14	Hmhz	S	25, 50	60	I: 2 s on/off	EEG band power	7/14 'responders' (sham as control)	3 electrode sites
Bell et al. (1992)	20, SB, RM	Hmhz	S	60, static	78	I: 2 s on/off	EEG band power	19/20 showed significant changes: most had increased power in 2 or more of 34 0.5Hz bands; 80% of participants showed responses to 60Hz, static or combined fields.	Pickup?
Bell et al. (1994b)	19, SB, RM	Hmhz	S	1.5, 10	20, 40	I: 2 s on/off	EEG band power	EEG altered at frequency of stimulation	Pickup?
Bell et al. (1994a)	10, SB, RM	Hmhz	S	10	100	I: 2 s on/off	EEG band power	10Hz spectral power reduced from occipital electrodes	Pickup?
Marino et al. (2004)	8, SB, RM	Hmhz	S	60	100	I: 2 s on/5 s off	EEG band power	Phase-space analysis showed 8/8 responders	
Carrubba et al. (2007a)	17, SB, RM	Coax	S	60	200	I: 2 s on/5 s off	EP latency, via recurrence analysis	16/17 responders	109–454 ms latency; 6 electrode sites; need to explain recurrence plots
Carrubba et al. (2007b)	8, SB, tested twice 1 week apart	Coax	C	60	100	I: 2 s on/5 s off	EP latency, via recurrence analysis	7/8 responded	?Number of electrodes given as 42 for above study?

(Continued)

TABLE 15.2 (Continued)

Human Volunteer Experiments Involving ELF Exposure with Electrophysiological Measurements

Author, Year	Number of Participants	Type of Coils	Orientation	Frequency	Field Strength(s) (µT)	Duration and Intermittency of Exposure	Measures	Outcomes (Effects of Exposure)	Notes
Carrubba et al. (2008)	15, SB, RM	Coax	C/S	30, 60	200	I: 0.05 s on/2.95 s off	EP latency, via recurrence analysis	EPs detected in all 15 participants, independently of frequency or field direction	109–504 ms latency
Carrubba et al. (2010)	22, SB, RM	Coax	S	60	1, 5	I: 2 s on/5 s off	EP latency, via recurrence analysis	EPs detected in all 22 participants, independent of strength	250 ms average latency
St Petersburg/Umea									
Lyskov et al. (1993a)	20, DB, RM	Hmhz	Head, S	45	1260	I, 1 s on/off, for 60 min vs C, 60 min	EEG spectra, Ω potentials	No clear RT effects, but increase in α and decrease in δ spectral power	Practice effect possible
Lyskov et al. (1998)	13	VDT	Head, mainly	60 or 72	Not measured, but 70 cm from monitor face	Not stated, but characteristic of VDT monitors	Steady-state Visual Evoked Potentials (from amplitude modulated light intensity)	SSVEP amplitude higher for 60 than 72 Hz	Prime interest: study of effects of light fluctuations rather than ELF fields

(Continued)

TABLE 15.2 (*Continued*)

Human Volunteer Experiments Involving ELF Exposure with Electrophysiological Measurements

Author, Year	Number of Participants	Type of Coils	Orientation	Frequency	Field Strength(s) (µT)	Duration and Intermittency of Exposure	Measures	Outcomes (Effects of Exposure)	Notes
U Hospital Zurich/UCLA									
Fuller et al. (1995)	7 epileptic patients	Coax (Hlmt)	Not stated	0	900–1,800	I, 20 s on/40 s off (typical)	No. of epileptiform discharges	6/7 patients showed higher 'spiking' during exposure	Delay of several s before 'spiking' begins
Fuller et al. (2003)	3 epileptic patients, RM	Hmhz	T	0	2,000	I, 60 s on/60 s off, also C	No. of epileptiform discharges	1/3 patients showed significant increase of firing rate	
London, Ontario									
Cook et al. (2004)	20, RM	Hmhz	T	Pulse sequences	±200	I, for 15 min	α-band (8–13 Hz) power	Post exposure, significant increase in α-band power for occipital sites	
Cook et al. (2005)	20	Hmhz	T	Pulse sequences	±200	I, for 15 min	α-band (8–13 Hz) power	During exposure, significant decrease in α-band power for occipital sites	Occurred during first 5 min of exposure
Legros et al. (2012)	73	Hmhz	S	60	1,800	C, 60 min	EEG band power, tremor, balance	No effects on EEG, but small increase in tremor amplitude and a decrease in standing balance oscillations (eyes shut).	Tremor result opposite to previously reported (Legros et al. 2006)
Liege, Belgium									
Crasson and Legros (2005)	18	Hlmt	GMF	50	100	C, 30 min	P300, in response to auditory 'oddball' task	No effects	

(Continued)

TABLE 15.2 (*Continued*)

Human Volunteer Experiments Involving ELF Exposure with Electrophysiological Measurements

Author, Year	Number of Participants	Type of Coils	Orientation	Frequency	Field Strength(s) (μT)	Duration and Intermittency of Exposure	Measures	Outcomes (Effects of Exposure)	Notes
Pisa, Italy									
Ghione et al. (2005)	40, DB, RM	Hmhz	T	50	40, 80	C, 90min	α-band (8–13 Hz) power, nociception	Doubling of α-band power for 80 μT, lowering of pain threshold for 40 μT	
Melbourne, Australia									
Cvetkovic and Cosic (2009)	33, DB, RM	Hmhz	S	50, 16.66, 13, 10, 8.33, 4	20	C, 2 min each	θ, α1, α2, β1, β2, γ	Lowered α-band power for 8.33 and 10 Hz; increased β-band power for 13 Hz exposures	EEG recorded after each exposure period; Bonferroni corrections applied
Rome, Italy									
Capone et al. (2009)	22, SB, RM	Hlmt	T	75, pulses 1.3 ms duration	1800	Duration not stated	Thresholds for specific EEG responses evoked by TMS stimulation	Increased 'Intercortical facilitation' threshold	Some concerns regarding statistical design (SCENIHR)

Key:

Number of participants: DB: double blind; SB: single blind (according to information provided); RM: repeated measures design.

Type of coils: Hmhz: Helmholtz coils; Coax: Coaxial coils; Hlmt: Helmet coils; VDT: Visual Display Terminal.

Orientation: S: Sagittal (L to R); C: Coronal (Front to back); T: Transverse (up and down); GMF: parallel to Geomagnetic field.

Duration/intermittency of exposure: I: Intermittent; C: Continuous.

relationships in the data, which is prone to picking up underlying contamination due to instrumental rather than biological sources. It would be useful if these findings could be independently confirmed by other laboratories.

A third group of human volunteer experiments involve the use of advanced imaging techniques to highlight brain regions involved in putative processing of responses to ELF stimulation (Table 15.3). The blood-oxygen level dependent (BOLD) signals are considered to represent local blood flow changes and hence level of neural activity. The results are interesting, but require independent verification or corroboration before concluding that magnetic fields are influencing cognition. The field strengths are close to the allowed limits and greater than those usually encountered in the environment by two orders of magnitude.

The rationale behind the exposure schemes vary: with the Shreveport group, the motivation is to try to identify an "EMF magnetic sense": other laboratories have been spurred by considering possible links with nociception studies (see below). In this regard, the review by Del Seppia et al. (2007) covers both human volunteer and experimental animal studies of possible modulation of pain perception by ELF fields and concludes that there is now a substantial body of evidence of consistent inhibitory effects on analgesia (in other words, made analgesic agents less effective). However, recent reviews of the literature of human volunteer studies (Barth et al. 2010, Cooket al. 2002, Di Lazzaro et al. 2013) conclude that studies so far do not provide convincing evidence that weak ELF magnetic fields affect cognitive processes.

Several epidemiological studies from the 1980s and 1990s examined whether those living close to electrical power transmission lines were more susceptible to mood disorders or more prone to suicide (see for example Beale et al. (1997), Perry et al. (1981)). More recent studies have been in relation to suicide risk among electrical workers (van Wijngaarden 2003, van Wijngaarden et al. 2000), with an estimate of magnetic field exposure based on job title and work history. Some reported odds ratios (ORs) were significantly high, especially among younger workers. The emphasis of epidemiological studies has now moved to specific neurological disease outcomes rather than effects on mood or behavior *per se*. For example, recent meta-analyses have examined occupational ELF field exposure and Amyotrophic Lateral Sclerosis (Zhou et al. 2012), Parkinson's disease (Huss et al. 2015) and these two diseases plus Alzheimer disease and other neurodegenerative diseases (Vergara et al. 2013). Since the workers included in such studies were likely to have suffered electrical shocks and been exposed to various chemicals, dusts and fumes in addition to exposure to ELF fields, it has not been possible to identify the causes of significantly raised ORs. The overall conclusion of recent reviews is that the evidence of a causative link between ELF fields (either magnetic or electric) and depression, suicide and neurodegenerative diseases is inconsistent and inconclusive (WHO 2007, SCENIHR 2015). Since the thrust of this chapter is to attempt to identify mechanisms whereby EMFs can lead to behavioral or cognitive effects, at this stage the epidemiological data is inadequate to do this, because it is unclear whether ELF fields are directly involved. A more complete list of relevant studies and a more in-depth analysis can be found in recent reviews (such as SCENIHR (2015), WHO (2007)), as well as Chapter 13 of this Volume.

15.3.2.3 Effects of Weak Fields on Laboratory Animals

In addition to the human volunteer experiments just reviewed, there is a large literature of studies on laboratory animals in relation to behavior and cognition. Space will only allow description of some of these, especially those that could serve to confirm or refute some

TABLE 15.3

Experiments Involving ELF Exposure Using Advanced Imaging Techniques

Author, Year	Number of Participants	Type of Coils	Orientation	Frequency	Field Strength(s) (μT)	Duration and Intermittency of Exposure	Measures	Outcomes (Effects of Exposure)	Notes
London, Ontario									
Robertson et al. (2010a)	31 (17 sham, 14 exposed), SB	MRIGC	T	Pulse sequence	200	Pulse sequence	fMRI (BOLD signals)	Responses to thermal pain stimulus: decrease in activity in the anterior cingulate and R insula after ELF exposure	
Robertson et al. (2010b)	6 + 10 exposed in addition to the above, SB	MRIGC	T	Pulse sequence	100, 1000	Pulse sequence	fMRI (BOLD signals)	Significant correlations between field strength and change in activity for anterior cingulate and the ipsilateral insula	Low r values for correlations: not corrected for multiple comparisons
Legros et al. (2015)	21 (11 sham, 10 exposed), DB	MRIGC	T	60	3000	C, 60 min	BOLD signals	Significant changes in task-induced functional brain activation, but not task performance	Changes occur after cessation of 60 Hz exposure. For finger-tapping part, only 9 exposed data usable.

Key:
Number of participants: RM: repeated measures design.
Type of coils: MRIGC: MRI Gradient Coils.
Orientation: T: Transverse (up and down).
Duration/intermittency of exposure: C: Continuous.

of the outcomes discussed in the previous section. The effects of (mainly) magnetic field exposure on behavioral and cognitive effects in laboratory animals has been extensively reviewed (SCENIHR 2015, WHO 2007). Essentially, the conclusion of these reviews is that most of the findings lack consistency, but there is evidence that (weak) "magnetic fields may modulate the functions of the opioid and cholinergic systems, and this is supported by the results of studies investigating the effects of analgesia and on the acquisition and performance of spatial memory tasks" (WHO 2007, p. 161).

Among early work, a group at Southwest Research Institute, San Antonio, exposed groups of baboons to mainly electric fields, but also to combined electric and magnetic fields. The threshold for electric field-related behavioral responses was determined to be 12 kV/m on average, but possibly lower (Orr et al. 1995a). The responses to combined fields were harder to interpret, however (Orr et al. 1995b). Other experiments, carried out earlier by a State University of New York group, were a series on a group of 10 monkeys, measuring various endpoints such as evoked EEG responses, and neurotransmitter levels over a 21-day period (Dowman et al. 1989, Seegal et al. 1989, Wolpaw et al. 1989). The animals were exposed to combined electrical and magnetic fields, up to 30 kV/m and 90 µT, respectively. Significant declines in dopamine and serotonin metabolites were recorded, along with decrease in the amplitudes of late components of the somatosensory evoked potentials in response to the stronger field levels. This was interpreted as possibly relating to an antagonistic effect of the fields on endogenous opiates, a concept which was subsequently investigated over several years by the London, Ontario group (Prato 2015). There appears to be some consistency in experiments from this and other groups (Del Seppia et al. 2007). Although the earlier experiments were with rodents, the bulk of these experiments involve the use of the land snail *Cepea nemoralis*. These have a relatively simple nervous system, but when placed on a mildly heated surface respond by foot retraction, the latency of which is lengthened by prior treatment with opiates. Magnetic fields of environmental relevance appear to reduce the analgesic effects of opiates and other related substances. The review by Del Seppia et al. (2007) highlights that effects have been reported from a wide range of intensities (1–9,000 mT), including complex mixes of frequencies. Reasonably consistent outcomes were obtained from around six different types of testing. Although pain sensitivity (nociception) and influences on pain inhibition are not direct effects on cognition, the involvement of neurotransmitter modulation and possible involvement of Ca^{++} ion and other messenger molecules (Del Seppia et al. 2007) has important ramifications for more general effects. The interaction mechanism between weak fields and initial biochemical events leading to this modulation remains speculative, although Prato (Prato 2015) has argued links to possible free radical effects.

Regarding spatial memory tasks (liked to cholinergic systems) many groups have studied rodent performance in mazes, in particular the Morris water maze, in which animals, swimming in water, have to remember the location of a hidden platform. Related forms of maze are the "radial arm maze" (where a reward is located at the end of a particular arm) or the "elevated plus maze" (which is a raised "plus" sign, with two open and two closed arms, where the open arms elicit anxiety in the animals). Several groups have conducted experiments using these types of apparatus, and the design, exposure details and outcomes are shown in Table 15.4. Although most groups report poorer performance associated with ELF exposure, three report improvements. The exposure times range from 5 min to over 2,000 h, with magnitudes from 5 to 10,000 µT (the latter hardly within the category of "weak"). Although improvements appear to be linked to chronic exposures, the same type of chronic exposure also seems to lead to detriments, and therefore, it is hard to come to a clear conclusion based on these studies.

TABLE 15.4

Experiments Involving ELF Exposure to Rodents Using Maze Tasks

Author, Year	Number, type of Animals	Type of Coils	Orientation	Frequency	Field Strength(s) μT	Duration and Intermittency of Exposure	Measures	Outcomes (Effects of Exposure)	Notes
London, Ontario									
Kavaliers et al. (1996)	3 × 5; 10 M	Hmhz	NS/EW	60	100	C, 5 min	Subsequent Water Maze task acquisition	Performance improved	Effect in ♀ animals, eliminating sex-difference observed in pre-exposure performance
Seattle, WA									
Lai (1996)	8 + 8 R	Hmhz	S/T	60	750	C, 45 min	Subsequent Radial Arm maze task	Performance poorer	Physostigmine reversed magnetic field effect
Lai et al. (1998)	10 + 9 R	Hmhz	S/T	60	1,000	C, 60 min	Subsequent Radial Arm maze task	No difference in performance, but swim speed slower	
Former NRPB, United Kingdom									
Sienkiewicz et al. (1996)	10 × 8 M	Hmhz	C	50	5, 50, 500, 5,000	C	Radial arm maze task during exposure	No differences, at any of the levels	
Sienkiewicz et al. (1998)	4 × (6 + 6) M	Hmhz	C	50	750	C, 45 min	Subsequent Radial Arm maze task	Acquisition time poorer, but no difference in accuracy	Partial replication of Lai (1996)

(Continued)

TABLE 15.4 (*Continued*)

Experiments Involving ELF Exposure to Rodents Using Maze Tasks

Author, Year	Number, type of Animals	Type of Coils	Orientation	Frequency	Field Strength(s) μT	Duration and Intermittency of Exposure	Measures	Outcomes (Effects of Exposure)	Notes
Semnan, Iran									
Jadidi et al. (2007)	3 × 11; 2 × 10; 2 × 7 R		?S	50	2,000, 8,000	C, 20 min	Subsequent Water Maze task acquisition and retention	Poorer retention for 8 mT, but no effects of 2 mT	
Budapest, Hungary									
Szemerszky et al. (2010)	2 × (8 + 8) R	Hmhz	C	50	500	C, 8 h/day, for 5 days or 24 h/day for 4–6 weeks	Elevated plus maze task, forced swim test	Enhanced floating time in swim test for longer exposure	Proopiomelanocortin elevation
Beijing, China									
He et al. (2011)	?, R	?	?	50	2,000	1 h/day or 4 h/day for 4 weeks	Water Maze task	Increase anxiety symptoms, but reduced latency of finding platform and improve long-term memory	

(*Continued*)

TABLE 15.4 (*Continued*)

Experiments Involving ELF Exposure to Rodents Using Maze Tasks

Author, Year	Number, type of Animals	Type of Coils	Orientation	Frequency	Field Strength(s) μT	Duration and Intermittency of Exposure	Measures	Outcomes (Effects of Exposure)	Notes
Istanbul, Turkey									
Korpinar et al. (2012)	38 + 38 R	?	?	50	10,000	C, 34 h/d for 21 days	Elevated plus-maze task	Significant reduction in stress and anxiety-related behavior (as measured by ratio of time in open arms to time in all arms)	
Suzhou, China									
Cui et al. (2012)	2 × (12 + 12 + 12) M	Rect. coil	C	50	100, 1,000	C, 4 h/day, 84 days	Subsequent performance in two versions of Water Maze task	Significant impairment at 1 mT (but not 0.1 mT) for at least one version of test	Biochemical analysis of hippocampus and striatum showed evidence of oxidative stress

(*Continued*)

TABLE 15.4 (Continued)

Experiments Involving ELF Exposure to Rodents Using Maze Tasks

Author, Year	Number, type of Animals	Type of Coils	Orientation	Frequency	Field Strength(s) µT	Duration and Intermittency of Exposure	Measures	Outcomes (Effects of Exposure)	Notes
Kunming, China									
Wang et al. (2013)	3 × 11 M	Rect. coil	C	50	2,000	C, 1 h/day, 12 days	Y-maze, Water Maze on subsequent days	Improved performance in Water Maze, but no difference in Y-maze	
Zhenjiang, China									
Duan et al. (2013)	5 × 10 M	Hmhz	?S/T	50	8,000	C, 4 h/day, 28 days	Subsequent Water Maze performance	Poorer learning and memory abilities	Lotus seedpod procyanidins reversed deficits, interpreted as oxygen free radical scavenging effect
Beijing, China									
Li et al. (2014)	4 × 10 R	Hmhz	?	50	100	C, 24 h/day, 90 days	Subsequent Water Maze performance	Improved spatial acquisition	See note on probe trial
Tokushima, Japan									
Kitaoka et al. (2013)	2 × 10 M	Round coils	C	50	3,000	C, 8 h/day, 25 days	Various tests	Poorer performance in swim/ light-dark transition tests	

Key:

Number, type of animals: R: rats; M: mice.

Type of coils: Hmhz: Helmholtz coils; Coax: Coaxial coils; Rect. Coil: Rectangular Coil.

Orientation: S: Sagittal (L to R); C: Coronal (Front to back); T: Transverse (Head to tail); NS/EW North South or East West orientation.

Duration/intermittency of exposure: C: Continuous.

In addition to the electrophysiological experiments on primates summarized above, evoked responses have also been investigated in rabbits (Bell et al. 1992). As with the experiments involving human volunteers, the responses seemed to occur with the same frequency characteristics as the stimulus, so the possibility of electrode pickup remains.

15.3.2.4 Effects of Weak Fields on Cellular Systems

Among the myriad of experiments in which cells and organ systems have been exposed to weak ELF magnetic fields there are those which link more directly to neurophysiological processes. In particular, some that mimic memory formation could help uncover a putative underlying mechanism. Some experiments have used rodent hippocampal slices, in which effects of pulsed magnetic fields on the long-term potentiation (LTP) effects of electrical stimulation have been studied (Ahmed and Wieraszko 2008, Wieraszko 2004). In these experiments the magnetic field magnitude is 15 mT, which is well above those normally encountered. However, the time rate of change (22 mT/s), which is applied over a very small chamber (1 cm diameter) corresponds to tissue fields of approximately 50 µV/m or less, which is well below ELF Basic Restrictions. The effect seems to be one of stimulation, both of excitatory and inhibitory processes. In a related experiment, (Komaki et al. 2014) studied the effects of 50 Hz, 0.1 mT magnetic fields (2 h/day for 90 days) on intact rats, in which LTP was studied subsequently, by lowering electrodes into the hippocampus under anesthesia. Both population spikes and magnitude of responses were enhanced in the exposed group. Other experiments, involving primary cultures of embryonal neurons exposed to 0.1 or 1 mT 50 Hz fields for 7 days (Di Loreto et al. 2009) reported higher levels of neuron vitality associated with the higher level of exposure. However, these and other experiments reviewed recently (SCENIHR 2015) do not provide any clues on how fields could interact with membrane processes or biochemical reactions.

15.3.2.5 Possible Interaction Mechanisms for Weak Fields Effects

Three candidate mechanisms were reviewed in (WHO 2007) to account for epidemiological and other evidence for possible low-level ELF effects. These were: effects on biogenic magnetite, induced electric fields in neural networks and effects on free radical pair dynamics or "free-radical lifetime" hypothesis. This latter mechanism, which underlies the magnetic sense for migratory birds, was reviewed in the weak static field section above. At the time of publication of the WHO 2007 review, it was thought that since the magnetic fields of ELF and static fields on free radicals was similar, it would be unlikely that ELF fields below 50 µT would be of biological significance. However, since then there has been further consideration of the possible transitions between energy levels. Whereas the Larmor frequency for the interaction between an unpaired electron and its nucleus in the earth's field is around 1.4 MHz (as remarked above), there are additional couplings possible between nuclei, with transition frequencies in the tens of Hz (Barnes and Greenebaum 2015), although these are possibly not strong enough to be of biological significance (Hore and Mouritsen 2016). More recently, Binhi and Prato (2017) have proposed a generalized interaction between biological entities with magnetic moments precessing in an AC/DC magnetic environment. However, Barnes and Greenebaum (2017) question how a stopping of precession as the effective field falls towards zero could affect a significant biological change. In response, Prato and Binhi (2017) argue that "motion peculiarities" could couple to changed biophysical events.

Since the evidence of the presence of significant amounts of magnetic particles in neural tissue in general (as opposed to specific locations, for example, the upper beak area of birds) is lacking, it appears unlikely that the mechanism underlying weak ELF fields (assuming they do exist) is due to this source. The lower limit of sensitivity of neural networks, on the other hand, was calculated to be around 1 mV/m (WHO 2007, McKinlay and Repacholi 2003), which is below the 50/60 Hz Basic Restriction in current standards. One of the constraints in such a mechanism is intrinsic fluctuations in membrane potentials, implying that fields below around 10 mV/m may be below the noise level (Wood 2008), unless specific signal enhancement mechanisms are in place (as there is for instance in fish electroreception, above).

15.4 Radiofrequency (RF) Fields

At high levels of RF exposure, cognitive and behavioral effects are a consequence of local or generalized temperature rise, leading to clinical hyperthermia. Experiments on both human volunteers and laboratory animals have contributed to an extensive database of physiological responses resulting from quantified RF dose, measured as specific absorption rate (SAR), which is directly related to local rise in temperature. Since a rise in body core temperature gives rise to compensatory mechanisms such as sweating and increased capillary blood flow (leading to greater heat convection and radiation), both humans and animals are able to continue functioning more or less normally until the range of compensation is exceeded. However, the feeling of discomfort can lead to reduced concentration and productivity. These experiments have been reviewed (D'Andrea et al. 2003, Adair and Black 2003 D'Andrea et al. (2007), examining, in particular, the behavioral issues of detection, aversion, and performance disruption. These considerations have been a major driver of determining the levels of Basic Restrictions for RF standards. These levels have remained in place for two decades and appear set to remain so (at least, below 6 GHz). The discussion for the remainder of this chapter will be on whether there could be nonthermal (or subtle thermal) effects below these levels affecting behavior or cognition. As in the case of ELF, the main lines of investigation have been: human volunteer studies; epidemiological studies; animal and in-vitro studies, with considerations of what possible mechanism could underlie such nonthermal effects. Again, it is not possible to be exhaustive in reviewing relevant literature. Lines of study have been selected to have direct bearing on cognitive processes: for those who require a more extensive coverage of the literature, this can be found in ICNIRP (1998), SCENIHR (2015), and Vecchia et al. (2009).

15.4.1 Effects of Weak RF Fields on Humans

15.4.1.1 Cognitive Performance and Event-Related Electroencephalogram Correlates

Human cognition encompasses many different processes and functions, most notably those related to attention, memory, decision-making, language, comprehension, and problem-solving. Since the majority of RF emitted by devices held near the head, such as mobile phones, is transmitted through the skull and reaches the brain, it has been suggested that exposure to such fields may influence cerebral activity, and therefore cognitive performance. Numerous studies have assessed this possible influence of RF exposure on cognition and behavior, with the most notable aspects of cognition all being addressed to at least some extent.

One of the most commonly assessed aspects of cognition is that of attention, which generally refers to the ability to actively concentrate and process information in our environment. Many studies have addressed different aspects and types of attention, such as performance on a vigilance task, complex visual search tasks, and in particular, measures of reaction time. Overall, results from these studies have been quite contradictory with impairments in attention (e.g., Eliyahu et al. 2006, Hamblin et al. 2004, Maier et al. 2004) and improvements in attention (e.g., Curcio et al. 2004, Preece et al. 1999, Verrender et al. 2016) both being shown. Furthermore, the large majority of studies have not shown any exposure-related changes to attention (e.g., Curcio et al. 2008, 2012, Hamblin et al. 2006, Russo et al. 2006).

In regard to memory, another commonly assessed aspect of cognition, the research has produced similarly inconsistent results. Memory refers to the way in which information is encoded, stored, and retrieved, and therefore forms an essential part of our daily information processing and learning. Although some studies have reported decrements in accuracy and performance in short-term, verbal, and working memory tasks during or following exposure to RF (Keetley et al. 2006, Krause et al. 2004, Leung et al. 2011 Sauter et al. 2015, Schmid et al. 2012a), a similar number of studies have reported improvements in these measures (Lass et al. 2002, Regel et al. 2007a,b, Verrender et al. 2016). Furthermore, as has been seen with the studies assessing attention, most studies have failed to show any effects of RF exposure on measures of memory (e.g., Krause et al. 2007, Preece et al. 1999, Wallace et al. 2012).

Although the majority of studies have focused on different aspects of attention and memory either during or following acute exposure to RF EMF in adults, there are some limited studies that have looked at other endpoints, longer exposures, and exposure in other samples such as children and adolescents. Gross motor task performance, such as finger movement, movement preparation, and psychomotor speed have all been shown to not be influenced by RF exposure (Curcio et al. 2008, Freude et al. 2000, Terao et al. 2006). Similarly, two studies have also looked at chronic or long-term exposure to RF, with neither reporting any effects (Besset et al. 2005, Fritzer et al. 2007). In regard to exposures on children and adolescents, although research is currently limited, results are similar to those reported for adults, with the majority of studies reporting no effects on measures of cognition (Haarala et al. 2005, Loughran et al. 2013, Preece et al. 2005, Riddervold et al. 2008). One study, however, did report impaired working memory performance in a 3G (but not 2G) RF exposure condition in a group of 13–15 year olds (Leung et al. 2011). Given the strong methodology employed in this study, and also that it is the only study to date that has accounted for floor and ceiling effects in memory performance, the possibility of subtle effects cannot be entirely ruled out and should be addressed in the future in children and adolescents.

In addition to these behavioral measures of cognition, event-related brain activity as measured by the EEG (e.g., event-related potentials (ERPs), event-related synchronization/ desynchronization (ERS/ERD) provides useful additional information regarding specific neural processes, and given that these are direct measures of neuronal function related to cognition, may be more sensitive at detecting exposure-related effects than behavioral measures. Indeed, a number of studies have investigated effects of RF exposure on early sensory (visual and auditory) and later cognitive ERP endpoints, and although some studies have reported subtle effects (e.g., Maby et al. 2005, 2006, Preece et al. 1998) when more appropriate methodologies have been employed (such as the use of double-blind study designs), no effects have been reported (e.g., Hamblin et al. 2006, Kleinlogel et al. 2008, Stefanics et al. 2008, Trunk et al. 2014).

Overall, a substantial amount of research has been performed related to possible effects of RF exposure on cognition, and although there have been some reports of subtle effects on different aspects of performance, behavior, and related neural activity, these studies have not been able to be replicated by larger studies with stronger methodologies, suggesting that cognitive functioning is likely not impacted by such RF exposures (Tables 15.5 and 15.6).

15.4.1.2 Electrical Brain Activity

Electrical brain activity, as measured by the EEG, is a non-invasive measurement that is recorded from electrodes placed on the scalp and reflects synchronous activity in relatively large populations of cortical neurons. It is commonly divided into discrete frequency ranges (delta: 1–4 Hz, theta: 4–8 Hz, alpha: 8–12 Hz, and beta: 12–30 Hz) which are also associated with different behavioral states (for example, sleep vs waking), making it particularly useful in the assessment of RF bioeffects. Due to early studies suggesting that different indices of the EEG may be influenced by RF exposure, a substantial amount of research has focused on this, both in relation to the awake resting EEG and the EEG during sleep.

15.4.1.2.1 Resting (awake) EEG

Resting EEG is commonly recorded for short durations under either eyes open or eyes closed conditions. The majority of research investigating the effects of RF exposure on resting EEG has been performed using eyes closed conditions, as alpha activity, the activity that has been of interest in this field, is attenuated with eyes being open.

Early studies tended to show no influence of RF exposure on alpha activity (Hietanen et al. 2000, Roschke and Mann 1997), however, these studies involved particularly short exposure durations with inadequate exposure and dosimetric information provided. Several studies from Switzerland followed up on this work and, using more rigorous methodology, were able to show a more consistent influence of mobile phone-like RF exposure on alpha EEG activity after exposure, an effect that was seen in both adults (Huber et al. 2002, Regel et al. 2007a) and children (Loughran et al. 2013). These studies have since been supported by numerous studies also showing RF exposure-related changes to EEG activity in the alpha frequency range (e.g., Curcio et al. 2005, Ghosn et al. 2015, Perentos et al. 2013), as well as two studies that used eyes open resting EEG to avoid possible ceiling effects (Croft et al. 2008, 2010).

Although most effects have been on alpha frequency activity, some studies have also reported effects on other frequency bands (e.g., D'Costa et al. 2003), but these results have not been replicated. Additionally, a limited number of studies have reported effects on inter-hemispheric coherence (e.g., Hountala et al. 2008, Vecchio et al. 2007, 2010), but again, these results are yet to be replicated and therefore interpretation remains unclear.

In summary, there is growing evidence that RF exposure, such as that emitted by mobile phones, is sufficient to influence EEG activity in the alpha frequency range (Table 15.7). Despite this, the evidence regarding effects on children, as well as the functional consequence for such changes to the EEG, remains limited.

15.4.1.2.2 Sleep Architecture and Sleep EEG

Sleep is an essential part of our health and wellbeing. It is a natural, periodically recurring state of reduced activity that is characterized by a reduction in consciousness, as well as by a number of specific changes in physiology, particularly in relation to brain activity.

TABLE 15.5

Human Volunteer Experiments Involving RF Exposure with Assessments of Cognition

Author, Year	Number of Participants	Type of Antenna	Orientation	Frequency	Field Strength(s)	Duration and Intermittency of Exposure	Measures	Outcomes (Effects of Exposure)	Notes
Berlin, Germany									
Freude et al. (1998)	16	GSM phone with extended antenna	Against the left ear	916.2 MHz	SAR$_{10g}$ 0.88 W/kg	About 13 min	Visual monitoring task (VMT) and simple finger movement task	No effect of exposure	
Freude et al. (2000)	16 in each of two experiments	GSM phone with extended antenna	Against the left ear	916.2 MHz	SAR$_{10g}$ 0.88 W/kg	About 6 min in the first and about 15 min in the second experiment	First experiment: VMT; Second experiment: VMT, simple finger movement task and two-stimulus task	No effect of exposure	
Bristol, United Kingdom									
Preece et al. (1999)	36	Mobile phone copy with quarter-wave antenna	Against right ear	Simulated GSM signal, 915 MHz; Analogue signal, 915 MHz	Mean output power 0.125 W; output power about 1 W	About 25–30 min	Attention and memory performance in 10 different tasks	Decrease in choice reaction times (stronger in the analogue condition)	
Preece et al. (2005)	18	GSM phone	Against the left ear	902 MHz	Average output power 0.25 W giving brain maximum SAR 0.28 W/kg	~30–35 min	Attention and memory performance in 10 different tasks	No effect of exposure	Participants were children (10–12 years)
Prague, Czech Republic									
Jech et al. (2001)	22	GSM signal emitted by a right ear phone	Close to the	900 MHz	SAR$_{10g}$ 0.06 W/kg	45 min	Sustained attention task (visual odd-ball paradigm)	Decrease in reaction times	Participants were patients with narcolepsy

(Continued)

TABLE 15.5 (*Continued*)

Human Volunteer Experiments Involving RF Exposure with Assessments of Cognition

Author, Year	Number of Participants	Type of Antenna	Orientation	Frequency	Field Strength(s)	Duration and Intermittency of Exposure	Measures	Outcomes (Effects of Exposure)	Notes
Tallinn, Estonia									
Lass et al. (2002)	100	EMF signal emitted by quarter wave antenna	10 cm from right side of the head	450 MHz pulse modulated at 7 Hz	Power density 1.58 W/m² SAR_{1g} 0.30 W/kg	10–20 min (varied between participants)	Attention, divided attention, and short-term memory tasks	Increase of accuracy only in the visual short-term memory task	Between subjects design (50 in the exposure and 50 in the sham group)
Rodina et al. (2005)	10	EMF signal emitted by quarter wave antenna	10 cm from right side of the head	450 MHz pulse modulated at 7 Hz	Power density 0.16 mW/cm² SAR_{1g} 0.35 W/kg	3–5 min (varied between participants)	Perception and awareness (visual masking task)	Decreased accuracy in exposure condition	
Turku, Finland									
Krause et al. (2000a)	24	GSM phone	Right side of head	902 MHz	SAR < 2 W/kg	About 30 min	Visual sequential letter memory task performance with varying working memory load (0-, 1-, and 2-back)	No effect of exposure	SAR not measured (data based on manufacturer information)
Krause et al. (2000b)	16	GSM phone	Right side of head	902 MHz	SAR < 2 W/kg	30 min	Auditory verbal memory task performance in encoding and retrieval activity	No effect of exposure	SAR not measured (data based on manufacturer information)
Krause et al. (2004)	24	GSM phone	Left side of head	902 MHz	SAR_{10g} 0.648 W/kg	30 min	Auditory verbal memory task performance in encoding and retrieval activity	Increased mean percentage of incorrect answers	

(*Continued*)

TABLE 15.5 (*Continued*)

Human Volunteer Experiments Involving RF Exposure with Assessments of Cognition

Author, Year	Number of Participants	Type of Antenna	Orientation	Frequency	Field Strength(s)	Duration and Intermittency of Exposure	Measures	Outcomes (Effects of Exposure)	Notes
Krause et al. (2007)	36 participants in each study	GSM phone antenna	~20 mm from right and left posterior temporal region	GSM-like and CW signals, 902 MHz	SAR_{10g} 0.74 W/kg	About 27 min for each side (auditory task) and about 40 min for each side (visual task)	First experiment: auditory verbal memory task; Second experiment: visual sequential letter memory task with varying working memory load (0-, 1-, 2- and 3-back)	No effect of exposure	
Koivisto et al. (2000b)	48	GSM phone	Against left ear	902 MHz	Average output power 0.25 W	About 60 min	Reaction time performance assessed in 12 tasks	Decrease of response times in simple reaction time and vigilance tasks; decrease of time needed in a mental arithmetic task. Fewer errors in vigilance task	
Haarala et al. (2003b)	64	GSM phone	Against left ear	902 MHz	SAR_{1g} 0.88 W/kg, peak value 1.2 W/kg	About 65 min	Cognitive functioning assessed in 9 tasks	No effect of exposure	
Koivisto et al. (2000a)	48	GSM phone	Against left ear	902 MHz	Average output power 0.25 W	About 30 min	Sequential letter memory task with varying working memory load (0-, 1-, 2-, and 3-back)	Decrease of response times with highest memory load for "targets"; no effect for non-targets	

(*Continued*)

TABLE 15.5 (*Continued*)

Human Volunteer Experiments Involving RF Exposure with Assessments of Cognition

Author, Year	Number of Participants	Type of Antenna	Orientation	Frequency	Field Strength(s)	Duration and Intermittency of Exposure	Measures	Outcomes (Effects of Exposure)	Notes
Haarala et al. (2004)	64	GSM phone	Against left ear	902 MHz	SAR_{10g} 0.99 W/kg, peak value 2.07 W/kg	About 65 min	Memory tasks with varying working memory load (0-,1-,2- and 3-back)	No effect of exposure	
Haarala et al. (2003a)	10	GSM phone	Against left ear	902 MHz	SAR_{10g} 0.99 W/kg	About 45 min	Memory task with varying working memory load (0-, 1-, 2- and 3-back)	No effect of exposure	
Aalto et al. (2006)	12	GSM phone	Against left ear	902 MHz	SAR_{10g} 0.74 W/kg	About 51 min	Simple working memory (1-back task)	No effect of exposure	
Haarala et al. (2005)	32	GSM phone	Against left ear	902 MHz	SAR_{10g} 0.99 W/kg	~50 min	Attention-vigilance and memory performance in eight tasks	No effect of exposure	Participants were children (10–14 years)
Haarala et al. (2007)	36	Pulsed and CW signal emitted by GSM phone	Against right or left ear	902 MHz	SAR_{10g} 0.74 W/kg, peak 1.18 W/kg	~45 min per side	Attention (simple reaction times, 10-choice reaction time, subtraction, verification and vigilance tasks) and short term memory tasks with varying load (0-,1-,2- and 3-back)	No effect of exposure	
Kwon et al. (2011)	13	GSM phone	Against right ear	902.4 MHz	SAR_{10g} 0.7 W/kg	33 min	Simple visual vigilance task (0-back task)	No effect of exposure	

(Continued)

TABLE 15.5 (*Continued*)

Human Volunteer Experiments Involving RF Exposure with Assessments of Cognition

Author, Year	Number of Participants	Type of Antenna	Orientation	Frequency	Field Strength(s)	Duration and Intermittency of Exposure	Measures	Outcomes (Effects of Exposure)	Notes
Kwon et al. (2012)	15	GSM phone	Against right ear	902.4 MHz	SAR_{10g} 0.7 W/kg (right exposure), 1.0 W/kg (left exposure), 0.7 W/kg (front exposure)	5 min, 3 times for each condition	Visual vigilance task (match-to sample 0-back task)	No effect of exposure	
Rome and L'Aquila, Italy									
Curcio et al. (2004)	20	GSM phone	1.5 cm from left ear	902.4 MHz	SAR_{10g} 0.5 W/kg	45 min	Vigilance, attention and mental arithmetic functioning (acoustic simple- and choice-reaction tasks, visual search task, and arithmetic descending subtraction task), assessed as speed and accuracy before, during (50% of volunteers) or after exposure (50% of volunteers)	Decrease of both simple- and choice-reaction times	
Curcio et al. (2008)	24	GSM phone	1.5 cm from right ear	902.40 MHz	SAR_{10g} 0.5 W/kg	15 min × 3 times	Psychomotor performance (acoustic simple reaction time task and sequential finger tapping task) assessed after exposure	No effect of exposure	

(Continued)

TABLE 15.5 (*Continued*)

Human Volunteer Experiments Involving RF Exposure with Assessments of Cognition

Author, Year	Number of Participants	Type of Antenna	Orientation	Frequency	Field Strength(s)	Duration and Intermittency of Exposure	Measures	Outcomes (Effects of Exposure)	Notes
Curcio et al. (2012)	12	GSM phone	1.5 cm from right ear	902.40 MHz	SAR_{10g} 0.5 W/kg	45 min	Attention assessed by somatosensory Go-No Go task before and after exposure	No effect of exposure	
Melbourne, Australia									
Hamblin et al. (2004)	12	GSM phone	Right side of head	894.6 MHz	Mean output power 0.25 W	60 min	Sustained attention task (auditory odd-ball paradigm)	Increase of reaction time	
Keetley et al. (2006)	120	GSM phone	Against left ear with antenna 1.5 ± 0.5 cm from head	900 MHz	Mean output power 0.23 W	About 90 min	Neuropsychological performance (8 tasks testing: learning, memory, attention, language, decision making, perception)	Impairment of simple- and choice-reaction times, of verbal memory task and of sustained attention task. Improvement of task switching/divided attention	
Hamblin et al. (2006)	120	GSM phone	Against right (n = 60) or left (n = 60) ear	895 MHz	SAR_{10g} 0.11 W/kg	30 min	Sustained attention tasks (auditory and visual odd-ball paradigm) assessed after exposure	No effect of exposure	

(Continued)

TABLE 15.5 (*Continued*)

Human Volunteer Experiments Involving RF Exposure with Assessments of Cognition

Author, Year	Number of Participants	Type of Antenna	Orientation	Frequency	Field Strength(s)	Duration and Intermittency of Exposure	Measures	Outcomes (Effects of Exposure)	Notes
Leung et al. (2011)	103	GSM (2G) handset; UMTS (3G) standard handset	Against left and right ear	894.6 MHz (GSM); 1900 MHz (UMTS)	SAR_{10g} 0.7 W/kg; SAR_{10g} 1.7 W/kg	~55 min	Sensory processing and working memory (auditory 3-stimulus oddball task and n-back task at varying cognitive load)	Reduced accuracy in n-back under 3G exposure, more evident in adolescents	Participants were different age groups: 41 adolescents (13–15 years); 42 young adults (19–40); 20 elderly (55–70 years). Effects independent of age
Magdeburg, Germany									
Hinrichs and Heinze (2004)	12	Mobile phone antenna emitting GSM-like signal	Against left ear	1870 MHz	SAR_{10g} 0.61 W/kg	30 min	Episodic memory task (encoding-retrieval paradigm), exposure during encoding phase	No effect of exposure	
Mainz, Germany									
Maier et al. (2004)	33	GSM signal emitted by patch antenna	2 m over the head	900 MHz	Power density 10 mW/m^2	30 min	Perceptual-attention assessed by auditory order threshold task before and after exposure	Decrease in performance	
Essex, United Kingdom									
Russo et al. (2006)	168	GMS and CW signal emitted by a phone	Over right (n = 42) or left (n = 42) ear	888 MHz	SAR_{10g} 1.4 W/kg	~35–40 min per side	Attention (simple- and choice-reaction time task, subtraction task and vigilant task)	No effect of exposure	Between subjects design

(*Continued*)

TABLE 15.5 (*Continued*)

Human Volunteer Experiments Involving RF Exposure with Assessments of Cognition

Author, Year	Number of Participants	Type of Antenna	Orientation	Frequency	Field Strength(s)	Duration and Intermittency of Exposure	Measures	Outcomes (Effects of Exposure)	Notes
Cinel et al. (2007)	168	GSM and CW signals emitted by a phone	Over right (n = 42) or left (n = 42) ear	888 MHz	SAR_{10g} 1.4 W/kg	40 min per side	Perceptual-attention (auditory order threshold task) assessed before and after exposure	No effect of exposure	Between subjects design
Eltiti et al. (2009)	88	Base station antenna emitting GSM like signal; and UMTS like signal	5 m from participant	Combined signal of 900 and 1,800 MHz frequency bands (GSM); 2,020 MHz (UMTS)	Power density 10 mW/m²	50 min	Attention and memory (digit symbol substitution, digit span and mental arithmetic tasks)	No effect of exposure	Half of the participants were IEI-EMF
Wallace et al. (2012)	48 volunteers with IEI-EMF; 132 healthy controls	TETRA signals emitted by antenna	4.95 m in front of participant irradiating upper legs and upwards	420 MHz	Power density 10 mW/m², mean SAR appr. 0.27 mW/kg	50 min	Working memory (Operation Span task), short term memory (Digit Span backward and forward), and attention (Letter Cancellation task)	No effect of exposure	Included participants with IEI-EMF
Montpellier, France									
Besset et al. (2005)	55	GSM phone	Against the preferred ear	900 MHz	SAR_{10g} 0.54 W/kg	120 min/day 5 day/week in 4 weeks	Information processing speed, attention capacity memory and executive function assessed by 22 tasks 4 times in a 45-day period	No effect of exposure	Between subjects design

(Continued)

TABLE 15.5 (*Continued*)

Human Volunteer Experiments Involving RF Exposure with Assessments of Cognition

Author, Year	Number of Participants	Type of Antenna	Orientation	Frequency	Field Strength(s)	Duration and Intermittency of Exposure	Measures	Outcomes (Effects of Exposure)	Notes
Vienna, Austria									
Schmid et al. (2005)	58	UMTS generic signal emitted by helical antenna	Left side of head	1,970 MHz	SAR_{10g} 0.037, 0.37 W/kg	~60 min	Visual perception (Critical Flicker and Fusion Frequency Test, Visual Pursuit Test, Tachistoscopic Traffic Test Mannheim, and Contrast Sensitivity Threshold)	No effect of exposure	
Unterlechner et al. (2008)	40	UMTS generic signal emitted by helical antenna	Left side of head	1,970 MHz	SAR_{10g} 0.037, 0.37 W/kg	90 min	Attention (simple-reaction time, vigilance and determination tasks, and Flicker and Fusion Frequency test)	No effect of exposure	
Zurich, Switzerland									
Regel et al. (2006)	33 volunteers with IEI-EMF; 84 healthy controls	UMTS base station-like signal emitted by antenna	Antenna 2 m from and targeting left back side of participants	2,140 MHz	Electric field strength 1 and 10 V/m; brain SAR_{10g} 0.45 mW/kg at 1 V/m, 0.045 mW/kg at 0.1 V/m	45 min	Attention (simple- and choice-reaction times tasks, and visual selective attention task) and short-term memory (n-back task)	No effect of exposure	Included participants with IEI-EMF

(*Continued*)

TABLE 15.5 (*Continued*)

Human Volunteer Experiments Involving RF Exposure with Assessments of Cognition

Author, Year	Number of Participants	Type of Antenna	Orientation	Frequency	Field Strength(s)	Duration and Intermittency of Exposure	Measures	Outcomes (Effects of Exposure)	Notes
Regel et al. (2007a)	24	GSM and CW signal emitted by planar patch antennas	115 mm from head at left side	900 MHz	SAR_{10g} 1 W/kg	30 min	Attention (simple- and choice-reaction times tasks) and working memory (n-back task)	Reduced reaction speed in the two working memory tasks (2- and 3-back) and increased accuracy in the one working memory task (3-back) for in last part of exposure (GSM exposure)	
Regel et al. (2007b)	15	GSM signal emitted by planar antenna	11.5 cm from left ear	900 MHz	SAR_{10g} 0.2, 5 W/kg	30 min	Attention (simple- and choice-reaction times tasks) and working memory (n-back task)	Dose-dependent reduced reaction speed for one working memory task (1-back) and increased accuracy in the first part of exposure to 0.2 W/kg for one working memory task (2-back)	
Schmid et al. (2012a)	30	GSM signals emitted by planar antenna	115 mm from left side of head	900 MHz, pulse modulated at 14 Hz or 217 Hz	SAR_{10g} 2 W/kg	30 min	Attention (simple reaction time task, 2-choice reaction time task) and memory (1-, 2-, 3-back tasks)	Decreased accuracy with 3-back memory task only with 14 Hz in the first part of exposure	

(*Continued*)

TABLE 15.5 (*Continued*)

Human Volunteer Experiments Involving RF Exposure with Assessments of Cognition

Author, Year	Number of Participants	Type of Antenna	Orientation	Frequency	Field Strength(s)	Duration and Intermittency of Exposure	Measures	Outcomes (Effects of Exposure)	Notes
Schmid et al. (2012b)	25	GSM pulse modulated signal emitted by planar antenna ; Pulsed magnetic field from Helmholtz coils over both sides, pulse frequency 2 Hz	115 mm from left side of head	900 MHz, pulse modulated at 2 Hz	SAR$_{10g}$ 2 W/kg; Peak magnetic flux density 0.70 mT	30 min	Attention (simple reaction time task, 2-choice reaction time task) and memory (1-, 2-, 3-back tasks)	Improved speed in one attention task (pulsed magnetic field exposure)	
Loughran et al. (2013)	22	GSM signal, Planar antenna	Left side of the head	900 MHz	SAR$_{10g}$ 1.33 W/ kg; 0.35 W/kg	30 min	Attention (simple reaction time task, 2-choice reaction time task) and working memory (1-, and 2—back tasks)	No effect of exposure	Participants were children (11–13 years)
Lustenberger et al. (2013)	16	Circular polarized antenna	Facing toward volunteer's forehead	Pulse modualted 900 MHz: 7 successive 7.1 ms pulses in	SAR$_{10g}$ averaged over burst 1.0 W/kg; averaged over	8 h during sleep, each 18-min period: 5 min 0.25-Hz burst	Psychomotor performance (finger sequence tapping task) after exposure during sleep	Decrease in performance to motor task	

(Continued)

TABLE 15.5 (Continued)

Human Volunteer Experiments Involving RF Exposure with Assessments of Cognition

Author, Year	Number of Participants	Type of Antenna	Orientation	Frequency	Field Strength(s)	Duration and Intermittency of Exposure	Measures	Outcomes (Effects of Exposure)	Notes
				500 ms bursts repeated every 4 s (0.25-Hz burst frequency) or every 1.25 s (0.8-Hz burst frequency)	8-h night exposure 0.15 W/kg	frequency, 1 min no exposure, 5 min 0.8-Hz burst frequency, 7 min no exposure			
Yavne, Israel									
Eliyahu et al. (2006)	36	GSM phone	Over right and left ears	890.2 MHz	Average output power 0.25 W	Two ~60 min exposures separated with 5 min break for each exposure condition.	Spatial and verbal recognition tasks, two spatial compatibility tasks	Increase in reaction time with left side exposure and left hand responses when compared to combined results for sham and right side exposures in one task	
Luria et al. (2009)	48	GSM phone	Over right and left ears	890.2 MHz	SAR 0.54–1.09 W/kg	50–60 min	Working memory assessed by spatial task	No effect of exposure	
Tokyo, Japan									
Terao et al. (2006)	16	Pulse modulated EMF signal emitted by mobile phone	Over right ear	800 MHz; 20 ms time division multiple access frame, 6.7 ms time slots	SAR_{10g} 0.05 ± 0.02 W/kg	30 min	Motor preparation (visuo-motor choice reaction time, movement time and accuracy) assessed before and after exposure	No effect of exposure	

(Continued)

TABLE 15.5 (*Continued*)

Human Volunteer Experiments Involving RF Exposure with Assessments of Cognition

Author, Year	Number of Participants	Type of Antenna	Orientation	Frequency	Field Strength(s)	Duration and Intermittency of Exposure	Measures	Outcomes (Effects of Exposure)	Notes
Terao et al. (2007)	10	Pulse modulated EMF signal emitted by mobile phone	Over right ear	800 MHz; 20 ms time division multiple access frame, 6.7 ms time slots	SAR_{10g} 0.05 ± 0.02 W/kg	30 min	3 saccade tasks (eye movement latency, speed, amplitude and task accuracy) and perceptual-attention performance assessed by reaction time to visual detection task before and after exposure	No effect of exposure	
Furubayashi et al. (2009)	11 volunteers with IEI-EMF; 43 healthy controls	W-CDMA base station like signals emitted by horn antenna	3 m behind participant	2,140 MHz	Electrical field strength 10 V/m, brain SAR_{10g} 0.0078 W/kg	30 min continuous and intermittent (randomly on and off at 5 min intervals)	Attention (choice reaction times) assessed after exposure	No effect of exposure	Included participants with IEI-EMF
Okano et al. (2010)	10	Mobile phone handset	Over left ear	1,950 MHz; 20 ms time division multiple access frame, 6.7 ms time slots	Mean output power 250 mW	30 min	Inhibitory cortical performance assessed by 4 oculomotor paradigms (eye movement latency, speed, amplitude, task accuracy of and partly frequency of saccades) before and after exposure	No effect of exposure	

(*Continued*)

TABLE 15.5 (*Continued*)

Human Volunteer Experiments Involving RF Exposure with Assessments of Cognition

Author, Year	Number of Participants	Type of Antenna	Orientation	Frequency	Field Strength(s)	Duration and Intermittency of Exposure	Measures	Outcomes (Effects of Exposure)	Notes
Umea, Sweden									
Wilén et al. (2006)	20 volunteers with IEI-EMF; 20 healthy controls	Signals from GSM test mobile phone emitted by a base station antenna	8.5 cm from right side of the head	900 MHz	SAR_{10g} 0.8 W/kg	30 min	Arousal/vigilance (critical flicker fusion threshold) and short-term memory (modified version of Sternberg test)	No effect of exposure	Included participants with IEI-EMF
Kiel, Germany									
Fritzer et al. (2007)	20	GSM signal emitted by 3 antennas	30 cm from the vertex of the head	900 MHz	SAR_{1g} 0.875 W/kg	8 h × 6 nights	Seven tests evaluating attention, learning and memory assessed before and after exposure	No effect of exposure	Between subjects design
Bern, Switzerland									
Kleinlogel et al. (2008b)	15	GSM base station-like signal emitted by broadband antenna; UMTS handset-like signal	Against left ear	900 MHz (GSM); 1,950 MHz (UMTS)	SAR_{10g} 1.0 W/kg; SAR_{10g} 0.1, 1.0 W/kg	Both 30 min	Attention assessed by continuous performance test	Increased errors in UMTS lowest level in one of two task conditions	

(Continued)

TABLE 15.5 (*Continued*)

Human Volunteer Experiments Involving RF Exposure with Assessments of Cognition

Author, Year	Number of Participants	Type of Antenna	Orientation	Frequency	Field Strength(s)	Duration and Intermittency of Exposure	Measures	Outcomes (Effects of Exposure)	Notes
Pecs, Hungary									
Stefanics et al. (2008)	36	Signals from UMTS mobile phone emitted by patch antenna	Over right ear	Not specified	SAR_{1g} 0.39 W/kg	20 min	Attention assessed by auditory oddball paradigm before and after exposure	No effect of exposure	
Trunk et al. (2014), Trunk et al. (2015)	25	Signals from UMTS mobile phone transmitted by a patch antenna	4–5 mm from right ear	1,947 MHz	SAR_{1g} 1.75 W/kg in brain 20 mm from the surface	15 min	Sustained attention task (visual odd-ball paradigm) and target probability processing (on RT from the same paradigm) assessed previous, during and after exposure	No effect of exposure	
Zentai et al. (2015)	19	Client unit 40 cm away from participant's nose, access point and control PC in an adjacent room	40 cm away from participant's nose	Wi-Fi exposure 2,453 MHz	SAR_{10g} 15.1 mW/kg (skin), 1.79 mW/kg (brain tissue)	60 min	Sustained attention (psychomotor vigilance test) assessed both during and after exposure	No effect of exposure	

(Continued)

TABLE 15.5 (Continued)

Human Volunteer Experiments Involving RF Exposure with Assessments of Cognition

Author, Year	Number of Participants	Type of Antenna	Orientation	Frequency	Field Strength(s)	Duration and Intermittency of Exposure	Measures	Outcomes (Effects of Exposure)	Notes
Aarhus, Denmark									
Riddervold et al. (2008)	40 adolescents; 40 adults	Three types of signals emitted by antenna-CW, signal modulated as UMTS, UMTS signal including all control features	Antenna 2.8 m from the participant	2,140 MHz	Electrical field strength 0.9–2.2 V/m	45 min	Attention, vigilance and memory (simple- and complex-reaction times tasks, Paired Associated Learning and Trail Making Test-B)	No effect of exposure	Included adolescent participants (15–16 years)
Riddervold et al. (2010)	53	TETRA handset	Against left side of the head	420 MHz	SAR_{10g} 2.0 W/kg	45 min	Vigilance, attention, working memory and executive functioning (Reaction Times, Corsi Span test, Digit Span test and Trail Making Test-B)	No effect of exposure	
Uppsala/Stockholm, Sweden									
Wiholm et al. (2009)	23 volunteers with IEI-EMF; 19 healthy controls	GSM signal emitted by patch antenna	Left side of head	884 MHz	SAR_{10g} 1.4 W/kg	150 min	Spatial memory and learning by Virtual Morris Water Task assessed before and after exposure	Improvement in performance in IEI-EMF group	Included participants with IEI-EMF

(Continued)

TABLE 15.5 (*Continued*)

Human Volunteer Experiments Involving RF Exposure with Assessments of Cognition

Author, Year	Number of Participants	Type of Antenna	Orientation	Frequency	Field Strength(s)	Duration and Intermittency of Exposure	Measures	Outcomes (Effects of Exposure)	Notes
Berlin, Germany									
Sauter et al. (2011)	30	Head mounted antenna emitting GSM signal; UMTS signal	Head mounted antenna	900 MHz; 1,966 MHz	SAR$_{10g}$ 2 W/kg	About 7 h 15 min per day, each condition on 3 days	Attention (divided attention, vigilance task, and selective attention) and working memory (0- and 2-back tasks)	No effect of exposure	
Eggert et al. (2014), Sauter et al. (2015)	30	Patch antenna	Left side of head	TETRA 385 MHz	SAR$_{10g}$ 1.5 W/kg (low), 6 W/kg (high)	150 min in each of 3 sessions for each condition	Clock visual monitoring task (Eggert et al. 2014); and divided attention, vigilance, selective attention, working memory (Sauter et al. 2015) for 35 total parameters assessed immediately before and after each exposure	Reduced variability of speed at vigilance task under low TETRA, faster but less accurate performance at 1-back task under high TETRA, faster performance at 2-back under low TETRA	
Wollongong, Australia									
Verrender et al. (2016)	36	GSM, planar antenna	Left side of head	920 MHz	Three conditions: SAR$_{10g}$ 0 W/kg (sham); 1 W/kg (low RF); 2 W/kg (high RF)	30 min	Visual discrimination task and a modified Sternberg working memory task, calibrated to individual performance levels	A significant decrease in reaction time (RT) in the Sternberg working memory task was found during exposure compared to sham	

TABLE 15.6

Human volunteer experiments involving RF exposure with event-related potential (ERP) measurements

Author, Year	Number of Participants	Type of Antenna	Orientation	Frequency	Field Strength(s)	Duration and Intermittency of Exposure	Measures	Outcomes (Effects of Exposure)	Notes
Berlin, Germany									
Freude et al. (1998)	16	GSM phone with extended antenna (fed by external generator)	Against the left ear	916.2 MHz	SAR_{10g} 0.88 W/kg	About 13 min	EEG (slow wave potentials, visual)	Decrease in slow brain potential during visual monitoring task, most prominent on right side	
Freude et al. (2000)	16 in each of two experiments	GSM phone with extended antenna (fed by external generator)	Against the left ear	916.2 MHz	SAR_{10g} 0.88 W/kg	About 6 min in the first and about 15 min in the second experiment	EEG (slow wave potentials, visual)	Decrease in slow brain potential amplitude during visual monitoring task in both experiments, most prominent at right side in the second experiment	
Prague, Czech Republic									
Jech et al. (2001)	22	GSM mobile phone	Right side of head	900 MHz	SAR_{10g} 0.06 W/kg	45 min	EEG (ERPs, visual)	Increased P3a amplitude and decreased N2 amplitude with one of three target variants	Participants were narcolepsy patients
Turku, Finland									
Krause et al. (2000a)	24	GSM phone	Right side of head	902 MHz	SAR < 2 W/kg	About 30 min	EEG (ERD and ERS)	ERD and ERS responses altered in the 6–8 and 8–10 Hz frequency bands	SAR not measured (data based on manufacturer information)

(Continued)

TABLE 15.6 (*Continued*)

Human volunteer experiments involving RF exposure with event-related potential (ERP) measurements

Author, Year	Number of Participants	Type of Antenna	Orientation	Frequency	Field Strength(s)	Duration and Intermittency of Exposure	Measures	Outcomes (Effects of Exposure)	Notes
Krause et al. (2000b)	16	GSM phone	Right side of head	902 MHz	SAR < 2 W/kg	About 30 min	EEG (ERD and ERS)	Increased EEG power in alpha range (8–10 Hz). ERD and ERS time course altered in all frequency bands	SAR not measured (data based on manufacturer information)
Krause et al. (2004)	24	GSM phone	Left side of head	902 MHz	SAR_{1g} 0.648 W/kg	About 30 min	EEG (ERD and ERS)	Decreased ERS in the 4–6 Hz frequency band during encoding and retrieval	
Krause et al. (2006)	15	GSM mobile phone	Left side of head	902 MHz	SAR_{1g} 1.4 W/kg	30 min	EEG (ERD and ERS)	Increased ERD and ERS responses during encoding (4–8 Hz) and during recognition (4–8, and 15 Hz)	Participants were children (10–14 years)
Krause et al. (2007)	72	GSM-like and CW signal emitted by mobile phone antenna	~20 mm from right and left posterior temporal regions	902 MHz	SAR_{1g} 0.74 W/kg	About 27 min (auditory task) and about 40 min (visual task) for each side	EEG (ERD and ERS)	Auditory: increased ERS (GSM and CW exposure), increased ERD (CW exposure) and decreased ERD (GSM exposure); Visual: increased ERD (GSM exposure)	All effects observed in the alpha frequency band

(*Continued*)

TABLE 15.6 (*Continued*)

Human volunteer experiments involving RF exposure with event-related potential (ERP) measurements

Author, Year	Number of Participants	Type of Antenna	Orientation	Frequency	Field Strength(s)	Duration and Intermittency of Exposure	Measures	Outcomes (Effects of Exposure)	Notes
Kwon et al. (2009)	17	GSM handset-like signal from generator emitted by mobile phone antenna	Against left and right ear	902 MHz	SAR_{10g} 0.82 W/kg	18 min (2 blocks GSM exposure, and 1 block sham, each block 6 min) to each ear	EEG (ERP: mismatch negativity (MMN), auditory)	No effect of exposure	
Kwon et al. (2010)	17	GSM handset	Against left and right ear	902 MHz	SAR_{10g} 0.82 W/kg	6 min RF EMF and 2 × 6 min sham at each side	EEG (ERP: mismatch negativity (MMN) and 3 others, auditory)	No effect of exposure	
Melbourne, Australia									
Hamblin et al. (2004)	12	GSM phone	Right side of head	894.6 MHz	Mean output power 0.25 W	60 min	EEG (visual and auditory ERPs)	Reduced N100 amplitude and latency and delayed P300 latency	
Hamblin et al. (2006)	120	GSM phone	Against right (n = 60) or left (n = 60) ear	895 MHz	SAR_{10g} 0.11 W/kg	30 min	EEG (visual and auditory ERPs)	No effect of exposure	
Leung et al. (2011)	103	GSM (2G) handset; UMTS (3G) standard handset	Against left and right ear	894.6 MHz (GSM); 1,900 MHz (UMTS)	SAR_{10g} 0.7 W/kg; SAR_{10g} 1.7 W/kg	About 55 min	EEG (ERD and ERS in alpha band and three ERP components)	Increased N1 amplitude during 2G exposure in one task, and delayed alpha ERD and ERS response during 2G and 3G exposures in the other task	Participants were different age groups: 41 adolescents (13–15 years); 42 young adults (19–40); 20 elderly (55–70 years). Effects independent of age (*Continued*)

TABLE 15.6 (Continued)

Human volunteer experiments involving RF exposure with event-related potential (ERP) measurements

Author, Year	Number of Participants	Type of Antenna	Orientation	Frequency	Field Strength(s)	Duration and Intermittency of Exposure	Measures	Outcomes (Effects of Exposure)	Notes
Magdeburg, Germany									
Hinrichs and Heinze (2004)	12	Mobile phone antenna emitting GSM-like signal	Against the left ear	1,870 MHz	SAR_{10g} 0.61 W/kg	30 min	Magneto-encephalography (MEG)	No effect of exposure	
Rennes, France									
Maby et al. (2005, 2006)	9 healthy volunteers; 6 epileptic patients	GSM mobile phone	Left side of head	900 MHz	SAR_{10g} 1.4 W/kg	Duration of exposure not specified	EEG (auditory evoked potentials (AEPs))	Variable exposure-related modifications to AEPs in both healthy and epileptic participants (changes in correlation coefficients, latencies, and amplitudes)	
Tokyo, Japan									
Yuasa et al. (2006)	12	TDMA mobile phone	Right side of head	800 MHz	Brain SAR_{10g} 0.02–0.05 W/kg	30 min	EEG (somatosensory evoked potentials)	No effects of exposure	
Inomata-Terada et al. (2007)	10 healthy volunteers; 2 multiple sclerosis patients	TDMA mobile phone	Left side of head	800 MHz	SAR_{10g} 0.05 ± 0.02 W/kg	30 min	EMP recorded before and after exposure using TMS	No effects of exposure	

(Continued)

TABLE 15.6 (*Continued*)

Human volunteer experiments involving RF exposure with event-related potential (ERP) measurements

Author, Year	Number of Participants	Type of Antenna	Orientation	Frequency	Field Strength(s)	Duration and Intermittency of Exposure	Measures	Outcomes (Effects of Exposure)	Notes
Rome and Isola Tiberina, Italy									
Ferreri et al. (2006)	15	GSM mobile phone	Left side of head	902.4 MHz	SAR 0.5 W/kg	45 min	Motor evoked potentials (MEP) recorded before and after exposure using transcranial magnetic stimulation (TMS)	No effects of exposure	
Vecchio et al. (2012a)	11	GSM mobile phone	Left side of the head	902.4 MHz	SAR_{10g} 0.5 W/kg	45 min	EEG (peak amplitude of alpha ERD)	High frequency alpha ERD amplitude lower in the post-exposure session when compared with sham	
Tombini et al. (2013)	10	GSM phone	Not specified	902.4 MHz	SAR 0.5 W/kg	45 min	MEP recorded before and after exposure using transcranial magnetic stimulation	Decreased MEP amplitude, increased cortical excitability and increased intra-cortical facilitation only after exposure on the opposite side to the location of the epileptic focus	Participants were focal epilepsy patients

(*Continued*)

TABLE 15.6 (Continued)

Human volunteer experiments involving RF exposure with event-related potential (ERP) measurements

Author, Year	Number of Participants	Type of Antenna	Orientation	Frequency	Field Strength(s)	Duration and Intermittency of Exposure	Measures	Outcomes (Effects of Exposure)	Notes
Pecs, Hungary									
Stefanics et al. (2008)	36	UMTS (3G) handset-like exposure emitted by planar antenna	Right side of head	No carrier frequency provided	Brain SAR_{1g} 1.75 W/kg	20 min	EEG (ERP, auditory)	No effect of exposure	
Trunk et al. (2014)	25	Signals from UMTS mobile phone emitted by patch antenna	Right side of head	1,947 MHz	SAR_{1g} 1.75 W/kg	15 min	EEG (ERP, visual)	No effect of exposure	
Bern, Switzerland									
Kleinlogel et al. (2008b)	15	GSM signal emitted by a broadband antenna; UMTS handset-like signal	Against left ear	900 MHz (GSM); 1,950 MHz (UMTS)	SAR_{10g} 1.0 W/kg; SAR_{10g} 0.1, 1 W/kg	30 min	EEG (ERP, visual and auditory)	No effect of exposure	

(Continued)

TABLE 15.6 (Continued)

Human volunteer experiments involving RF exposure with event-related potential (ERP) measurements

Author, Year	Number of Participants	Type of Antenna	Orientation	Frequency	Field Strength(s)	Duration and Intermittency of Exposure	Measures	Outcomes (Effects of Exposure)	Notes
Bari, Italy									
Di Tommaso et al. (2010)	10	GSM handset-like exposure	At left side of head	900 MHz	Maximum local SAR 0.5 W/kg	10 min	EEG (initial contingent negative variation, auditory)	Reduced initial contingent negative variation amplitude and habituation index during both exposures	
Milan, Italy									
Parazzini et al. (2009)	59	UMTS mobile phone	Against test ear	1,947 MHz	Max SAR 0.069 W/kg	20 min, concurrent speech signal	EEG (ERP, auditory)	No effect of exposure	
Parazzini et al. (2010)	52	Signals from UMTS mobile phone transmitted by patch antenna	Against test ear	1,947 MHz	SAR_{1g} 1.75 W/kg	20 min, concurrent speech signal	EEG (ERP, auditory)	No effect of exposure	

TABLE 15.7

Human Volunteer Experiments Involving RF Exposure with Resting EEG Measurements

Author, Year	Number of Participants	Type of Antenna	Orientation	Frequency	Field Strength(s)	Duration and Intermittency of Exposure	Measures	Outcomes (Effects of Exposure)	Notes
Mainz, Germany									
Roschke and Mann (1997)	34	GSM handset-like signal	40 cm from subjects head	900 MHz	Peak output power 8 W, average power density 0.05 mW/cm² (0.5 W/m²)	3.5 min	EEG (1–15 Hz) recorded with eyes closed during exposure	No effect of exposure	
Helsinki, Finland									
Hietanen et al. (2000)	19	Three analogue phones; two GSM phones	1 cm from subjects head	Analogue phones (900 MHz); GSM phones (900 and 1,800 MHz)	Peak output power 1–2 W [Not specified for each phone]	20 min	EEG (1.5–25 Hz) recorded with eyes closed during exposure	Decrease in absolute power in the delta band for one of the analogue exposures, however, no difference was seen in the relative power of the same band	
Zurich, Switzerland									
Huber et al. (2002)	16	GSM and CW signals, planar antenna	11.5 cm from left side of head	900 MHz, pulse modulated at 2, 8, 217 and 1,736 Hz; CW, 900 MHz	SAR$_{10g}$ 1 W/kg	30 min	EEG (1–25 Hz)	EEG spectral power was increased in the alpha frequency range after GSM exposure	

(Continued)

TABLE 15.7 (Continued)

Human Volunteer Experiments Involving RF Exposure with Resting EEG Measurements

Author, Year	Number of Participants	Type of Antenna	Orientation	Frequency	Field Strength(s)	Duration and Intermittency of Exposure	Measures	Outcomes (Effects of Exposure)	Notes
Regel et al. (2007a)	24	GSM and CW signals, planar antenna	11.5 cm from left side of head	900 MHz	SAR_{10g} 1 W/kg	30 min	EEG (5–14 Hz) recorded with eyes open and closed before and 0, 30, and 60 min after exposure	Higher alpha power (10.5–11 Hz) 30 min after the GSM exposure and lower alpha power (12 Hz) 60 min after GSM exposure (all eyes closed). No effects for eyes open or following the CW exposure	
Loughran et al. (2013)	22	GSM signal, Planar antenna	Left side of the head	900 MHz	SAR_{10g} 1.33 W/kg, 0.35 W/kg	30 min	EEG (alpha) recorded with eyes closed before and 0, 30, and 60 min after exposure	Increased EEG spectral power in the alpha band (12–12.5 Hz) immediately (0 min) following exposure at 0.035 W/kg	Participants were children (11–13 years)
Melbourne, Australia									
Perentos et al. (2007)	12	Two different signals emitted by a model handset: GSM-like and CW	Left side of head	GSM (2, 8, 217, 1736 Hz); CW, 900 MHz	SAR_{10g} 1.56 W/kg	15 min	EEG (2–32 Hz) recorded with eyes closed before, during and after exposure	No effects of exposure	

(Continued)

TABLE 15.7 (*Continued*)

Human Volunteer Experiments Involving RF Exposure with Resting EEG Measurements

Author, Year	Number of Participants	Type of Antenna	Orientation	Frequency	Field Strength(s)	Duration and Intermittency of Exposure	Measures	Outcomes (Effects of Exposure)	Notes
D'Costa et al. (2003)	10	GSM phone	Phone horizontally behind head with antenna 2 cm from head	900 MHz	(1) Mean output power 0.25 W; (2) Standby mode	5 × 5-min real and 5 × 5-min sham	EEG (1–18 Hz) recorded with eyes closed during exposure	Decreases in alpha and beta bands in 0.25 W condition	
Croft et al. (2008)	120	GSM handset-like signal	Half participants received left and half right side exposure	894.6 MHz, pulse modulated at 217 Hz	SAR_{10g} 0.67 W/kg	30 min	EEG (8–12 Hz) recorded with eyes open during and after exposure	Increased alpha activity during exposure	
Croft et al. (2010)	103	GSM (2G) handset ; UMTS (3G) standard handset	Against left and right ear	894.6 MHz (GSM); 1,900 MHz (UMTS)	SAR_{10g} 0.7 W/kg; SAR_{10g} 1.7 W/kg	About 55 min	EEG (alpha: 8–12 Hz) recorded with eyes open before, during and after exposure	Increased alpha power during 2G exposure in the young adults. No effect of 2G on adolescents or elderly, and no effect of 3G on any of the age groups	Participants were different age groups: 41 adolescents (13–15 years); 42 young adults (19–40); 20 elderly (55–70 years). Effects independent of age
Perentos et al. (2013)	72	Signals emitted by specially constructed handset	Against right ear	900 MHz	SAR_{10g} 0.06 W/kg pulse modulated RF; SAR_{10g} 1.95 W/kg CW RF; ELF (pulsed as per RF condition), 25 µT: 7.77 µA/m²	20 min per condition	EEG (8–12.75 Hz) recorded with eyes closed before, during, and after exposure	Reduced alpha activity in both the PM and CW conditions compared to sham	

(Continued)

TABLE 15.7 (*Continued*)

Human Volunteer Experiments Involving RF Exposure with Resting EEG Measurements

Author, Year	Number of Participants	Type of Antenna	Orientation	Frequency	Field Strength(s)	Duration and Intermittency of Exposure	Measures	Outcomes (Effects of Exposure)	Notes
Tallinn, Estonia									
Hinrikus et al. (2004)	20	Quarter-wave antenna	10 cm from left side of head	450 MHz, pulse modulated at 7 Hz	SAR 0.0095 W/kg	Approx. 22 min (1 min on/1 min off)	EEG (4–38 Hz) recorded with eyes closed during exposure	No effect of exposure	
Hinrikus et al. (2008b)	13	Quarter-wave antenna	10 cm from left side of head	450 MHz, pulse modulated at 7, 14, and 21 Hz separately	SAR$_{1g}$ 0.30 W/kg	10 min per modulation (1 min on/1 min off)	EEG (4–38 Hz) recorded with eyes closed during exposure	For the 14 and 21 Hz modulations, alpha (8–13 Hz) and beta (15–20 Hz) frequencies were both increased in the first half-period of the exposure interval (30 s)	
Hinrikus et al. (2008a)	19, 13, 15, and 19 across 4 different studies	Quarter-wave antenna	10 cm from left side of head	450 MHz, pulse modulated at 7 Hz (group 1), 14 and 21 Hz (group 2), 40 and 70 Hz (group 3), 217 and 1000 Hz (group 4)	SAR$_{1g}$ 0.30 W/kg	20 min per modulation (1 min on/1 min off, except 7 Hz (group 1): 20 min (1 min on/1 min off)	EEG (4–38 Hz) recorded with eyes closed during exposure	Significant changes in EEG power for some individuals at all modulation frequencies except 1,000 Hz	

(*Continued*)

TABLE 15.7 (*Continued*)

Human Volunteer Experiments Involving RF Exposure with Resting EEG Measurements

Author, Year	Number of Participants	Type of Antenna	Orientation	Frequency	Field Strength(s)	Duration and Intermittency of Exposure	Measures	Outcomes (Effects of Exposure)	Notes
Hinrikus et al. (2011)	14 in each of two studies	PM signal emitted by quarter-wave antenna	10 cm from left side of head	450 MHz; (1) PM at 7, 14, and 21 Hz; (2) PM at 40 and 70 Hz	SAR$_{1g}$ 0.303 W/kg	(1) PM at 7, 14, and 21 Hz, 30 min; (2) PM at 40 and 70 Hz, 20 min; 10 min per modulation (1 min on/1 min off)	EEG (4–42 Hz) recorded with eyes closed during exposure in two groups during exposure	Increased EEG power at between 7 and 35 Hz across modulations	
Rome, L'Aquila, and Isola Tiberina, Italy									
Curcio et al. (2005)	20	GSM mobile phone	1.5 cm from left side of head	902.4 MHz	Max SAR 0.5 W/kg	45 min	EEG (1–24 Hz) recorded with eyes closed during (n = 10) and after exposure (n = 10)	Increased EEG alpha power	
Curcio et al. (2015)	12	GSM mobile phone	1.5 cm from the side of the head that the epileptic focus was on	902.4 MHz	SAR$_{10g}$ 0.5 W/kg	45 min	EEG (spiking count, spectral power (0.5–60 Hz), and coherence (0.5–100 Hz)) recorded with eyes closed before, during, and after exposure	Compared to sham, increased gamma activity in parieto-occipital and temporal areas, and increased instantaneous interhemispheric coherence in beta frequency band	Participants were epileptic patients

(*Continued*)

TABLE 15.7 (*Continued*)

Human Volunteer Experiments Involving RF Exposure with Resting EEG Measurements

Author, Year	Number of Participants	Type of Antenna	Orientation	Frequency	Field Strength(s)	Duration and Intermittency of Exposure	Measures	Outcomes (Effects of Exposure)	Notes
Vecchio et al. (2007)	10	GSM mobile phone	1.5 cm from left side of head	902.4 MHz	No SAR mentioned	45 min	EEG (coherence; about 2–12 Hz) recorded with eyes closed before and after exposure	Decreased alpha (8–12 Hz) coherence at frontal areas and increased alpha (8–10 Hz) coherence at temporal areas	
Vecchio et al. (2010)	16 elderly volunteers; 15 young volunteers	GSM mobile phone	1.5 cm from left side of head	902.4 MHz	SAR_{10g} 0.5 W/kg	45 min	EEG (coherence in about 2–12 Hz) recorded with eyes closed before and after exposure	Compared with the young, the elderly subjects showed an increase of inter-hemispheric coherence in the alpha frequency range (8–12 Hz) at both frontal and temporal regions during exposure	
Vecchio et al. (2012b)	10 epileptic volunteers; 15 age- and sex-matched controls	GSM mobile phone	1.5 cm from left side of head	902.4 MHz	SAR_{10g} 0.5 W/kg	45 min	EEG (coherence in about 2–12 Hz) recorded with eyes closed before and after exposure	Compared to control group, increased inter-hemispheric coherence in epileptic patients in frontal and temporal regions in the alpha frequency range (8–12 Hz) following exposure	Included participants who were epileptic patients

(*Continued*)

TABLE 15.7 (*Continued*)

Human Volunteer Experiments Involving RF Exposure with Resting EEG Measurements

Author, Year	Number of Participants	Type of Antenna	Orientation	Frequency	Field Strength(s)	Duration and Intermittency of Exposure	Measures	Outcomes (Effects of Exposure)	Notes
Athens, Greece									
Hountala et al. (2008)	19 and 20 volunteers across 2 studies	Dipole antenna	Positioned 20 cm from right ear	Study 1: 900 MHz (not modulated); Study 2: 1,800 MHz (not modulated)	(1) mean output power 64 mW; (2) mean output power 128 mW	Exposure duration approximately 45 min	EEG (coherence in theta, alpha, and beta bands) recorded with eyes closed during exposure	EEG coherence was reduced in males with 1,800 MHz exposure and increased in females with both 900 MHz and 1,800 MHz exposures	
Bern, Switzerland									
Kleinlogel et al. (2008a)	15	Signals emitted by broadband antenna; GSM base station-like; UMTS handset-like	Against left ear	900 MHz (GSM); 1950 MHz (UMTS)	SAR_{10g} 1 W/kg; SAR_{10g} 0.1, 1 W/kg	30 min	EEG (1–32 Hz) recorded with eyes closed during exposure	No effect of exposure	

(Continued)

TABLE 15.7 (*Continued*)

Human Volunteer Experiments Involving RF Exposure with Resting EEG Measurements

Author, Year	Number of Participants	Type of Antenna	Orientation	Frequency	Field Strength(s)	Duration and Intermittency of Exposure	Measures	Outcomes (Effects of Exposure)	Notes
Amiens, France									
Ghosn et al. (2015)	26	GSM mobile phone	Against left ear	900 MHz	SAR_{10g} 0.49 W/kg	26 min 15 sec	EEG (8–12 Hz) recorded with eyes closed and open before, during, and after exposure	Reduced alpha activity during and after exposure (eyes closed)	
Pecs, Hungary									
Trunk et al. (2015)	25	Signals from UMTS mobile phone transmitted by a patch antenna	Antenna 4–5 mm from right ear	1947 MHz	SAR_{1g} 1.75 W/kg in brain 20 mm from the surface	15 min	EEG (8–70 Hz) recorded during exposure in the pre-target period of an ERP task	No effect of exposure	

These changes occur in a cyclical fashion throughout the night, giving rise to several measures, such as sleep latency, total sleep duration, and sleep efficiency, which are collectively referred to as sleep architecture. These measures of sleep architecture, as well as the underlying changes in EEG, have high intra-individual reliability, which makes sleep a particularly sensitive measure in which to investigate potential bioeffects.

A series of initial studies from Germany, in which participants were exposed to RF throughout sleep, produced conflicting results, with a first study (Mann and Roschke 1996) reporting reduced sleep latency, reduced rapid eye movement (REM) sleep, and increased EEG power (1–20 Hz), all results which were unable to be replicated in two subsequent studies (Wagner et al. 2000, Wagner et al. 1998). However, further to these conflicting results, inadequate information regarding exposure dosimetry also made interpretation of these studies difficult.

Given the suggestion of a possible influence of RF on sleep and the sleep EEG, research from Switzerland followed up on these results, performing several studies with stronger methodologies. An initial study showed that all-night intermittent RF exposure induced increased EEG power in the alpha and sleep spindle frequency ranges (8–15 Hz) during non-REM sleep (Borbely et al. 1999). This study was followed by several studies in which similar results were found using exposure prior to sleep (Huber et al. 2000, 2002, Regel et al. 2007b, Schmid et al. 2012a,b). Importantly, these results were also subsequently replicated in Australia in a study with a rigorous methodology and largest sample size to date (Loughran et al. 2005).

Although effects on the sleep EEG have been shown consistently following RF exposure, the frequency range of the EEG in which these effects occurs has differed somewhat between studies. It is well known that alpha and sleep spindle activity varies across individuals, which may be one possible explanation for these slight differences across studies, and indeed a subsequent study on differential responsivity across individuals suggests that effects are sensitive to individual variability and that previous results are not due to chance (Loughran et al. 2012).

Studies looking at the interaction of RF with sleep have also suggested that effects may be dose-dependent (Regel et al. 2007b), and to date have only been shown to occur with pulse-modulated exposures compared to continuous wave exposures (Huber et al. 2002, Regel et al. 2007b). It is also important to note that some studies have failed to find effects of RF exposure on the EEG, however, the majority of these null effects can also be explained by differences in methodologies employed, such as the use of patient samples (Jech et al. 2001) and ill-defined or markedly different or lower exposures to those employed by previous studies reporting effects (e.g., Hung et al. 2007, Lustenberger et al. 2013). Furthermore, although some studies have reported minor changes to different aspects of sleep architecture following RF exposure, these have been inconsistent, unable to be replicated, and interpreted as being most likely due to chance.

Overall, there is substantial evidence that RF exposures influence the sleep EEG in the alpha and sleep spindle frequency ranges (Table 15.8). Despite these consistent effects, it still remains unknown what the mechanism of interaction between RF and brain activity is, and unlike other areas of bioelectromagnetic research, similar studies have not been performed in children and adolescents and therefore conclusions regarding effects on younger populations cannot yet be made.

15.4.1.3 Epidemiological Studies with Behavioral Outcomes

Although most epidemiological studies of health effects associated with RF exposure have been directed towards nervous system cancers, a number have considered behavior.

TABLE 15.8

Human Volunteer Experiments Involving RF Exposure with Sleep EEG Measurements

Author, Year	Number of Participants	Type of Antenna	Orientation	Frequency	Field Strength(s)	Duration and Intermittency of Exposure	Measures	Outcomes (Effects of Exposure)	Notes
Mainz, Germany									
Mann and Marino (1996)	12	GSM handset	40 cm from head	900 MHz	Average power density 0.05 mW/ cm^2 (0.5 W/m^2)	8 h	EEG (1–20 Hz, sleep architecture) recorded during 8 h night-time sleep	Decreased sleep latency, decreased REM sleep percentage, and increased EEG power density during REM sleep in all frequency bands	
Wagner et al. (1998)	22	GSM handset-like signal emitted by a circular polarized antenna	40 cm from head	900 MHz	SAR 0.3 W/kg, average power density 0.2 W/m^2	8 h	EEG (1–15 Hz, sleep architecture) recorded during 8 h night-time sleep	No effect of exposure	
Wagner et al. (2000)	20	GSM handset-like signal emitted by a circular polarized antenna	40 cm from head	900 MHz	Average power density 50 W/m^2 (SAR$_{10g}$ < 2 W/kg)	8 h	EEG (1–15 Hz, sleep architecture) recorded during 8-h night-time sleep	No effect of exposure	
Zurich, Switzerland									
Borbely et al. (1999)	24	GSM base station-like signal emitted by array of 3 half-wave antennas	30 cm from head behind bed	900 MHz	SAR$_{10g}$ 1 W/kg	All night intermittent exposure (15 min on, 15 min off, for 8 h)	EEG (1–25 Hz, sleep architecture) recorded during 8-h night-time sleep	Waking after sleep onset reduced; EEG spectral power increased during NREM sleep (8–15 Hz)	

(Continued)

TABLE 15.8 (Continued)

Human Volunteer Experiments Involving RF Exposure with Sleep EEG Measurements

Author, Year	Number of Participants	Type of Antenna	Orientation	Frequency	Field Strength(s)	Duration and Intermittency of Exposure	Measures	Outcomes (Effects of Exposure)	Notes
Huber et al. (2000)	16	GSM base station-like signal emitted by a planar antenna	11.5 cm from head, left and right exposures in separate sessions	900 MHz	SAR_{10g} 1 W/kg	30 min	EEG (1–25 Hz, sleep architecture) recorded during 3-h daytime sleep episode	EEG spectral power increased during NREM sleep (9.75–11.25 and 12.25–13.25 Hz)	
Huber et al. (2002)	16	GSM and CW signals; both emitted by planar antenna	11.5 cm from left side of head	GSM and CW, 900 MHz	SAR_{10g} 1 W/kg	30 min	EEG (1–25 Hz, sleep architecture) recorded during 8-h night-time sleep episode	EEG spectral power increased during NREM sleep (12.25–13.5 Hz) for GSM condition	
Regel et al. (2007b)	15	GSM signal emitted by planar antenna	11.5 cm from left ear	900 MHz	SAR_{10g} 0.2, 5 W/kg	30 min	EEG (1–25 Hz, sleep architecture) recorded during 8 h sleep episode	Increased spectral power in fast spindle frequency range during NREM (13.5–13.75 Hz) sleep following the 5 W/kg exposure	
Schmid et al. (2012a)	30	GSM signals emitted by planar antenna	115 mm from left side of head	900 MHz, pulse modulated at 14 Hz or 217 Hz	SAR_{10g} 2 W/kg	30 min	EEG (0.75–20 Hz, sleep architecture) recorded during 8 h sleep episode	Increased spectral power in spindle frequency range during NREM (12.75–13.25 Hz) and stage 2 (11.25, 12.75–13 Hz) sleep following the 14 Hz PM exposure. Increased spectral power in REM sleep (11.75–12.25 Hz) following the 217 Hz exposure	

(Continued)

TABLE 15.8 (*Continued*)

Human Volunteer Experiments Involving RF Exposure with Sleep EEG Measurements

Author, Year	Number of Participants	Type of Antenna	Orientation	Frequency	Field Strength(s)	Duration and Intermittency of Exposure	Measures	Outcomes (Effects of Exposure)	Notes
Schmid et al. (2012b)	23	GSM signal emitted by planar antenna; Pulsed magnetic field from Helmholtz coils over both sides	115 mm from left side of head	900 MHz, pulse modulated at 2 Hz (GSM); Pulsed magnetic field at 2 Hz	SAR_{10g} 2 W/kg; Peak magnetic flux density 0.70 mT	30 min	EEG (0.75–20 Hz, sleep architecture) recorded during 8 h sleep episode	NREM and stage 2 sleep: increased spectral power in spindle frequency range following PM RF (13.75–15.25 Hz), and increased delta and theta power following both exposure conditions (1.5–9 Hz) REM sleep: increased spectral power in alpha range (7.75–12.25 Hz) following PM RF, and increased power in lower delta (0.75–1.5 Hz) in REM sleep following pulsed magnetic field	
Lustenberger et al. (2013)	16	Circular polarized antenna	Facing toward volunteer's forehead	Pulse modualted 900 MHz: 7 successive 7.1 ms pulses in 500 ms bursts repeated every 4 s (0.25-Hz burst frequency) or every 1.25 s (0.8-Hz burst frequency)	SAR_{10g} averaged over burst 1.0 W/kg; averaged over 8-h night exposure 0.15 W/kg	8 h during sleep; each 18-min period: 5 min 0.25-Hz burst frequency, 1 min no exposure, 5 min 0.8-Hz burst frequency, 7 min no exposure	EEG (0.75–15 Hz, sleep architecture), event-related spectral power (1–4 Hz) and inter-trial coherence recorded during 8-h sleep episode	Decrease of total sleep time, reduced sleep efficiency, and increased waking after sleep onset during exposure. Higher slow wave activity (0.75–4.5 Hz) in the 4th NREM sleep episode during exposure. Increased event-related spectral power in the slow wave activity range in the inter-burst interval and increased phase-locking of the EEG signal in the 4th NREM sleep episode	

(*Continued*)

TABLE 15.8 (*Continued*)

Human Volunteer Experiments Involving RF Exposure with Sleep EEG Measurements

Author, Year	Number of Participants	Type of Antenna	Orientation	Frequency	Field Strength(s)	Duration and Intermittency of Exposure	Measures	Outcomes (Effects of Exposure)	Notes
Lustenberger et al. (2015)	19	Pulse modulated RF signal emitted by planar antenna	110 mm from left side of head	900 MHz, pulse modulated at 2 Hz	SAR_{10g} 2 W/kg	30 min	EEG (0.75–20 Hz, sleep architecture) recorded during 8 h sleep episode	No effect of exposure	
Melbourne, Australia									
Loughran et al. (2005)	50	GSM mobile phone	Right side of the head	894.6 MHz	SAR_{10g} 0.674 W/kg	30 min	EEG (11.5–14 Hz, sleep architecture) recorded during sleep	Increased EEG power during NREM sleep (11.5–12.25 Hz) and decreased REM sleep latency	
Loughran et al. (2012)	20	GSM mobile phone	Right side of the head	894.6 MHz	SAR_{10g} 0.674 W/kg	30 min	EEG (11.5–14 Hz, sleep architecture) recorded during sleep	Increase of sleep EEG power (11.5–12.25 Hz) at the beginning of NREM sleep. This increase was more prominent in those that had shown an increase previously compared to those that had originally decreased. The effect was greater in females	Participants were those who had participated in Loughran et al (2005)
Prague, Czech Republic									
Jech et al. (2001)	22	Signals from GSM mobile phone	Close to the right side of the head	900 MHz	SAR_{10g} 0.06 W/kg	45 min	EEG (latencies in alpha extinction, theta onset, sleep and spindle appearance) recorded during sleep	No effect of exposure	Participants were narcolepsy patients

(Continued)

TABLE 15.8 (Continued)

Human Volunteer Experiments Involving RF Exposure with Sleep EEG Measurements

Author, Year	Number of Participants	Type of Antenna	Orientation	Frequency	Field Strength(s)	Duration and Intermittency of Exposure	Measures	Outcomes (Effects of Exposure)	Notes
Magdeburg, Germany									
Hinrichs et al. (2005)	14	GSM signal emitted by a flat panel antenna	1.5 m from participants head	1800 MHz, PM 1736 Hz	Estimated SAR_{10g} 0.072 W/kg	All night (duration not specified)	EEG (1.5–30 Hz, sleep architecture) recorded during night time sleep	No effect of exposure	
Loughborough, United Kingdom									
Hung et al. (2007)	10	GSM mobile phone (controlled by GSM900 base-station simulator located in another room)	2 cm from right ear	900 MHz	SAR_{10g} talk mode: 0.13 W/kg, listen mode: 0.015 W/kg, standby: < 0.001 W/kg	Not specified	EEG (1–4 Hz, latency of sleep onset and stage 2 sleep) recorded during a 90 min daytime nap	Sleep latency delayed after talk mode exposure; delta EEG power (1–4 Hz) increased 10 min after listen mode and sham exposures, 20 min after standby exposure and at no period after talk mode	
Berlin, Germany									
Danker-Hopfe et al. (2011)	30	GSM handset-like signal; WCDMA handset-like signal	Both emitted by head-worn antenna at side of head	900 MHz (GSM); 1966 MHz (WCDMA)	SAR_{10g} 2 W/kg	8 h × 3 nights for each condition	EEG (sleep architecture) recorded during 8 h sleep episode	No effect of exposure on sleep architecture (spectral analysis not reported)	

(Continued)

TABLE 15.8 (Continued)

Human Volunteer Experiments Involving RF Exposure with Sleep EEG Measurements

Author, Year	Number of Participants	Type of Antenna	Orientation	Frequency	Field Strength(s)	Duration and Intermittency of Exposure	Measures	Outcomes (Effects of Exposure)	Notes
Uppsala/Stockholm, Sweden									
Lowden et al. (2011)	71	GSM handset-like signal emitted by a micropatch antenna	Headset at left side of head	884 MHz, PM 2, 8, 217, 1736 Hz	SAR$_{10g}$ 1.4 W/kg	3 h	EEG (0.5–16 Hz, sleep architecture) recorded during 7 h sleep episode	Duration of stage 2 sleep increased, stage 4 and slow wave sleep decreased. EEG power increased during first 30 min (0.5–1.5, 5.75–10.5 Hz), first hour (7.5–11.75 Hz) and second hour (4.75–8.25 Hz) of stage 2 sleep	Study included participants reporting symptoms from RF exposure; more than half of the participants were excluded from spectral analysis
Fukushima and Tokyo, Japan									
Nakatani-Enomoto et al. (2013)	19	Mobile phone, W-CDMA-like signal	15 mm from left side of the head	1950 MHz	SAR$_{10g}$ in head 1.52 W/kg, SAR$_{10g}$ in brain 0.13 W/kg	3 h	EEG (0.5–29.9 Hz, sleep architecture) recorded during overnight sleep episode (6.5–8 h)	No effect of exposure	

See Chapter 14 in this volume for further details of relevant studies. In laboratory studies, the RF exposure (to the head in particular) can be carefully controlled. In population-based epidemiological studies, on the other hand, the estimation of individual exposure remains problematical, since many of these studies have relied on crude estimates, such as distance to base stations or recollection of calls made as an exposure metric. Some studies have used "dose phones" in which participants have used specially modified handsets to collect individualized call data. However, these still have limitations in representing actual SAR values in the head (Inyang et al. 2010). Adolescents who are frequent users of mobile phones tend to have faster response times because of the mental exercise operating the phone gives, rather than due to RF exposure (Abramson et al. 2009, Thomas et al. 2010).

15.4.2 Effects of RF fields on Laboratory Animals (*In-vivo* Exposure)

Many of the experiments involving laboratory animals have looked at aversion behavior at thermal levels of exposure, and these have assisted in determining the Basic Restrictions referred to above. Nevertheless, some have involved lower levels of exposure, resulting in SAR values unlikely to cause significant temperature changes. As with the case of ELF exposure, a useful technique for assessing behavioral effects in laboratory animals (rodents in particular) is studying performance in a maze. No differences were found in performance in an 8-arm maze for mice exposed to GSM radiation compared to controls (Sienkiewicz et al. 2000). In a related study (Cobb et al. 2000), exposure to ultra-wideband electromagnetic pulses, produced no clear behavioral changes in rat pups exposed either pre- or postnatally, although some significant changes in some of the end-points were noted, likely (according to the authors) to be a consequence of the large number of comparisons made. Another group (Dubreuil et al. 2002) found that rats exposed to GSM-type RF (90 min, with a head-SAR of 1 or 3.5 W/kg) showed no differences in spatial learning tasks in a radial arm maze or a Morris water maze. Young male rats were studied for behavioral and post-mortem histological tests after exposure to two levels of RF (0.3 and 3 W/kg) or sham (Kumlin et al. 2007), for 2 h/day for 25 days. In general, no significant changes were noted, however in the water-maze test, slight improvements in learning and memory were recorded. More recently, changes in Morris water maze performance was noted (Tang et al. 2015) in response to exposure to GSM-type radiation (2 W/kg in the head, 3 h/day for 14 or 28 days). Specifically, the frequency of crossing platforms and the percentage of time spent in the target quadrant were lower for 28 day exposure compared to 14 day and sham exposure. In addition, evidence for blood-brain barrier (BBB) damage was also noted. Further experiments investigating RF in relation to BBB are described below. Offspring of exposed and sham-exposed GSM-type RF were tested, when reaching adulthood, for a range of measures of learning and cognition (Bornhausen and Scheingraber 2000). No significant differences were found, for the SAR values in the dams estimated to be in the range 17.5–75 mW/kg.

Other investigations have measured levels of neurotransmitter in brain tissue obtained immediately post-sacrifice following RF exposure. Levels of the neurotransmitter Gamma-amino-butyric acid (GABA) and related compounds in rat cerebellum have been studied (Mausset et al. 2001), at both low (4 W/kg) and high (32 W/kg) SAR values (exposed or sham-exposed for 2 h prior to sacrifice). A diminution in cerebellar GABA content was noted, but it was not possible to eliminate local heating as the mechanism. In further experiments (Bouji et al. 2012), endpoints relating to inflammatory processes were assessed (with a SAR of 6 W/kg), with effects appearing to be age-related.

In a study designed to elucidate possible involvement of heat-shock proteins (HSPs) following RF exposure, Yang et al. (2012) compared the gene expression patterns and immunochemistry of HSP 27 and HSP 70 between exposed and sham-exposed rats. The exposure consisted of pulsed 2.45 GHz RF (pulse duration 20 ms, 500 pps and averaged SAR of 6 W/kg, for 20 min prior to sacrifice). Significantly increased HSP expression was observed, but it was unclear whether this was purely a consequence of the relatively high SAR employed in the experiment.

BBB permeability has been the subject of several studies involving exposure of rodents to GSM-type RF. A Scandinavian group (Nittby et al. 2009) has presented evidence for increased albumin extravasation (indicating increased BBB permeability), following 2 h/day exposure for 14 days (exposure: 0, 0.12, and 120 mW/kg). However, experiments performed by an Australian group have shown no significant changes (Finnie and Blumbergs 2004, Finnie et al. 2001, 2002, 2006a). This latter group also showed no change in expression of genes such as C-fos or HSP, nor did they find changes in levels of the protein products (Finnie et al. 2006b, 2009). In these experiments, exposure was for 22 h/day for around 300 days. In experiments by another group, rats were exposed to 0.9 and 1.8 GHz continuous-wave for 20 min (at SARs of 1.46 and 4.26 mW/kg respectively) and the BBB permeability assessed via an Evans Blue marker, to indicate possible albumen extravasation (Sirav and Seyhan 2011). The results showed no extravasation in female rats, but conversely, significant extravasation was found for male rats, for both frequency values.

A number of investigations have studied whether RF exposure can be protective against the development or progression of Alzheimer's disease (AD). The Arendash group have been pre-eminent in pursuing this possibility and of the potential of RF as a therapeutic agent for AD in humans. The first evidence was from a study published in 2010, but with much supportive evidence from that group since then (Arendash 2016). However, the exposure used in the mice studies was similar to a mobile phone handset, whereas the exposure proposed for human therapy is "transcranial electromagnetic treatment" (TEMT), whose characteristics are not fully specified. Other studies are divided in their support for the hypothesis that RF affects AD. Jeong et al. (2015) present behavioral and gene expression data to conclude that 1.95 GHz RF protects against cognitive deficits in mice engineered to exhibit AD-like pathology. However, the same group were unable to find RF-related differences in a subsequent study, run over a 3-month rather than an 8-month period (Son et al. 2016). Similarly no effects were reported by Park et al. (2017), although this was study of a cell culture with exposure in vitro for only 3 days, rather than much longer periods *in-vivo*, as is the case with the Arendash work. However, experiments on mice predisposed to developing Alzheimer's-like cognitive deficits showed evidence of improved performance in maze and other cognitive tests (Flex field activity; two-compartment box test) (Banaceur et al. 2013). Here, the exposure was to 2.4 GHz, for 2 h/day for 30 days, with an estimated SAR of 1.6 W/kg, when comparing transgenic with wild-type mice. In an experiment in which rats were exposed for 2 h/day for 10 months (Dasdag et al. 2012), significant changes were reported in "protein carbonyl" but not in beta amyloid protein or malondialdehyde. On the other hand, in an experiment involving Electromagnetic Pulses (Jiang et al. 2013) on rats, subsequent observations were of performance in a Morris water maze and post-mortem measurement of expression of beta amyloid proteins and measures of oxidative stress. This exposure consisted of intense electric fields of 50 kV/m at 100 pps, with numbers of pulses ranging from 0 to 10^4. The results showed evidence of impaired cognition and memory, with increased oxidative stress. However, although the apparatus was designed to eliminate arcing, it was not possible to assess whether painful sensations were actually experienced. A follow-up study

(Jiang et al. 2016) involved exposure over an 8-month period and further showed increase in beta-amyloid content in the hippocampus.

In passing, in relation to epidemiological studies into AD, a significant reduction in the risk of hospitalization for Alzheimer's disease was noted among heavy mobile phone users in a Danish study (Schuz et al. 2009). However, in view of the possible self-selection bias, it is not possible to draw definitive conclusions.

A number of animal studies in general have provided insufficient details of RF dosimetry to allow for meaningful analysis, so the SAR estimates cannot be confirmed. A few have used mobile phone handsets in "listening" (rather than transmitting) mode as an RF source. Surprisingly, most of these have reported significant alterations in biological endpoints. Whatever has caused these changes is most therefore likely to be something other than RF.

In summary, *in-vivo* studies of RF on animal cognition and performance and studies on possible effects on BBB permeability, HSP expression, neurotransmitter release and a role in the progression of AD lack consistency and do not provide any elucidation of possible mechanisms involved putative human laboratory experiments.

15.4.3 Effects of RF Fields on Nervous System Models: *In-Vitro* Exposure

In an elegant *in-vitro* experiment, the dynamics of rat hippocampal Long-Term Potentiation (related to memory formation in the intact animal) was studied using a strip-line RF applicator, allowing simultaneous measurement of neural electrical activity (Tattersall et al. 2001). Significant SAR-dependent changes were noted in population spike amplitudes, although the changes in temperature were not detectable using direct measurement.

15.4.4 Effects of RF Fields on Animal Magnetoreception

A number of investigators have studied the effects of RF fields on direction-finding abilities of migratory birds. For example, robins were shown to be disorientated both by single-frequency and broadband RF exposures (Ritz et al. 2004). Here the magnitude of the RF magnetic field was 0.085 µT for 0.1–10 MHz broadband and 0.47 µT for the single 7 MHz frequency. Later studies showed disruption specifically at the Larmor frequency corresponding to the Earth's field (Ritz et al. 2009, Thalau et al. 2005), which was 1.315 MHz at the location of the experiment (with a magnitude of 0.015 µT. Some studies showed that both 1.315 and 7 MHz fields caused disruption (Wiltschko et al. 2015). More recent studies, again at the local Larmor frequency show disruption in both garden warblers (Kavokin et al. 2014) and cockroaches (Vacha et al. 2009). Broadband RF fields (2 kHz to 9 MHz) were shown, in double-blinded trials to be disruptive to direction-finding in robins (Engels et al. 2014, Schwarze et al. 2016). The second study was interesting, in that it found that narrow-band RF at the Larmor frequency (1.315 MHz) was unable to cause disruption (unlike the studies just discussed) but that on the other hand, the broadband exposure was very effective at doing this. The review of (Hore and Mouritsen 2016) gives further discussion of these (and other related) studies and gives some justification on the basis of modelled singlet-triplet interconversion frequencies of why an enhanced broadband response might be expected and questions whether the earlier experiments using nominally single frequencies had in fact included extra frequencies inadvertently. There appear to be no reports of direction-finding disruption above 10 MHz, although there has been speculation that if the biological compass is based on magnetite rather than retinal pigments, absorption in the GHz region would be possible (Kirschvink 1996).

15.5 Idiopathic Environmental Intolerance due to EMF (IEI-EMF)

Certain individuals report symptoms which they associate with being in proximity of electrical appliances, electricity supply infrastructure and telecommunications systems such as mobile phone handsets and base stations. These individuals suffer from what is called Idiopathic Environmental Intolerance due to EMF (IEI-EMF), or more commonly referred to as electromagnetic hypersensitivity (EHS). Although there remains no medical diagnosis for EHS (i.e., it is a self-diagnosed condition), reports of individuals experiencing unpleasant and debilitating symptoms when near such EMF-emitting devices have now been prevalent for some time (WHO 2004).

In general, EHS can be defined as a condition in which sufferers report a variety of symptoms that they attribute to being caused by EMF exposure. The symptoms reported are wide and varied, but commonly include things such as headaches, fatigue and sleeping difficulties, tingling and burning sensations in the skin, tinnitus, nausea, as well as a variety of cognitive-type problems such as memory or concentration difficulties. The type of symptoms experienced, the frequency and duration of symptoms, and the trigger for these symptoms also varies widely among sufferers of EHS. Despite this, devices and infrastructure using the RF and ELF frequency ranges have arguably been the most frequently attributed sources responsible for triggering EHS.

Although with the development of modern telecommunication technologies the prevalence of those suffering from EHS has seemed to rise, the reporting of symptoms associated with EMF is certainly not a new thing. Many years ago, several studies investigated self-reported facial skin symptoms in relation to exposure to electric fields from visual display units. However, despite this spate of research, neither laboratory nor epidemiological studies were able to show substantiated evidence of adverse health effects from the EMF that emanates from such visual display units (COMAR, 1997). As technology has developed, so too have the reports of symptoms from EMF-emitting devices, with modern devices and technologies such as mobile phones, Wi-Fi, and smart meters now being connected by sufferers as the sources of their sensitivity.

Research has responded to this, with many epidemiological and laboratory studies specifically focusing on exposures from these modern devices in an attempt to better understand this condition. In regard to epidemiological studies, two recently reported significant associations between exposure to RF EMF and symptoms. In the first, Hutter et al. (2006) found a relationship between the level of exposure to a base station signal and several symptoms (headache, cold hands and feet, difficulty concentrating) in a sample of people living near ten selected mobile phone base stations across Austria. Similarly, Abdel-Rassoul et al. (2007) conducted a study in Egypt and reported a higher prevalence of neuropsychiatric complaints (such as headaches, depressive symptoms, memory, and sleep problems) in a sample of people living near a base station when compared to matched controls. Despite these two reports of associations between RF EMF exposure and symptoms, the majority of epidemiological studies addressing this issue have actually failed to show any significant association between exposure and symptoms; in addition, epidemiological studies of higher quality and with more sophisticated exposure measurements rarely indicate any association (Roosli et al. 2010).

The situation is also similar when it comes to laboratory studies, which offer a more powerful method for detecting any possible relationship between exposure and symptoms. Typically, these human provocation studies have involved subjecting EHS sufferers to both active and sham exposures and testing whether symptoms are triggered more under conditions of EMF than sham, or whether those with EHS are better able to detect the presence of EMF than those without the condition (Verrender et al. 2017). One early study suggested a reduction in wellbeing associated with a universal mobile telecommunications system (UMTS) exposure signal (Zwamborn et al. 2003), however, a subsequent report from the Health Council of the Netherlands highlighted several limitations of this study and concluded that no health or wellbeing-related interpretations could be made and that replication was required (Health Council of the Netherlands, 2004). In general, the results from further laboratory studies have also not been able to provide evidence for any links between exposure to mobile phone and base station RF EMF exposures and symptoms experienced (Roosli et al. 2010, Rubin et al. 2010). Where studies have reported an association, methodological confounds have been present, making the results unreliable and also explaining why such associations have not been able to be replicated (Rubin et al. 2010). Additionally, many studies have also shown that sham exposures are sufficient to produce symptoms in EHS sufferers, providing further evidence that there is no relationship with EMF exposure and reinforcing the possibility of a nocebo effect being at play, where the person's expectations or perceptions of how EMF might affect them induces symptoms (Rubin et al. 2010, Verrender et al. 2017).

EHS is a complex condition that, to date, still has no medical or scientific basis. Research has consistently failed to find any association between EMF exposure and reported symptoms, suggesting that a phenomena outside of the physical interaction of EMF and the body is at play in this condition, however further studies are needed before any firm conclusions are made regarding the aetiology of EHS.

15.6 Conclusions

At sufficiently high fields, behavioral effects are manifested, not all of them deficits. For static magnetic fields, MRI workers need to be aware of sensations of vertigo and nystagmus that can lead to nausea. For static and ELF electric fields, the annoyance of spark discharges can affect performance and concentration. Migratory birds and other organisms possess a "magnetic sense" whose origin is still not entirely explained, but free radical and magnetite hypotheses have a firm theoretical and experimental basis. Electroreception is finely tuned in some fish and other organisms (including mammals) but no evidence of electroreception in humans and only limited evidence of a magnetic sense in humans.

For ELF magnetic fields, there are definite and reasonably well-understood effects from neural stimulation following strong fields from TMS, but there is growing evidence that weaker fields associated with tDCS and DBS can also modulate electrophysiology. Human studies of EEG seem to suggest significant changes, but these are hard to interpret in the light of conflicting results, in some respects. Some of the reported effects are constituent within a single laboratory, but have not been independently replicated or corroborated. The experiments involving tests of cognition are largely inconsistent; however, those using advanced imaging techniques are perhaps better placed to identify possible effects. Animal studies (including tests of memory using mazes) give little clarification, with the possible exception of work into nociception and analgesia. Assuming low-level effects do exist, the free radical lifetimes hypothesis appears to offer the "best explanation," but the amplification of weak field effects in neural networks is still a possibility. Epidemiological studies in which cognitive endpoints were assessed seem to offer little clarity into whether or not low-level ELF effects occur.

RF fields have also been extensively studied. Cognitive testing outcomes lack consistency, but electrophysiological measures such as EEG activity, both in waking and in sleep, has shown relatively consistent effects. Despite this, *in-vivo* and *in-vitro* testing for effects in animals has shown little support for human laboratory findings, although this has not been as extensively investigated. Free radical effects offer an explanation of possible influences of broadband RF effects on bird direction-finding, but in frequency ranges below around 10 MHz. The possible beneficial effects of RF in the treatment of Alzheimer's disease currently rely on the results from one laboratory and replication studies are needed.

In regard to EHS, epidemiological cross-sectional studies have not been able to provide evidence of an association between EMF and EHS symptoms, and provocation studies have not been able to show that the symptoms reported by EHS sufferers are caused by exposure to EMF.

References

Aalto, S., C. Haarala, A. Bruck, H. Sipila, H. Hamalainen, and J. O. Rinne. 2006. Mobile phone affects cerebral blood flow in humans. *J Cereb Blood Flow Metab* 26(7):885–890.

Abdel-Rassoul, G., O. A. El-Fateh, M. A. Salem, A. Michael, F. Farahat, M. El-Batanouny, and E. Salem. 2007. Neurobehavioral effects among inhabitants around mobile phone base stations. *Neurotoxicology* 28(2):434–440.

Abramson, M. J., G. P. Benke, C. Dimitriadis, I. O. Inyang, M. R. Sim, R. S. Wolfe, and R. J. Croft. 2009. Mobile telephone use is associated with changes in cognitive function in young adolescents. *Bioelectromagnetics* 30(8):678–686.

Adair, E. R., and D. R. Black. 2003. Thermoregulatory responses to RF energy absorption. *Bioelectromagnetics* (Suppl 6):S17–S38. DOI:10.1002/bem.10133.

Ahmed, Z., and A. Wieraszko. 2008. The mechanism of magnetic field-induced increase of excitability in hippocampal neurons. *Brain Res* 1221:30–40.

Arendash, G. W. 2016. Review of the evidence that transcranial electromagnetic treatment will be a safe and effective therapeutic against Alzheimer's disease. *J Alzheimers Dis* 53(3):753–771.

Baker, R. R. 1989. *Human Navigation and Magnetoreception*. Manchester: Manchester University Press.

Banaceur, S., S. Banasr, M. Sakly, and H. Abdelmelek. 2013. Whole body exposure to 2.4 GHz WIFI signals: effects on cognitive impairment in adult triple transgenic mouse models of Alzheimer's disease (3xTg-AD). *Behav Brain Res* 240:197–201.

Barnes, F., and B. Greenebaum. 2017. Comments on Vladimir Binhi and Frank Prato's A physical mechanism of magnetoreception: Extension and analysis. *Bioelectromagnetics* 38(4):322–323.

Barnes, F. S., and B. Greenebaum. 2015. The effects of weak magnetic fields on radical pairs. *Bioelectromagnetics* 36(1):45–54.

Barth, A., I. Ponocny, E. Ponocny-Seliger, N. Vana, and R. Winker. 2010. Effects of extremely low-frequency magnetic field exposure on cognitive functions: results of a meta-analysis." *Bioelectromagnetics* 31(3):173–179.

Beale, I. L., N. E. Pearce, D. M. Conroy, M. A. Henning, and K. A. Murrell. 1997. Psychological effects of chronic exposure to 50 Hz magnetic fields in humans living near extra-high-voltage transmission lines. *Bioelectromagnetics* 18(8):584–594.

Begall, S., E. P. Malkemper, J. Cerveny, P. Nemec, and H. Burda. 2013. Magnetic alignment in mammals and other animals. *Mammalian Biol* 78(1):10–20.

Bell, G. B., A. A. Marino, and A. L. Chesson. 1992. Alterations in brain electrical activity caused by magnetic fields: Detecting the detection process. *Electroencephalogr Clin Neurophysiol* 83(6):389–397.

Bell, G. B., A. A. Marino, and A. L. Chesson. 1994a. Frequency-specific blocking in the human brain caused by electromagnetic fields. *Neuroreport* 5(4):510–512.

Bell, G. B., A. A. Marino, and A. L. Chesson. 1994b. Frequency-specific responses in the human brain caused by electromagnetic fields. *J Neurol Sci* 123(1–2):26–32.

Bell, G. B., A. A. Marino, A. L. Chesson, and F. A. Struve. 1991. Human sensitivity to weak magnetic fields. *Lancet* 338(8781):1521–1522.

Bell, G., A. Marino, A. Chesson, and F. Struve. 1992. Electrical states in the rabbit brain can be altered by light and electromagnetic fields. *Brain Res* 570(1–2):307–315.

Berlim, M. T., F. Van den Eynde, and Z. J. Daskalakis. 2013. Efficacy and acceptability of high frequency repetitive transcranial magnetic stimulation (rTMS) versus electroconvulsive therapy (ECT) for major depression: A systematic review and meta-analysis of randomized trials. *Depress Anxiety* 30(7):614–623.

Bertucci, P. 2006. Revealing sparks: John Wesley and the religious utility of electrical healing. *Br J Hist Sci* 39(142 Pt 3):341–362.

Besset, A., F. Espa, Y. Dauvilliers, M. Billiard, and R. de Seze. 2005. No effect on cognitive function from daily mobile phone use. *Bioelectromagnetics* 26(2):102–108.

Binhi, V. N., and F. S. Prato. 2017. A physical mechanism of magnetoreception: Extension and analysis. *Bioelectromagnetics* 38(1):41–52.

Borbely, A. A., R. Huber, T. Graf, B. Fuchs, E. Gallmann, and P. Achermann. 1999. Pulsed high-frequency electromagnetic field affects human sleep and sleep electroencephalogram. *Neurosci Lett* 275(3):207–210.

Bornhausen, M., and H. Scheingraber. 2000. Prenatal exposure to 900 MHz, cell-phone electromagnetic fields had no effect on operant-behavior performances of adult rats. *Bioelectromagnetics* 21(8):566–574.

Bouji, M., A. Lecomte, Y. Hode, R. de Seze, and A. S. Villegier. 2012. Effects of 900 MHz radiofrequency on corticosterone, emotional memory and neuroinflammation in middle-aged rats. *Exp Gerontol* 47(6):444–451.

Capone, F., M. Dileone, P. Profice, F. Pilato, G. Musumeci, G. Minicuci, F. Ranieri, R. Cadossi, S. Setti, P. A. Tonali, and V. Di Lazzaro. 2009. Does exposure to extremely low frequency magnetic fields produce functional changes in human brain? *J Neural Transm (Vienna)* 116(3):257–265.

Carrubba, S., C. Frilot, 2nd, A. L. Chesson, Jr., and A. A. Marino. 2007a. Evidence of a nonlinear human magnetic sense. *Neuroscience* 144(1):356–367.

Carrubba, S., C. Frilot, 2nd, A. L. Chesson, Jr., and A. A. Marino. 2010. Numerical analysis of recurrence plots to detect effect of environmental-strength magnetic fields on human brain electrical activity. *Med Eng Phys* 32(8):898–907.

Carrubba, S., C. Frilot, A. L. Chesson, and A. A. Marino. 2007b. Nonlinear EEG activation evoked by low-strength low-frequency magnetic fields. *Neurosci Lett* 417(2):212–216.

Carrubba, S., C. Frilot, A. L. Chesson, Jr., C. L. Webber, Jr., J. P. Zbilut, and A. A. Marino. 2008. Magnetosensory evoked potentials: Consistent nonlinear phenomena. *Neurosci Res* 60(1):95–105.

Cinel, C., A. Boldini, R. Russo, and E. Fox. 2007. Effects of mobile phone electromagnetic fields on an auditory order threshold task. *Bioelectromagnetics* 28(6):493–496.

Cobb, B. L., J. R. Jauchem, P. A. Mason, M. P. Dooley, S. A. Miller, J. M. Ziriax, and M. R. Murphy. 2000. Neural and behavioral teratological evaluation of rats exposed to ultra-wideband electromagnetic fields. *Bioelectromagnetics* 21(7):524–537.

COMAR (IEEE Committee on Radiation and Man). 1997. Biological and health effects of electric and magnetic fields from video display terminals. *IEEE Engineering in Medicine and Biology Magazine* 16(3):87–92.

Cook, C. M., A. W. Thomas, L. Keenliside, and F. S. Prato. 2005. Resting EEG effects during exposure to a pulsed ELF magnetic field. *Bioelectromagnetics* 26(5):367–376.

Cook, C. M., A. W. Thomas, and F. S. Prato. 2002. Human electrophysiological and cognitive effects of exposure to ELF magnetic and ELF modulated RF and microwave fields: a review of recent studies. *Bioelectromagnetics* 23(2):144–157.

Cook, C. M., A. W. Thomas, and F. S. Prato. 2004. Resting EEG is affected by exposure to a pulsed ELF magnetic field. *Bioelectromagnetics* 25(3):196–203.

Cook, M. R., C. Graham, H. D. Cohen, and M. M. Gerkovich. 1992. A replication study of human exposure to 60-Hz fields: Effects on neurobehavioral measures. *Bioelectromagnetics* 13(4):261–285.

Corbacio, M., S. Brown, S. Dubois, D. Goulet, F. S. Prato, A. W. Thomas, and A. Legros. 2011. Human cognitive performance in a 3 mT power-line frequency magnetic field. *Bioelectromagnetics* 32(8):620–633.

Crasson, M., and J. J. Legros. 2005. Absence of daytime 50 Hz, 100 microT(rms) magnetic field or bright light exposure effect on human performance and psychophysiological parameters. *Bioelectromagnetics* 26(3):225–233.

Crasson, M., J. J. Legros, P. Scarpa, and W. Legros. 1999. 50 Hz magnetic field exposure influence on human performance and psychophysiological parameters: Two double-blind experimental studies. *Bioelectromagnetics* 20(8):474–486.

Crasson, M., J. J. Legros, and M. Timsit-Berthier. 1996. A double-blind evaluation of 50 Hz magnetic fields effects on human cognitive tasks, event-related potentials and neuroendocrine parameters. In C.C. Ogura, C.Y. Koga and M. Schimokochi (Eds.) *Recent Advances in Event-Related Brain Potential Research*, pp. 530–535. Belgium: Elsevier.

Croft, R. J., D. L. Hamblin, J. Spong, A. W. Wood, R. J. McKenzie, and C. Stough. 2008. The effect of mobile phone electromagnetic fields on the alpha rhythm of human electroencephalogram. *Bioelectromagnetics* 29(1):1–10.

Croft, R. J., S. Leung, R. J. McKenzie, S. P. Loughran, S. Iskra, D. L. Hamblin, and N. R. Cooper. 2010. Effects of 2G and 3G mobile phones on human alpha rhythms: Resting EEG in adolescents, young adults, and the elderly. *Bioelectromagnetics* 31(6):434–444.

Cui, Y., Z. Ge, J. D. Rizak, C. Zhai, Z. Zhou, S. Gong, and Y. Che. 2012. Deficits in water maze performance and oxidative stress in the hippocampus and striatum induced by extremely low frequency magnetic field exposure. *PLoS One* 7(5):e32196.

Curcio, G., M. Ferrara, L. De Gennaro, R. Cristiani, G. D'Inzeo, and M. Bertini. 2004. Time-course of electromagnetic field effects on human performance and tympanic temperature. *Neuroreport* 15(1):161–164.

Curcio, G., M. Ferrara, F. Moroni, G. D'Inzeo, M. Bertini, and L. De Gennaro. 2005. Is the brain influenced by a phone call? An EEG study of resting wakefulness. *Neurosci Res* 53(3):265–270.

Curcio, G., E. Mazzucchi, G. Della Marca, C. Vollono, and P. M. Rossini. 2015. *Electromagnetic* fields and EEG spiking rate in patients with focal epilepsy. *Clin Neurophysiol* 126(4):659–666.

Curcio, G., D. Nardo, M. G. Perrucci, P. Pasqualetti, T. L. Chen, C. Del Gratta, G. L. Romani, and P. M. Rossini. 2012. Effects of mobile phone signals over BOLD response while performing a cognitive task. *Clin Neurophysiol* 123(1):129–136.

Curcio, G., E. Valentini, F. Moroni, M. Ferrara, L. De Gennaro, and M. Bertini. 2008. Psychomotor performance is not influenced by brief repeated exposures to mobile phones. *Bioelectromagnetics* 29(3):237–241.

Cvetkovic, D., and I. Cosic. 2009. Alterations of human electroencephalographic activity caused by multiple extremely low frequency magnetic field exposures. *Med Biol Eng Comput* 47(10):1063–1073.

Czech-Damal, N. U., A. Liebschner, L. Miersch, G. Klauer, F. D. Hanke, C. Marshall, G. Dehnhardt, and W. Hanke. 2012. Electroreception in the Guiana dolphin (Sotalia guianensis). *Proc Biol Sci* 279(1729):663–668.

D'Andrea, J. A., E. R. Adair, and J. O. de Lorge. 2003. Behavioral and cognitive effects of microwave exposure. *Bioelectromagnetics* (Suppl 6):S39–S62.

D'Andrea, J. A., J. M. Ziriax, and E. R. Adair. 2007. Radio frequency electromagnetic fields: mild hyperthermia and safety standards. *Prog Brain Res* 162:107–135.

D'Costa, H., G. Trueman, L. Tang, U. Abdel-rahman, W. Abdel-rahman, K. Ong, and I. Cosic. 2003. Human brain wave activity during exposure to radiofrequency field emissions from mobile phones. *Australas Phys Eng Sci Med* 26(4):162–167.

Danker-Hopfe, H., H. Dorn, A. Bahr, P. Anderer, and C. Sauter. 2011. Effects of electromagnetic fields emitted by mobile phones (GSM 900 and WCDMA/UMTS) on the macrostructure of sleep. *J Sleep Res* 20(1 Pt 1):73–81.

Dasdag, S., M. Z. Akdag, G. Kizil, M. Kizil, D. U. Cakir, and B. Yokus. 2012. Effect of 900 MHz radio frequency radiation on beta amyloid protein, protein carbonyl, and malondialdehyde in the brain. *Electromagn Biol Med* 31(1):67–74.

de Vocht, F., T. Stevens, P. Glover, A. Sunderland, P. Gowland, and H. Kromhout. 2007. Cognitive effects of head-movements in stray fields generated by a 7 Tesla whole-body MRI magnet. *Bioelectromagnetics* 28(4):247–255.

Del Seppia, C., S. Ghione, P. Luschi, K. P. Ossenkopp, E. Choleris, and M. Kavaliers. 2007. Pain perception and electromagnetic fields. *Neurosci Biobehav Rev* 31(4):619–642.

Delhez, M., J. J. Legros, and M. Crasson. 2004. No influence of 20 and 400 microT, 50 Hz magnetic field exposure on cognitive function in humans. *Bioelectromagnetics* 25(8):592–598.

Di Lazzaro, V., F. Capone, F. Apollonio, P. A. Borea, R. Cadossi, L. Fassina, C. Grassi, M. Liberti, A. Paffi, M. Parazzini, K. Varani, and P. Ravazzani. 2013. A consensus panel review of central nervous system effects of the exposure to low-intensity extremely low-frequency magnetic fields. *Brain Stimul* 6(4):469–476.

Di Loreto, S., S. Falone, V. Caracciolo, P. Sebastiani, A. D'Alessandro, A. Mirabilio, V. Zimmitti, and F. Amicarelli. 2009. Fifty hertz extremely low-frequency magnetic field exposure elicits redox and trophic response in rat-cortical neurons. *J Cell Physiol* 219(2):334–343.

Di Tommaso, D., and N. H. de Leeuw. 2010. Structure and dynamics of the hydrated magnesium ion and of the solvated magnesium carbonates: Insights from first principles simulations. *Phys Chem Chem Phys* 12(4):894–901.

Diebel, C. E., R. Proksch, C. R. Green, P. Neilson, and M. M. Walker. 2000. Magnetite defines a vertebrate magnetoreceptor. *Nature* 406(6793):299–302.

Dowman, R., J. R. Wolpaw, R. F. Seegal, and S. Satya-Murti. 1989. Chronic exposure of primates to 60-Hz electric and magnetic fields: III. Neurophysiologic effects. *Bioelectromagnetics* 10(3):303–317.

Duan, Y., Z. Wang, H. Zhang, Y. He, R. Lu, R. Zhang, G. Sun, and X. Sun. 2013. The preventive effect of lotus seedpod procyanidins on cognitive impairment and oxidative damage induced by extremely low frequency electromagnetic field exposure. *Food Funct* 4(8):1252–1262.

Dubreuil, D., T. Jay, and J. M. Edeline. 2002. Does head-only exposure to GSM-900 electromagnetic fields affect the performance of rats in spatial learning tasks? *Behav Brain Res* 129(1–2):203–210.

Eggert, T., H. Dorn, C. Sauter, A. Marasanov, M. L. Hansen, A. Peter, G. Schmid, T. Bolz, and H. Danker-Hopfe. 2015. Terrestrial Trunked Radio (TETRA) exposure and its impact on slow cortical potentials. *Environ Res* 143(Pt A):112–122.

Eliyahu, I., R. Luria, R. Hareuveny, M. Margaliot, N. Meiran, and G. Shani. 2006. Effects of radiofrequency radiation emitted by cellular telephones on the cognitive functions of humans. *Bioelectromagnetics* 27(2):119–126.

Eltiti, S., D. Wallace, A. Ridgewell, K. Zougkou, R. Russo, F. Sepulveda, and E. Fox. 2009. Short-term exposure to mobile phone base station signals does not affect cognitive functioning or physiological measures in individuals who report sensitivity to electromagnetic fields and controls. *Bioelectromagnetics* 30(7):556–563.

Engels, S., N. L. Schneider, N. Lefeldt, C. M. Hein, M. Zapka, A. Michalik, D. Elbers, A. Kittel, P. J. Hore, and H. Mouritsen. 2014. Anthropogenic electromagnetic noise disrupts magnetic compass orientation in a migratory bird. *Nature* 509(7500):353–356.

Ferreri, F., G. Curcio, P. Pasqualetti, L. De Gennaro, R. Fini, and P. M. Rossini. 2006. Mobile phone emissions and human brain excitability. *Ann Neurol* 60(2):188–196.

Fettiplace, R., and C. M. Hackney. 2006. The sensory and motor roles of auditory hair cells. *Nat Rev Neurosci* 7(1):19–29.

Finger, S., and M. Piccolino. 2011. *The Shocking History of Electric Fishes from Ancient Epochs to the Birth of Electrophysiology.* Oxford: Oxford University Press.

Finnie, J. W., and P. C. Blumbergs. 2004. Mobile telephones and brain vascular leakage. *Pathology* 36:96–97.

Finnie, J. W., P. C. Blumbergs, Z. Cai, J. Manavis, and T. R. Kuchel. 2006a. Effect of mobile telephony on blood-brain barrier permeability in the fetal mouse brain. *Pathology* 38(1):63–65.

Finnie, J. W., P. C. Blumbergs, J. Manavis, T. D. Utteridge, V. Gebski, R. A. Davies, B. Vernon-Roberts, and T. R. Kuchel. 2002. Effect of long-term mobile communication microwave exposure on vascular permeability in mouse brain. *Pathology* 34(4):344–347.

Finnie, J. W., P. C. Blumbergs, J. Manavis, T. D. Utteridge, V. Gebski, J. G. Swift, B. Vernon-Roberts, and T. R. Kuchel. 2001. Effect of global system for mobile communication (GSM)-like radiofrequency fields on vascular permeability in mouse brain. *Pathology* 33(3):338–340.

Finnie, J. W., Z. Cai, P. C. Blumbergs, J. Manavis, and T. R. Kuchel. 2006b. Expression of the immediate early gene, c-fos, in fetal brain after whole of gestation exposure of pregnant mice to global system for mobile communication microwaves. *Pathology* 38(4):333–335.

Finnie, J.W., G. Chidlow, P. C. Blumbergs, J. Manavis, and Z. Cai. 2009. Heat shock protein induction in fetal mouse brain as a measure of stress after whole of gestation exposure to mobile telephony radiofrequency fields. *Pathology* 41(3):276–279.

Fitzgerald, P. B., K. Hoy, S. McQueen, J. J. Maller, S. Herring, R. Segrave, M. Bailey, G. Been, J. Kulkarni, and Z. J. Daskalakis. 2009. A randomized trial of rTMS targeted with MRI based neuro-navigation in treatment-resistant depression. *Neuropsychopharmacology* 34(5):1255–1262.

Fitzpatrick, R., D. Burke, and S. C. Gandevia. 1994. Task-dependent reflex responses and movement illusions evoked by galvanic vestibular stimulation in standing humans. *J Physiol* 478(Pt 2):363–372.

Fleissner, G., E. Holtkamp-Rotzler, M. Hanzlik, M. Winklhofer, N. Petersen, and W. Wiltschko. 2003. Ultrastructural analysis of a putative magnetoreceptor in the beak of homing pigeons. *J Comp Neurol* 458(4):350–360.

Foley, L. E., R. J. Gegear, and S. M. Reppert. 2011. Human cryptochrome exhibits light-dependent magnetosensitivity. *Nat Commn* 2:356, DOI:10.1038/ncomms1364.

Freude, G., P. Ullsperger, S. Eggert, and I. Ruppe. 1998. Effects of microwaves emitted by cellular phones on human slow brain potentials. *Bioelectromagnetics* 19(6):384–387.

Freude, G., P. Ullsperger, S. Eggert, and I. Ruppe. 2000. Microwaves emitted by cellular telephones affect human slow brain potentials. *Eur J Appl Physiol* 81(1–2):18–27.

Fritzer, G., R. Goder, L. Friege, J. Wachter, V. Hansen, D. Hinze-Selch, and J. B. Aldenhoff. 2007. Effects of short- and long-term pulsed radiofrequency electromagnetic fields on night sleep and cognitive functions in healthy subjects. *Bioelectromagnetics* 28(4):316–325.

Fuller, M., J. Dobson, H. G. Wieser, and S. Moser. 1995. On the sensitivity of the human brain to magnetic fields: evocation of epileptiform activity. *Brain Res Bull* 36(2):155–159.

Fuller, M., C. L. Wilson, A. L. Velasco, J. R. Dunn, and J. Zoeger. 2003. On the confirmation of an effect of magnetic fields on the interictal firing rate of epileptic patients. *Brain Res Bull* 60(1–2):43–52.

Furubayashi, T., A. Ushiyama, Y. Terao, Y. Mizuno, K. Shirasawa, P. Pongpaibool, A. Y. Simba, K. Wake, M. Nishikawa, K. Miyawaki, A. Yasuda, M. Uchiyama, H. K. Yamashita, H. Masuda, S. Hirota, M. Takahashi, T. Okano, S. Inomata-Terada, S. Sokejima, E. Maruyama, S. Watanabe, M. Taki, C. Ohkubo, and Y. Ugawa. 2009. Effects of short-term W-CDMA mobile phone base station exposure on women with or without mobile phone related symptoms. *Bioelectromagnetics* 30(2):100–113.

Ghione, S., C. Del Seppia, L. Mezzasalma, and L. Bonfiglio. 2005. Effects of 50 Hz electromagnetic fields on electroencephalographic alpha activity, dental pain threshold and cardiovascular parameters in humans. *Neurosci Letters* 382(1–2):112–117.

Ghosn, R., L. Yahia-Cherif, L. Hugueville, A. Ducorps, J. D. Lemarechal, G. Thuroczy, R. de Seze, and B. Selmaoui. 2015. Radiofrequency signal affects alpha band in resting electroencephalogram. *J Neurophysiol* 113(7):2753–2759.

Glover, P. M., I. Cavin, W. Qian, R. Bowtell, and P. A. Gowland. 2007. Magnetic-field-induced vertigo: a theoretical and experimental investigation. *Bioelectromagnetics* 28(5):349–361.

Graham, C., H. D. Cohen, M. R. Cook, J. W. Phelps, M. M. Gerkovich, and S. S. Fotopopolous. 1987. A double-blind evaluation of 60-Hz field effects on human performance. In L. E. Anderson (Ed.) *Interaction of Biological Sytems with Static and ELF Electric and Magnetic Fields.* Springfield, VA: NTIS.

Graham, C., M. R. Cook, H. D. Cohen, and M. M. Gerkovich. 1994. Dose response study of human exposure to 60 Hz electric and magnetic fields. *Bioelectromagnetics* 15(5):447–463.

Haarala, C., S. Aalto, H. Hautzel, L. Julkunen, J. O. Rinne, M. Laine, B. Krause, and H. Hamalainen. 2003a. Effects of a 902 MHz mobile phone on cerebral blood flow in humans: A PET study. *Neuroreport* 14(16):2019–2023.

Haarala, C., M. Bergman, M. Laine, A. Revonsuo, M. Koivisto, and H. Hamalainen. 2005. Electromagnetic field emitted by 902 MHz mobile phones shows no effects on children's cognitive function. *Bioelectromagnetics* (Suppl 7):S144–S150

Haarala, C., L. Bjornberg, M. Ek, M. Laine, A. Revonsuo, M. Koivisto, and H. Hamalainen. 2003b. Effect of a 902 MHz electromagnetic field emitted by mobile phones on human cognitive function: A replication study. *Bioelectromagnetics* 24(4):283–288.

Haarala, C., M. Ek, L. Bjornberg, M. Laine, A. Revonsuo, M. Koivisto, and H. Hamalainen. 2004. 902 MHz mobile phone does not affect short term memory in humans. *Bioelectromagnetics* 25(6):452–456.

Haarala, C., F. Takio, T. Rintee, M. Laine, M. Koivisto, A. Revonsuo, and H. Hamalainen. 2007. Pulsed and continuous wave mobile phone exposure over left versus right hemisphere: Effects on human cognitive function. *Bioelectromagnetics* 28(4):289–295.

Hamblin, D. L., R. J. Croft, A. W. Wood, C. Stough, and J. Spong. 2006. The sensitivity of human event-related potentials and reaction time to mobile phone emitted electromagnetic fields. *Bioelectromagnetics* 27(4):265–273.

Hamblin, D. L., A. W. Wood, R. J. Croft, and C. Stough. 2004. Examining the effects of electromagnetic fields emitted by GSM mobile phones on human event-related potentials and performance during an auditory task. *Clin Neurophysiol* 115(1):171–178.

Hart, V., P. Novakova, E. P. Malkemper, S. Begall, V. Hanzal, M. Jezek, T. Kusta, V. Nemcova, J. Adamkova, K. Benediktova, J. Cerveny, and H. Burda. 2013. Dogs are sensitive to small variations of the Earth's magnetic field. *Front Zoology* 10:80, DOI:10.1186/1742–9994-10–80.

He, L. H., H. M. Shi, T. T. Liu, Y. C. Xu, K. P. Ye, and S. Wang. 2011. Effects of extremely low frequency magnetic field on anxiety level and spatial memory of adult rats. *Chin Med J (Engl)* 124(20):3362–3366.

Health Council of the Netherlands. 2004. *TNO Study on the Effects of GSM and UMTS Signals on Well-Being and Cognition: Review and Recommendations for Further Research.* The Hague: Health Council of the Netherlands.

Heinrich, A., A. Szostek, F. Nees, P. Meyer, W. Semmler, and H. Flor. 2011. Effects of static magnetic fields on cognition, vital signs, and sensory perception: A meta-analysis. *J Magn Reson Imaging* 34(4):758–763.

Hietanen, M., T. Kovala, and A. M. Hamalainen. 2000. Human brain activity during exposure to radiofrequency fields emitted by cellular phones. *Scand J Work Environ Health* 26(2):87–92.

Hinrichs, H., and H. J. Heinze. 2004. Effects of GSM electromagnetic field on the MEG during an encoding-retrieval task. *Neuroreport* 15(7):1191–1194.

Hinrichs, H., H-J. Heinze, and M. Rotte. 2005. Human sleep under the influence of a GSM 1800 electromagnetic far field. *Somnologie* 9: 185–191.

Hinrikus, H., M. Bachmann, and J. Lass. 2011. Parametric mechanism of excitation of the electroencephalographic rhythms by modulated microwave radiation. *Int J Radiat Biol* 87(11):1077–1085.

Hinrikus, H., M. Bachmann, J. Lass, D. Karai, and V. Tuulik. 2008a. Effect of low frequency modulated microwave exposure on human EEG: Individual sensitivity. *Bioelectromagnetics* 29(7):527–538.

Hinrikus, H., M. Bachmann, J. Lass, R. Tomson, and V. Tuulik. 2008b. Effect of 7, 14 and 21 Hz modulated 450 MHz microwave radiation on human electroencephalographic rhythms. *Int J Radiat Biol* 84(1):69–79.

Hinrikus, H., M. Parts, J. Lass, and V. Tuulik. 2004. Changes in human EEG caused by low level modulated microwave stimulation. *Bioelectromagnetics* 25(6):431–440.

Hore, P. J., and H. Mouritsen. 2016. The radical-pair mechanism of magnetoreception. *Annu Rev Biophys* 45:299–344.

Hountala, C. D., A. E. Maganioti, C. C. Papageorgiou, E. D. Nanou, M. A. Kyprianou, V. G. Tsiafakis, A. D. Rabavilas, and C. N. Capsalis. 2008. The spectral power coherence of the EEG under different EMF conditions. *Neurosci Lett* 441(2):188–192.

Huber, R., T. Graf, K. A. Cote, L. Wittmann, E. Gallmann, D. Matter, J. Schuderer, N. Kuster, A. A. Borbely, and P. Achermann. 2000. Exposure to pulsed high-frequency electromagnetic field during waking affects human sleep EEG. *Neuroreport* 11(15):3321–3325.

Huber, R., V. Treyer, A. A. Borbely, J. Schuderer, J. M. Gottselig, H. P. Landolt, E. Werth, T. Berthold, N. Kuster, A. Buck, and P. Achermann. 2002. Electromagnetic fields, such as those from mobile phones, alter regional cerebral blood flow and sleep and waking EEG. *J Sleep Res* 11(4):289–295.

Hung, C. S., C. Anderson, J. A. Horne, and P. McEvoy. 2007. Mobile phone 'talk-mode' signal delays EEG-determined sleep onset. *Neurosci Lett* 421(1):82–86.

Huss, A., T. Koeman, H. Kromhout, and R. Vermeulen. 2015. Extremely low frequency magnetic field exposure and Parkinson's disease–A systematic review and meta-analysis of the data. *Int J Environ Res Public Health* 12(7):7348–7356.

Hutter, H. P., H. Moshammer, P. Wallner, and M. Kundi. 2006. Subjective symptoms, sleeping problems, and cognitive performance in subjects living near mobile phone base stations. *Occup Environ Med* 63(5):307–313.

ICNIRP. 1998. Guidelines on limits of exposure to time-varying electric, magnetic and electromagnetic fields (1 Hz -300 GHz). *Health Phys* 74:494–522.

ICNIRP. 2003. Exposure to static and low frequency electromagnetic fields, biologcial effects and health consequences (0–100 kHz). In R. Matthes, P. Vecchia, A. F. McKinlay, B. Veyret and J.H. Bernhardt (Eds.) *Static and Low Frequency Review – 2003*. Munich: International Commission for Non-Ionizing Radiation Protection.

ICNIRP. 2010. Guidelines on limits of exposure to time-varying electric, magnetic and electromagnetic fields (1 Hz -100 kHz). *Health Physics* 99:818–836.

IEEE. 2002. *IEEE Standard for Safety Levels with Respect to Human Exposure to Electromagnetic Fields, 0–3 kHz.* edited by Standards Coordinating Committee 28. New York: IEEE.

Inomata-Terada, S., S. Okabe, N. Arai, R. Hanajima, Y. Terao, T. Frubayashi, and Y. Ugawa. 2007. Effects of high frequency electromagnetic field (EMF) emitted by mobile phones on the human motor cortex. *Bioelectromagnetics* 28(7):553–561.

International Commission on Non-Ionizing Radiation Protection. 2009. Guidelines on limits of exposure to static magnetic fields. *Health Phys* 96(4):504–514.

Inyang, I., G. Benke, C. Dimitriadis, P. Simpson, R. McKenzie, and M. Abramson. 2010. Predictors of mobile telephone use and exposure analysis in Australian adolescents. *J Paediatr Child Health* 46(5):226–233.

Jadidi, M., S. M. Firoozabadi, A. Rashidy-Pour, A. A. Sajadi, H. Sadeghi, and A. A. Taherian. 2007. Acute exposure to a 50 Hz magnetic field impairs consolidation of spatial memory in rats. *Neurobiol Learn Mem* 88(4):387–392.

Jech, R., K. Sonka, E. Ruzicka, A. Nebuzelsky, J. Bohm, M. Juklickova, and S. Nevsimalova. 2001. Electromagnetic field of mobile phones affects visual event related potential in patients with narcolepsy. *Bioelectromagnetics* 22(7):519–528.

Jeong, Y. J., G-Y. Kang, J. H. Kwon, H-D. Choi, J-K. Pack, N. Kim, Y-S. Lee, H-J. Lee. 2015. 1950 MHz electromagnetic fields ameliorate Aβ pathology in Alzheimer's disease mice. *Curr Alzheimer Res* 12:481–492.

Jiang, D. P., J. H. Li, J. Zhang, S. L. Xu, F. Kuang, H. Y. Lang, Y. F. Wang, G. Z. An, J. Li, and G. Z. Guo. 2016. Long-term electromagnetic pulse exposure induces Abeta deposition and cognitive dysfunction through oxidative stress and overexpression of APP and BACE1. *Brain Res* 1642:10–19.

Jiang, D. P., J. Li, J. Zhang, S. L. Xu, F. Kuang, H. Y. Lang, Y. F. Wang, G. Z. An, J. H. Li, and G. Z. Guo. 2013. Electromagnetic pulse exposure induces overexpression of beta amyloid protein in rats. *Arch Med Res* 44(3):178–184.

Johnsen, S., and K. J. Lohmann. 2005. The physics and neurobiology of magnetoreception. *Nat Rev Neurosci* 6(9):703–712.

Kalmijn, A. D. 2000. Detection and processing of electromagnetic and near-field acoustic signals in elasmobranch fishes. *Philos Trans R Soc Lond B Biol Sci* 355(1401):1135–1141.

Kangarlu, A., R. E. Burgess, H. Zhu, T. Nakayama, R. L. Hamlin, A. M. Abduljalil, and P. M. Robitaille. 1999. Cognitive, cardiac, and physiological safety studies in ultra high field magnetic resonance imaging. *Magn Reson Imaging* 17(10):1407–1416.

Karipids, K. 2017. Static electric and magnetic field hazards. In A.W. Wood and K. Karipidis (Eds.) *Non-Ionizing Radiation Protection*, pp. 341–356. Hoboken, NJ: Wiley.

Kattnig, D. R., I. A. Solov'yov, and P. J. Hore. 2016. Electron spin relaxation in cryptochrome-based magnetoreception. *Phy Chem Chem Phy* 18(18):12443–12456.

Kavaliers, M., K. P. Ossenkopp, F. S. Prato, D. G. Innes, L. A. Galea, D. M. Kinsella, and T. S. Perrot-Sinal. 1996. Spatial learning in deer mice: sex differences and the effects of endogenous opioids and 60 Hz magnetic fields. *J Comp Physiol A* 179(5):715–724.

Kavokin, K., N. Chernetsov, A. Pakhomov, J. Bojarinova, D. Kobylkov, and B. Namozov. 2014. Magnetic orientation of garden warblers (Sylvia borin) under 1.4 MHz radiofrequency magnetic field. *J R Soc Interface* 11(97):20140451.

Kazantzis, N., J. Podd, and C. Whittington. 1998. Acute effects of 50 Hz, 100 microT magnetic field exposure on visual duration discrimination at two different times of the day. *Bioelectromagnetics* 19(5):310–317.

Keetley, V., A. Wood, H. Sadafi, and C. Stough. 2001. Neuropsychological sequelae of 50 Hz magnetic fields. *Int J Radiat Biol* 77(6):735–742.

Keetley, V., A. W. Wood, J. Spong, and C. Stough. 2006. Neuropsychological sequelae of digital mobile phone exposure in humans. *Neuropsychologia* 44(10):1843–1848.

Kirschvink, J. L. 1996. Microwave absorption by magnetite: A possible mechanism for coupling non-thermal levels of radiation to biological systems. *Bioelectromagnetics* 17(3):187–194.

Kitaoka, K., M. Kitamura, S. Aoi, N. Shimizu, and K. Yoshizaki. 2013. Chronic exposure to an extremely low-frequency magnetic field induces depression-like behavior and corticosterone secretion without enhancement of the hypothalamic-pituitary-adrenal axis in mice. *Bioelectromagnetics* 34(1):43–51.

Kleinlogel, H., T. Dierks, T. Koenig, H. Lehmann, A. Minder, and R. Berz. 2008. Effects of weak mobile phone - electromagnetic fields (GSM, UMTS) on event related potentials and cognitive functions. *Bioelectromagnetics* 29(6):488–497.

Kleinlogel, H., T. Dierks, T. Koenig, H. Lehmann, A. Minder, and R. Berz. 2008a. Effects of weak mobile phone - electromagnetic fields (GSM, UMTS) on well-being and resting EEG. *Bioelectromagnetics* 29(6):479–487.

Kleinlogel, H., T. Dierks, T. Koenig, H. Lehmann, A. Minder, and R. Berz. 2008b. Effects of weak mobile phone - electromagnetic fields (GSM, UMTS) on event related potentials and cognitive functions. *Bioelectromagnetics* 29(6):488–497.

Koivisto, M., C. M. Krause, A. Revonsuo, M. Laine, and H. Hamalainen. 2000a. The effects of electromagnetic field emitted by GSM phones on working memory. *Neuroreport* 11(8):1641–1643.

Koivisto, M., A. Revonsuo, C. Krause, C. Haarala, L. Sillanmaki, M. Laine, and H. Hamalainen. 2000b. Effects of 902 MHz electromagnetic field emitted by cellular telephones on response times in humans. *Neuroreport* 11(2):413–415.

Komaki, A., A. Khalili, I. Salehi, S. Shahidi, and A. Sarihi. 2014. Effects of exposure to an extremely low frequency electromagnetic field on hippocampal long-term potentiation in rat. *Brain Res* 1564:1–8.

Komeili, A. 2012. Molecular mechanisms of compartmentalization and biomineralization in magnetotactic bacteria. *FEMS Microbiol Rev* 36(1):232–255.

Korpinar, M. A., M. T. Kalkan, and H. Tuncel. 2012. The 50 Hz (10 mT) sinusoidal magnetic field: effects on stress-related behavior of rats. *Bratisl Lek Listy* 113(9):521–524.

Krause, C. M., C. H. Bjornberg, M. Pesonen, A. Hulten, T. Liesivuori, M. Koivisto, A. Revonsuo, M. Laine, and H. Hamalainen. 2006. Mobile phone effects on children's event-related oscillatory EEG during an auditory memory task. *Int J Radiat Biol* 82(6):443–450.

Krause, C. M., C. Haarala, L. Sillanmaki, M. Koivisto, K. Alanko, A. Revonsuo, M. Laine, and H. Hamalainen. 2004. Effects of electromagnetic field emitted by cellular phones on the EEG during an auditory memory task: A double blind replication study. *Bioelectromagnetics* 25(1):33–40.

Krause, C. M., M. Pesonen, C. Haarala Bjornberg, and H. Hamalainen. 2007. Effects of pulsed and continuous wave 902 MHz mobile phone exposure on brain oscillatory activity during cognitive processing. *Bioelectromagnetics* 28(4):296–308.

Krause, C. M., L. Sillanmaki, M. Koivisto, A. Haggqvist, C. Saarela, A. Revonsuo, M. Laine, and H. Hamalainen. 2000a. Effects of electromagnetic fields emitted by cellular phones on the electroencephalogram during a visual working memory task. *Int J Radiat Biol* 76(12):1659–1667.

Krause, C. M., L. Sillanmaki, M. Koivisto, A. Haggqvist, C. Saarela, A. Revonsuo, M. Laine, and H. Hamalainen. 2000b. Effects of electromagnetic field emitted by cellular phones on the EEG during a memory task. *Neuroreport* 11(4):761–764.

Kumlin, T., H. Iivonen, P. Miettinen, A. Juvonen, T. van Groen, L. Puranen, R. Pitkaaho, J. Juutilainen, and H. Tanila. 2007. Mobile phone radiation and the developing brain: behavioral and morphological effects in juvenile rats. *Radiat Res* 168(4):471–479.

Kurokawa, Y., H. Nitta, H. Imai, and M. Kabuto. 2003. No influence of short-term exposure to 50-Hz magnetic fields on cognitive performance function in human. *Int Arch Occup Environ Health* 76(6):437–442.

Kwon, M. K., J. Y. Choi, S. K. Kim, T. K. Yoo, and D. W. Kim. 2012. Effects of radiation emitted by WCDMA mobile phones on electromagnetic hypersensitive subjects. *Environ Health* 11:69.

Kwon, M. S., and H. Hamalainen. 2011. Effects of mobile phone electromagnetic fields: critical evaluation of behavioral and neurophysiological studies. *Bioelectromagnetics* 32(4):253–272.

Kwon, M. S., M. Huotilainen, A. Shestakova, T. Kujala, R. Naatanen, and H. Hamalainen. 2010. No effects of mobile phone use on cortical auditory change-detection in children: An ERP study. *Bioelectromagnetics* 31(3):191–199.

Kwon, M. S., T. Kujala, M. Huotilainen, A. Shestakova, R. Naatanen, and H. Hamalainen. 2009. Preattentive auditory information processing under exposure to the 902 MHz GSM mobile phone electromagnetic field: A mismatch negativity (MMN) study. *Bioelectromagnetics* 30(3):241–248.

Lai, H. 1996. Spatial learning deficit in the rat after exposure to a 60 Hz magnetic field. *Bioelectromagnetics* 17(6):494–496.

Lai, H., M. A. Carino, and I. Ushijima. 1998. Acute exposure to a 60 Hz magnetic field affects rats' water-maze performance. *Bioelectromagnetics* 19(2):117–122.

Lass, J., V. Tuulik, R. Ferenets, R. Riisalo, and H. Hinrikus. 2002. Effects of 7 Hz-modulated 450 MHz electromagnetic radiation on human performance in visual memory tasks. *Int J Radiat Biol* 78(10):937–944.

Legros, A., M. Corbacio, A. Beuter, J. Modolo, D. Goulet, F. S. Prato, and A. W. Thomas. 2012. Neurophysiological and behavioral effects of a 60 Hz, 1,800 muT magnetic field in humans. *Eur J Appl Physiol* 112(5):1751–1762.

Legros, A., P. Gaillot, and A. Beuter. 2006. Transient effect of low-intensity magnetic field on human motor control. *Med Eng Phys* 28(8):827–836.

Legros, A., J. Modolo, S. Brown, J. Roberston, and A. W. Thomas. 2015. Effects of a 60 Hz Magnetic Field Exposure Up to 3000 muT on human brain activation as measured by functional magnetic resonance imaging. *PLoS One* 10(7):e0132024.

Lepsien, J., K. Muller, D. Y. von Cramon, and H. E. Moller. 2012. Investigation of higher-order cognitive functions during exposure to a high static magnetic field. *J Magn Reson Imaging* 36(4):835–840.

Leung, S., R. J. Croft, R. J. McKenzie, S. Iskra, B. Silber, N. R. Cooper, B. O'Neill, V. Cropley, A. Diaz-Trujillo, D. Hamblin, and D. Simpson. 2011. Effects of 2G and 3G mobile phones on performance and electrophysiology in adolescents, young adults and older adults. *Clin Neurophysiol* 122(11):2203–2216.

Levin, M. 2014a. Endogenous bioelectrical networks store non-genetic patterning information during development and regeneration. *J Physiol* 592(11):2295–2305.

Levin, M. 2014b. Molecular bioelectricity: how endogenous voltage potentials control cell behavior and instruct pattern regulation in vivo. *Mol Biol Cell* 25(24):3835–3850.

Li, Y., C. Zhang, and T. Song. 2014. Disturbance of the magnetic field did not affect spatial memory. *Physiol Res* 63(3):377–385.

Loughran, S. P., D. C. Benz, M. R. Schmid, M. Murbach, N. Kuster, and P. Achermann. 2013. No increased sensitivity in brain activity of adolescents exposed to mobile phone-like emissions. *Clin Neurophysiol* 124(7):1303–1308.

Loughran, S. P., R. J. McKenzie, M. L. Jackson, M. E. Howard, and R. J. Croft. 2012. Individual differences in the effects of mobile phone exposure on human sleep: Rethinking the problem. *Bioelectromagnetics* 33(1):86–93.

Loughran, S. P., A. W. Wood, J. M. Barton, R. J. Croft, B. Thompson, and C. Stough. 2005. The effect of electromagnetic fields emitted by mobile phones on human sleep. *Neuroreport* 16(17):1973–1976.

Lovsund, P., P. A. Oberg, S. E. Nilsson, and T. Reuter. 1980. Magnetophosphenes: A quantitative analysis of thresholds. *Med Biol Eng Comput* 18(3):326–334.

Lowden, A., T. Akerstedt, M. Ingre, C. Wiholm, L. Hillert, N. Kuster, J. P. Nilsson, and B. Arnetz. 2011. Sleep after mobile phone exposure in subjects with mobile phone-related symptoms. *Bioelectromagnetics* 32(1):4–14.

Lu, J., and H. M. Fishman. 1995a. Ion channels and transporters in the electroreceptive ampullary epithelium from skates. *Biophys J* 69(6):2467–2475.

Lu, J., and H. M. Fishman. 1995b. Localization and function of the electrical oscillation in electroreceptive ampullary epithelium from skates. *Biophys J* 69(6):2458–2466.

Luria, R., I. Eliyahu, R. Hareuveny, M. Margaliot, and N. Meiran. 2009. Cognitive effects of radiation emitted by cellular phones: the influence of exposure side and time. *Bioelectromagnetics* 30(3):198–204.

Lustenberger, C., M. Murbach, R. Durr, M. R. Schmid, N. Kuster, P. Achermann, and R. Huber. 2013. Stimulation of the brain with radiofrequency electromagnetic field pulses affects sleep-dependent performance improvement. *Brain Stimul* 6(5):805–811.

Lustenberger, C., M. Murbach, L. Tushaus, F. Wehrle, N. Kuster, P. Achermann, and R. Huber. 2015. Inter-individual and intra-individual variation of the effects of pulsed RF EMF exposure on the human sleep EEG. *Bioelectromagnetics* 36(3):169–77.

Lyskov, E. B., J. Juutilainen, V. Jousmaki, J. Partanen, S. Medvedev, and O. Hanninen. 1993a. Effects of 45-Hz magnetic fields on the functional state of the human brain. *Bioelectromagnetics* 14(2):87–95.

Lyskov, E. B., S. V. Medvedev, Z. A. Aleksanian, and T. E. Safonova. 1994. Anthropogenic ultra-low frequency magnetic field and the process of skill formation. Possible negative effect. *Fiziol Cheloveka* 20(6):28–33.

Lyskov, E., J. Juutilainen, V. Jousmaki, O. Hanninen, S. Medvedev, and J. Partanen. 1993b. Influence of short-term exposure of magnetic field on the bioelectrical processes of the brain and performance. *Int J Psychophysiol* 14(3):227–231.

Lyskov, E., V. Ponomarev, M. Sandstrom, K. H. Mild, and S. Medvedev. 1998. Steady-state visual evoked potentials to computer monitor flicker. *Int J Psychophysiol* 28(3):285–290.

Maby, E., B. Jeannes Rle, and G. Faucon. 2006. Scalp localization of human auditory cortical activity modified by GSM electromagnetic fields. *Int J Radiat Biol* 82(7):465–472.

Maby, E., R. Le Bouquin Jeannes, G. Faucon, C. Liegeois-Chauvel, and R. De Seze. 2005. Effects of GSM signals on auditory evoked responses. *Bioelectromagnetics* 26(5):341–350.

Maier, R., S. E. Greter, G. Schaller, and G. Hommel. 2004. The effects of pulsed low-level EM fields on memory processes. *Z Med Phys* 14(2):105–112.

Mann, K., and J. Roschke. 1996. Effects of pulsed high-frequency electromagnetic fields on human sleep. *Neuropsychobiology* 33(1):41–47.

Marino, A. A., E. Nilsen, A. L. Chesson, Jr., and C. Frilot. 2004. Effect of low-frequency magnetic fields on brain electrical activity in human subjects. *Clin Neurophysiol* 115(5):1195–1201.

Mausset, A. L., R. de Seze, F. Montpeyroux, and A. Privat. 2001. Effects of radiofrequency exposure on the GABAergic system in the rat cerebellum: Clues from semi-quantitative immunohisto-chemistry. *Brain Res* 912(1):33–46.

McCaig, C. D., A. M. Rajnicek, B. Song, and M. Zhao. 2005. Controlling cell behavior electrically: current views and future potential. *Physiol Rev* 85(3):943–978.

McKinlay, A., and M. Repacholi. 2003. Weak electric field effects in the body. In A. McKinlay and M. Repacholi (Eds.) *Radiation Protection Dosimetry*, pp. 290–400. Ashford: Nuclear Technology Publishing.

Mian, O. S., P. M. Glover, and B. L. Day. 2015. Reconciling magnetically induced vertigo and nystagmus. *Front Neurol* 6:201.

Mian, O. S., Y. Li, A. Antunes, P. M. Glover, and B. L. Day. 2013. On the vertigo due to static magnetic fields. *PLoS One* 8(10):e78748.

Mouritsen, H. 2012. Sensory biology: Search for the compass needles. *Nature* 484(7394):320–321.

Mouritsen, H., and P. J. Hore. 2012. The magnetic retina: Light-dependent and trigeminal magneto-reception in migratory birds. *Curr Opin Neurobiol* 22(2):343–352.

Nadeem, M., T. Thorlin, O. P. Gandhi, and M. Persson. 2003. Computation of electric and magnetic stimulation in human head using the 3-D impedance method. *IEEE Trans Biomed Eng* 50(7):900–907.

Nakajima, K., K. Zhu, Y. H. Sun, B. Hegyi, Q. Zeng, C. J. Murphy, J. V. Small, Y. Chen-Izu, Y. Izumiya, J. M. Penninger, and M. Zhao. 2015. KCNJ15/Kir4.2 couples with polyamines to sense weak extracellular electric fields in galvanotaxis. *Nat Commun* 6:8532.

Nakatani-Enomoto, S., T. Furubayashi, A. Ushiyama, S. J. Groiss, K. Ueshima, S. Sokejima, A. Y. Simba, K. Wake, S. Watanabe, M. Nishikawa, K. Miyawaki, M. Taki, and Y. Ugawa. 2013. Effects of electromagnetic fields emitted from W-CDMA-like mobile phones on sleep in humans. *Bioelectromagnetics* 34(8):589–598.

Nevelsteen, S., J. J. Legros, and M. Crasson. 2007. Effects of information and 50 Hz magnetic fields on cognitive performance and reported symptoms. *Bioelectromagnetics* 28(1):53–63.

Nitsche, M. A., L. G. Cohen, E. M. Wassermann, A. Priori, N. Lang, A. Antal, W. Paulus, F. Hummel, P. S. Boggio, F. Fregni, and A. Pascual-Leone. 2008. Transcranial direct current stimulation: State of the art 2008. *Brain Stimul* 1(3):206–223.

Nittby, H., A. Brun, J. Eberhardt, L. Malmgren, B. R. Persson, and L. G. Salford. 2009. Increased blood-brain barrier permeability in mammalian brain 7 days after exposure to the radiation from a GSM-900 mobile phone. *Pathophysiology* 16(2–3):103–112.

Nolte, C. M., D. W. Pittman, B. Kalevitch, R. Henderson, and J. C. Smith. 1998. Magnetic field conditioned taste aversion in rats. *Physiol Behav* 63(4):683–688.

Nuccitelli, R. 2003. A role for endogenous electric fields in wound healing. *Curr Top Dev Biol* 58:1–26.

Okano, T., Y. Terao, T. Furubayashi, A. Yugeta, R. Hanajima, and Y. Ugawa. 2010. The effect of electromagnetic field emitted by a mobile phone on the inhibitory control of saccades. *Clin Neurophysiol* 121(4):603–611.

Orr, J. L., W. R. Rogers, H. D. Smith. 1995a. Detection thresholds for 60 Hz Electric Fields by non-human primates. *Bioelectromagnetics* 16(Supplement S3):23–34.

Orr, J.L., W. R. Rogers, H.D. Smith. 1995b. Exposure of baboons to combined 60 Hz electric and magnetic fields does not produce work stoppage or affect operant performance on a match-to-sample task. *Bioelectromagnetics* 16(Supplement S3):61–70.

Pagnin, D., V. de Queiroz, S. Pini, and G. B. Cassano. 2004. Efficacy of ECT in depression: A meta-analytic review. *J ECT* 20(1):13–20.

Parazzini, M., M. E. Lutman, A. Moulin, C. Barnel, M. Sliwinska-Kowalska, M. Zmyslony, I. Hernadi, G. Stefanics, G. Thuroczy, and P. Ravazzani. 2010. Absence of short-term effects of UMTS exposure on the human auditory system. *Radiat Res* 173(1):91–97.

Parazzini, M., F. Sibella, M. E. Lutman, S. Mishra, A. Moulin, M. Sliwinska-Kowalska, E. Woznicka, P. Politanski, M. Zmyslony, G. Thuroczy, F. Molnar, G. Kubinyi, G. Tavartkiladze, S. Bronyakin, I. Uloziene, V. Uloza, E. Gradauskiene, and P. Ravazzani. 2009. Effects of UMTS cellular phones on human hearing: Results of the European project EMFnEAR. *Radiat Res* 172(2):244–251.

Park, J., J. H. Kwon, N. Kim, and K. Song. 2017. Effects of 1950 MHz radiofrequency electromagnetic fields on Abeta processing in human neuroblastoma and mouse hippocampal neuronal cells. *J Radiat Res*: 59:18–26.

Pascual-Leone, A., V. Walsh, and J. Rothwell. 2000. Transcranial magnetic stimulation in cognitive neuro-science–virtual lesion, chronometry, and functional connectivity. *Curr Opin Neurobiol* 10(2):232–237.

Patullo, B. W., and D. L. Macmillan. 2010. Making sense of electrical sense in crayfish. *J Exp Biol* 213(4):651–657.

Perentos, N., R. J. Croft, R. J. McKenzie, and I. Cosic. 2013. The alpha band of the resting electroencephalogram under pulsed and continuous radio frequency exposures. *IEEE Trans Biomed Eng* 60(6):1702–1710.

Perentos, N., R. J. Croft, R. J. McKenzie, D. Cvetkovic, and I. Cosic. 2007. Comparison of the effects of continuous and pulsed mobile phone like RF exposure on the human EEG. *Australas Phys Eng Sci Med* 30(4):274–280.

Perlmutter, J. S., and J. W. Mink. 2006. Deep brain stimulation. *Annu Rev Neurosci* 29:229–257.

Perry, F. S., M. Reichmanis, A. A. Marino, and R. O. Becker. 1981. Environmental power-frequency magnetic fields and suicide. *Health Phys* 41(2):267–277.

Petri, A. K., K. Schmiedchen, D. Stunder, D. Dechent, T. Kraus, W. H. Bailey, and S. Driessen. 2017. Biological effects of exposure to static electric fields in humans and vertebrates: A systematic review. *Environ Health* 16(1):41.

Pettigrew, J. D. 1999. Electroreception in monotremes. *J Exp Biol* 202(Pt 10):1447–1454.

Pickard, W. F. 1988. A model for the acute electrosensitivity of cartilaginous fishes. *IEEE Trans Biomed Eng* 35(4):243–249.

Podd, J., J. Abbott, N. Kazantzis, and A. Rowland. 2002. Brief exposure to a 50 Hz, 100 microT magnetic field: Effects on reaction time, accuracy, and recognition memory. *Bioelectromagnetics* 23(3):189–195.

Podd, J. V., C. J. Whittington, G. R. Barnes, W. H. Page, and B. I. Rapley. 1995. Do ELF magnetic fields affect human reaction time? *Bioelectromagnetics* 16(5):317–323.

Polk, C., and E. Postow. 1996. *Handbook of Biological Effects of Electromagnetic Fields*, 2nd Edition. Boca Raton, FL: CRC Press.

Prato, F. S. 2015. Non-thermal extremely low frequency magnetic field effects on opioid related behaviors: Snails to humans, mechanisms to therapy. *Bioelectromagnetics* 36(5):333–348.

Prato, F. S., and V. N. Binhi. 2017. Response to comments by Frank Barnes and Ben Greenebaum on "A physical mechanism of magnetoreception: Extension and analysis. *Bioelectromagnetics* 38(4):324–325.

Preece, A. W., S. Goodfellow, M. G. Wright, S. R. Butler, E. J. Dunn, Y. Johnson, T. C. Manktelow, and K. Wesnes. 2005. Effect of 902 MHz mobile phone transmission on cognitive function in children. *Bioelectromagnetics* (Suppl 7):S138–S143.

Preece, A. W., G. Iwi, A. Davies-Smith, K. Wesnes, S. Butler, E. Lim, and A. Varey. 1999. Effect of a 915-MHz simulated mobile phone signal on cognitive function in man. *Int J Radiat Biol* 75(4):447–456.

Preece, A. W., K. A. Wesnes, and G. R. Iwi. 1998. The effect of a 50 Hz magnetic field on cognitive function in humans. *Int J Radiat Biol* 74(4):463–470.

Regel, S. J., J. M. Gottselig, J. Schuderer, G. Tinguely, J. V. Retey, N. Kuster, H. P. Landolt, and P. Achermann. 2007a. Pulsed radio frequency radiation affects cognitive performance and the waking electroencephalogram. *Neuroreport* 18(8):803–807.

Regel, S. J., S. Negovetic, M. Roosli, V. Berdinas, J. Schuderer, A. Huss, U. Lott, N. Kuster, and P. Achermann. 2006. UMTS base station-like exposure, well-being, and cognitive performance. *Environ Health Perspect* 114(8):1270–1275.

Regel, S. J., G. Tinguely, J. Schuderer, M. Adam, N. Kuster, H. P. Landolt, and P. Achermann. 2007b. Pulsed radio-frequency electromagnetic fields: Dose-dependent effects on sleep, the sleep EEG and cognitive performance. *J Sleep Res* 16(3):253–258.

Repacholi, M. H., and B. Greenebaum. 1999. Interaction of static and extremely low frequency electric and magnetic fields with living systems: Health effects and research needs. *Bioelectromagnetics* 20(3):133–160.

Riddervold, I. S., S. K. Kjaergaard, G. F. Pedersen, N. T. Andersen, O. Franek, A. D. Pedersen, T. Sigsgaard, R. Zachariae, L. Molhave, and J. B. Andersen. 2010. No effect of TETRA hand portable transmission signals on human cognitive function and symptoms. *Bioelectromagnetics* 31(5):380–390.

Riddervold, I. S., G. F. Pedersen, N. T. Andersen, A. D. Pedersen, J. B. Andersen, R. Zachariae, L. Molhave, T. Sigsgaard, and S. K. Kjaergaard. 2008. Cognitive function and symptoms in adults and adolescents in relation to rf radiation from UMTS base stations. *Bioelectromagnetics* 29(4):257–267.

Rieke, F., and D. A. Baylor. 1998. Single-photon detection by rod cells of the retina. *Rev Modern Phy* 70(3):1027–1036.

Ritz, T., P. Thalau, J. B. Phillips, R. Wiltschko, and W. Wiltschko. 2004. Resonance effects indicate a radical-pair mechanism for avian magnetic compass. *Nature* 429(6988):177–180.

Ritz, T., R. Wiltschko, P. J. Hore, C. T. Rodgers, K. Stapput, P. Thalau, C. R. Timmel, and W. Wiltschko. 2009. Magnetic compass of birds is based on a molecule with optimal directional sensitivity. *Biophys J* 96(8):3451–3457.

Roberts, D. C., V. Marcelli, J. S. Gillen, J. P. Carey, C. C. Della Santina, and D. S. Zee. 2011. MRI magnetic field stimulates rotational sensors of the brain. *Curr Biol* 21(19):1635–1640.

Robertson, J. A., N. Juen, J. Theberge, J. Weller, D. J. Drost, F. S. Prato, and A. W. Thomas. 2010a. Evidence for a dose-dependent effect of pulsed magnetic fields on pain processing. *Neurosci Lett* 482(2):160–162.

Robertson, J. A., J. Theberge, J. Weller, D. J. Drost, F. S. Prato, and A. W. Thomas. 2010b. Low-frequency pulsed electromagnetic field exposure can alter neuroprocessing in humans. *J R Soc Interface* 7(44):467–473.

Rodina, A., J. Lass, J. Riipulk, T. Bachmann, and H. Hinrikus. 2005. Study of effects of low level microwave field by method of face masking. *Bioelectromagnetics* 26(7):571–577.

Roosli, M., P. Frei, E. Mohler, and K. Hug. 2010. Systematic review on the health effects of exposure to radiofrequency electromagnetic fields from mobile phone base stations. *Bull World Health Organ* 88(12):887–896F.

Roschke, J., and K. Mann. 1997. No short-term effects of digital mobile radio telephone on the awake human electroencephalogram. *Bioelectromagnetics* 18(2):172–176.

Rubin, G. J., R. Nieto-Hernandez, and S. Wessely. 2010. Idiopathic environmental intolerance attributed to electromagnetic fields (formerly 'electromagnetic hypersensitivity'): An updated systematic review of provocation studies. *Bioelectromagnetics* 31(1):1–11.

Russo, R., E. Fox, C. Cinel, A. Boldini, M. A. Defeyter, D. Mirshekar-Syahkal, and A. Mehta. 2006. Does acute exposure to mobile phones affect human attention? *Bioelectromagnetics* 27(3):215–220.

Sauter, C., H. Dorn, A. Bahr, M. L. Hansen, A. Peter, M. Bajbouj, and H. Danker-Hopfe. 2011. Effects of exposure to electromagnetic fields emitted by GSM 900 and WCDMA mobile phones on cognitive function in young male subjects. *Bioelectromagnetics* 32(3):179–190.

Sauter, C., T. Eggert, H. Dorn, G. Schmid, T. Bolz, A. Marasanov, M. L. Hansen, A. Peter, and H. Danker-Hopfe. 2015. Do signals of a hand-held TETRA transmitter affect cognitive performance, well-being, mood or somatic complaints in healthy young men? Results of a randomized double-blind cross-over provocation study. *Environ Res* 140:85–94.

SCENIHR. 2015. (Scientific Committee on Emerging and Newly Identified Health Risks). *Opinion on Potential Health Effects of Exposure to Electromagnetic Fields (EMF)*. Luxembourg: European Commission. DG Health and Food Safety.

Schaap, K., L. Portengen, and H. Kromhout. 2016. Exposure to MRI-related magnetic fields and vertigo in MRI workers. *Occup Environ Med* 73(3):161–166.

Scheich, H. 1983. Biophysics of electroreception. In W. Hoppe, W. Lohmann, H. Markl and H. Ziegler (Eds.) *Biophysics*, pp. 764–776. Berlin and New York: Springer-Verlag.

Schmid, M. R., S. P. Loughran, S. J. Regel, M. Murbach, A. Bratic Grunauer, T. Rusterholz, A. Bersagliere, N. Kuster, and P. Achermann. 2012a. Sleep EEG alterations: Effects of different pulse-modulated radio frequency electromagnetic fields. *J Sleep Res* 21(1):50–58.

Schmid, M. R., M. Murbach, C. Lustenberger, M. Maire, N. Kuster, P. Achermann, and S. P. Loughran. 2012b. Sleep EEG alterations: Effects of pulsed magnetic fields versus pulse-modulated radio frequency electromagnetic fields. *J Sleep Res* 21(6):620–629.

Schmid, G., C. Sauter, R. Stepansky, I. S. Lobentanz, and J. Zeitlhofer. 2005. No influence on selected parameters of human visual perception of 1970 MHz UMTS-like exposure. *Bioelectromagnetics* 26(4):243–250.

Schuz, J., G. Waldemar, J. H. Olsen, and C. Johansen. 2009. Risks for central nervous system diseases among mobile phone subscribers: a Danish retrospective cohort study. *PLoS One* 4(2):e4389.

Schwarze, S., N. L. Schneider, T. Reichl, D. Dreyer, N. Lefeldt, S. Engels, N. Baker, P. J. Hore, and H. Mouritsen. 2016. Weak broadband electromagnetic fields are more disruptive to magnetic compass orientation in a night-migratory songbird (Erithacus rubecula) than strong narrowband fields. *Front Behav Neurosci* 10:55.

Seegal, R. F., J. R. Wolpaw, and R. Dowman. 1989. Chronic exposure of primates to 60-Hz electric and magnetic fields: II. Neurochemical effects. *Bioelectromagnetics* 10(3):289–301.

Siebner, H. R., G. Hartwigsen, T. Kassuba, and J. C. Rothwell. 2009. How does transcranial magnetic stimulation modify neuronal activity in the brain? Implications for studies of cognition. *Cortex* 45(9):1035–1042.

Sienkiewicz, Z. J., R. P. Blackwell, R. G. Haylock, R. D. Saunders, and B. L. Cobb. 2000. Low-level exposure to pulsed 900 MHz microwave radiation does not cause deficits in the performance of a spatial learning task in mice. *Bioelectromagnetics* 21(3):151–158.

Sienkiewicz, Z. J., R. G. E. Haylock, and R. D. Saunders. 1996. Acute exposure to power-frequency magnetic fields has no effect on the acquisition of a spatial learning task by adult male mice. *Bioelectromagnetics* 17(3):180–186.

Sienkiewicz, Z. J., R. G. E. Haylock, and R. D. Saunders. 1998. Deficits in spatial learning after exposure of mice to a 50 Hz magnetic field. *Bioelectromagnetics* 19(2):79–84.

Singer, J. H., L. Lassova, N. Vardi, and J. S. Diamond. 2004. Coordinated multivesicular release at a mammalian ribbon synapse. *Nat Neurosci* 7(8):826–833.

Sirav, B., and N. Seyhan. 2011. Effects of radiofrequency radiation exposure on blood-brain barrier permeability in male and female rats. *Electromagn Biol Med* 30(4):253–260.

Son, Y., Y-J. Jeong, J. H. Kwon, H-D. Choi, J-K. Pack, N. Kim, Y-S. Lee, H-J. Lee. 2016. 1950 MHz radiofrequency electromagnetic fields do not aggravate memory deficits in 5xFAD mice. *Bioelectromagnetics* 37:391–399.

Stefanics, G., G. Thuroczy, L. Kellenyi, and I. Hernadi. 2008. Effects of twenty-minute 3G mobile phone irradiation on event related potential components and early gamma synchronization in auditory oddball paradigm. *Neuroscience* 157(2):453–462.

Sterling, P., and G. Matthews. 2005. Structure and function of ribbon synapses. *Trends Neurosci* 28(1):20–29.

Stollery, B. T. 1986. Effects of 50 Hz electric currents on mood and verbal reasoning skills. *Br J Ind Med* 43(5):339–349.

Stollery, B. T. 1987. Effects of 50 Hz electric currents on vigilance and concentration. *Br J Ind Med* 44(2):111–118.

Szemerszky, R., D. Zelena, I. Barna, and G. Bardos. 2010. Stress-related endocrinological and psychopathological effects of short- and long-term 50Hz electromagnetic field exposure in rats. *Brain Res Bull* 81(1):92–99.

Tang, J., Y. Zhang, L. Yang, Q. Chen, L. Tan, S. Zuo, H. Feng, Z. Chen, and G. Zhu. 2015. Exposure to 900 MHz electromagnetic fields activates the mkp-1/ERK pathway and causes blood-brain barrier damage and cognitive impairment in rats. *Brain Res* 1601:92–101.

Tattersall, J. E., I. R. Scott, S. J. Wood, J. J. Nettell, M. K. Bevir, Z. Wang, N. P. Somasiri, and X. Chen. 2001. Effects of low intensity radiofrequency electromagnetic fields on electrical activity in rat hippocampal slices. *Brain Res* 904(1):43–53.

Terao, Y., T. Okano, T. Furubayashi, and Y. Ugawa. 2006. Effects of thirty-minute mobile phone use on visuo-motor reaction time. *Clin Neurophysiol* 117 (11):2504–2511.

Terao, Y., T. Okano, T. Furubayashi, A. Yugeta, S. Inomata-Terada, and Y. Ugawa. 2007. Effects of thirty-minute mobile phone exposure on saccades. *Clin Neurophysiol* 118(7):1545–1556.

Thalau, P., T. Ritz, K. Stapput, R. Wiltschko, and W. Wiltschko. 2005. Magnetic compass orienta-tion of migratory birds in the presence of a 1.315 MHz oscillating field. *Naturwissenschaften* 92(2):86–90.

Thomas, S., G. Benke, C. Dimitriadis, I. Inyang, M. R. Sim, R. Wolfe, R. J. Croft, and M. J. Abramson. 2010. Use of mobile phones and changes in cognitive function in adolescents. *Occup Environ Med* 67(12):861–866.

Thoss, F., and B. Bartsch. 2003. The human visual threshold depends on direction and strength of a weak magnetic field. *J Comp Physiol A Neuroethol Sens Neural Behav Physiol* 189(10):777–779.

Thut, G., and A. Pascual-Leone. 2010. A review of combined TMS-EEG studies to characterize last-ing effects of repetitive TMS and assess their usefulness in cognitive and clinical neurosci-ence. *Brain Topogr* 22(4):219–232.

Tiller, J., and R. Lyndon. 2003. *Electroconvulsive Therapy: An Australasian Guide*. Melbourne: Australian Postgraduate Medicine.

Tombini, M., G. Pellegrino, P. Pasqualetti, G. Assenza, A. Benvenga, E. Fabrizio, and P. M. Rossini. 2013. Mobile phone emissions modulate brain excitability in patients with focal epilepsy. *Brain Stimul* 6(3):448–454.

Trunk, A., G. Stefanics, N. Zentai, I. Bacskay, A. Felinger, G. Thuroczy, and I. Hernadi. 2014. Lack of interaction between concurrent caffeine and mobile phone exposure on visual target detection: An ERP study. *Pharmacol Biochem Behav* 124:412–420.

Trunk, A., G. Stefanics, N. Zentai, I. Bacskay, A. Felinger, G. Thuroczy, and I. Hernadi. 2015. Effects of concurrent caffeine and mobile phone exposure on local target probability processing in the human brain. *Sci Rep* 5:14434.

Ueno, S., and M. Sekino. 2015. *Biomagnetics: Principles and Applications of Biomagnetic Stimulation and Imaging*. Boca Raton, FL: CRC Press.

Unterlechner, M., C. Sauter, G. Schmid, and J. Zeitlhofer. 2008. No effect of an UMTS mobile phone-like electromagnetic field of 1.97 GHz on human attention and reaction time. *Bioelectromagnetics* 29(2):145–153.

Vacha, M., T. Puzova, and M. Kvicalova. 2009. Radio frequency magnetic fields disrupt magnetore-ception in American cockroach. *J Exp Biol* 212(Pt 21):3473–3477.

van Nierop, L. E., P. Slottje, M. J. van Zandvoort, F. de Vocht, and H. Kromhout. 2012. Effects of mag-netic stray fields from a 7 tesla MRI scanner on neurocognition: a double-blind randomised crossover study. *Occup Environ Med* 69(10):759–766.

van Wijngaarden, E. 2003. An exploratory investigation of suicide and occupational exposure. *J Occup Environ Med* 45(1):96–101.

van Wijngaarden, E., D. A. Savitz, R. C. Kleckner, J. Cai, and D. Loomis. 2000. Exposure to electro-magnetic fields and suicide among electric utility workers: A nested case-control study. *West J Med* 173(2):94–100.

Vecchia, P., R. Matthes, G. Ziegelberger, J. C. Lin, R. Saunders, and A. J. Swerdlow. 2009. *Exposure to High Frequency Electromagnetic Fields, Biological Effects and Health Consequences (100 kHz–300 GHz)*. Oberschleißheim: ICNIRP.

Vecchio, F., C. Babiloni, F. Ferreri, P. Buffo, G. Cibelli, G. Curcio, S. van Dijkman, J. M. Melgari, F. Giambattistelli, and P. M. Rossini. 2010. Mobile phone emission modulates inter-hemi-spheric functional coupling of EEG alpha rhythms in elderly compared to young subjects. *Clin Neurophysiol* 121(2):163–171.

Vecchio, F., C. Babiloni, F. Ferreri, G. Curcio, R. Fini, C. Del Percio, and P. M. Rossini. 2007. Mobile phone emission modulates interhemispheric functional coupling of EEG alpha rhythms. *Eur J Neurosci* 25(6):1908–1913.

Vecchio, F., P. Buffo, S. Sergio, D. Iacoviello, P. M. Rossini, and C. Babiloni. 2012a. Mobile phone emission modulates event-related desynchronization of alpha rhythms and cognitive-motor performance in healthy humans. *Clin Neurophysiol* 123(1):121–128.

Vecchio, F., M. Tombini, P. Buffo, G. Assenza, G. Pellegrino, A. Benvenga, C. Babiloni, and P. M. Rossini. 2012b. Mobile phone emission increases inter-hemispheric functional coupling of electroencephalographic alpha rhythms in epileptic patients. *Int J Psychophysiol* 84(2):164–171.

Vergara, X., L. Kheifets, S. Greenland, S. Oksuzyan, Y. S. Cho, and G. Mezei. 2013. Occupational exposure to extremely low-frequency magnetic fields and neurodegenerative disease: A meta-analysis. *J Occup Environ Med* 55(2):135–146.

Verrender, A., S. P. Loughran, V. Anderson, L. Hillert, G. J. Rubin, G. Oftedal, and R. J. Croft. 2017. IEI-EMF provocation case studies: A novel approach to testing sensitive individuals. *Bioelectromagnetics* 39(2):132–143.

Verrender, A., S. P. Loughran, A. Dalecki, R. McKenzie, and R. J. Croft. 2016. Pulse modulated radiofrequency exposure influences cognitive performance. *Int J Radiat Biol* 92(10):603–610.

Wagner, P., J. Roschke, K. Mann, J. Fell, W. Hiller, C. Frank, and M. Grozinger. 2000. Human sleep EEG under the influence of pulsed radio frequency electromagnetic fields. Results from polysomnographies using submaximal high power flux densities. *Neuropsychobiology* 42(4):207–212.

Wagner, P., J. Roschke, K. Mann, W. Hiller, and C. Frank. 1998. Human sleep under the influence of pulsed radiofrequency electromagnetic fields: A polysomnographic study using standardized conditions. *Bioelectromagnetics* 19(3):199–202.

Wallace, D., S. Eltiti, A. Ridgewell, K. Garner, R. Russo, F. Sepulveda, S. Walker, T. Quinlan, S. Dudley, S. Maung, R. Deeble, and E. Fox. 2012. Cognitive and physiological responses in humans exposed to a TETRA base station signal in relation to perceived electromagnetic hypersensitivity. *Bioelectromagnetics* 33(1):23–39.

Walsh, V., and A. Cowey. 2000. Transcranial magnetic stimulation and cognitive neuroscience. *Nat Rev Neurosci* 1(1):73–79.

Wang, X., K. Zhao, D. Wang, W. Adams, Y. Fu, H. Sun, X. Liu, H. Yu, and Y. Ma. 2013. Effects of exposure to a 50 Hz sinusoidal magnetic field during the early adolescent period on spatial memory in mice. *Bioelectromagnetics* 34(4):275–284.

Weiss, J., R. C. Herrick, K. H. Taber, C. Contant, and G. A. Plishker. 1992. Bio-effects of high magnetic fields: A study using a simple animal model. *Magn Reson Imaging* 10(4):689–694.

Wiholm, C., A. Lowden, N. Kuster, L. Hillert, B. B. Arnetz, T. Akerstedt, and S. D. Moffat. 2009. Mobile phone exposure and spatial memory. *Bioelectromagnetics* 30(1):59–65.

Wilén, J., A. Johansson, N. Kalezic, E. Lyskov, and M. Sandstrom. 2006. Psychophysiological tests and provocation of subjects with mobile phone related symptoms. *Bioelectromagnetics* 27(3):204–214.

Whittington, C. J., J. V. Podd, and B. R. Rapley. 1996. Acute effects of 50 Hz magnetic field exposure on human visual task and cardiovascular performance. *Bioelectromagnetics* 17(2):131–137.

WHO. 2004. *Workshop on electromagnetic hypersensitivity.* October 25–27, Prague, Czech Republic: World Health Organisation.

WHO. 2007. *Extremely Low Frequency Fields*, Environmental Health Criteria No. 238, Environmental Health Criteria Monographs. Geneva: World Health Organisation.

Wieraszko, A. 2004. Amplification of evoked potentials recorded from mouse hippocampal slices by very low repetition rate pulsed magnetic fields. *Bioelectromagnetics* 25(7):537–544.

Wiltschko, R., P. Thalau, D. Gehring, C. Niessner, T. Ritz, and W. Wiltschko. 2015. Magnetoreception in birds: The effect of radio-frequency fields. *J R Soc Interface* 12(103).

Wiltschko, R., and W. Wiltschko. 2012. Magnetoreception. In C. Lopez-Larrera (Ed.) *Sensing in Nature*, Austin, TX: Landes Bioscience.

Winklhofer, M., and J. L. Kirschvink. 2010. A quantitative assessment of torque-transducer models for magnetoreception. *J R Soc Interface* 7(Suppl 2):S273–S289.

Wolpaw, J. R., R. F. Seegal, and R. Dowman. 1989. Chronic exposure of primates to 60-Hz electric and magnetic fields: I. Exposure system and measurements of general health and performance. *Bioelectromagnetics* 10(3):277–288.

Wood, A. W. 2008. Extremely low frequency (ELF) electric and magnetic field exposure limits: Rationale for basic restrictions used in the development of an Australian standard. *Bioelectromagnetics* 29(6):414–428.

Xu, Y., S. Wu, G. Di, P. Ling, J. Jiang, and H. Bao. 2016. Influence of static electric field on cognition in mice. *Bioengineered* 7(4):241–245.

Yang, X. S., G. L. He, Y. T. Hao, Y. Xiao, C. H. Chen, G. B. Zhang, and Z. P. Yu. 2012. Exposure to 2.45 GHz electromagnetic fields elicits an HSP-related stress response in rat hippocampus. *Brain Res Bull* 88(4):371–378.

Yuasa, K., N. Arai, S. Okabe, Y. Tarusawa, T. Nojima, R. Hanajima, Y. Terao, and Y. Ugawa. 2006. Effects of thirty minutes mobile phone use on the human sensory cortex. *Clin Neurophysiol* 117(4):900–905.

Zentai, N., A. Csatho, A. Trunk, S. Fiocchi, M. Parazzini, P. Ravazzani, G. Thuroczy, and I. Hernadi. 2015. No Effects of acute exposure to Wi-Fi electromagnetic fields on spontaneous EEG activity and psychomotor vigilance in healthy human volunteers. *Radiat Res* 184(6):568–577.

Zhou, H., G. Chen, C. Chen, Y. Yu, and Z. Xu. 2012. Association between extremely low-frequency electromagnetic fields occupations and amyotrophic lateral sclerosis: A meta-analysis. *PLoS One* 7(11):e48354.

Zwamborn, A. P. M., S. H. J. A. Vossen, B. J. A. M. van Leersum, M. A. Ouwens, and W. N. Makel. 2003. Effects of Global Communication system radio-frequency fields on Well Being and Cognitive Functions of human subjects with and without subjective complaints. In *TNO-Report FEL-03-C148*. TNO Physics and Electronics Laboratory.

Index

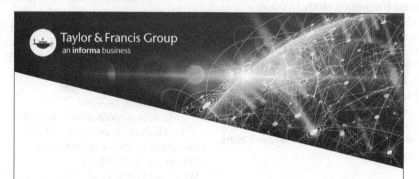